A tailored education experience —

Sherpath book-organized collections

Sherpath is the digital teaching and learning technology designed specifically for healthcare education.

ELSEVIER

Sherpath book-organized collections offer:

Objective-based, digital lessons, mapped chapter-by-chapter to the textbook, that make it easy to find applicable digital assignment content.

Adaptive quizzing with personalized questions that correlate directly to textbook content.

Teaching materials that align to the text and are organized by chapter for quick and easy access to invaluable class activities and resources.

Elsevier ebooks that provide convenient access to textbook content, even offline.

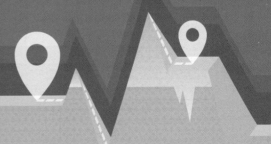

**VISIT
myevolve.us/sherpath**
today to learn more!

21-CS-0280 TM/AF 6/21

BRIEF CONTENTS

Eighth Edition

Conceptual Foundations

The Bridge to Professional Nursing Practice

ELIZABETH E. FRIBERG, DNP, RN
Associate Professor Emerita, General Faculty
University of Virginia School of Nursing
Charlottesville, Virginia

KAREN J. SAEWERT, PHD, RN, CPHQ, ANEF
Clinical Professor
Chair, Mary Killeen Program for Educational Excellence
Edson College of Nursing and Health Innovation
Arizona State University
Phoenix, Arizona

ELSEVIER

Elsevier
3251 Riverport Lane
St. Louis, Missouri 63043

CONCEPTUAL FOUNDATIONS: THE BRIDGE TO PROFESSIONAL
NURSING PRACTICE, EIGHTH EDITION

ISBN: 978-0-323-84713-1

Notice

Practitioners and researchers must always rely on their own experience and knowledge in evaluating and using any information, methods, compounds or experiments described herein. Because of rapid advances in the medical sciences, in particular, independent verification of diagnoses and drug dosages should be made. To the fullest extent of the law, no responsibility is assumed by Elsevier, authors, editors or contributors for any injury and/or damage to persons or property as a matter of products liability, negligence or otherwise, or from any use or operation of any methods, products, instructions, or ideas contained in the material herein.

Previous editions copyrighted 2020, 2011, 2007, and 2001.

Director, Content Development: Laurie Gower
Senior Content Strategist: Sandra Clark
Content Development Specialist: Brooke Kannady
Publishing Services Manager: Deepthi Unni
Project Manager: Sheik Mohideen K
Design Direction: Bridget Hoette

Printed in India

Last digit is the print number: 9 8 7 6 5 4 3 2

Working together
to grow libraries in
developing countries

www.elsevier.com • www.bookaid.org

CONTRIBUTORS

Rebeca M. Almanza, MBA, LPN, CPHQ
Director, Quality Training
Centene
Chicago, Illinois

Marianne Baernholdt, PhD, MPH, RN, FAAN
Sadie Heath Cabaniss Professor and Dean
University of Virginia School of Nursing
Charlottesville, Virginia

Salina Bednarek, EdD, MSN/Ed, RN, CNE
Senior Director, Prelicensure Nursing Programs
Edson College of Nursing and Health Innovation
Arizona State University
Phoenix, Arizona

Cathy Campbell, PhD, RN
Associate Professor
Acute and Specialty Care
University of Virginia School of Nursing
Charlottesville, Virginia

Regina M. DeGennaro, DNP, CNS, AOCN, CNL
Professor
Acute and Specialty Care
University of Virginia School of Nursing
Charlottesville, Virginia

Beth Epstein, PhD, RN, HEC-C, FAAN
Associate Professor, School of Nursing
Associate Professor, Center for Biomedical Ethics and
    Humanities
University of Virginia
Charlottesville, Virginia

Elizabeth E. Friberg, DNP, RN
Associate Professor Emerita, General Faculty
University of Virginia School of Nursing
Charlottesville, Virginia

Tammy Hall, MSN, RN, RDMS
Clinical Instructor
Family and Community
University of North Carolina at Greensboro School of Nursing
Greensboro, North Carolina

Susan E. Harrell, DNP, RN, PMHNP-BC
Associate Professor, Doctor of Behavioral Health Program
College of Health Solutions
Arizona State University
Phoenix, Arizona

Elizabeth Hundt, PhD, RN, NP-C, ACNS-BC
Assistant Professor
Acute and Specialty Care
University of Virginia School of Nursing
Charlottesville, Virginia

Arleen W. Keeling, PhD, RN, FAAN
Emeritus Centennial Distinguished Professor
University of Virginia School of Nursing
Charlottesville, Virginia

Andrew Kopolow, MPA, MSW, CPHQ, PMP, CLSSMBB, FNAHQ
Associate Director, Operational Excellence
Quality Optimization & Insights, United Healthcare
Minnetonka, Minnesota;
Assistant Program Director, Healthcare Quality and Safety
Adjunct Faculty, Jefferson College of Population Health
Thomas Jefferson University
Philadelphia, Pennsylvania

Gerri Lamb, PhD, RN, FAAN
Research Professor, Edson College of Nursing and Health
    Innovation
Founding Director, ASU Center for Advancing
    Interprofessional Practice, Education and Research
Arizona State University
Phoenix, Arizona

Frances R. Maynard, PhD, MBE, APN
Associate Professor
Rutgers University School of Nursing
Newark, New Jersey

Brenda C. Morris, EdD, MS, RN, CNE
Clinical Professor
Edson College of Nursing and Health Innovation
Arizona State University
Phoenix, Arizona

Victoria Petermann, RN, BSN, PhD(c)
PhD Candidate
University of North Carolina at Chapel Hill School of Nursing
Hillsborough, North Carolina

Aliria M. Rascón, PhD, RN, CCRN-K
Clinical Associate Professor
Director, Global Health Collaboratory
Edson College of Nursing and Health Innovation
Arizona State University
Phoenix, Arizona

Richard Ridge, PhD, MBA, RN, NEA-BC
Assistant Professor
Family, Community & Mental Health Systems
University of Virginia School of Nursing
Charlottesville, Virginia

Karen J. Saewert, PhD, RN, CPHQ, ANEF
Clinical Professor
Chair, Mary Killeen Program for Educational Excellence
Edson College of Nursing and Health Innovation
Arizona State University
Phoenix, Arizona

Heidi C. Sanborn, DNP, RN, CNE
Senior Director, Postlicensure Programs
Edson College of Nursing and Health Innovation
Arizona State University
Phoenix, Arizona

Donna L. Schminkey, PhD, MPH, RN, CNM
Associate Professor
School of Nursing, College of Health and Behavioral Studies
James Madison University
Harrisonburg, Virginia

Barbara Shellian, RN, MN
Director, Rural Health
Calgary Zone
Alberta Health Services
Canmore, Alberta, Canada

Audrey E. Snyder, PhD, RN, ACNP-BC, FAANP, FAEN, FAAN
Professor and Associate Dean of Experiential Learning and
    Innovation
School of Nursing
University of North Carolina Greensboro
Greensboro, North Carolina;
Nurse Practitioner
Hospitalist-Palliative Medicine
Cone Health
Greensboro, North Carolina

Sandra P. Thomas, PhD, RN, FAAN
Professor
College of Nursing
University of Tennessee—Knoxville
Knoxville, Tennessee

Debra C. Wallace, PhD, RN, FAAN
Professor
School of Nursing
University of North Carolina at Greensboro
Greensboro, North Carolina

Malinda L. Whitlow, DNP, FNP-BC, RN
Associate Professor
Family, Community & Mental Health Systems
University of Virginia School of Nursing
Charlottesville, Virginia

Gretchen Wiersma, DNP, RN, CNE, CHSE
Assistant Professor
Family, Community & Mental Health Systems
University of Virginia School of Nursing
Charlottesville, Virginia

Daniel T. Wilson, MLS
Deputy Director for Collections & Library Services
Claude Moore Health Sciences Library
University of Virginia
Charlottesville, Virginia

CONTRIBUTORS TO PREVIOUS EDITION

The editors wishes to thank the following individuals who contributed chapters or profiles in practice to the previous edition of this text:

Edie D. Barbero, PhD, RN, PMHNP-B

Camille Burnett, PhD, MPH, APHN-BC, DSW

Sarah W. Craig, PhD, RN, CCNS, CCRN-K, CHSE, CNE

Allyson Duffy, PhD, RN

Vicki S. Good, DNP, RN, CENP, CPPS

Kathryn Laughon, PhD, RN, FAAN

Lacy Phillips, MSN, RN

Teresa M. Stephens, PhD, RN, CNE

Carolyn M. Wellford, BAA, BSN, RN

Ishan C. Williams, PhD

REVIEWERS

Debra Bacharz, PhD, MSN, RN
Professor of Nursing
University of St. Francis
Joliet, Illinois

D. Kathaleen Guilkey, MSN, BSN, RN
Clinical Instructor
University of Kansas School of Nursing
Kansas City, Kansas

Allison Sayre, MSN, DNP, RN, CNE
Associate Professor of Nursing
West Virginia University at Parkersburg
Parkersburg, West Virginia

Charlene Z. Velasco, PhD, RN
Professor of Nursing
St. Johns River State College
Orange Park, Florida

The eighth edition of *Conceptual Foundations: The Bridge to Professional Nursing Practice* brings many changes in chapter contributing authors and chapter approach, the addition of four new chapters, and some major revisions to other chapters to address the impact of the *Future of Nursing 2020–2030; Healthy People 2030;* nursing regulation licensure, examination and certification; nursing education redesign initiatives of academic accreditation associations and competency-based education strategies; and major changes to the *Publication Manual of the American Psychological Association 7th edition.* Additionally, many chapters address the impact of the SARS COVID-19 pandemic as it applies to the concept the chapter addresses. Previous contributors of chapters are acknowledged altogether at the end of this preface. The work of the previous contributors provided a foundation on which new chapters were based, expanded, or revised to reflect major impacts since our last edition and into the future. Our new contributing authors eagerly took on the task of updating and verifying existing work while presenting the material in a creative or fresh format to encourage student engagement. We have added four new chapters that differentiate on evidence-based practice; interprofessional collaboration; diversity, inclusion, and equity; and trauma-informed care, all areas in which nursing provides significant leadership. As we go to press, we have made every effort to integrate the most current information on the *transforming health care delivery system, related legislation/regulations,* and *the changing roles for nurses.* It continues to be a period of dynamic change.

Since 2020 and the release of the seventh edition of this text, the profession and practice of nursing have faced many challenges, launched new initiatives, and taken leadership roles in various aspects of health care and health care service delivery. The 1965 American Nurses Association (ANA) recommendation that the minimum educational preparation for professional nurses be at a baccalaureate level, the Institute of Medicine's (IOM) *The Future of Nursing: Leading Change, Advancing Health* (2010), and the Carnegie Foundation for the Advancement of Teaching's *Educating Nurses: A Call for Radical Transformation* (2010) led the way to nursing education redesign and elevated practice level opportunities. Educational pathways to increase the number of professional nurses and advanced practice nurses have created multiple models for professional entry and advancement. The creation of a Doctor of Nursing Practice as a terminal practice doctorate established parity with other health care professions. (A summary of these initiatives to transform nursing education is provided in Chapter 2.) Nursing workforce challenges and other national agendas, such as patient and workforce safety; health care quality, cost, and access; and health care delivery reform, have created a demand for professional nurses in a variety of health care delivery settings and academia. Workforce challenges related to the SARS COVID-19 pandemic have provided leadership opportunities and staffing, illness burden, and resilience concerns. On the national agenda side, we have transitioned to *Healthy People 2030, The Future of Nursing 2020–2030: Charting a Path to Achieve Health Equity,* and ongoing nursing shortage and workforce diversity initiatives, among a few. The demands of practice complexity, professional career advancement, and nurse/faculty shortages provide the stimulus for many associate degree and diploma program graduates to consider educational advancement. New academic progression models and terminal doctoral practice parity models have increased the options for nurses' professional development and career advancement.

The first edition of *Conceptual Foundations* targeted the RN-BSN student by focusing on the context, dimensions, and themes of professional nursing practice. The *context* of professional nursing practice sheds meaning on the nursing profession and the conditions that must be present for societal recognition of nursing as a profession from historical aspects to the future *NOW* within the evidence-based reality of current policy climates. The *dimensions* of professional practice are the spatial influences on professional nursing practice that may evolve over time, such as the economic issues, team-based interprofessional collaboration, clinical reasoning, ethical comportment, legal aspects, information management, and competency-based teaching and learning principles. *Themes* in professional nursing practice reflect a sampling of nursing leadership areas of interest as the profession assumes its societal role as a recognized and trusted profession in a changing health care delivery infrastructure. Since the first edition, nursing programs other than completion programs have used this text in foundational courses at the baccalaureate and graduate levels. We believe that the content of this eighth edition remains relevant for use in these programs, but we have retained language targeted at a postlicensure audience seeking to advance professional careers.

APPROACH

The rapid changes in the health care delivery system continue to influence nursing education and practice. With the passage of a landmark health care reform initiative and the explosion of health care technology and informatics, professional nursing has provided extensive leadership and received public role recognition for its contributions. From planning and delivery to patient/workforce safety, consumer/patient-centric services, quality improvement, cost containment, community-based services, health promotion, disease prevention, palliative care, and end-of-life care, nursing has emerged as the pivotal coordinator and leader to ensure high-quality care at reasonable cost. During the SARS COVID-19 pandemic, nurses demonstrated their leadership and innovation skills to provide patient-centric, compassionate care. Now more than ever, nurses need strong foundations in the political, legal, economic, population, systems, and ethical aspects of health care in general and nursing care specifically. Additionally, nurses need to embrace the concepts of compassionate care and resilience for self and others. Nursing is also critical to advancing the diversity, inclusion, and equity challenges of the health care delivery system. This text provides that foundation and relates those general concepts to the professional practice of nursing.

Nursing education programs have diverse student populations that span multiple ages and cultural and life experience parameters that bring a richness and depth to their educational advancement. Many are adult learners with increased capacity for critical thinking and self-directed learning. Others are advancing their education while working or raising a family. Some are pursuing their advanced education using distance-learning pedagogies. *Conceptual Foundations* provides a meaningful and diverse conceptual approach to nursing practice that encourages exploration of original theorists, critical analysis of issues and concepts, and applicability to diverse client populations and clinical settings. The text frames the professional practice of nursing by using a variety of subject matter experts for concepts relevant to current and future nursing practice.

The editors recognize that multiple educational pathways exist toward professional nursing education and practice, including a variety of entry-level and seamless academic progression models. These pathways are explored in more depth in Chapter 2. The American Association of Colleges of Nursing (AACN) and the National League for Nursing (NLN) are key stakeholders in the nursing education arena and provide programmatic guidance frameworks for determining the content of nursing education programs and ultimate competencies of graduates from those programs. However, this text has *not* organized its content to *map* to any specific nursing education guidance framework. Instead, we have approached the text content from the previously discussed framework of *context, dimensions,* and *themes.* This provides flexibility for nursing educators to utilize the text in a variety of educational pathways to fit their institution's adopted educational framework and philosophy. Chapter titles provide sufficient information to crosswalk to both guidance frameworks.

The reader will find both *client* and *patient* terminology used, at times interchangeably, to reflect changes in nursing practice and delivery settings. Although philosophically we think a distinction exists, to maintain the flow of the content, we allowed authors the liberty to use these terms interchangeably.

ORGANIZATION

The text is divided into three parts: *Part I, Context of Professional Nursing Practice,* explores a brief history of professional nursing in the United States, academic progression pathways, development of professional identity (beyond socialization), evidence-based practice, select theories and frameworks for professional nursing practice, and health policy and planning within the nursing practice environment. Chapter 1, "A Brief History of the Professionalization of Nursing in the United States," examines the historical aspect of nursing and its relevance to current practice by engaging students in a flow of issues, instead of using the typical timeline approach, and framing a future professional nursing vision. Chapter 2, "Academic Progression," frames the current discussions around the need for nurses to practice at their highest level of academic preparation and training to meet the demands of a rapidly changing health care delivery system and higher complexity of care. Chapter 3, "Beyond Professional Socialization," takes an expanded approach, moving students into discussions of professional identity formation consistent with the IOM reports on the *Future of Nursing* (2010, 2021) and the Carnegie report on *Educating Nurses* (2010). Chapter 4, "Fostering a Spirit of Inquiry: The Role of Nurses in Evidence-Based Practice," a new chapter, addresses evidence-based practice as a problem-solving approach to clinical decision-making. The chapter examines its relationship to the Quintuple Aim and explores its place in the clinical scholarship continuum. Chapter 5, "Theories and Frameworks for Professional Nursing Practice," provides links to the classic works of original theorists using their own words while updating these concepts with current research applications in nursing. Chapter 6, "Health Policy and Planning and the Nursing Practice Environment," provides a framework for understanding health policy, factors that influence health policy, the complex legislative process, health policy implementation and regulation, stakeholder diversity, and leadership concepts involved. Additionally, the chapter summarizes major historical policy eras and their impact on nursing practice.

Part II, Dimensions of Professional Nursing Practice, explores economic issues; interprofessional collaboration; "thinking like a nurse" (critical thinking, clinical reasoning, and the nursing process); continuum of teaching and learning principles; legal aspects of nursing practice; ethical dimensions of nursing and health care (day-to-day ethics); information management; and diversity, equity, and inclusion challenges in health and illness. Economic issues that currently drive health care delivery and practice reform, including current and future nursing practice, are presented in Chapter 7, "Economic Issues in Nursing and Health Care," in a manner that engages students in the complexities of the current economic climate. Chapter 8, "Nurse as Interprofessional Collaborator," a new chapter, speaks to effectively navigating the interprofessional context of health care to provide safe, effective, patient-centered, timely, efficient, and equitable quality care delivery to individuals, families, communities, and populations through collaboration and teamwork. Chapter 9, "Think Like a Nurse," explores the relationships among critical thinking disposition, clinical reasoning, and the nursing decision-making process, including the outcomes of clinical judgment. Chapter 10, "The Continuum of Learning and Teaching in Nursing," a new chapter, presents a high-level exploration of learning and teaching as foundational to nursing across roles, settings, and spheres of influence (community, client, and colleagues). Chapter 11, "Legal Aspects of Nursing Practice," provides a basic understanding of statutory, public, and private law and covers topics such as licensure, delegation, practice acts, and the recent issue of criminalization of practice errors in a format that makes these legal aspects easily accessible to the student and reflects practice in a high-technology environment. Chapter 12, "Ethical Dimensions of Nursing and Health Care," identifies resources and strategies to address everyday practice problems, defines key terms in ethics language, and provides an ethical framework for use in day-to-day practice at four professional levels: patient, unit, organization, and national/global. Chapter 13, "Information Management," distinguishes among informatics, information management, and information literacy and discusses the need for controlled vocabulary searching in evidence-based practice using answerable clinical questions. Chapter 14, "Diversity, Equity, and Inclusion: Impact on Health Care and Nursing Care Strategies," a new chapter, contextualizes culture in the health care setting and describes theories to guide culture and health care. Additionally, this chapter emphasizes culture as a social determinant of health (SDOH) and addresses challenges and barriers to providing equitable and inclusive care.

Part III, Themes in Professional Nursing Practice, explores subjects and topics in which professional nursing is demonstrating leadership, such as health and health promotion, genetics and genomics, global rural health, violence against women, telehealth, patient safety, palliative care, and end-of-life care, resilience, and compassionate care. Chapter 15, "Health and Health Promotion," emphasizes preventive services; the concepts of behavioral and lifestyle change; self-efficacy; environmental, socioeconomic, behavioral, and psychological factors related to wellness; and the *Healthy People 2030* agenda. Chapter 16, "Genetics and Genomics in Professional Nursing," provides a foundation for the rapid developments in this area and nursing's role, especially in the family history pedigree and referral for genetic testing and counseling. With a fresh perspective and contribution from professional peers in Canada, Chapter 17, "Global Rural Nursing Practice," explores the new local and international rural context of nursing practice and the impact of SDOH. Chapter 18, "Trauma-Informed Care," a new chapter, focuses on competencies needed to recognize trauma and respond with strengths-based service delivery of trauma-informed care practices. Chapter 19, "Telehealth," focuses on nurses' role in emerging interventions using telehealth technology to address access and improve outcomes for patient care, including policy implications and evaluations of local capability. Chapter 20, "Health Care Quality and Safety," uses the Donabedian Model (structure, process, outcome) to frame discussion of dimensions of health care quality and safety relevant to nursing and collaborative team-based health professions' practice and care delivery, knowledge, and empowerment.

New Chapter 21, "Palliative Care: Compassionate Care Across Settings of Care," provides a foundation for understanding the underlying concepts related to specialty care in these areas. Additionally, new Chapter 22, "The Wisdom of Self-Care, Well-Being, and Resilience in Nursing," explores these concepts from both patient and practitioner perspectives. Finally, we have added a section for **Appendices A and B** that summarize national policy statement drivers that impact the nursing profession and delivery of health care services.

PEDAGOGY

Each chapter is organized to direct the attention of the student or faculty reader and developed in a similar format. Chapters begin with learning *Objectives* related to the chapter topic. The text includes an opening *Introduction* to explain the approach of the chapter and closes with a *Summary* of the chapter content. *Salient Points* emphasize the major take-away concepts from each chapter to help students develop a *sense of discernment and prioritization* about the content. This models a way of thinking about implications for practice. Chapter content flows from the general concept to application in nursing practice. *Key Terms* are presented in *italics*, and definitions are embedded in the text for reading ease. The structure of text chapters allows for significant flexibility in sequencing of topics and is *not* intended to be read in sequential order. The nature of the content creates the need for cross-references of topics addressed by multiple chapters. The editors provide those cross-references where they are most useful to the reader. Boxes, tables, and figures are used throughout for emphasis and provide a visual reinforcement for important content. *Internet links* are embedded within the text *or* provided in *Website Resources* lists when websites other than those referenced in the chapter may be useful for both students and faculty. *Critical Reflection Exercises* are provided at the end of each chapter to expand the student's exploration of key concepts, reflect on practice implications, and stimulate further group discussions. Critical reflection is necessary for accountable professional practice now and in the future in an ever-changing practice environment. We refrain from the use of superficial bulleted presentations because we wish to engage students in a context that provides opportunities for critical thinking and reflection, stimulating deeper learning. We also refrain from the use of color or excessive inclusion of photos or figures (except for Chapter 1) because this significantly increases the cost of producing the text, which would reflect in higher text fees for students.

References, either classic or current (within the past 5 years), are provided for all citations. The authors have chosen to reference classic works where appropriate to instill in students a sense of the richness of nursing's body of knowledge that supports current professional practice. References except for texts are largely accessible to students and faculty through DOIs or active weblinks at the time of production in APA Style 7th edition. Evidence-based and research-based references are largely current except where a classic reference is better suited. We have retained our practice of providing classic references for major theorists and use of the actual theorist's language and words in describing their theories. This practice provides the opportunity for students and faculty to experience their work first-hand and refer to their original writings. Current research and evidence-based application are integrated throughout the content.

The text format approach challenges the reader to discover new knowledge or reframe prior learning on a more conceptual and universally applicable level in professional practice. The contextual, dimensional, and theme-based approach provides a comprehensive source text for exploring foundational concepts of professional nursing practice targeted to transition or completion programs but applicable in a variety of educational programs. Nursing practice as it is today and will be in the future is supported by these foundational concepts and the ever-expanding nursing knowledge base that flows from them.

SPECIAL FEATURES

The website http://evolve.elsevier.com/Friberg/bridge/ provides student resources as well as these instructor resources: TEACH for Nurses (a faculty Instruction Manual), Test Bank, Image Collection, PowerPoint presentations, Answers to Case Studies, and Generic Issues and Trends Next Generation NCLEX®-Style Cases and Answers.

Student resouces include Review Question and Case Studies.

To the dedicated nurses and their families globally who paid the ultimate price caring for people during the SARS COVID-19 pandemic and nurses burdened with the physical and mental residuals after contracting SARS COVID-19.

Dedicated in memory of
Mary Gunther, PhD, RN
Associate Professor
College of Nursing
University of Tennessee—Knoxville
10/29/1946–7/19/2021
Contributor to *Conceptual Foundations: The Bridge to Professional Nursing Practice* since the 3rd edition.

Dedicated in honor of a remarkable mentor
Mary L. Killeen, PhD, RN
Professor Emerita and Former Senior
Associate Dean for Evaluation and
Educational Excellence, Edson
College of Nursing and Health
Innovation
Arizona State University
Phoenix, Arizona
Contributor to *Conceptual Foundations: The Bridge to Professional Nursing Practice* for the 3rd and 4th editions.

CONTENTS

Conceptual Foundations

The Bridge to Professional Nursing Practice

PART I

Context of Professional Nursing Practice

1

A Brief History of the Professionalization of Nursing in the United States

Elizabeth Hundt, PhD, RN, NP-C, ACNS-BC and
Arlene Wynbeek Keeling, PhD, RN, FAAN

 http://evolve.elsevier.com/Friberg/bridge/

OBJECTIVES

At the completion of this chapter, the reader will be able to:

- Describe the relevance of the study of history to clinical practice and health policy in the 21st century.
- Discuss late 19th- and 20th-century contributions to the professionalization of the nursing role in American society.
- Describe entry into practice and the transition of nursing education from the hospital to collegiate programs.

- Discuss the role of nursing in health promotion and disease prevention.
- Discuss the development of advanced clinical practice nursing and doctoral education for nurses from the 1960s to the present and the context in which these developments occurred.

INTRODUCTION

No occupation can be intelligently followed or correctly understood unless it is, at least to some extent, illumined by the light of history interpreted from the human standpoint.

(Dock & Stewart, 1938)

Writing in the early 20th century, historian and nurse activist Lavinia Dock wrote these words, testifying to the importance of knowing one's history. For nurses, studying their history provides the novice with a sense of identity within the profession. Indeed, as nurse historian Olga Church once noted: "Graduates of nursing programs who have not been exposed to their heritage have not been properly oriented to the profession" (Church, 1987, p. 1). Writing in 1995, scholars Arlene Keeling and Mary Ramos agreed with these positions, arguing that studying nursing history not only provides nursing students with a sense of professional identity but also a useful methodological

research skill and a context for evaluating information (Keeling & Ramos, 1995).

More recently, historians have argued that "History infuses health reform debates [and] provides a critically important perspective if we are to understand and address contemporary health system problems" (D'Antonio & Fairman, 2010, p. 113). Adding to the argument for the inclusion of history in nursing's heavily science-based curricula, Toman and Thifault (2012) examined the ways in which students who use primary source historical data during their nursing education begin to use more complex, critical analyses of health care issues—skills that will serve them well as practicing nurses.

In spite of these strong and evidence-based recommendations, the study of nursing history has all but been eliminated from most nursing curricula. That may change in the near future, due to the American Association of Colleges of Nursing (AACN) recent statements in their newly released revisions to The Essentials (AACN, 2021, April 6) about including history in the nursing undergraduate curriculum.

Because of the complicated breadth and depth of the history of nursing in the United States (see Keeling et al., 2017, for a more complete analysis), this chapter provides only select historical highlights, supporting student learning with historical information based on primary source documents. Its purpose is to provide the reader with an overview of the history of modern nursing in the United States from the middle of the 19th century to today. Topics include Florence Nightingale's influential nursing practice in the United Kingdom and the spread of her ideas about nursing education from Britain to the United States, issues surrounding the development of professional and educational standards for nurses, the influence of science and technology on the development of nursing, the diversification of the nursing workforce to include men and minorities, and the rise of advanced practice programs and doctoral education for nurses. These events and topics did not happen in isolation from the history of medicine and the health care system. Therefore that context is considered, as well as how nursing has shaped—and has been shaped by—a confluence of social, political, and economic factors.

Nursing has indeed evolved over the course of more than 150 years since the inception of the first Nightingale schools in the United States, but it has not done so without facing significant challenges. Many of these challenges persist today, including issues surrounding gender, race, socioeconomic status, educational requirements for entry into practice, professional licensure, nursing shortages, wars, and pandemics.

British Influences on American Nursing, 1860–1873

Historically women have been charged with providing physical care to those who are sick or injured. In the 19th century, women's work as the primary caregiver was accepted as a natural extension of their role as homemaker. To assist with that role, in 1859 Florence Nightingale published *Notes on Nursing: What It Is and What It Is Not.* In the preface of this book, Nightingale explained that her notes on nursing were "meant simply to give hints for thought to women who have personal charge of the health of others. Every woman or at least almost every woman has, at one time or another of her life, charge of the personal health of somebody, whether child or invalid—in other words, every woman is a nurse" (Nightingale, 1859, p. 8).

In England, that nursing role would be formalized in the first Nightingale school for nurses established at St. Thomas Hospital in 1860, after Nightingale returned from the Crimean War (1853–1856), fully aware that specific training was required to create professional nurses. News of the St. Thomas School spread to the United States; soon the school would be recognized as the "Nightingale model" of nursing education. Its premise was that the image of nursing needed to change to attract educated women to the profession.

The Nightingale model had female pupil nurses (ostensibly well-educated and refined women) training on hospital wards under the direction of a lady nurse superintendent. The model not only provided hospitals with an inexpensive and skilled workforce but also gave working-class women an opportunity for employment outside the home. For many working-class women, nursing was an alternative to factory work. (See Susan Reverby's *Ordered to Care* for more on this.)

Based on the Nightingale model, the first nurse training schools opened in the United States in 1873. The first was at Bellevue Hospital in New York City, followed within months by the Connecticut Hospital in New Haven and Massachusetts General Hospital's "Boston Training School for Nurses" in Boston.

The training in these hospital-based schools was arduous, requiring long days of patient service on the wards, after which students attended classes, some taught by physicians, others by head nurses. In addition to providing bedside care to patients, students performed housekeeping tasks, prepared meals, cleaned the wards and operating rooms, sterilized instruments, and assisted physicians with dressing changes. In exchange for these 2 to 3 years of intense ward work, pupil nurses acquired the necessary knowledge and skills to find employment as private duty nurses after graduation. In fact, most graduates worked outside the hospital in patients' homes until the 1930s.

Later that would change as the number of hospitals in the United States continued to grow and patients entered them for care. In 1873, fewer than 200 hospitals existed in the entire United States. In a relatively short time, hospitals proliferated. To staff them with pupil nurses, many opened training schools. By 1900 the United States had 432 hospital-based nursing schools (Roberts, 1954). By the early 1920s, that number had risen to more than 1700 (Keeling et al., 2018, p. 163) (Fig. 1.1).

Despite the proliferation of nurse training programs in the late 19th century, few admitted minority women. One exception was Mary Eliza Mahoney, who was the first African-American nurse to receive formal nurse training, graduating from the New England Hospital for Women and Children training school in August 1879. Indeed, racial segregation in higher education afforded few minority women the opportunity to pursue a career in nursing. In response, between 1886 and 1893 several schools for

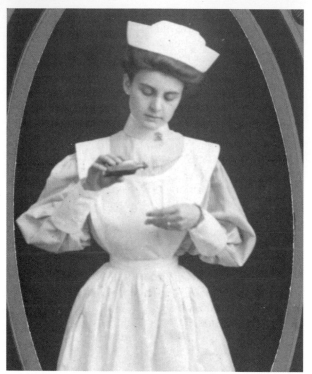

Fig. 1.1 Graduate Nurse Pouring Medicine, Circa 1900. (Courtesy, Eleanor Crowder Bjoring Center for Nursing Historical Inquiry, The University of Virginia.)

Blacks opened. These included: Howard University in Washington, DC; Provident Hospital School of Nursing in Chicago, Illinois; Tuskegee Institute Nurse Training School in Tuskegee, Alabama; Spelman Seminary in Atlanta, Georgia; and Dixie Hospital Training School in Hampton, Virginia (Keeling et al., 2018).

Describing the importance of the Dixie School in Virginia, its founder, White nurse Alice M. Bacon, made clear that "the colored woman [sic], with a Hampton education behind her, can be trained into as good a nurse as any white woman" (Bacon, 1892, p. 108). However, that is not to say that the African-American nursing students had an equivalent experience to White pupils working at such hospitals as Massachusetts General with its access to Harvard-trained physicians. The first Dixie Hospital nursing class faced many challenges, including the lack of a dormitory, a paucity of physician lectures, and little or no pay. Nonetheless, the students, clad in their gray uniforms and white aprons, provided competent and compassionate care to the sick (Keeling et al., 2018). While Bacon may have sounded condescending in her initial remarks, her conclusion was correct: the Dixie nurses were as good as any other graduates.

Unfortunately, racial bias and segregation of medical and nursing services persisted through much of the 20th century. As Canadian nurse Ethel Johns noted in her 1925 report on Black schools of nursing, commissioned by the Rockefeller Foundation: "No matter how high her personal and professional qualifications may be, certain doors remain closed to the African American nurse" (Johns, 1925, p. 6). It was a reality that would not change until the 1940s, when the Bolton Act mandated the integration of nursing schools during World War II.

Professionalism Through Organization and Licensure

Meanwhile, in the early years of the 20th century, nursing had a long way to go before it would be considered a profession. Superintendents of nursing, responsible for student learning within nurse training schools, soon expressed their concern about the demands on students to serve as staff in hospital wards. To address this issue, Isabel Hampton, Superintendent of the Johns Hopkins Hospital School of Nursing, assembled superintendents of America's largest schools at the 1893 Chicago World's Fair. Her goal was to raise and standardize requirements for the training of nurses (Draper, 1893/1949).

In January 1894, the superintendents created the Society of Superintendents of Training Schools for Nurses of the United States and Canada (later renamed the National League for Nursing Education [NLNE] in 1912). The goals of the Society of Superintendents were "to promote fellowship of members, to establish and maintain a universal standard of training, and to further the best interests of the nursing profession" (American Society of Superintendents of Training Schools for Nurses, 1897, p. 4). Shortly thereafter the national government released data revealing that there were almost 109,000 "untrained nurses and midwives competing with 12,000 graduate nurses" for nursing positions (US Bureau of Census, 1900, p. xxiii).

While the NLNE was concerned with the educational standards for nurses, the Nurses' Associated Alumnae of the United States and Canada (renamed the American Nurses Association [ANA] in 1912) focused on achieving legal recognition for trained nurses. Their goal was to protect the public from nurses who lacked formal training by requiring state licensure for nurses who had graduated from schools that met specific standards. Superintendent Isabel Hampton argued in support of educational standards and licensure, noting that at that time a trained nurse meant "anything, everything, or next to nothing" (Hampton, 1893/1949, p. 5).

Thus the Nurses' Associated Alumnae, composed of alumnae associations from established schools of nursing, quickly moved to set up state organizations so nurses could undertake the necessary political lobbying for the enactment of state registration laws. Their mission was to "strengthen the union of nursing organizations, to elevate nursing education, [and] to promote ethical standards" for the profession (Nurses' Associated Alumnae of the United States, 1902/2007, p. 766). Their goal was to "achieve legal recognition of nursing as a profession and provide a means for distinguishing trained nurses from those who purported to be but whose preparation for the practice of nursing fell short of standards" (Daisy, 1996, p. 35).

In March 1903, the Nurses' Associated Alumnae efforts resulted in nurse registration legislation in North Carolina. Later that same year, New Jersey, New York, and Virginia followed. These acts defined for the public that a "registered nurse" had attended an acceptable nursing program and passed a board examination. However, still lacking were national educational standards and an agreed-upon definition of professional nursing practice.

After the enactment of nurse licensure, leaders of the profession created state nursing boards and empowered them to use their legal authority to protect the public from unfit nurses. Ironically, women who lacked the legal right to vote in 1910 aided 27 states in enacting nurse registration laws. By 1923, all states in the nation, along with Hawaii and the District of Columbia, had enacted nurse registration laws (Bullough, 1975).

NURSING PRACTICE IN EARLY 20TH-CENTURY AMERICA

Employment opportunities for graduate nurses in the early 20th century were, for the most part, limited to caring for ill persons in the patient's home; hospitals were seen as places where patients turned if they had no one else to care for them. With the exception of head nurses and nurse anesthetists, nursing students staffed the hospital. Most nursing school graduates eagerly donned their white uniforms, caps, and nursing pins and joined a "registry," allowing them to practice as private duty nurses in patients' homes. Nurse registries, operated by hospitals, professional organizations, or private businesses, provided sites where the public could acquire the services of these private duty nurses. Families could contract for the services of a nurse for a day or a few hours to care for their loved ones either at home or in the hospital (Whelan, 2005).

Although physicians' orders were required, private duty in the home provided graduate nurses with the venue and the opportunity to break away from the rigid hospital routine and allowed for a more autonomous practice. These nurses provided care to patients with contagious diseases such as pneumonia and typhoid fever, aided women after childbirth, and supported patients with fractures, infected wounds, strokes, and mental diseases. Private duty nurses lived with and worked for their patients, providing 24-hour care, often for weeks at a time (Stoney, 1919).

For the most part, middle- and upper-class households employed private duty nurses. Graduate nurses were generally pleased with their role as private duty nurses, but their employment was seasonal and sporadic. Because of the onslaught of contagious diseases in the cold months of the year, winters were busy and summers slow. The average annual income of a private duty nurse in the late 1910s was approximately $950, a sum that sustained her but left little savings for future needs (Reverby, 1987). Nonetheless, the trend toward private duty prevailed. By the 1920s, 70% to 80% of graduates worked as private duty nurses.

However, during the early 20th century, new medical discoveries led the public to hospitals for the latest in scientific care. To deal with the increasing hospital census in the 1920s, nursing superintendents were pressured to admit more students into school programs. In turn, the increase of nursing students resulted in an increase of graduate nurses, thus creating a surplus. In 1926 the ANA and NLNE grew concerned about the economic plight of graduate nurses and authorized a comprehensive study of the working conditions of graduate nurses. The study, later known as the *Burgess Report*, documented that registered nurses faced widespread underemployment and harsh working conditions (Burgess, 1928). Another survey, conducted by Janet Geister, underscored the private duty nurses' economic plight. According to Geister, 80% of nurses' patient cases lasted only 1 day. This level of employment earned them approximately $31.26 a week, or 49 cents an hour—less than the income of scrubwomen, who earned 50 cents an hour (Geister, 1926).

With the collapse of the stock market in 1929 and the subsequent economic depression that enveloped the United States, even the lowest-paying jobs for private duty nurses disappeared. Private duty nursing became a luxury few could afford. This reality, combined with the fact that patients would soon prefer the scientific medical care offered in hospitals, would lead to changes in the profession. In the 1930s many graduate nurses would turn to hospitals for work. However, before that, urbanization, immigration, and industrialization would also impact the nursing profession.

The Progressive Era and Public Health Nursing

At the turn of the 20th century, the United States was undergoing major social changes. Urbanization, industrialization, and the influx of European immigrants, especially into the northeastern section of the country, soon resulted in overcrowded tenement slums, filthy streets, and poor working conditions. Soon communicable diseases ran rampant. Something had to be done, and Americans were soon advocating for progressive social reform.

One young nurse, Lillian Wald, saw the conditions on the lower East Side of New York City as her opportunity to care for the poor and to establish a role for nursing in the community. According to Wald, the needs of the newly arrived immigrants were limitless.

> *There were nursing infants, many of them with the summer bowel complaint that sent infant mortality soaring during the hot months; there were children with measles, not quarantined; there were children with ophthalmia, a contagious eye disease; there were children scarred with vermin bites; there were adults with typhoid; there was a case of puerperal septicemia, lying on a vermin-infested bed without sheets or pillow cases; a family consisting of a pregnant mother, a crippled child and two others living on dry bread; a young girl dying of tuberculosis amid the very conditions that had produced the disease.*
>
> **(Wald, quoted in Duffus, 1938, p. 43)**

In response to these conditions, in 1895 Wald and her colleague Mary Brewster founded the Henry Street Settlement House and Henry Street Visiting Nurse Services. Based on Progressive Era ideals, HSS nurses provided immigrants with nursing care and social services. Convinced that the sickness they saw was part of a larger set of social problems, Wald and her colleagues provided a wide range of social services, including safe places for children to play, sterilized milk, free medicines, meals, and referrals for infants to attend baby camps in the countryside. Their goal was to promote health and prevent disease in the poverty-stricken immigrants. The visiting nurses' work quickly expanded to include new services, most notably school nursing, industrial nursing, tuberculosis nursing, and infant welfare nursing. Later Wald joined forces with the Metropolitan Life Insurance Company to send nurses into the homes of the company's customers when they became ill (Keeling, 2007).

In 1912, Wald founded the National Organization for Public Health Nursing (NOPHN)—nursing's first specialty organization. That year there were approximately 3000 public health nurses working throughout the United States—in both urban and rural areas (Gardner, 1936). The major goals of the NOPHN were to develop adequate numbers of public health nurses to meet the needs of the public and to link the emerging field of public health nursing to preventive medicine (Brainard, 1922).

In response to abysmal working conditions in the plethora of factories spreading throughout the country, Wald undertook a survey of industrial workers' health needs (1908–1911). Her work led to the creation of an industrial

nursing branch of the NOPHN. Industrial nurses staffed corporate welfare departments for major industries such as textile factories. Nurses lived and worked in mill villages and provided care to workers and entire families, treating infectious diseases, respiratory ailments, and injuries. They also gave health demonstrations and provided prenatal and postnatal care for mothers. Standing orders from a supervising mill or community physician covered the diverse services the nurses provided (Craig, 2015).

The creation of the federally based Children's Bureau in 1912 and the passage of the Maternal and Infant Act (Sheppard-Towner) in 1921 reflected the federal government's growing concern for the health of women and children during the Progressive Era. Public health nurses served as the backbone of new initiatives under the Sheppard-Towner Act, traveling to remote areas in their states to bring clinics and health services to those most in need (Keeling et al., 2018) (Fig. 1.2). Although the federal programs experienced opposition, especially from physicians, in the 8 years of their existence, the programs demonstrated the effectiveness of nurses in the screening of patients and referring them to physicians. The programs also brought health education to thousands of American families (Meckel, 1990).

At the turn of the 20th century, the main focus of the American Red Cross (ARC) was relief and provision of nursing services during wartime and natural disasters. However, in the mid-1910s the organization established the Town and Country Nursing Service (1913–1918) to meet the needs of communities in peacetime. The Town and Country nurses collaborated with local agencies to give direct nursing care to patients and deliver health education to the community. Trained nurses qualified for the nursing

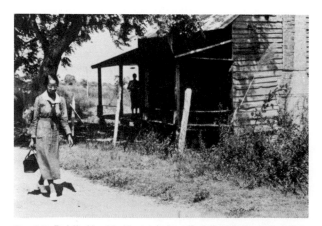

Fig. 1.2 Public Health Nurse Infant Feeding Demonstration. (Public domain, National Library of Medicine.)

service after completion of a 4-month course on public health and hands-on experience with a public health nurse at an official visiting nurses' association (Lewenson, 2015).

The development of public health nursing was important to the nation and to the nursing profession because it brought essential health services to the public. It also provided nurses with unique opportunities to integrate epidemiological knowledge and sanitation practices—as well as medical science—into the care and education of the public. Outside the hospital, public health nurses expanded the domain of nursing practice to include individuals, families, and communities.

Nurses in War

Just as Nightingale's work in the Crimea was an impetus for instituting a training school for nurses in England, the provision of nursing care by American women during the US Civil War (1861–1865) was the impetus for the establishment of nurse training programs in the United States. After the firing on Fort Sumter, thousands of women from both Northern and Southern states volunteered their services to care for the injured, sick, and dying soldiers in homes, in hospitals, and on battlefields. In the Union, many women volunteered to work under Dorothea Dix. Others, like Mary Ann Bickerdyke, reported directly to President Abraham Lincoln as she worked on the battlefields of the west. In the Confederacy, White women organized private wayside hospitals and worked in makeshift warehouse hospitals, often accompanied by their slaves (Maling, 2007).

Indeed a diverse group of volunteers offered to nurse the sick and wounded during the war. Throughout the Confederacy, hundreds of Black men (both slave and free) served as nurses (Maling, 2007). American poet Walt Whitman nursed the wounded and facilitated soldiers' correspondence home. African-American women Harriet Tubman, Sojourner Truth, and Susie King Taylor ministered to soldiers and worked to improve camp conditions for Black military units (Keeling et al., 2018). In addition, Catholic nuns and Lutheran deaconesses provided care to the soldiers. In 1863, Ann Bradford Stokes, an emancipated slave, volunteered with the Sisters of St. Joseph to care for Union soldiers on the hospital transport ship *Red Rover* (King, 1998). Together, these *volunteer* women demonstrated the effectiveness of skilled nursing on improving the care of sick and injured soldiers.

It would not be until 1898, during the Spanish American War, that *trained* nurses were used in the military. During this war, trained nurses volunteered to serve in the army to care for injured and sick soldiers. This experience helped to convince military physicians and Congress that trained female nurses should become permanent members of the nation's defense forces. It set the stage for the creation of the Army Nurse Corps in 1901 and the Navy Nurse Corps in 1908 (Keeling et al., 2018).

Both the Army Nurse Corps and the Navy Nurse Corps would serve in World War I during the next decade. From the start, nursing leaders cooperated with the federal government in a major recruitment and mobilization campaign; in the spring of 1917, when the United States entered the war, the shortage of nursing personnel was profound. As part of that effort, the ARC, led by Jane Delano, conducted an ambitious campaign to recruit trained nurses to serve in the 50 Base Hospitals that were being set up by major hospitals and universities.

The leaders of the nursing profession insisted on the use of properly trained nurses, despite the fact that many society women, eager to help in the environment of patriotic fervor, wished to volunteer. A dual solution was reached: an innovative program was begun at Vassar College for college-educated women to become nurses in a shorter period of time, and the Army School of Nursing was established. Both programs were designed to increase the supply of trained nurses for the military (Clappison, 1964).

During World War I, even nurses who were properly trained faced challenges once they arrived near the battlefields. In France, tested by harsh weather and a continuous influx of casualties from the front, nurses soon became exhausted. Air raids at night further disrupted their sleep, while shortages of help and supplies caused additional stress. Then, in the late spring and early fall of 1918, a deadly variant of influenza struck and thousands of soldiers fell ill. By October 1918, more than 6000 American soldiers had already died of the flu in France (Fig. 1.3). By the end of the war, thousands more had succumbed, despite the best efforts of nursing and medical staff (Keeling et al., 2018, p. 199).

Hospitals Become Businesses

After World War I, hospitals continued to grow in both number and size. Between 1925 and 1929, more than $890 million was spent on their construction. The use of x-rays, the introduction of new drugs such as sulfa and insulin, and the reliance on laboratory tests such as urinalysis and the complete blood count revolutionized modern medicine, just as the introduction of aseptic techniques and developments in anesthesia had revolutionized surgery at the turn of the 20th century (Howell, 1996).

Modern obstetrics, with its promise of scopolamine-induced "twilight sleep" to reduce the pain of childbirth, brought women who previously had their babies at home into hospitals. Over the course of the next few decades, the addition of pediatric, psychiatric, and physical therapy services, as well as the introduction of private patient

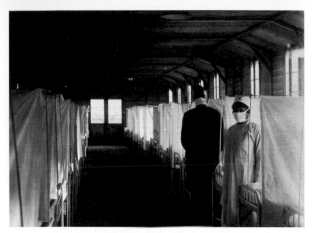

Fig. 1.3 Influenza Ward, World War I, France. (Public domain, National Library of Medicine.)

rooms, enhanced the hospital's image and attracted thousands of new patients into hospitals (Roren, 1930). Indeed, the first half of the 20th century saw America's appreciation of the benefits of scientific medicine.

With the growth of hospitals, the social and economic status of staff physicians and hospital directors also increased. However, the status of nurses did not increase, and nursing administrators continued their struggle to convince hospitals that graduate nurses, rather than nursing students, should be responsible for patient care. Meanwhile nurse educators urged that students spend more time in formal classroom instruction. This struggle continued even after the Goldmark Report, commissioned by the Rockefeller Foundation in the early 1920s, revealed shocking deficiencies in the education of nursing students (Goldmark, 1923).

It would take the stock market crash of 1929 and the subsequent national economic depression of the 1930s to change the hospital staffing situation. Indeed, the economic depression that gripped the United States caused serious financial, social, and health problems for the nation. Business failures and unemployment spread; by 1932, 25% of working Americans had lost their jobs (Blum, 1981). As fewer and fewer patients were able to pay for private duty nurses, physicians, or medical and surgical procedures, hospital administrators were forced to examine the costs of providing care. Maintaining a nursing school was expensive, and many small hospitals had to close their schools. In fact, 570 training programs were closed during the 1930s (Roberts, 1954). To keep the remaining nursing schools intact, their budgets were seriously curtailed and students' education was further compromised.

At the same time, large hospitals, especially municipal hospitals, experienced a large influx of patients seeking charitable care. The Social Security Act of 1935, with its financial aid for the elderly and its Title V health care benefits for disabled children, had provided some relief, but it was not until the development of Blue Cross, a revolutionary prepaid health insurance plan (Numbers, 1978), that hospitals found a solution. Health insurance plans for workers able to pay for future hospitalizations helped to ensure the financial stability of hospitals that accepted Blue Cross payments.

However, members of the American Medical Association (AMA) rejected the new Blue Cross health plan, characterizing it as "economically unsound, unethical and inimical to the public interests" (Kimball, 1934, p. 45). In spite of the AMA's opposition, Blue Cross proved to be attractive to patients and hospitals. Moreover, because it filled hospital beds with paying patients, it was formally endorsed by the AHA in 1937. As a hospital official noted, "Blue Cross was sired by the Depression and mothered by hospitals out of desperate economic necessity" (Sommers & Sommers, 1961).

As the economy slowly improved in the late 1930s, it soon became evident, especially to physicians, that additional graduate nurses were needed to provide patients with safe and effective nursing care. This realization, coupled with new sources of income from health insurance and government relief programs and the availability of unemployed private duty nurses willing to work for minimum wages, led to administrators hiring graduate nurses (Fitzpatrick, 1975). In turn, the increase in the numbers of registered nurses on hospital staffs—from 4000 positions in 1929 to 28,000 in 1937 and to more than 100,000 by 1941—improved the quality of patient services.

Paradoxically, graduate nurses also introduced a new professional tension within the hospital system (Cannings & Lazonick, 1975). Hospital administrators, accustomed to a docile and inexpensive student workforce, considered graduate nursing services costly and only partially necessary. In addition, administrators and physicians saw registered nurses as potential threats because they were less compliant than students. The nurses used their own judgment in providing patient care, basing their decisions on their professional knowledge and experiences rather than simply following physician orders.

Tensions resulted. As independent practitioners working in private homes, the nurses had worked autonomously to give the quality of care they thought patients needed. Now, as staff nurses working in the hospital setting, they were part of a bureaucracy that demanded loyalty to physicians and the hospital itself rather than to patients. In addition, the hospitals' employment of subsidiary nursing and housekeeping staff added managerial tasks to the nurses' responsibilities. Moreover, the strict institutional control of their clinical practice reminded them of the exploitation, harsh discipline, and regimentation they had experienced in their training schools (Flood, 1981).

However, given the economic realities of the Great Depression (1929–1939), graduate nurses and hospitals began an uneasy working alliance. Learning how to interact successfully with professional graduates rather than a student workforce challenged hospital administrators and nursing superintendents, who struggled to establish personnel policies that professional nurses would accept. Nonetheless, for the most part, hospitals offered registered nurses "low pay, long hours, split shifts, authoritarian supervision, and rigid rules" (Reverby, 1987, p. 192).

By the 1950s, hospitals had become the major employers of nurses. As such, they gained the power to set nursing wages and working conditions and often thwarted nurses in their quest for adequate compensation and the right to participate in hospital decisions regarding patient care (Reverby, 1987). Likely fueled by their lack of autonomy and their plight as subservient members of a hierarchical hospital system, nurses identified education as a potential pathway to leadership.

Collegiate Nursing Education: The Early Years

Throughout the early years of the 20th century, some nurse educators advocated for the nursing superintendents, faculty, and public health nurses to have postgraduate education in institutions of higher learning. As early as 1899, Teachers College at Columbia University offered a postdiploma hospital economics program. Nurse leaders Mary Adelaide Nutting and Isabel Stewart directed this program and offered innovative courses in administration, education, and public health nursing to thousands of nurses from the United States and abroad (Christy, 1969).

In 1909 the University of Minnesota established the first permanent *undergraduate* nursing education program in the United States. However, for most students, admission to college was prohibited by cost and the time required to complete the program. Thus enrollment in these institutions remained low compared with diploma programs. By 1923, only 17 collegiate schools nationwide offered 5-year degree programs. Although the profession had made some progress toward collegiate status, it still lacked the social endorsement and financial support that had paved the way for medical education to move into universities.

Medical education experienced a very different trajectory from nursing. Large financial endowments, primarily from the Rockefeller, Carnegie, and Commonwealth foundations, had propelled medical education into the mainstream of university education. Data from the famous 1910 Abraham Flexner Report had demonstrated inadequacies in medical education, acting as a catalyst for reform. The Rockefeller General Education Board alone funneled more than $91 million into medical schools (Starr, 1982).

Although nursing leaders sought similar assistance for nursing education, only the Rockefeller Foundation was persuaded to endow the establishment of two university-based nursing schools—Yale in 1924 and Vanderbilt in 1930 (Abrams, 1993). Annie Goodrich, a noted nursing educator, directed the first independent nursing collegiate school at Yale University. This baccalaureate program was based on the premise that nursing concepts pertinent to acute illness, the psychosocial dimensions of illness, and public health principles were essential components of educational programs for professional nurses (Sheahan, 1979).

By 1935, sufficient numbers of collegiate programs provided the catalyst for the organization of the Association of Collegiate Schools of Nursing, an organization whose mission was to establish collegiate nursing programs in American universities. Its early members strongly maintained that nursing could not develop into a profession until it could generate scientifically sound nursing knowledge that could sustain the practice of nursing (Stewart, 1943). Although this group later disbanded, in 1969 a small group of deans of collegiate and university programs established the Conference of Deans of Colleges and University Schools of Nursing, known today as the AACN (Keeling et al., 2009). The AACN continues to play an essential role in nursing education, research, and health policy. Ironically, however, the nursing profession continues to allow many pathways into practice and has yet to reach a consensus about the educational qualifications needed by entry-level practicing nurses.

World War II

The United States' entry into World War II, after the bombing of Pearl Harbor in December of 1941, immediately increased the demand for skilled nurses. Indeed, both military and civilian nurses were needed. To meet the increased demands, the federal government created two new programs: the ARC volunteer nurse's aides program in 1941 and the Cadet Nurse Corps in 1943 (Johnston, 1966; Keeling et al., 2018).

The loss of professional and nonprofessional staff to the military and defense industry left hospitals and public health agencies in need of auxiliary help to care for citizens at home. Through a joint venture with the Office of Civilian Defense and the ARC, more than 200,000 women volunteered to become certified nurse's aides and work under nursing supervision to provide patient care. This venture proved to be an important step in the stratification of nursing into registered, practical, and aide levels (Keeling et al., 2018).

In 1943 Frances Payne Bolton, a congresswoman from Ohio, sponsored a bill that authorized the US Public Health Service to establish the Cadet Nurse Corps. This was the most significant federally sponsored program to increase the supply of professional nurses in the 1940s. The bill subsidized the education of students who agreed, on graduation, to serve in military or civilian health agencies for the duration of the war (Fig. 1.4). Students were provided tuition, fees, and books, plus a monthly stipend throughout their training. Participating schools also received funds for instructional facilities and postgraduate education for their nursing faculty.

Although the Cadet Corps accepted students for only 2 years (July 1943–October 1945), almost 170,000 cadets entered 1125 participating schools, and two-thirds of them graduated. The program recruited a large number of graduates to the profession and led to major changes in nursing education. The government's requirements of a modified program, including policies of nondiscrimination on the basis of race and marital status, allowed an opportunity to redesign nursing education. In addition, because nursing school directors rather than hospital administrators were required to administer the federal funds, the actual costs of the nursing program and the services provided to hospitals by students became known. Armed with this information, nursing directors were better equipped to negotiate with administrators for funds to upgrade their programs after the war (Brueggemann, 1992).

Diversity in the Professional Nursing Workforce

Unlike their predecessors, nursing leaders during World War II attempted to remedy the shortage of nursing personnel by employing people belonging to two groups that had been previously excluded from mainstream nursing: men and African-American women. Since their inception in the late 19th century, most nursing schools had excluded men and African-American women from admission, based on racial discrimination and restrictive policies. To ensure that African-American patients received medical care and that African-American physicians and nurses had opportunities to become professionals, separate African-American hospitals and schools had been created in the late 1800s (Gamble, 1989). African-American graduates of these programs faced further discrimination as registered nurses because many hospitals and community health agencies refused to employ them, citing objections from White patients to being cared for by African-American nurses. African-American nurses faced additional discrimination when they attempted to join most of the state associations of the ANA. To overcome such overt and covert forms of discrimination, the National Association of Colored Graduate Nurses (NACGN) was formed in 1908. The NACGN fought for almost 50 years to end the social, economic, and professional injuries inflicted on African-American graduate nurses (Staupers, 1951). It would not be until 1945 that discriminatory policies would change.

Stirred by patriotism, many young African-American women had entered the Cadet Nurse Corps because that program prohibited discrimination based on race. However, throughout World War II the Army Nurse Corps maintained restrictive racial quotas, whereas the Navy Nurse Corps excluded all African Americans. By 1944, public opinion had turned against the armed services' discriminatory policies, and in January 1945 both corps lifted their racial restrictions and accepted African-American female nurses into their ranks.

When World War II came to an end, the presence of many more African-American registered nurses, many of whom were graduates of the Cadet Nurse Corps, caused state nurses associations to remove racial barriers to membership. General integration into the ANA was hastened in 1948, when its House of Delegates granted individual

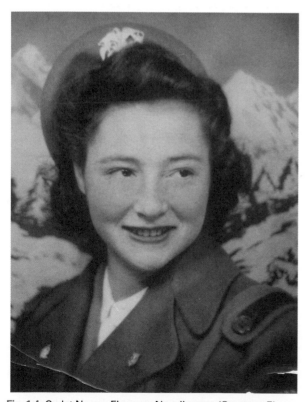

Fig. 1.4 **Cadet Nurse, Florence Noodleman.** (Courtesy, Eleanor Crowder Bjoring Center for Nursing Historical Inquiry, The University of Virginia.)

membership to African-American nurses barred from their state associations and called for the establishment of biracial integration at district and state levels. In 1950 only two state associations retained racial restrictions, allowing the NACGN to announce its dissolution. By 1952, all state nurses' associations had removed racial discriminatory policies for ANA membership. Unfortunately, the end of overt racial discrimination against African-American nurses did not eradicate the more subtle and entrenched forms of prejudice. For Black nurses, the struggle to be fully accepted as professionals by patients, hospitals, and fellow health care colleagues continued. This deep-seated discrimination led to the emergence of the National Black Nurses Association in 1971. As was its predecessor (the NACGN), the National Black Nurses Association was (and continues to be) committed to acting as an advocate for the improvement of the health care for Blacks and to ensuring that African-American nurses participate fully in the nursing profession and the larger health care system (Carnegie, 1995).

Male Nurses

The long-standing bias against male nurses that was present in the opening decades of the 20th century was based on society's belief that nursing was a feminine skill and therefore men should not be nurses (Nurses' Associated Alumnae of the United States, 1902/2007). In the late 19th and early 20th centuries, most men who wanted to be nurses attended all-male programs sponsored by religious groups or affiliated with psychiatric hospitals. Some hospital administrators hired male graduate nurses but often treated them as orderlies rather than as nursing professionals (Craig, 1940; Keeling et al., 2018).

Within the military, male nurses faced a more entrenched form of discrimination than did their African-American female nurse counterparts. Tradition and sentiment had long dictated that nursing was a woman's field, and when Congress established the nurse corps, it had mandated that *only women* could be appointed as military nurses. Male nursing students and graduates were subject to the Selective Service Act draft but most volunteered for service rather than waiting to be drafted. Once in, male nurses were denied professional nursing status; most served as enlisted personnel in health-related positions (Rose, 1947). It would not be until 1955, after the Korean conflict, that Congress passed legislation allowing the appointment of male nurses as reserve officers in the Army, Navy, and Air Force Nurse Corps (Sarnecky, 1999).

Post–World War II Era

America emerged from World War II profoundly changed as a people, society, and country. After years of war, with the rationing of resources and lack of individual choices, Americans wanted better lives for themselves and their families. In particular, they wanted quality health care and educational opportunities. In response to citizens' needs, the federal government formulated new health priorities and policies and funded health initiatives. One of the first of these was the Hospital Survey and Reconstruction Act (the Hill-Burton Act) of 1946, which began to provide federal funds for hospital construction and new health centers. Over the next decade these funds significantly expanded and updated the nation's hospitals, increased bed capacity, and transformed hospitals into scientific and technical medical centers (Risse, 1999).

At midcentury, the public's growing belief in the power of modern medicine was sustained by impressive advances in pharmacology, medicine, and surgery. Penicillin, one of the earliest "miracle drugs," successfully treated serious infections and, in preventing postoperative infections, opened the door to radically new surgical procedures (Fig. 1.5).

The dramatic advances in pharmacology, medical sciences, and technology enticed health professionals and patients alike to believe in the possibility that humans might conquer all diseases. The public encouraged the federal government to continue its large appropriations for medical research, education, and services (Stevens, 1989).

The Nursing Shortage

With a rise in the number and size of hospitals, the postwar "baby boom" (78 million children were born between 1946 and 1964), and an increase in the incidence of chronic

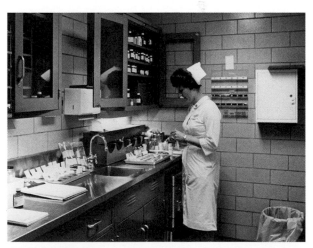

Fig. 1.5 Medication Nurse, Circa 1950s. (Courtesy, Eleanor Crowder Bjoring Center for Nursing Historical Inquiry, The University of Virginia.)

disease, the nation's demand for nurses increased dramatically after World War II. Demand for hospital beds was at an all-time high. The problem was that there were not enough nurses; many female nurses turned to a career in homemaking, leaving the nursing workforce.

Faced with a serious nursing shortage, hospital administrators were forced to restrict admissions. They also had to seek solutions, initially focusing on acquiring more nurses rather than on creating ways to improve the education of nurses (Lynaugh & Brush, 1996). Other strategies to address the shortage followed. These included the employment of ward clerks, the use of volunteers, practical nurses, and aides to help nurses provide patient care, the initiation of team nursing, the importation of foreign nurses, and improvement in nurses' salaries and working conditions.

Federal funding for nursing education remained modest until 1964, when Congress passed the Nurse Training Act in response to pressure from the AMA and the American Hospital Association about the need for nurses. This landmark legislation awarded $242.6 million for nursing student scholarships, loans, recruitment, school construction and maintenance, and special educational projects (Kalisch & Kalisch, 1995). The success of these initiatives helped to diminish the nation's shortages of nurses. Between 1950 and 1967, the number of registered nurses rose by 67%, the number of practical nurses rose by 134%, and the number of nursing aides/assistants rose by 244% (US Public Health Service, 1976).

NURSING IN INSTITUTIONS OF HIGHER EDUCATION

Baccalaureate Programs

In addition to other legislation after the war, in 1946 Congress passed the GI Bill of Rights, enabling veterans to acquire vocational training or a college education (Kiester, 1994). Nurse veterans took advantage of the opportunity to enroll in college programs and earned degrees in nursing education and administration. The increased enrollment provided a new direction for collegiate nursing programs. Beginning in the 1950s, entry-level baccalaureate nursing programs were opened to high school graduates throughout the nation. In 1962, 178 colleges offered undergraduate degrees in nursing, and the pool of baccalaureate-educated nurses, essential to the creation of advanced nursing educational programs, dramatically expanded (Brown, 1978).

Community College Programs

The severity of the nursing shortage in the postwar years encouraged faculty to develop new entry-level nursing programs. In 1951, nurse educator Mildred Montag proposed an innovative program to prepare nurse technicians in 2-year associate degree (AD) community colleges. A 5-year study of AD programs found that their graduates were able to pass state nursing licensure examinations. They demonstrated an adequate level of clinical nursing competency and were employed as graduate nurses (Haase, 1990).

The results of this study launched the AD educational movement. Securing funding from the Nurse Training Act of 1964, community colleges opened AD programs at a phenomenal rate. From 1952 to 1974, the number of AD programs in the country doubled every 4 years. During one period, new programs opened at the rate of one per week (Rines, 1977).

Several important goals were attained by the AD programs' success. A new pool of students, including men, married women with children, and older-than-typical undergraduates, were now able to choose nursing careers. The AD graduates helped to minimize the nursing shortages of the 1970s and 1980s; this encouraged hospital directors to close their expensive 3-year diploma programs and let colleges and universities educate nurses. Soon diploma education disappeared in most states (Lynaugh & Brush, 1996). In 2014 the National League for Nursing's Annual Survey of Schools of Nursing, Academic Year 2013–2014, reported that AD programs (58.4%) remain the major point of entry into nursing, followed by baccalaureate degree programs (40%), of the total of 1869 nursing programs surveyed (National League for Nursing, 2014).

Although AD education opened nursing education to a broader student population, the existence of three entry-level educational programs—diploma, associate, and baccalaureate degree, all leading to registered nurse licensure and beginning positions—has led to confusion among the public and the profession as to the exact requirements for a credential as a professional nurse. However, what is becoming clearer with recent research is that Bachelor of Science in Nursing (BSN)-prepared graduates give care that is evidence based and improves patient outcomes. Today there is a focus on hospitals hiring more nurses prepared at the BSN level.

Graduate Programs

In the mid-1950s the need for nurses prepared at the graduate level to direct nursing service departments and teach in baccalaureate programs encouraged faculty to develop more master's-level programs. These earlier programs focused on preparing educators and administrators rather than clinicians. However, in the 1960s, as the pace of medical innovation increased and new clinical subspecialties such as cardiology, nephrology, and oncology came into existence, master's programs shifted their focus to preparing clinical nurse specialists (CNSs) and nurse practitioners (NPs).

Although nurses have earned doctoral degrees since the mid-1920s, most of them acquired their education in related disciplines such as education and sociology. In the late 1960s, aided by funds from the federal government, doctoral nursing programs began to appear (Grace, 1978). Nursing doctoral programs provided the profession with the rigorous academic credentials it needed to develop its unique disciplinary knowledge and prepare its future researchers and scholars. Questions about the nature of nursing, its mission and goals, and the scope of nurses' roles drove nurse educators to consider the answers to these questions and present them in a more coherent whole. These questions grew out of an interest in changes in the educational preparation of nurses from diploma to baccalaureate programs and concerns about what to include or exclude in curricula and what nurses needed to learn to function as nurses (Meleis, 2004).

To begin to answer questions about the discipline of nursing, schools and colleges of nursing were incorporated into institutions of higher education devoted to scholarly inquiry and research. One of these was Columbia University Teachers College. Many of the prominent nursing leaders of the 1950s took courses in education and administration at Teachers College. Some of these nursing leaders received a doctoral degree in education (EdD).

Teachers College also can be credited with the birth of nursing theory (Omery et al., 1995). The earliest nursing theories were similar to system and physiological models. These models reflected the paradigm that was strongly supported by the field of education at the time: the received view of science. Other disciplines considered these tenets to be *one* way of gaining knowledge in the sciences; however, education—and therefore nursing—held that these tenets were the *only* way. Nurses then adopted this paradigm as truth. This view was not without its problems; as nurses restricted themselves to objective data based on quantitative methods of inquiry, they simultaneously restricted knowledge development in the discipline (Telford, 2004). Only later did the profession's leaders incorporate other ways of knowing, including clinical expertise, qualitative methods, and historical research.

RISE OF ADVANCED PRACTICE NURSING IN CLINICAL SETTINGS

Acute Care Nurse Specialist

Advances in medical science and technology through the latter half of the 20th century radically changed the practice of medicine and the treatment of hospitalized patients. However, the newly constructed hospitals, with their private rooms and long hallways, caused new problems for an already short-handed nursing staff, because patients could no longer be seen from a central nurses' station. Moreover, many nurses were unskilled and unfamiliar with the new treatments and new technologies. As a result, nurse and physician teams initiated the concept of the intensive care unit (ICU), a large room in which the hospital's most experienced and competent nurses could work with critically ill patients. Within these new units, the care of the critically ill changed, as did the nurses' role. Their success paved the way for the creation of acute care nurse specialist roles.

An example of one of these units was the coronary care unit (CCU). Influenced by research on the success of cardiopulmonary resuscitation and cardiac defibrillation and interested in using electronic monitoring technology for improving the care of cardiac patients, physicians and nurses opened CCUs to manage patients with acute myocardial infarction. Supported by federal appropriations for medical research, CCUs proliferated. Central to the coronary care specialist movement was the nurses' drive toward independent practice, nurse-derived standards of care, and a collegial relationship with the units' physicians. Working together, nurses and physicians shared the emerging clinical knowledge for managing critically ill patients. They mastered new medical technology and wrote standard "order sets," educating nurses to identify changes in cardiac rhythms and to treat patients without waiting for physicians' orders. Gaining acceptance as essential members of the CCU team, nurses stretched the boundaries of nursing practice and laid the foundation for a more autonomous practice for other master's-prepared nurses (Keeling, 2004).

As these highly specialized nurses realized their need for continuing education, ICU nurses formed national specialty organizations, including the AACN in 1969, renamed the American Association of Critical Care Nurses in 1972. These organizations established practice standards and developed continuing education programs and certification for their respective emerging clinical specialties. The success of ICU nurses paved the way for the creation of many subspecialty units (including units for neonatology, burns, renal dialysis, and oncology) and marked a significant advance in the scope of practice for nurses and opportunities for professional growth.

Primary Care Nurse Practitioners

At the same time that acute care specialist roles were emerging in hospitals, the primary care NP movement crystallized. The idea of an advanced practice role for pediatric nurses, the rise of medical specialization, the concurrent shortage of primary care physicians (especially in rural areas), and the public's demand for improved access to health care all helped foster the movement.

In 1965 Loretta Ford and Henry Silver opened the first pediatric NP program at the University of Colorado. This collaborative project, designed by a nurse and a pediatrician, prepared professional nurses to provide well childcare and manage the care of children with common childhood illnesses. Its success would lead to federal funding for the education of NPs in other clinical areas.

Similar to acute care specialists, primary care NPs developed organizations that created certification requirements and clinical standards. However, because NPs assumed diagnostic and treatment responsibilities outside the confines of the hospital, they also set in place legal certification at the state level and began to seek prescriptive authority (for more on this see Keeling, 2007).

By the 1970s NPs were employed in a variety of primary care settings, including physicians' offices, clinics, and schools (Fig. 1.6). In addition, some practiced in hospitals in subspecialty areas such as nephrology, oncology, and neonatology. In the early 1990s, in response to the growing shortage of medical residents in subspecialty areas and the need to manage patients with increasingly complex medical needs (e.g., heart and lung transplants), acute care nurse practitioner (ACNP) programs began to develop across the nation. Currently, numerous ACNPs work in acute care hospitals in various subspecialties—some as "nurse hospitalists." In addition, states are requiring that NPs have the proper educational requirements (e.g., ACNP vs. primary care NP) related to their specific job requirements and scope of practice. Moreover, many are requiring the Doctor of Nursing Practice (DNP).

Clinical Nurse Leader and Doctor of Nursing Practice

At the turn of the 21st century, the development of a new role for nurses came about as a response to growing patient care needs and the changing health care delivery environment. In February 2004, the AACN Board of Directors approved a new model of nursing practice and nursing education at the master's level—the CNL (AACN, 2004a). The CNL, a generalist master's-prepared clinician, was to provide care in all health care settings at the point of care. He or she was to be accountable for client care outcomes by coordinating, delegating, and

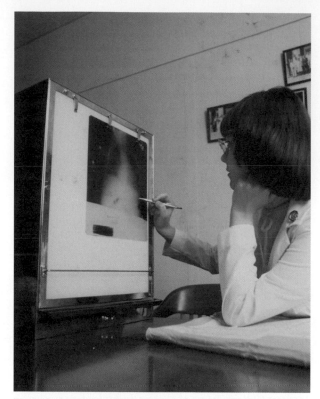

Fig. 1.6 Nurse Practitioner Student Reading X-Ray. (Courtesy, Eleanor Crowder Bjoring Center for Nursing Historical Inquiry, The University of Virginia.)

supervising the care provided by the health care team. The CNL was not considered to be an advanced practice nurse. According to AACN, if the education of the *generalist* nurse was elevated to the master's degree level, it was reasonable to assume that *specialty* education and the education of those individuals prepared for the highest level of nursing practice would occur at the doctoral level. Thus the DNP degree was proposed. It would be a terminal doctorate, equivalent to a PhD but with a focus on practice rather than research. It would be a degree, not a new "role."

The *practice-focused* doctoral degree was not a new idea. The first such program, offering the Nursing Doctorate (ND), was established at Case Western Reserve University in 1979 and offered an entry-level nursing degree. Since then, numerous practice-focused doctoral programs were begun throughout the country (AACN, 2004b). According to AACN's 2020–2021 survey of 964 nursing programs nationally (91.2% response rate), there are now 407 DNP programs currently enrolling students at schools of nursing nationwide. DNP programs are now available in all 50 states plus the District of Columbia (AACN, 2022, June, p. 10). In the future, the DNP will be the requisite preparation for all advanced practice nursing roles, including the NP, CNS, certified nurse midwife, and certified registered nurse anesthetist (CRNA). Advanced practice nursing care will be needed if the United States is to provide equal access to care for patients in both rural and urban areas—care that is today often provided in volunteer nursing and medical clinics (Fig. 1.7).

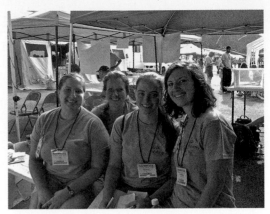

Fig. 1.7 Nurses in Regional Area Medical Clinic, Virginia, Circa 2010. (Courtesy, Eleanor Crowder Bjoring Center for Nursing Historical Inquiry, The University of Virginia.)

SUMMARY

This chapter provides a brief overview of the history of American nursing from the middle of the 19th century to the present day. Highlights include the effect of Florence Nightingale's ideas about nursing and nurse training, issues surrounding the development of professional and educational standards for nurses, the role of nurses in war, and the development of CNS, NP, and doctoral programs for nurses. These events and topics did not happen in isolation; rather they occurred in the context of the development of the practice of medicine and the rise of science and the health care system. Therefore the chapter discusses how nursing was influenced by these events and how nursing has also shaped its own progress.

The chapter also discusses the challenges the profession has faced in the past 150 years. Many of the issues that nurses faced in the past persist today. Among these are the issues of equal opportunity for all races, genders, and classes, and professional consensus about the educational requirements for entry into practice.

The context in which the nursing profession exists is also still a consideration as the world faces the implications of a global society and the challenges of emerging pandemic diseases, persistent wars, and continuing nursing shortages. The future of nursing will likely continue to demand nursing care that is innovative, efficient, cost-effective, and responsive to human needs in all settings. As in the past, nursing leaders' decisions today are already shaping the profession's future. Those decisions can be better made with an understanding of the profession's past.

SALIENT POINTS

- The first hospital-based nurse training schools, built on the apprenticeship model of learning, had the dual task of providing care to patients and educating students to become professional nurses.
- Nursing state licensure, begun in 1903, is important because it protects the public and defines the role and scope of nursing practice.
- Nurses have played a major role in providing essential health services to the community for more than a century, especially for the poor and chronically ill.
- During World War II, the US Public Health Service Cadet Nurse Corps attracted thousands of students to the profession and provided essential nursing services in civilian hospitals.
- Nursing, still a predominately White and female-oriented profession, needs to continue to recruit outside of this domain.
- Associate degree programs, begun in 1952, opened the nursing profession to a more diverse population than had existed with diploma and baccalaureate education.
- Advanced clinical practice nurses, as acute care nurses and NPs, expanded the boundaries of the profession.
- Graduate programs prepared nursing educators, directors, clinical specialists, researchers, and administrative leaders needed by the health care system and society.
- The CNL role and the DNP degrees continue to evolve.

CRITICAL REFLECTION EXERCISES

1. Discuss how the past informs the present in relation to two of the following current issues:
   - Nurses practicing to the full extent of their education and experiences
   - Nurses practicing as full partners in redesigning health care in the United States
   - Diversity in gender, race, and class in the nursing profession
   - Disaster and pandemic preparedness and response
   - Access to health care
   - Health promotion and disease prevention
   - Health service delivery value (Quintuple Aim)
   - Aging of the population
   - Increase in chronic diseases
   - Emerging technologies
   - Expanding knowledge and information in the sciences and nursing profession
   - Nursing education mobility/progression models

REFERENCES

Abrams, S. E. (1993). Brilliance and bureaucracy: Nursing and changes in the Rockefeller Foundation, 1915–1930. *Nursing History Review, 1,* 119–138.

American Association of Colleges of Nursing. (2004a, March 29). *Dialogue with the board: AACN clinical leader project* [Power-Point slides]. https://www.aacnnursing.org/Portals/42/CNL/Spring04Dialogue.pdf

American Association of Colleges of Nursing. (2004b). *AACN position statement on the practice doctorate in nursing.* http://www.aacn.nche.edu/DNP/DNPPositionStatement.htm

American Association of Colleges of Nursing. (2021, April 6). *The Essentials: Core competencies for professional nursing education.* https://www.aacnnursing.org/Portals/42/AcademicNursing/pdf/Essentials-2021.pdf

American Association of Colleges of Nursing. (2022, June). *State of the Doctor of Nursing Practice Education in 2022.* https://www.aacnnursing.org/Portals/42/News/Surveys-Data/State-of-the-DNP-Summary-Report-June-2022.pdf

American Society of Superintendents of Training Schools for Nurses. (1897). *First and second annual reports.* https://www.nursing.upenn.edu/live/files/795-nin-annual-report-1-2

Bacon, A. (1892). Report on Dixie Hospital and Training School for Nurses. *Southern Workman, 22,* 108.

Blum, J. (1981). The end of an era. In J. Blum (Ed.), *The national experience* (pp. 652–669). Harcourt Brace Jovanovich.

Brainard, A. M. (1922). *The evolution of public health nursing.* Saunders.

Brown, J. (1978). Master's education in nursing, 1945–1969. In M. L. Fitzpatrick (Ed.), *Historical studies in nursing* (pp. 104–130). Teachers College.

Brueggemann, D. (1992). *The United States Cadet Nurse Corps 1943–1948: The Nebraska experience* (Unpublished master's thesis) University of Nebraska.

Bullough, B. (1975). The first two phases in nursing licensure. In B. Bullough (Ed.), *The law and the expanding nurse's role* (pp. 7–21). Appleton-Century-Crofts.

Burgess, M. (1928). *Nurses, patients and pocketbooks.* National League for Nursing Education, Committee on the Grading of Nursing Schools.

Cannings, K., & Lazonick, W. (1975). The development of the nursing labor force in the United States: A basic analysis. *International Journal of Health Services, 5*(2), 185–216. https://doi.org/10.2190/UE7W-VQLR-KR1M-CD5H

Carnegie, M. E. (1995). *The path we tread: Blacks in nursing, 1854–1984.* Jones & Bartlett.

Christy, T. E. (1969). *Cornerstone for nursing education.* Teachers College.

Church, O. (1987). Historiography in nursing research. *Western Journal of Nursing Research, 9*(2), 275–279. https://doi.org/10.1177/019394598700900211

Clappison, G. B. (1964). *Vassar's rainbow division 1918.* Graphic.

Craig, L. (1940). Opportunities for men nurses. *American Journal of Nursing, 40*(1), 667–670.

Craig, S. (2015). Nursing in Schoolfield Mill Village: Cotton and welfare. In J. Kirchgessner, & A. W. Keeling (Eds.), *Nursing rural America: Perspectives from the early 20th century* (pp. 53–67). Springer.

Daisy, C. (1996). *Keeping the flame: The influence of Agnes Ohlson on licensure and registration for nurses: 1936–1963* (Unpublished doctoral dissertation). University of Texas.

D'Antonio, P., & Fairman, J. (2010). Guest editorial: History matters. *Nursing Outlook, 58*(2), 113–114. https://www.doi.org/10.1016/j.outlook.2010.01.004

Dock, L. D., & Stewart, I. (1938). *A short history of nursing* (4th ed.). Putnam.

Draper, E. A. (1893/1949). Necessity of an American Nurses' Association. In J. S. Billings, & H. M. Hurd (Eds.), *Nursing of the sick* (pp. 149–153). McGraw-Hill.

Duffus, R. L. (1938). *Lillian Wald, neighbor and crusader.* Macmillan.

Fitzpatrick, M. L. (1975). Nurses in American history. Nursing and the great depression. *American Journal of Nursing, 75*(12), 2188–2190.

Flood, M. (1981). *The troubling expedient: General staff nursing in United States hospitals in the 1930s: A means to institutional, educational, and personal ends* (Unpublished doctoral dissertation). University of California.

Gamble, V. (1989). *Making a place for ourselves.* Oxford University.

Gardner, M. S. (1936). *Public health nursing* (3rd ed.). Macmillan.

Geister, J. M. (1926). Hearsay and facts in private duty. *American Journal of Nursing, 26*, 515–528.

Goldmark, J. (1923). *Nursing and nursing education in the United States: Report of the committee for the study of nursing education*. Macmillan.

Grace, H. K. (1978). The development of doctoral education in nursing: In historical perspective. *Journal of Nursing Education, 17*(4), 17–27.

Haase, P. T. (1990). *The origins and rise of associate degree nursing education*. Duke University Press.

Hampton, I. A. (1893/1949). Educational standards for nurses. In *Nursing of the sick* (pp. 1–12). McGraw-Hill. Reprinted from Billings, J. S., & Hurd, H. M. (Eds.). (1894). *Hospitals, dispensaries and nursing: Papers and discussions in the International Congress of Charities, Correction, and Philanthropy, Section III, Chicago, IL, June 12th to 17th, 1893. Part III, Nursing of the sick*. Johns Hopkins University Press.

Howell, J. D. (1996). *Technology in the hospital: Transforming patient care in the early twentieth century*. Johns Hopkins University Press.

Johns, E. (1925). *A study of the present status of the Negro woman in nursing, 1925* (pp. 29–41). Rockefeller Foundation records, Rockefeller Archive Center.

Johnston, D. F. (1966). *History and trends of practical nursing*. Mosby.

Kalisch, P. A., & Kalisch, B. J. (1995). *The advance of American nursing* (3rd ed.). Lippincott.

Keeling, A. W. (2004). Blurring the boundaries between medicine and nursing: Coronary care nursing, circa the 1960s. *Nursing History Review: Official Journal of the American Association for the History of Nursing, 12*, 139–164.

Keeling, A. W. (2007). *Nursing and the privilege of prescription, 1893–2000*. Ohio State University Press.

Keeling, A. W., Hehman, M. C., & Kirchgessner, J. C. (2018). *History of professional nursing in the United States: Toward a culture of health*. Springer.

Keeling, A. W., Kirchgessner, J., & Brodie, B. (2009). *A history of the American Association of Colleges of Nursing*. AACN.

Keeling, A. W., & Ramos, M. C. (1995). The role of nursing history in preparing nursing for the future. *Nursing and Health Care Perspectives on Community: Official Publication of the National League for Nursing, 16*(1), 30–34.

Kiester, E. Jr. (1994). The GI Bill may be the best deal ever make by Uncle Sam. *Smithsonian, 25*(8), 128–139.

Kimball, J. F. (1934). Prepayment plan of hospital care. *American Hospital Association Bulletin, 8*, 45.

King, L. Y. (1998). In search of women of African descent who served in the Civil War Union Navy. *Journal of Negro History, 83*(4), 302–309.

Lewenson, S. (2015). Town and Country nursing: Community participation and nurse recruitment. In J. Kirchgessner & A. W. Keeling (Eds.), *Nursing rural America: Perspectives from the early 20th century* (pp. 1–19). Springer.

Lynaugh, J. E., & Brush, B. L. (1996). *American nursing: From hospitals to health systems*. Blackwell.

Maling, B. (2007). *Women providing nursing care in Charlottesville during the American Civil War, 1861–1865*. Windows in Time:

The Newsletter of the Eleanor C. Bjoring Center for Nursing Historical Inquiry (University of Virginia), *15*(1), 6–10.

Meckel, R. A. (1990). *Save the babies*. Johns Hopkins University Press.

Meleis, A. I. (2004). *Theoretical nursing development & progress*. Lippincott Williams & Wilkins.

National League for Nursing. (2014). *Annual survey of schools of nursing. Academic year 2013–2014*. https://www.nln.org/news/research-statistics/newsroomnursing-education-statistics/annual-survey-of-schools-of-nursing-academic-year-2013-2014-2862bd5c-7836-6c70-9642-ff00005f0421

Nightingale, F. (1859). *Notes on nursing: What it is and what it is not*. D. Appleton and Company (1860).

Numbers, R. (1978). The third party: Health insurance in America. In J. Leavitt & R. Numbers (Eds.), *Sickness and health in America* (pp. 142–145). University of Wisconsin.

Nurses' Associated Alumnae of the United States. (1902/2007). Proceedings of the fifth annual convention. In C. O'Lynn, & R. E. Tranbarger (Eds.), *Men in nursing: History, challenges, and opportunities* (pp. 743–809). Springer.

Omery, A., Kasper, C. E., & Page, G. G. (1995). *In search of nursing science*. Sage.

Reverby, S. (1987). *Ordered to care*. Cambridge University Press.

Rines, A. R. (1977). Associate degree education: History, development, and rationale. *Nursing Outlook, 25*, 496–501.

Risse, G. B. (1999). *Mending bodies, saving souls: History of hospitals*. Oxford University Press.

Roberts, M. (1954). *American nursing: History and interpretation*. Macmillan.

Roren, R. (1930). *The public's investment in hospitals (Committee on the Costs of Medical Care, Publication No. 7)*. The University of Chicago Press.

Rose, J. (1947). Men nurses in military service. *American Journal of Nursing, 47*, 147–148.

Sarnecky, M. (1999). *History of the Army Nurse Corps*. University of Pennsylvania Press.

Sheahan, D. (1979). *The social origins of American nursing and its movement into the university* (Unpublished doctoral dissertation). New York University.

Sommers, H., & Sommers, A. (1961). *Patients and health insurance*. Brookings Institution.

Starr, P. (1982). *The social transformation of American medicine*. Basic Books.

Staupers, M. K. (1951). Story of the National Association of Colored Graduate Nurses. *American Journal of Nursing, 51*(4), 221–222.

Stevens, R. (1989). *In sickness and in wealth*. Basic Books.

Stewart, I. (1943). *The education of nurses*. Macmillan.

Stoney, E. (1919). *Practical points in nursing*. Saunders.

Telford, J. (2004). *The liberation of the minds and practices of nurses: The evolution and adoption of the received view to enlightenment in nursing science, circa 1873–present* (Unpublished).

Toman, C., & Thifault, M. C. (2012). Historical thinking and the shaping of nursing identity. *Nursing History Review: Official Journal of the American Association for the History of Nursing, 20*, 184–204. https://doi.org/10.1891/1062-8061.20.184

U.S. Bureau of Census. (1900). *Special reports: Occupation roles, and gender*. U.S. Government Printing Office.

U.S. Public Health Service. (1976). *The consumer and health planners*. U.S. Government Printing Office.

Wald, L. D. (1938). *The house on Henry street*. Henry Holt.

Whelan, J. C. (2005). A necessity in the nursing world: The Chicago nurses professional registry, 1918–1950. *Nursing History Review, 13*, 49–76.

FURTHER READING IN NURSING HISTORY

Cockerham, A., & Keeling, A. W. (2012). *Rooted in the mountains, reaching to the world: Stories of nursing and midwifery at Kentucky's Frontier School, 1939–1989*. Butler Books.

Keeling, A. W., Hehman, M., & Kirchgessner, J. (2017). *History of professional nursing in the United States: Towards a culture of health*. Springer.

Keeling, A. W., & Wall, B. (2015). *Nurses and disasters: Global, historical cases*. Springer.

Wall, B. (2015). *Into Africa: A transnational history of Catholic missions and social change*. Rutgers University Press.

Wall, B. M., & Keeling, A. W. (2011). *Nurses on the frontline: When disaster strikes, 1878–2010*. Springer.

2

Academic Progression

Salina Bednarek, EdD, MSN/Ed, RN, CNE and
Elizabeth E. Friberg, DNP, RN

 http://evolve.elsevier.com/Friberg/bridge/

OBJECTIVES

At the completion of this chapter, the reader will be able to:

- Discuss the vision of a transformed 21st-century health care delivery system and nursing's expanded role.
- Analyze the key recommendations of select Institute of Medicine (IOM) *Quality Chasm* reports and trends on health care transformation.
- Analyze the key messages of the Robert Wood Johnson Foundation's *Future of Nursing: Leading Change, Advancing Health* (2011) report and the report's impact on the nursing profession and academic progression.
- Analyze the key conclusions of the National Academies of Science, Engineering, and Medicine's (NASEM's)

The Future of Nursing 2020–2030: Charting a Path to Achieving Health Equity report and the report's impact on the nursing workforce.
- Engage in identifying current barriers and obstacles to academic progression and potential solutions.
- Reflect on your academic strategy for achieving higher levels of education in either direct- or indirect-care roles in advanced nursing practice.
- Reflect on the value and professional opportunities of expanding advanced nursing practice and nurse scientist roles.

INTRODUCTION

The health care industry is not merely changing. With a focus on population and community health, patient-centered care, treatment innovation, data analytics, health care technology, and patient and practitioner experiences, the health care system is being dramatically transformed. As the health care system is transformed, practice is transformed; therefore health care practitioner education must also be transformed. Nursing, as the largest segment of health care practitioners, has a large responsibility for elevating the educational levels of all nurses—a transformational reality at best. Nursing opportunities will open and expand. Our health care model will be dramatically different in the next decade and beyond. Simultaneously, educating nurses about the realities of today's practice and their anticipated future practice requires a strategy for academic progression that is reasonable, relevant, realistic, flexible, affordable, and seamless. Similar issues are experienced worldwide, but this chapter focuses on academic

progression generically and seamless academic progression specifically. The following definitions are used:

- *Academic progression* is defined as educational articulation models that promote lifelong learning through the attainment of academic credentials (Organization for Associate Degree Nursing [OADN] & American Nurses Association [ANA], 2015).
- *Seamless academic progression* encompasses the concept of advancement from one educational facility to another in an orderly and clearly charted plan so that one can acquire sequential degrees without the repetition of coursework or cumbersome prerequisite coursework (OADN & ANA, 2015).

LOOKING BACK

Chapter 1 (A Brief History of the Professionalization of Nursing in the United States) explores the historical perspectives of the US nursing profession's response to societal events over the years to meet the health care needs of individuals, families, communities, and populations across the lifespan. Dr. Mildred Montag sought to decrease the length of time to "entry into practice" in the early 1950s by creating an option to achieve an associate degree in nursing (2-year degree) to alleviate a critical shortage of nurses, in lieu of diploma programs (3-year degree), the dominant choice for entry into practice at the time, and baccalaureate programs for professional nurses (4-year degree) (OADN & ANA, 2015). This strategy allowed the profession to move nursing education from within a hospital environment to collegiate and higher education settings while meeting the need for more nurses. The associate degree in nursing expanded quickly, and diploma programs began to close. Nursing demonstrated its strength and ability to innovatively fill the workforce need and meet the health care needs of society. However, this innovation contributed to the multiplicity of pathways available to enter the nursing profession. The innovative associate degree to baccalaureate degree in nursing (Bachelor of Science in Nursing [BSN]) progression pathways originally envisioned in the 1950s are explained in Box 2.1. Because the academic progression from the associate degree in nursing to the BSN vision was not realized in the early 1950s, the discontinuities and misalignments of institutional policies that impeded a smooth academic progression and career path for students were perpetuated in the years that followed.

In 1964, and reaffirmed in 2000, the ANA voted to continue to work toward baccalaureate education as the educational foundation for professional nursing (OADN & ANA, 2015). In a 2010 policy statement, the Tri-Council for Nursing, an alliance representing the ANA, the American Association of Colleges of Nursing (AACN), the American Organization of Nurse Executives (AONE), and the National League for Nursing (NLN), supported the development of a "highly educated nursing workforce" and advocated for the educational advancement of registered nurses (RNs) as a critical component of safe and effective patient care consistent with the Institute of Medicine's (IOM's) goals (OADN & ANA, 2015).

For students, understanding the concepts of **lifelong learning** and **career advancement** to higher levels of nursing practice is challenging. In their classic work, Pittman et al. (2014) stated that the absence of smooth transition points, salary differentiation, and professional distinctions in perceived abilities across academic preparations contributed to a student's lack of appreciation for the rewards and relevancy of pursuing advanced education. The concept of academic progression was embraced by higher education, but the approach to best align and coordinate nursing education varied. Many of these issues persist today.

National conversations for transforming the US health care delivery system and health professionals' education were initiated with the IOM's landmark *Quality Chasm* report series launched following the IOM's *1998 National Roundtable on Health Care Quality* report. The initial report explored the "burden of harm" classified as underuse, overuse, and misuse, and stated the quality of care was the problem not the prevailing and piloted models of care at

---

BOX 2.1   Types of 1950's Innovative Academic Models for Associate Degree to Bachelor of Science in Nursing Progression*

Community College Baccalaureate is a bachelor's degree conferred by a community college that is authorized to do so.

Competency-Based Curriculum is defined by the Learning Collaborate on Advanced Education Transformation, which is part of the Center to Champion Nursing in America, as a process in which education partners, who generally represent different educational approaches and backgrounds, develop a shared understanding and a common goal and framework. The scope of the curriculum reaches beyond core competencies and focuses on knowledge, attitudes, and skills that encompass professional nursing practice. The curriculum is not standardized, but the model *aims to reach standardized outcomes*.

Dual Enrollment is the concept of a student enrolling concurrently in two separate academic institutions at the same time, often studying in two related programs.

Statewide Curriculum Programs are educational collaboratives between universities and community colleges that enable students to transition automatically and seamlessly from an associate degree to a Bachelor of Science in Nursing program, with all schools sharing curriculum, simulation facilities, and faculty. Faculty workload is reduced, and the schools make more efficient and greater use of resources. Implementation of such programs requires *formal articulation agreements* between community colleges and universities, adjustments of prerequisite and nursing curricula, and buy-in from legislative bodies and institutions.

*Organization for Associate Degree Nursing and American Nurses Association, 2015.

that time (IOM, 1997). *To Err is Human* focused on building a safer health care system and the relationship between quality and safety as a system issue and not a human error issue (IOM, 2000). *Crossing the Quality Chasm* further explored quality as a system property defining improvement aims for a new care environment using evidence, information technology, reimbursement incentives, workforce preparation, and safety strategies to assess, analyze, and mitigate risk (IOM, 2001). *Transforming Health Professions Education* (IOM, 2003a) for a new care environment defined core competencies for ALL health professions to establish a common language (provide patient-centered care, work in interdisciplinary teams, use evidence-based practice, apply quality improvement, and utilize informatics). The 2003 report also proposed using oversight processes (accreditation, certification, and licensure) to drive curriculum and practice reform that demonstrated competency (a public safety issue). This report established the foundation for the many present day initiatives, such as removing practice barriers, developing academic-practice partnerships, reimbursement reform, interdisciplinary education and practice, and leadership change. *Priority Areas for National Action* (IOM, 2003b) addressed the issue of translating knowledge into clinical practice and identified more than 20 priority areas that formed the basis of the *National Healthcare Quality Report*. *Patient Safety* (IOM, 2004) established the need for a national health information infrastructure providing immediate access to complete patient information and decision-support tools. *Quality Through Collaboration* (IOM, 2005) focused on the needs of rural health and defined core health services as primary care, emergency medical services, hospital care, long-term care, mental health and substance abuse services, oral health care, and public health services. This report also addressed the recruitment and retention of health care professionals and telehealth. As we move from one study report to the next, we can see how the vision for a 21st-century health care system unfolds—and with it—the complexity of care demands for the health care professionals increases and expands. This vision demands an increase in the quality and safety of services and drives the need for changing how we educate health care practitioners and how they ultimately practice. Chapter 20 (Health Care Quality and Safety) explores the concepts of health care quality and safety in more depth. A summary of the aforementioned IOM 1997–2002 reports can be found in the Appendices of this text.

It is beyond the scope of the chapter to review the research related to the relationship between a higher educated nursing workforce and improved patient-care outcomes in quality and safety in hospitals. The evidence is strong, and institutions have committed to employing an increasingly educated nursing workforce to achieve their aspirational institutional outcomes and reduce errors in care delivery. With the passing of health care reform legislation in 2010 (the Affordable Care Act [ACA]), an opportunity was presented to improve the US health care system's ability to deliver health care for all, that is high quality, patient centered, evidence based and affordable, and optimizes care outcomes. Aspects of the ACA are discussed in Chapter 6 (Health Policy and Planning and the Nursing Practice Environment).

The *Future of Nursing* 2010–2020, the first landmark report, investigated the expanded role nurses would need to play with the increasing demand for safe, high-quality, and effective health care (IOM, 2010). The investigators stated that nurses should practice to the full extent of their education and training (Key Message #1). Looking into the future, recognizing the increasing aging and diversity of the population, ever-increasing technology advances, and the rapidly changing health care delivery system, the investigators concluded that nurses should achieve higher levels of education and training through an improved education system that supports *seamless academic progression* (Key Message #2). In addition, the investigators stated that nurses should be **full** partners with physicians and other health professionals in redesigning health care in the United States—reflecting the need for *parity* in education preparation (Key Message #3).

In 2010, the IOM called for updating and adapting curriculum to meet the demands of the **new delivery system** with emphasis on **prevention**, **wellness**, **care coordination,** and **improved outcomes** for undergraduate nursing programs. At the graduate level, the IOM stated the **Doctor of Nursing Practice (DNP)** is a complement to other health care professions' practice doctorates. **Advanced practice registered nurses (APRNs)** serve as nurse practitioners (NPs), certified nurse-midwives (CNMs), clinical nurse specialists (CNSs), and certified registered nurse anesthetists (CRNAs). In addition to the course work in areas such as **advanced health assessment**, **advanced pharmacology**, and **advanced pathophysiology**; content in **health promotion**, **disease prevention**, **differential diagnosis**, and **disease management** was required to meet the needs of the aging population with increased chronic disease morbidities, complex health challenges, and increased **primary care** needs. The IOM also addressed the need for demonstrating **continuing competence** and **lifelong learning** as well as **interprofessional education** initiatives. Creating a **seamless academic progression framework** was also viewed as necessary to support increasing the **diversity of the nursing workforce** because it allows students to advance their education/careers in a step-wise fashion while working as a nurse and balancing personal and family needs.

Launched in 2007, The Center to Champion Nursing in America (CCNA), a national initiative of the Robert Wood Johnson Foundation (RWJF), American Association of Retired People (AARP), and its Foundation, provided a technical assistance framework for the **Future of Nursing (FON): Campaign for Action.** They launched state-based organizations called Action Coalitions in 50 states and the District of Columbia as the foundation for implementing the 2010 IOM FON recommendations, including a **Learning Collaborative on Advancing Education Transformation** of state, national nursing leaders, and stakeholders. The CCNA identified four models encompassing common practices and strategies that showed significant promise: shared curriculum, competency-based or outcomes-based curriculum, registered nurse (RN)-BSN degree conferred by community colleges, and accelerated options such as RN-Master of Science in Nursing (MSN) programs. These programs are like those envisioned in the 1950s, when the associate degree entry point was implemented. Partnerships across university and community colleges, practice partners, and regulatory/legislative arenas were critical to overcoming resistance to change. Because funding support to initiate and sustain change was critical, CCNA directly shared funding resources through their website. These activities ultimately proposed a set of national standards for prerequisites/corequisites and BSN foundational courses, while promoting open-source sharing, solution-targeted activities, and an extensive support network in support of academic progression.

MOVING FORWARD

In 2012, the RWJF created and funded the **Academic Progression in Nursing (APIN)** program that awarded nine state-level grants to FON-Action Coalitions to develop academic models to create a more highly educated and diverse nursing workforce and remove barriers to academic progression. APIN work concluded in June 2017, and a next-generation collaborative was created. APIN became and is now called **National Education Progression in Nursing (NEPIN)**. The collaborative is jointly led by OADN, Health Impact, and the Washington Center for Nursing, along with a Leadership Alliance of nursing stakeholders across the country. Their mission has evolved to foster collaboration to ensure that nurses have access to higher levels of education and achievement. The OADN Foundation serves as the fiduciary support for the collaborative (NEPIN, n.d.).

The coalition has multiple facets, and the NEPIN Advisory Alliance is the operative arm of the organization. The Advisory Alliance's Special Interest Groups (SIGs) work on programs such as (a) associate degree to BSN progression data analysis; (b) incumbent nurse (currently licensed)

barriers to progression recommendations for employers and nursing leaders; (c) roles of equity, achievement, and thriving in progression; (d) development of the NEPIN Quality Designation; (e) exploration of alternatives for clinical education and training; and (f) career progression mentoring (NEPIN, n.d.). In addition, the RWJF launched the **State Implementation Program (SIP)** for 31 State Action Coalition 2-year matching grants, 20 of which focused on education initiatives.

In 2011 the NLN released a vision statement on APIN Education supporting the need for curriculum reform/reconceptualization and promotion of academic progression to meet the needs of an ever-changing and dynamic health system (NLN, 2011). In a subsequent 2021 value statement, the NLN expanded on its statement highlighting the need for a growing workforce by also addressing the growing shortage of faculty to provide the education for this future nursing workforce (NLN, 2021).

Nursing leaders in the ANA and OADN released a 2015 Joint Position Statement on Academic Progression to Meet the Needs of the Registered Nurse, the Health Care Consumer, and the US Health Care System (OADN & ANA, 2015), committing to collaborate with health care leaders, policymakers, academic institutions, and other stakeholders to support the adoption of innovative and emerging strategies to achieve the IOM recommendation of seamless academic progression and 80% of nurses with a baccalaureate degree target by 2020.

The Josiah Macy Jr. Foundation addressed this issue as well in its 2017 annual report. With a focus on competency-based education on the horizon, the Macy Foundation asserted that all programs must address and redesign curricula and included five recommendations: conducting system redesign, creating a continuum of education, providing training and practice, implementing a robust assessment system, enabling technologies, and continuing outcomes evaluation. These recommendations address the key issues related to program cost, program time constraints, program completion designation, and nurse educator role in the evolving focus on competency rather than specific courses (Josiah Macy Jr. Foundation, 2017).

The academic progression model that showed the greatest potential to achieve the IOM proposed target of 80% of the nursing workforce holding a baccalaureate or higher degree by 2020 was the *intentional academic partnership model* between the existing community college infrastructure and the university infrastructure. This model proved to be flexible across many other model variations. Successful programs aligned curriculum and supportive infrastructure, as well as promoted a close academic collaboration with practice partner support. The proportion of students that progress directly from an associate degree in nursing to a BSN degree in integrated progressive pathways has increased to 80%, a substantial improvement from nonintegrated pathways. However, even with intentional partnership models in place, unless students were incentivized to complete their BSN through specific aspects of program design or employer incentives (funding, scheduling, format, or academic support services), achievement of the 80% BSN workforce was not achieved.

As of 2021, 59% of RNs had a baccalaureate or higher and 37,852 employed nurses hold a doctoral degree, up from 8267 in 2009 and 22,454 in 2016 (Campaign for Action, 2021). The IOM goal was to double the number of nurses with a doctorate by 2020; this goal has been exceeded. Because of the slow progress toward the "80 in 20" goal for baccalaureate or higher by 2020, Spetz (2018) presented a projection model that helped identify the key reasons indicating that progress has been slow. Although more than half of entry-level RNs have associate degrees in nursing and many want to obtain a BSN, there is not a sufficient capacity level in BSN or RN-to-BSN programs to reach the IOM recommendation in the foreseeable future. Only 11 states have reached at least 60% of RNs with a baccalaureate or higher. The reluctance to pursue higher education persists for the same reasons identified earlier in this chapter. Despite doubling the growth of RN-to-BSN graduates, increasing the capacity of RN-to-BSN programs that are part-time, easy to access, geographically available, financially manageable, and efficient may be the only solution to achieve the IOM recommendations.

A complicating factor in meeting the IOM recommendation of an 80% baccalaureate-prepared nursing workforce by 2020 is the projections of the US Bureau of Labor Statistics (USBLS). The USBLS's Quick Facts (2022, April 18) reports that nurses held 3,080,100 jobs in 2020. This represents the size of the occupation at approximately 3 million. Of these near 3 million jobs, 60.5% were in hospitals (state, local, and private); 17.8% were in ambulatory service settings (physicians' offices, home health care, outpatient care settings); 6% were in nursing/residential care facilities; 5% were in government employment, including the military; and 3% were in educational services (state, local, and private). The USBLS projects a 9% growth rate for the nursing occupation between 2020 and 2030, an increase of 276,800 jobs. The average increase across all occupations is 8%. Nursing is growing much faster than other occupations. The USBLS notes the rapid growth is related to increased emphasis on preventive care, growing rates of individuals with chronic conditions, and the demand for health care services from the baby-boom population who are living longer with more active lifestyles. This employment growth is compounded by the need to replace experienced nurses who will retire over the coming decade.

Policy initiatives may encourage nurses to achieve higher levels of education. For example, the federal Health Resources and Services Administration (HRSA) programs (HRSA website) provide equitable health care to people who are geographically isolated and economically or medically disadvantaged. In addition, HRSA fosters health care workforce training and health care infrastructure support for advancing telehealth through scholarships, loans, and repayment programs. Recently, HRSA added two new programs to fund training for clinical faculty as preceptors and training of RNs to address and respond to social determinants of health factors to improve health equity. Despite the increased demand for baccalaureate-prepared nurses as a value proposition, the convergence of a nursing shortage, growing demand for health care services, and a hot employment market, there is a decline in nurses pursuing higher education. This may affect patient care quality, nurse leadership, and other professional nursing factors. In December 2017, the New York State Education Department (Commissioner's Regulation §64.1.c.1 Professional Study of Nurses) passed the "BSN in 10" law, which required all RNs who entered into practice as an associate degree RN to achieve their BSN within 10 years to retain their license. However, the trade-off of pressuring RNs to achieve a baccalaureate may backfire in higher nurse employment vacancy rates. National policies and local employer initiatives are needed to address the increasing nurse workforce shortage, increasing demand for health care services, and reducing the cost and complexity of pursuing higher nursing education.

In 2021, the IOM, now named the National Academies of Science, Engineering, and Medicine (NASEM) published an updated FON report for 2020 to 2030. The original course content areas noted in 2010 for APRNs were **advanced health assessment**, **advanced pharmacology**, **advanced pathophysiology**; **health promotion**, **disease prevention**, **differential diagnosis**, **disease management**; and **primary care**. In 2021, the content areas were expanded to include **population health, environmental health, trauma-informed care, and health equity**. Competencies associated with **decision-making**, **quality improvement**, **systems thinking**, and **team leadership** remain for prelicensure through the doctoral level as well as the need to demonstrate **continuing competence, lifelong learning**, and **interprofessional education and collaboration**. To accomplish these objectives, NASEM added education needs to provide a better understanding of experience with **care management, quality improvement methods, systems-level change management, population health, social determinants of health, health equity, and reconceptualization of the expanded role of nurses** in a transformed health care system. Therefore accrediting, licensing, and certifying organizations must move in the direction of mandating core skills competencies (competency-based education, licensure, and stackable credentialing) that complement academic degree completion and align with licensing examinations. The NASEM more directly calls for state and federal programs to support the academic progression of socioeconomically disadvantaged students (NASEM, 2021). The report encourages partnership between entry-level and higher degree nursing programs to create a more seamless experience. Creating a **seamless academic progression framework** was also viewed as necessary to support increasing the **diversity of the nursing workforce** because it allows students to advance their education/careers in a step-wise fashion while working as a nurse and balancing personal and family needs. The important role of the associate degree entry point in decreasing education financial burden in progression models is important to note. Innovative models such as concurrent enrollment programs, where a student attends associate degree nursing program courses while simultaneously attending baccalaureate program coursework create a bridge to advanced education while tending to the financial burden of pursuing higher degrees. In addition, nursing education needs to prepare nurses for practice in a **variety of settings** other than acute care, including public and community health, behavioral health, primary care, long-term care, geriatrics, and school health. The transformed health care delivery system will rely heavily on these and other alternative settings that predominately employ nurses today. A summary of the FON 2020–2030 recommendations can be found in the Appendices of the text. Many of these content areas are discussed in various chapters to provide an opportunity to explore them in a more contextualized depth.

THE *NOW* FUTURE

Although the emphasis has been placed on nurses achieving higher levels of education and training through increasing the number of entry-level RNs who pursue a baccalaureate degree, academic progression does not end there. Understanding how we got to this point is important. If we do not grasp the significance of a transformed health care system and the demands it will place on health care practitioners, especially nurses at the point of care, we will not be able to see into the future and appreciate the need for a more highly educated workforce to address the complexity of care, care management needs of patients and families, promotion of wellness, and demands for primary care. This major transformation in care and care delivery will significantly change what we understand as the health care environment today.

Preparing the future nursing workforce to navigate a highly complex, diverse, and growing health care system has never been more important than it is today. RNs have been at the forefront of the response to the COVID-19 pandemic from its start, experiencing undocumented landscape changes as nurses struggled with burnout, trauma, alarming rates of death, and leaving the profession altogether. We are rebounding from changed health care environments while at the same time trying to propel a profession forward. Academic progression to the highest levels of graduate education is critical for nursing to provide leadership in this transformation, especially in the areas of community health, behavioral health, primary care, long-term care, geriatrics, and school health. Expanding knowledge and skills in community-based delivery services; use of data particularly that related to social determinants of health, health equity, and program design; implementation and evaluation of critical value-based assets for advanced practice nursing at its highest level as collaborative partners and leaders of health care teams will all be essential. Making the work of nurses visible is critical to assuming leadership and determining the value of nursing services.

This is OUR time as nurses to demonstrate that nursing can respond and contribute to NAM FON 2020–2030 vision; fulfill the promise of practicing to the full extent of our education and training; and contribute as full partners, with physicians and other health professions in redesigning US health care. The FON directly calls for state and federal programs to support the academic progression of socioeconomically disadvantaged students, including community and tribal colleges in rural and urban underserved areas (NASEM, 2021). In addition, the report states that we should eliminate policies, procedures, curricular content, and clinical experiences that promote structural racism, cultural racism, and discrimination of any kind.

It is not an easy decision to pursue additional education. Many competing factors play into that decision. As students with a desire to move forward with your academic pursuits, you have an opportunity to demand that barriers and obstacles be removed to facilitate your academic progression; *desire* and *access* need to go hand-in-hand. As students or potential students, let your institutions know what you might require to move forward to facilitate your academic journey. Plan for that journey. Have a vision of the endpoint you want to achieve.

Specialty practice at a graduate-level is an advanced nursing education opportunity. APRN, nurse informaticist, nurse ethicist, public health nurse, public policy nurse, clinical nurse leader, or nurse administrator are all advanced nursing specialty roles. Nurse educators may require additional training in the science of teaching and learning. At a doctoral level, the practice doctorate (DNP) or a research doctorate (Doctor of Philosophy [PhD]) is the highest level of nursing practice and opens a wide array of professional opportunities. Progression models continue to evolve. Using the resources identified, students/nurses can keep abreast of these new evolving models such as degree completion programs such as RN-Master's degree, accelerated baccalaureate, master's, and doctoral nursing degrees, as well as changes in licensure/regulatory, accreditation, and certification requirements for ongoing demonstration of knowledge and skill competencies.

Career coaching (Koppi, 2018) is the development of a resourceful partnership with a coach to close the gap between the present and the future toward envisioning possible futures and taking next steps. According to Koppi, it is grounded in positive psychology and appreciative inquiry. In partnership with another individual, the coach, in a thought-provoking way, helps the individual to explore what concrete steps can be used to achieve a particular goal or objective. Although career coaching is designed to help transition you to new roles or settings, a nurse can seek out role models in both their work or academic settings to receive coaching on academic progression related to future nursing opportunities across the continuum of health care delivery and into emerging career paths that require advanced education, specialization, or alternative practice settings. This is especially true if a nurse is considering management or leadership pathways where business and leadership skills are required. Advanced technology skills are also increasingly required in the transformed health care system.

SUMMARY

Educating for today's practice and tomorrow's needs promises to be challenging. Preparing the current and future nursing workforce to navigate a highly complex, diverse, and growing health care system has never been more important than it is today. Academic progression is essential not only for the growth of the profession but for the health and security of our nation. The nursing profession must become increasingly diverse and highly educated to be considered an equal, valued, and integral partner.

To continue to be integral partners, a more diverse and highly educated nursing profession is necessary. Health care quality is impacted by a nursing workforce's resilience, level of academic preparation, seamless academic progression protocols, effective academic-practice partnerships, and data infrastructure to support resource allocation.

SALIENT POINTS

- Health care delivery is changing, and with it how nurses will practice into the future.
- If nursing practice changes, so must nursing education programs that produce new nurses and support a nurse's academic progression to advanced academic degrees.
- A reformulated and innovative nursing education infrastructure is needed to accommodate both accelerated and stepped approaches to meeting the diverse student needs and learning styles across geographic regions in a cost-effective manner.

- A more highly educated and diverse nursing workforce is needed to meet the needs of society, patients, and 21st-century health care delivery system.
- Advanced skills and knowledge competencies will be required to demonstrate the competency to practice into the future.
- A variety of nursing educational pathways will be required to meet NASEM's vision and recommendations.

CRITICAL REFLECTION EXERCISES

1. Articulate the relationship between health care delivery reform, health care system transformation, nursing's full participation in the health care team, and required changes in nursing education.
2. Share a recent academic and/or professional learning experience and its impact on your desire to pursue higher levels of education in advanced nursing practice. What insights (reflections) do you have about the impact of this experience?

3. What personal and professional transformations can you envision for your academic journey and life-long learning in your professional nursing career. Write a personal plan reflecting your academic progression plan/career trajectory. What was your entry point to nursing? Reflect on your desire to progress from a generalist level of professional practice to a specialist level of professional practice and ultimately the highest level of professional nursing practice.

REFERENCES

Campaign for Action. (2021). *Transforming nursing education* [Report]. https://campaignforaction.org/wp-content/up-loads/2021/02/Dashboard-Indicator-Updates_Fall-2021.pdf

Institute of Medicine. (1997). *National roundtable on health care quality* [Report]. National Academies Press. https://doi.org/10.17226/9439

Institute of Medicine. (2000). *To err is human: Building a safer healthcare system* [Report]. National Academies Press. https://doi.org/10.17226/9728

Institute of Medicine. (2001). *Crossing the quality chasm* [Report]. National Academies Press. https://doi.org/10.17226/10027

Institute of Medicine. (2003a). *Health professions education: A bridge to quality*. National Academies Press. https://doi.org/10.17226/10681

Institute of Medicine. (2003b). *Priority areas for national action: Transforming health care quality*. In K. Adams & J. M. Corrigan (Eds.), National Academies Press. https://doi.org/10.17226/10593

Institute of Medicine. (2004). *Patient safety: Achieving a new standard for care*. National Academies Press. https://doi.org/10.17226/10863

Institute of Medicine. (2005). *Quality through collaboration: The future of rural health*. National Academies Press. https://doi.org/10.17226/11140

Institute of Medicine. (2010). *The future of nursing: Leading change, advancing health*. National Academies Press. https://doi.org/10.17226/12956

Josiah Macy Jr. Foundation. (2017). *Annual report*. January 22, 2022. https://macyfoundation.org/assets/reports/publications/jmf2017_annual_report_webpdf.pdf

Koppi, S. (2018, May 1). *Career coaching: A new paradigm for student-centered career services*. National Association of Colleges and Employees. https://www.naceweb.org/career-development/organizational-structure/career-coaching-a-new-paradigm-for-student-centered-career-services/

National Academies of Science, Engineering, and Medicine (NASEM). (2021). *The future of nursing 2020–2030: Charting a path to achieve health equity*. National Academies Press. https://doi.org/10.17226/25982

National Education Progression in Nursing. (n.d.). May 10, 2022. https://nepincollaborative.org/

National League for Nursing. (2011, January). *Academic progression in nursing education: A living document from the National League of Nursing* [NLN Vision Series]. https://www.nln.org/docs/default-source/uploadedfiles/about/nlnvision_1.pdf?sfvrsn=67074931_3

National League for Nursing. (2021, November 9). *NLN value statement on workforce demands of the future: The educational imperative*. https://www.nln.org/detail-pages/news/2022/01/12/nln-value-statement-on-workforce-demands-of-the-future-the-educational-imperative

Organization for Associate Degree Nursing and American Nurses Association (ANA). (2015, July 21). *Joint position statement on academic progression to meet the needs of the registered nurse, the health care consumer, and the U.S. health care system* [Position Statement]. https://www.nursingworld.org/~490461/globalassets/practiceandpolicy/nursing-excellence/ana-position-statements/nursing-practice/academic-progression-ana-and-oadn-joint-position-statement-07-27-2015.pdf

Pittman, P. M., Kurtzman, E. T., & Johnson, J. E. (2014). Academic progression models in nursing: Design decisions faced by administrators in four case studies. *Journal of Nursing Education, 53*(6), 329–335. https://doi.org/10.3928/01484834-20140520-03

Spetz, J. (2018). Projections of progress toward the 80% bachelor of science in nursing recommendation and strategies to accelerate change. *Nursing Outlook, 66*(4), 394–400. https://doi.org/10.1016/j.outlook.2018.04.012

U.S. Bureau of Labor Statistics. (2022, April 18). *Occupational outlook handbook: Registered nurses*. [Quick facts] July 20, 2022. https://www.bls.gov/ooh/healthcare/registered-nurses.htm

3

Beyond Professional Socialization

Karen J. Saewert, PhD, RN, CPHQ, ANEF

 http://evolve.elsevier.com/Friberg/bridge/

OBJECTIVES

At the completion of this chapter, the reader will be able to:
- Contrast professional socialization with professional identity formation.
- Discuss the key messages of the National Academy of Medicine (NAM) (formerly Institute of Medicine) reports: *The Future of Nursing: Leading Change, Advancing Health* and *The Future of Nursing 2020–2030: Charting a Path to Achieve Health Equity,* as it relates to professional identity formation.
- Engage in identifying personal commitments to advance professional identity formation.
- Reflect on a recent academic and/or professional learning experience and its effect on beliefs about self-development and professional engagement.
- Recognize nurse colleagues who integrate *innovation catalyst, interprofessional collaborator, engaged stakeholder, expert learner, knowledge worker, agent of inquiry, voice for action, assimilator,* and/or *reflective practitioner* in their way of being a nurse.

INTRODUCTION

Nursing is at a pivotal point in its trajectory and is not alone in the quest of defining its professional identity.
Joseph et al. (2021, p. 27)

Professional identity formation reveals shifts in self-understanding that occur as a nurse carries out multifaceted responsibilities to society, recipients of care, colleagues, and self (Simmonds et al., 2020). Knowledge, values, skills, behaviors, and norms relevant and appropriate to professional nursing practice are acquired over time through interactive and repetitive processes. Like any life experience, professional identity formation is a process, not an event, nested within everyday experience (Crigger & Godfrey, 2011). The processes of learning and incorporating aspects of a profession into one's professional identity are collectively termed *socialization*. Professional socialization is a complex process that reflects four critical attributes: learning, interaction, development, and adaptation (Dinmohammadi et al., 2013). Educational programs, role models, and field experiences serve as precursors to these attributes that can either have positive or negative consequences for a nurse's professional development.

Nursing education is strong in ways of teaching that effectively assist students to develop a deep sense of professional identity, commit to the values of the profession, and act with ethical comportment (Benner et al., 2010). Thus, socialization begins in the basic nursing program educational setting and continues throughout one's professional nursing career. Fostering and encouraging a more focused growth of professional identity is also influenced by organizational culture and practice environments (Crigger & Godfrey, 2014).

Benner et al. (2010) hold that rather than being taught knowledge and skills to perform nursing care, students must learn to *be* nurses through powerful and integrative learning experiences. Nursing is not something that is simply done but is rather an embodied state of being. Within this identity, the professional nurse integrates scientific knowledge (cognitive apprenticeship), judgment and know-how (skill apprenticeship), and ethics (ethical comportment apprenticeship) daily in unique and changing situations. Fluid use of these three apprenticeships is essential for practice excellence (Handwerker, 2012).

This process is reactivated at a number of junctures: (1) when a new graduate leaves the educational setting and begins professional nursing practice; (2) when an experienced nurse changes work settings, either within the same organization or in a new organization; and (3) when a nurse undertakes new roles, such as returning to school or assuming a leadership role. At all of these junctures, socialization involves personal change, as a new professional self-identity is reformed or redefined. Consequently, nurses are either in the process of developing a growing sense of professional identity and flourishing or failing to expand their notion of professional identity (Crigger & Godfrey, 2011).

LOOKING BACK

Although historical continuity gives shape, context, and perspective to nursing's values and responsibilities as the largest group of health care providers in the health care arena (Fairman, 2012), new technologies and evolving roles demand continuous adaptation (Lai & Lim, 2012) and more autonomous practitioners (Eckhardt, 2002). However, it is important not to fail to *build* on the past in the rush toward innovation while at the same time let go of past difficulties (Lee & Fawcett, 2013).

The personal and social components of professional identity are not easily separated; it is *personal* because of the self-identification a nurse has as a member of a group and it is *social* in that it involves the definition of a group (Fitzgerald & Clukey, 2021). Relinquishing preconceptions, letting go of expectations, and acclimating to the realities of the profession and health care is essential to the success of professional identity development (Goodolf, 2018). Embracing new ideas means having the courage to let go of familiar processes, which in turn may mean letting go of familiar tasks and roles so patients receive the benefit of each nurse's professional role (Battié, 2013).

A robust understanding of the professional identity of nursing—at both the individual and disciplinary level—empowers nurses to (1) assume a professional identity that reflects a more responsible and equitable role, (2) challenge the traditional way nurses perceive themselves and are perceived by others, and (3) develop a more relevant notion of professional identity (Crigger & Godfrey, 2014). Nurses share a responsibility for understanding and communicating the direction that nursing and health care are taking, critical to nursing's visibility, credibility, clout, and momentum to lead (not follow) into the future (Cardillo, 2011). It is also crucial to the continuous development of the professional discipline of nursing that its members embrace not only their role as members of the professional discipline, but also embrace continuous changes in self, others, and the knowledge and practice of the discipline (Lee & Fawcett, 2013).

MOVING FORWARD

The Future of Nursing 2020–2030: Charting a Path to Achieve Health Equity and *The Future of Nursing: Leading Change, Advancing Health* are the largest comprehensive studies of the nursing profession published by the National Academy of Medicine (NAM) (formerly Institute of Medicine) since 1983. The original 2011 and follow-up 2015 NAM reports call for fundamental transformation of the nursing profession in practice, education, and leadership (Rutherford-Hemming & Lioce, 2018). These landmark reports have had and will continue to have a profound effect on nursing education, practice, and research (Chard, 2013). The key messages and related recommendations affirm and encourage professional nurses to practice fully, achieve higher levels of education, become full partners in providing and reforming health care, and develop an infrastructure for workforce data collection (Institute of Medicine, 2010). These influential reports call for broad changes in the nursing profession for the benefit of society and patients, the ultimate recipients of these transformations (Thibault, 2011). Incorporating the key messages of these reports and using the reports as an evidence-based blueprint for change will require a commitment from all stakeholders in a shared vision for a better health care system (Chard, 2013).

THE *NOW* FUTURE

Now is the time to develop a more relevant notion of professional identity and bring forward words that better explain the contemporary view of nursing and collectively move us forward in responding to the recommendations (Crigger & Godfrey, 2011). Nurses are at the forefront of advancing evidence-based solutions and leading innovation in this time of COVID-19, unparalleled global health concerns, and an atmosphere of accelerating change (Goodolf & Godfrey, 2021).

The NAM continues to identify nurses as key leaders in driving the reform and work to be done to reshape health care delivery in the United States. It is important that all nurses become educated and knowledgeable about these reports, understand the implications for the future of the discipline, identify ways that individual nurses can get involved in implementing the recommendations, and educate others on what needs to be done (Battié, 2013).

STATE OF BEING TRANSFORMATION

Being a professional nurse is a dynamic process—one with many possibilities for action, influence, and transformation. Every nurse—from bedside to the boardroom—has a role in transforming nursing (Thibault, 2011). The personal and social components of professional identity are not easily separated; it is personal because of the self-identification a nurse has as a member of a group and it is social in that it involves the definition of a group (Fitzgerald & Clukey, 2021).

Although not exhaustive or exclusive, these possibilities include nurse as *innovation catalyst, interprofessional collaborator, engaged stakeholder, expert learner, knowledge worker, agent of inquiry, voice for action, assimilator,* and/or *reflective practitioner.*

NURSE AS INNOVATION CATALYST

Nurses, with the capacity for lifelong and expert learning, are preparing for new challenges and opportunities by moving beyond the *process* of professional socialization to *learning* that promotes new capabilities to *see, do,* and *be* anchored in the fundamental purposes of nursing. It is essential for nurses to function optimally and influence change. For this to happen, a strong, confident, and flexible professional identity is essential (Joseph et al., 2021).

NURSE AS INTERPROFESSIONAL COLLABORATOR

The process of developing a professional identity requires mutual respect, collaborative partnerships, and supportive networks. Interprofessional education is one strategy to strengthen nursing education and enhance the role of nurses as collaborative leaders in the health care system (see Chapter 8: Nurse as Interprofessional Collaborator). For nurses to practice at the highest level for which they are educated, for there to be uniformly high standards for nursing education, and for nurses to successfully partner with physicians and other health professionals in redesigning our health care system, rigorous, structured interprofessional education experiences can be one of the tools used in accomplishing these goals (Thibault, 2011).

Improved systems are frequently the result of collaboration among health care professionals who are first committed to improving their own practice; accordingly, insights into improved systems begin in a nurse's own practice (Armstrong & Sherwood, 2012). The increased complexity of providing patient care demands an educational process that includes how to "be" a nurse in an interprofessional environment, develops the nurse's

ability to make clinical judgments (see Chapter 9: Think Like a Nurse—Essential Thinking Skills for Professional Nurses), uses and coordinates interdisciplinary approaches to care, yet focuses on the specific needs of the patient (Thibault, 2011). It is in the "being" that nurses have the voice and strength of advocacy and systems-level change and the capacity to serve as champions for patient-, family-, and community-based perspectives in an interprofessional environment (Bleich, 2013).

NURSE AS EXPERT LEARNER, KNOWLEDGE WORKER, AND AGENT OF INQUIRY

Many students entering RN-BSN programs already have a strong sense of clinical competence and a variety of diverse practice-based experiences but may enroll without a clear understanding of nursing as a professional discipline and what it means to be a member of a professional discipline (Lee & Fawcett, 2013). Increasing the competency and education of the nursing workforce is a new necessity in keeping with the shifting standards of all health care professions that may require changing individual beliefs about self-development and professional engagement on the never-ending road to professionalism in nursing (Bleich, 2013; Morris & Faulk, 2012). This process and adaptation of learning is one by which nurses continually seek new information, receive clarity on the information, synthesize the new information into practice, and prepare to learn new information again (Candela, 2012).

Patient care is but one part of the overall system through which nurses can direct their energy and articulate their position as full partners in redesigning health care (Chard, 2013). This knowledge can come from many sources that can enhance evidence-based practice in nursing care delivery (see Chapter 4: Fostering a Spirit of Inquiry—The Role of Nurses in Evidence-Based Practice).

NURSE AS ASSIMILATOR AND REFLECTIVE PRACTITIONER

Collaboration with and between practice and education is essential to operationalizing innovation and instituting change. Without forward movement in both practice and education it will be difficult to accept and institute change. Sullivan (2005), as cited by Day (2011), identified three high-level professional apprenticeships that form the background to all the Carnegie Foundation studies of professional education: the cognitive apprenticeship (knowledge base required for practice), the skills-based apprenticeship (judgment and know-how), and the apprenticeship of ethical comportment (professional behavior), with assimilation of these apprenticeships essential to integrated professional performance and practice.

Reflection becomes essential to systematic thinking about our actions and responses in a manner that allows transformed perspective and reframing for determination of future actions and responses (Sherwood & Horton-Deutsch, 2012). Integrating reflective practices into nursing education and professional development has a significant effect on the quality of work processes and their outcomes by considering what we know, believe, and value (Horton-Deutsch & Sherwood, 2008; Sherwood & Horton-Deutsch, 2012).

NURSE AS ENGAGED STAKEHOLDER AND VOICE FOR ACTION

Nurses have remained too silent in a system that favors other health professionals—so much so that among some people there is a public image that we exist in service to these other health care disciplines, patients, and their family members and in care delivery models and processes that favor labor-intensive efforts (Bleich, 2013).

The need for a full partnership and the large responsibility it carries will require individual nurses to enhance their leadership skills and competencies and position themselves as advocates for patient care, professional nursing, and effective health care policy (Chard, 2013). Nurses and supportive stakeholders have a blueprint for meeting the public's need to promote health, mitigate illness, and enhance quality-of-life care (Bleich, 2013). Although the reports reinforce the need for all nurses to make a personal commitment to lifelong learning and education so they are increasingly well prepared for their roles in a reformed health care system, each nurse must consider personal and professional goals and find a part of this process that means something to him or her and become involved (Battié, 2013).

SUMMARY

How will you lead from where you stand?

The process of professional identity formation shapes the answer to this question today, tomorrow, and further into the future. The willingness to embrace continuous change in self, others, and the knowledge and practice of the nursing profession supports the fundamental and evidence-based changes needed in practice, education, and leadership. How nurses individually and collectively give voice to and leverage the key messages and related recommendations of the landmark reports fundamentally influences how the current and future state of health care will ultimately be delivered, reformed, and improved. Fostering intraprofessional and interprofessional mutual respect is essential to building critical collaborative partnerships and supportive networks needed to accomplish the important work ahead.

Find meaning and make a personal commitment to one's personal and professional goals. Prepare by looking back, moving forward, and bringing the *now* future into focus. Become involved and consider one's role as an *innovation catalyst, interprofessional collaborator, engaged stakeholder, expert learner, knowledge worker, agent of inquiry, voice for action, assimilator,* and/or *reflective practitioner.*

Through self-knowledge and awareness, become open to *new ways of thinking, new ways of doing,* and *new ways of being.* In doing so, emerge stronger in one's sense of professional identity.

SALIENT POINTS

- Socialization to professional nursing is an interactive and lifelong process that includes internalization of its attitudes, behaviors, skills, and values.
- Professional identity formation transcends the socialization process; nursing is not something that is simply done but is rather an embodied state of being.
- The National Academy of Medicine's messages and recommendations focus on advancing the profession of nursing to enhance the preparation of nurses to function to the full extent of their education in an envisioned and transformed health care system.

- Every nurse has a professional role and responsibility to participate in realizing the vision and reality of *The Future of Nursing: Leading Change, Advancing Health* and *The Future of Nursing 2020–2030: Charting a Path to Achieve Health Equity* reports and recommendations.
- Being a nurse is a dynamic process. Possibilities exist for nurses to integrate *innovation catalyst, interprofessional collaborator, engaged stakeholder, expert learner, knowledge worker, agent of inquiry, voice for action, assimilator,* and/or *reflective practitioner* in ways of being a nurse.

CRITICAL REFLECTION EXERCISES

1. Specify five commitments you are willing to make to advance your professional identity formation. What resources will you need to fulfill the identified commitments and overcome any obstacles you may encounter?

2. Consider an action you can take and/or have taken as a member of the professional nursing community to advance a key message of the National Academy of Medicine reports. What is/was the catalyst for selection of this action?

3. Share a recent academic and/or professional learning experience and its effect on your beliefs about self-development and professional engagement. What insights do you have about the effect of this experience?

4. What personal and professional transformations can you envision making to enhance the integration of

innovation catalyst, interprofessional collaborator, engaged stakeholder, expert learner, knowledge worker, agent of inquiry, voice for action, assimilator, and/or *reflective practitioner* in your way of being a nurse? Share the rationale for your choice(s).

5. Do you know nurse colleagues who integrate *innovation catalyst, interprofessional collaborator, engaged stakeholder, expert learner, knowledge worker, agent of inquiry, voice for action, assimilator,* and/or *reflective practitioner* in their way of being a nurse? Consider asking them to share their personal and professional transformation story. Reflect on these stories as you carve out your own journey.

REFERENCES

Armstrong, G., & Sherwood, G. D. (2012). Reflection and mindful practice: A means to quality and safety. In G. D. Sherwood & S. Horton-Deutsch (Eds.), *Reflective practice: Transforming education and improving outcomes* (pp. 21–39). Sigma Theta Tau International.

Battié, R. N. (2013). The IOM Report on the Future of Nursing: What perioperative nurses need to know. *AORN, 98*(3), 227–234. https://doi.org/10.1016/j.aorn.2013.07.007

Benner, P. A., Sutphen, M., Leonard, V., & Day, L. (2010). *Educating nurses: A call for radical transformation.* Jossey-Bass.

Bleich, M. R. (2013). The Institute of Medicine Report on the Future of Nursing: A transformational blueprint. *AORN, 98*(3), 214–217. https://doi.org/10.1016/j.aorn.2013.07.008

Candela, L. (2012). From teaching to learning: Theoretical foundations. In D. M. Billings & J. A. Halstead (Eds.), *Teaching in nursing: A guide for faculty* (4th ed., pp. 202–243). Saunders.

Cardillo, D. (2011, November–December). Nursing: The future is yours! *National Student Nurses' Association, 58*(5), 36–38. Cardillo/NSNA Imprint 2011.

Chard, R. (2013). The personal and professional impact of the Future of Nursing report. *AORN, 98*(3), 273–280. https://doi.org/10.1016/j.aorn.2013.01.019

Crigger, N., & Godfrey, N. (2011). *The making of nurse professionals: A transformational, ethical approach.* Jones & Bartlett.

Crigger, N., & Godfrey, N. (2014). From the inside out: A new approach to teaching professional identity formation and professional ethics. *Journal of Professional Nursing, 30*(5), 376–382. https://doi.org/10.1016/j.profnurs.2014.03.004

Day, L. (2011). Using unfolding case studies in a subject-centered classroom. *Journal of Nursing Education, 50*(8), 447–452. https://doi.org/10.3928/01484834-20110517-03

Dinmohammadi, M., Peyrovi, H., & Mehrdad, N. (2013). Concept analysis of professional socialization in nursing. *Nursing Forum, 48*(1), 26–34. https://doi.org/10.1111/nuf.12006

Eckhardt, J. A. (2002). Effects of program design on the professional socialization of RN-BSN students. *Journal of Professional Nursing, 18*(3), 157–164. https://doi.org/10.1053/jpnu.2002.125476

Fairman, J. (2012). History for the future (of nursing). *Nursing History Review, 20*(1), 10–13. https://doi.org/10.1891/1062-8061.20.10

Fitzgerald, A., & Clukey, L. (2021). Professional identity in graduating nursing students. *Journal of Nursing Education, 60*(2), 74–80. https://doi.org/10.3928/01484834-20210120-04

Goodolf, D. M. (2018). Growing a professional identity: A grounded theory of baccalaureate nursing students. *Journal of Nursing Education, 57*(12), 705–711. https://doi.org/10.3928/01484834-20282229-02

Goodolf, D. M., & Godfrey, N. (2021). A think tank in action: Building new knowledge about professional identity. *Journal of Professional Nursing, 37*(2), 493–499. https://doi.org/10.1016/j.profnurs.2020.10.007

Handwerker, S. (2012). Transforming nursing education: A review of current curricular practice in relation to Benner's latest work. *International Journal of Nursing Education Scholarship, 9*(1), 1–16. https://doi.org/10.1515/1548-923X.2510

Horton-Deutsch, S., & Sherwood, G. D. (2008). Reflection: An educational strategy to develop emotionally competent nurse leaders. *Journal of Nursing Management, 16*(8), 946–954. https://doi.org/10.1111/j.1365-2834.2008.00957.x

Institute of Medicine. (2010). *FON Report Brief. The future of nursing: Leading change, advancing health.* https://nap.nationalacademies.org/resource/12956/Future-of-Nursing-2010-Report-Brief.pdf

Joseph, M. L., Edmonson, C., Godfrey, N., Liebig, D., & Weybrew, K. (2021). The nurse leader's role: A conduit for professional identify formation and sustainability. *Nurse Leader*, *19*(1), 27–32. https://doi.org/10.1016/j.mnl.2020.10.001

Lai, P. K., & Lim, P. H. (2012). Concept of professional socialization in nursing. *International e-Journal of Science [Research Note]. Medicine & Education*, *6*(1), 31–35. [Lai & Lim Research Note 2012.]

Lee, R. C., & Fawcett, J. (2013). The influence of the metaparadigm of nursing on professional identity development among RN-BSN students. *Nursing Science Quarterly*, *26*(1), 96–98. https://doi.org/10.1177/0894318412466734

Morris, A. H., & Faulk, D. R. (2012). *The road to professionalism: Transformative learning for professional role development. Transformative learning in nursing: A guide for nurse educators* (pp. 91–103). Springer.

Rutherford-Hemming, T., & Lioce, L. (2018). State of interprofessional education in nursing: A systematic review. *Nurse Educator*, *43*(1), 9–13. https://doi.org/10.1097/NNE.0000000000000405

Sherwood, G. D., & Horton-Deutsch, S. (2012). Turning vision into action. In G. D. Sherwood & S. Horton-Deutsch (Eds.), *Reflective practice: Transforming education and improving outcomes* (pp. 3–19). Sigma Theta Tau International.

Simmonds, A., Nunn, A., Gray, M., Hardie, C., Mayo, S., Peter, E., & Richard, J. (2020). Pedagogical practices that influence professional identity formation in baccalaureate nursing education: A scoping review. *Nurse Education Today*, *93*, 1–8. https://doi.org/10.1016/j.nedt.2020.104516

Sullivan, W. (2005). *Work and integrity: The crisis and promise of professionalism in America* (2nd ed.). Jossey-Bass.

Thibault, G. E. (2011). Interprofessional education: An essential strategy to accomplish the Future of Nursing goals. *Journal of Nursing Education*, *50*(6), 313–317. https://doi.org/10.3928/01484834 20110519-03

Fostering a Spirit of Inquiry: The Role of Nurses in Evidence-Based Practice

Brenda C. Morris, EdD, MS, RN, CNE

e http://evolve.elsevier.com/Friberg/bridge/

OBJECTIVES

At the completion of this chapter, the reader will be able to:
- Explain evidence-based practice (EBP) and its relationship to the Quintuple Aim: improving the health of populations, reducing the costs of care, improving the patient experience (quality and safety), enhancing clinician well-being, and improving health equity.
- Contrast EBP, evaluation/quality improvement, and research.
- Discuss strategies to foster a spirit of inquiry.
- Contrast EBP models.
- Describe the steps in the EBP process.
- Apply EBP to a clinical situation.

INTRODUCTION

The professional foundations for evidence-based practice (EBP) and fostering a spirit of inquiry lie within the American Nurses Association's (ANA, 2015) *Code of Ethics for Nurses with Interpretative Statements (the Code)*. Provisions 1 and 2 of *the Code* call upon nurses to incorporate patient preferences and the right to self-determination in the clinical decision-making process, which is congruent with one of the guiding principles for EBP. Provision 3 of *the Code* charges nurses with protecting the health and safety of the patient (ANA, 2015). Using EBP allows nurses to use the best available evidence to inform patient care decisions, thus promoting the health and safety of the patient. Provision 7 of *the Code* directs nurses to advance the profession through research and scholarly inquiry, which sets expectations for nurses to develop a spirit of inquiry to expand the body of nursing knowledge and apply the best evidence to inform nursing practice (ANA, 2015).

The EBP movement has gained tremendous momentum over the past two decades due to forces within our society that call for cost-effective, value-based, evidence-based, high-quality, and safe care that increases patient satisfaction. One of these forces is the introduction of a pay-for-performance (P4P) model where health insurers reimburse for health care services based upon the health care organization meeting predetermined outcomes related to cost, quality, safety, and patient satisfaction. Additionally, initiatives such as the American Nurses Credentialing Center's (ANCC) Magnet Recognition Program recognize health care organizations that "provide high quality nursing care and demonstrate a sustained commitment to EBP" (Polit & Beck, 2022, p. 2). These forces continue to propel the EBP movement forward. Additional information on the economic drivers of P4P and ANCC Magnet Recognition impacts can be found in Chapter 7, Economic Issues in Nursing and Health Care, and Chapter 20, Health Care Quality and Safety.

WHAT IS EVIDENCE-BASED PRACTICE?

EBP is a problem-solving approach to clinical decision-making that involves the use of the best available evidence, clinical expertise, and patient preferences and values to improve outcomes (Melnyk & Fineout-Overholt, 2019). Another term that may be used interchangeably to describe EBP is evidence-informed practice. The ANA (2015) describes evidence-informed practice as a decision-making approach that combines the best available research, practice expertise, clinical or experiential insights, ethics, patient preferences, cultural backgrounds, and community values to make patient care decisions. Similarities within these problem-solving approaches are that they use multiple sources of current, credible evidence including research, clinical expertise, and patient preferences and values to make the best decisions for practice.

Historically, some health care professionals were taught to prioritize research evidence and clinician expertise, at the risk of minimizing the influence of patient preferences and values in making clinical decisions. This approach to decision-making was flawed because it did not consider whether the prescribed intervention was acceptable to the patient and was one that they could implement. In the current health care environment, all health care providers are mandated to provide patient-centric care and consider patient preferences and values as a driving focus of care delivery. When using an EBP approach, the patient's preferences and values are as important as the clinician's expertise and the research evidence in making clinical care decisions. To illustrate this point, let's examine a situation in which the research evidence and the clinician expertise suggest prescribing an expensive medication to a patient to treat a chronic health condition. The patient shares that they cannot afford to buy the expensive medication and asks the provider if there is another effective, less expensive medication available. The clinician, guided by the EBP approach, honors the patient's preferences and collaborates with them to identify another medication that is effective in treating the condition and is affordable to the patient. The result of this approach is that the patient can treat their health condition because they were prescribed a medication they can afford, increasing the likelihood of achieving better patient outcomes, better care, and a more satisfying patient experience.

WHY IS EVIDENCE-BASED PRACTICE IMPORTANT?

EBP leads to better care, better outcomes, lower costs, and greater nursing staff satisfaction (Alves, 2021; Cullen et al., 2020; Melnyk et al., 2021). EBP incorporates patient preferences, clinician expertise, and current, relevant research evidence. It is challenging for health care providers to stay current with the latest research evidence, because of the rapid pace of new advances in health care, which leads to current practices or traditions becoming outdated.

EBP is critical to the provision of health care that is grounded in science and not tradition. Individuals are at risk for receiving suboptimal care resulting in poor

outcomes when care is based on tradition or "how we've always done it" because the tradition may not be supported by current evidence. The length of time it takes to change practice is too long. Khan et al. (2021) examined the amount of time it takes to implement EBPs in cancer prevention and screening. They found that on average it took 15 years to implement an EBP change from the time the research was published. It will be important to implement EBP changes at a quicker pace to achieve the quintuple aim. Additionally, the healthcare costs are higher in the United States when compared to other industrialized nations. Thus, we need to ensure that we are using effective interventions that are based on evidence to use health care resources wisely (see Chapter 7: Economic Issues in Nursing and Health Care).

RELATIONSHIPS AMONG EVIDENCE-BASED PRACTICE AND THE QUINTUPLE AIM: IMPROVED POPULATION HEALTH, REDUCED COST, IMPROVED PATIENT EXPERIENCE, ENHANCED CLINICIAN WELL-BEING, AND IMPROVED HEALTH EQUITY

Efforts to improve the value in providing health care relate to advancing the Institute for Healthcare Improvement's Quintuple Aim, which is improving the health of populations, reducing the costs of care, improving the patient experience, enhancing clinician well-being, and improving health equity (Nundy et al., 2022). The use of evidence from research, EBP, and quality improvement (QI) studies provides the foundations to achieve the Quintuple Aim and improve health care for all.

Several studies demonstrate the positive effects of EBP on advancing the quintuple aim. Melnyk et al. (2021) examined the relationships between EBP culture and mentorship with nurse job satisfaction and nurse intent to stay, which are dimensions of clinician well-being. They found that EBP culture positively impacts nurse job satisfaction. Additionally, EBP mentorship positively impacts nurse intent to stay in their current position. Alves (2021) conducted an integrative review of 15 studies that evaluated the effects of EBP mentorship programs on organizational readiness for EBP, clinician readiness to implement EBP, and client outcomes. They found that EBP mentorship programs increased clinician readiness to implement EBP and increased organizational readiness for EBP. Cullen et al. (2020) examined the effect of using an EBP change champion program on the incidence of catheter-associated urinary tract infections. They found that the use of an EBP nursing care bundle combined with EBP change champions reduced the incidence of catheter-associated urinary tract infections.

CLINICAL SCHOLARSHIP CONTINUUM: EVIDENCE-BASED PRACTICE, QUALITY IMPROVEMENT, AND NURSING RESEARCH

"Nurses' active involvement in clinical scholarship is necessary to advance the nursing profession and improve patient outcomes" (Carter et al., 2017, p. 266). As such, it is important for nurses to understand the clinical scholarship continuum, the similarities and differences among the types of systematic inquiry, and the nurses' role in advancing the knowledge of the discipline.

One type of scholarly inquiry is research which uses a systematic process to gather and interpret data to answer questions or solve problems. Research can be quantitative or qualitative. The aims of quantitative research are to use empirical data to describe, explore, predict, or explain phenomenon. A goal of quantitative research is for the findings to be generalizable to the larger population, whereas the aim of qualitative research is to identify, describe, or explain phenomenon to better understand the human experience. Nursing research examines problems relevant to nursing practice and it generates the evidence that is used to guide nursing practice. Steps in the research process include identifying a question or problem for study, then determining the population/sample, the intervention (if applicable), and how data will be collected and analyzed, and how the findings will be shared with others.

EBP uses evidence from research, clinician expertise, and patient preferences to improve outcomes. Research studies that address therapy/intervention questions are most likely to "provide the most direct evidence for EBP" (Polit & Beck, 2022, p. 13). Therapy/intervention questions are used to understand the effectiveness of "actions, treatments, products, or processes" (Polit & Beck, 2022, p. 11). An example of a therapy/intervention question is "Does participation in a yoga therapy program reduce anxiety in adolescent girls?" Evidence from other types of research studies that address diagnosis and assessment, prognosis, and etiology questions may also guide EBP efforts.

Common steps in the EBP process include identifying a clinical question, searching for the best evidence, appraising the evidence, integrating the evidence with clinician expertise and patient preferences, applying the evidence to clinical practice, evaluating the outcome of practice change, and disseminating the findings. Melnyk and Fineout-Overholt (2019) incorporate an additional initial step, which is fostering a spirit of inquiry.

The goal of QI is to use data-driven efforts to improve clinical care, patient outcomes, or processes within a health care organization (Carter et al., 2017; Polit & Beck, 2022).

The first step in the QI process is to identify a problem or process for improvement based on the health care organization's internal data. Once a problem has been identified, the QI team may use the Plan-Do-Study-Act (PDSA) cycle to address the problem. As part of this process, the team will plan and implement interventions and strategies to address the problem, collect baseline data for outcome comparisons, study the data to see if a positive improvement occurred, and act to either sustain the positive improvement or repeat the PDSA cycle if there were minimal or no improvements to the outcomes.

The similarities among these approaches to clinical scholarship include that they all use a systematic approach to inquiry, aim to improve outcomes, and begin by identifying a problem. The primary differences among these approaches relate to the generalizability of findings, the use of evidence, the integration of clinician expertise and patient preferences in the decision-making process, and requirements to follow human subjects' protections. QI studies are dependent on context and, while transferable, they may have limited generalizability of their findings to organizations external to where the QI project was undertaken, whereas the findings from nursing research and EBP may be generalized to larger populations. Another difference is that EBP appraises research evidence for application to a clinical question.

Nurses are involved in different levels of clinical scholarship based upon their educational preparation and experience. For example, baccalaureate-prepared nurses are educated to be consumers of research, to use EBP to guide their nursing practice, and participate in the clinical scholarship by being a part of an EBP, QI, or research team. Nurses who hold a graduate degree in nursing or a related discipline may lead EBP or QI projects, or research studies, in addition to being a consumer of research and using EBP to guide their practice. Nurses who hold a research-focused doctoral degree, such as a PhD, are prepared to conduct original research studies and generate new knowledge for the nursing profession.

STEPS IN THE EVIDENCE-BASED PRACTICE PROCESS

Cultivate a Spirit of Inquiry Along With an Evidence-Based Practice Culture and Environment

There are individual behaviors and traits as well as institutional culture and environments that support a spirit of inquiry. Individual behaviors and traits consistent with a spirit of inquiry are routinely displaying a sense of inquisitiveness and demonstrating a willingness to question current clinical practices or traditions (Melnyk & Fineout-Overholt, 2019). Some nurses naturally exhibit a spirit of inquiry, whereas others learn the behaviors and develop the traits associated with a spirit of inquiry such as asking questions about their patient's care and questioning institutional or unit-based practices or traditions. For an individual to cultivate a spirit of inquiry, they need to be in a culture and environment that supports EBP. For example, if a nurse receives positive feedback and support when demonstrating a spirit of inquiry by questioning institutional practices or traditions, they will be more likely to continue to engage in this practice. However, if a nurse receives negative feedback and no support in this circumstance, they will be less likely to question institutional practice or traditions in the future.

There are certain characteristics of cultures and environments that support EBP and cultivate a spirit of inquiry. These institutions provide resources to advance EBP, such as access to EBP mentors, librarians, computers, databases, and time to search for evidence. Additionally, these institutions make their commitment to EBP visible in their philosophy and mission statements, as well as criteria for nurses' performance evaluation and nurses' professional advancement (e.g., career ladder).

There are several models of EBP. Usually, the health care organization will select an EBP model for use within their organization. The models used most frequently by Magnet-designated hospitals in the United States are the Iowa Model of EBP, the John Hopkins Nursing EBP Model, and the Advancing Research Through Close Collaboration Model (Speroni et al., 2020). The nurses should be familiar with the EBP model selected for use by their health care organization.

Identify a Problem and Write a Clinical Question

Some of the first steps in the EBP process are for the nurse to identify a practice problem and write a clinical question. Additional information about formulating a clinical question can be found in Chapter 13, Information Management.

As part of this process, the nurse will substantiate that the problem exists or the magnitude of the problem. Some models, such as the Iowa Model of EBP, use triggering issues or opportunities to identify the problem. Examples of triggering issues or opportunities include issues identified by the client; organizational, state, or national initiatives; accreditation requirements; or new data or evidence (Iowa Model Collaborative et al., 2017). Once the problem has been identified, a clinical question that defines the population (P), intervention or issue or interest (I), the comparison intervention (C), and the outcome (O) will be formed.

Some clinical questions also include a timeframe (T). The abbreviation PICO or PICO(T) may be used to refer to clinical questions.

Search for the Evidence

Once the clinical question has been identified, it's time to search for current, relevant evidence. To begin this step, the research databases that will be used to conduct the search for evidence will be identified. It is a good idea to start the search by using primary databases that focus on medical and nursing literature, such as the Cumulative Index to Nursing and Allied Health Record (CINAHL) or MEDLINE. Controlled vocabularies (i.e., search terms, search headings, or key words) are used to identify potential sources of evidence. If the search terms are too broad, the search may reveal too many sources of evidence, thus necessitating the need to limit the search. The most common ways to limit the search are to use Boolean operators (i.e., and/or) to combine search terms, or to use limitation parameters, such as year published or language published or resource type (e.g., article, book, etc.). The evidence should be reviewed to ensure that it addresses the clinical question, including the population, intervention, and outcome. There are different types of evidence, including clinical practice guidelines, synthesized evidence, research studies (e.g., randomized controlled trials, experimental or quasi-experimental studies, qualitative studies), and gray literature (e.g., dissertations, conference proceedings, governmental reports). Additional information about searching literature databases can be found in Chapter 13, Information Management.

Appraise the Evidence

Appraising evidence involves two aspects: evaluating the level of evidence and assessing the quality of evidence.

Levels of Evidence. Evaluation of the level of evidence is frequently accomplished by using an evidence hierarchy or a level of evidence scale. Evidence hierarchies evaluate evidence sources that address therapy/intervention questions according to their risk of bias (Polit & Beck, 2022), although there are evidence hierarchies for research studies that address other types of research questions. Usually, evidence hierarchies are depicted as a pyramid, with the highest or least biased evidence at the top, which is also referred to as Level I evidence. For example, a systematic review of randomized controlled trials is usually ranked as Level I evidence for therapy/intervention questions, indicating that this type of study has the lowest risk of bias, whereas a single randomized controlled trial is ranked as Level II evidence and a nonrandomized quasi-experimental study is ranked as Level III evidence for therapy/intervention questions. Additional information about appraising the evidence can be found in Chapter 13, Information Management.

Quality of Evidence. A common misconception is that the level of evidence indicates the quality of evidence (Polit & Beck, 2022). The level of evidence only evaluates the study's risk of bias, whereas the quality of evidence is determined through a critical appraisal process which involves an objective assessment of the study's strengths and limitations. This process is usually accomplished by answering appraisal questions to evaluate different aspects of the research study. For example, a critical appraisal of a study to inform EBP is usually focused on the clinical application of the study, the research methods and findings, and "whether the evidence is accurate, sound, and clinically relevant" (Polit & Beck, 2022, p. 48).

Implement the Evidence

The next step in the EBP process is to develop a plan for implementation. The plan incorporates clinician expertise by identifying who the clinical experts are and then gathers information from them about what interventions have worked or have not worked in the past to address the problem. Additionally, the clinical experts are asked about their experiences/knowledge of the proposed intervention. A similar process is used to obtain information about the patient's preferences. The implementation plan may be modified based upon the information obtained from the clinical experts and/or the patients. The plan describes how the proposed EBP practice change will be implemented. Specifically, the "who, what, when, and how" dimensions of the practice change will be identified. It is also recommended that a change theory, such as Lewin's theory of change, be used to guide EBP implementation.

Evaluate the Outcomes

The last step in the EBP process is to evaluate if the outcome was met. Data will be collected and analyzed. If the outcome was met, plans to sustain the practice change will be implemented, whereas if the outcome was not met, plans to modify the practice change or, to phase out the practice change, will be implemented.

EVIDENCE-BASED PRACTICE MODELS

This section presents several frameworks and models that are used to guide the implementation of evidence to practice. The difference between a framework and a model is that a framework is intended to "provide a frame of reference, for organizing thinking, as a guide for what to focus on, and for interpretation" (Rycroft-Malone & Bucknall, 2010, pp. 27–28), whereas models are "more specific, narrower in scope, and more precise" (Rycroft-Malone & Bucknall, 2010, p. 28). Models frequently specify a sequence of steps to follow to implement the model, as well as decision points to facilitate application of evidence to practice. (See Box 4.1 for key features of each of the EBP Models.)

Advancing Research and Clinical Practice Through Close Collaboration

In 1999, the Advancing Research and Clinical Practice through Close Collaboration (ARCC©) model was conceptualized as an approach to combine research and clinical practice to improve health care quality and patient outcomes (Melnyk & Fineout-Overholt, 2002). The model was formalized in 2005 and refined in 2017. The aim of the model is to change the organizational culture to support EBP, thereby improving patient outcomes, decreasing health care costs, and increasing clinician job satisfaction (Melnyk et al., 2017). The model accomplishes this goal by assessing culture and organizational readiness for EBP, identifying facilitators and barriers to EBP, and using EBP mentors and mentorship to increase the implementation of EBP.

A key feature of the model is the use of EBP mentors, who are usually advanced-practice nurses, to guide EBP implementation and facilitate organizational culture change. The model is designed for use by individual clinicians, teams, health care organizations, or clinical settings. The EBP teams may be interprofessional or uni-professional. Baccalaureate-prepared nurses serve as members of the EBP team, whereas advanced-practice nurses serve as team leaders and change agents. The model uses different sources of evidence, including research evidence, clinical expertise, and patient preference.

Iowa Model of Evidence-Based Practice to Promote Quality Care

In 1994, the Iowa Model of Research-Based Practice to Promote Quality Care was conceptualized to guide clinicians in the use of research to improve health care outcomes. The model was renamed in 2001 to the Iowa Model of EBP to Promote Quality Care, which reflected the evolution in practice from research utilization to EBP. The model was again revised in 2017 to reflect feedback from users and changes in the health care system, such as the availability of synthesized evidence, initiatives to adopt EBP, the expansion of interprofessional practice, and enhanced patient engagement (Iowa Model Collaborative et al., 2017).

BOX 4.1   Characteristics of Evidence-Based Practice Models

Advancing Research and Clinical Practice Through Close Collaboration (ARCC©)
- Change organizational culture and promote evidence-based practice (EBP) readiness
- Individual or team-based
- EBP mentors and mentorship increase implementation of EBP
- Remove barriers to EBP

Iowa Model of Evidence-Based Practice to Promote Quality Care
- Step-wise model with decision-points
- Team-based
- Triggering issues or opportunities to identify practice problem
- Organizational change

Johns Hopkins Nursing Evidence-Based Practice (JHNEBP)
- Step-wise model
- Team-based
- Practice, evidence, translation (PET) process for EBP implementation
- Interrelationships between inquiry, practice, and learning
- Organizational change

Knowledge to Action (KTA) Framework
- Relationship between knowledge creation and knowledge users
- Individual or team-based
- Organizational change

Model for Evidence-Based Practice Change
- Step-wise model
- Individual or team-based
- Change management embedded in EBP steps
- Organizational change

Promoting Action on Research Implementation in Health Services (PARIHS)
- Framework
- Individual or team-based
- Interaction among factors (evidence, context, facilitation) promotes successful EBP implementation
- Organizational change

Stetler Model of Evidence-Based Practice
- Step-wise model practitioner oriented
- Individual or team-based
- Practitioner oriented
- Integrates critical thinking

The model uses a step-wise approach to guide inter-professional or uni-professional teams through the EBP process. The first step in the model is to identify triggering issues or opportunities such as clinical or patient-identified issues, organizational initiatives, new data or evidence, and accrediting or regulatory agency requirements (Iowa Model Collaborative et al., 2017). Next, the clinicians will state the clinical question or purpose of the EBP project. Then, they will determine if the clinical question or purpose is a priority for the organization. A team will be formed if the question or purpose is a priority for the organization. If it is not a priority, then the team will consider another issue or opportunity. Once the team is formed, they will assemble, appraise, and synthesize the whole body of evidence, and then determine if there is sufficient evidence to continue with the EBP project; if the evidence is insufficient, then the team may conduct research to obtain new evidence. Once the team has decided to continue the EBP project, they will design and pilot the practice change. As part of this process, the team will obtain patient preferences as they relate to the practice change, develop an implementation plan, and collect baseline and postpilot data. Next, the team will determine if the change is appropriate for implementation into practice. Once the practice change is deemed appropriate, a sustainability plan will be developed and implemented. The final step in the model is the dissemination of results.

Johns Hopkins Nursing Evidence-Based Practice Model

The Johns Hopkins Nursing Evidence-Based Practice Model (JHNEBP) was created in 2002 to address a gap in the utilization of best evidence to nursing practice. The model has undergone two revisions since its inception to reflect changes in the health care system and feedback from clinicians using the model (Dang & Dearholt, 2017). The goal of the model is to help nurses apply best evidence into practice, thereby improving client outcomes. The model has three interrelated components: inquiry, practice, and learning. Inquiry launches the EBP process and is defined as an "effort to question, examine, and collect information about a problem, an issue, or a concern" (Dang & Dearholt, 2017, p. 37). During the inquiry component, nurses seek to identify "whether current practice reflects the best available evidence" (Dang & Dearholt, 2017, p. 44). The second interrelated component of the model is practice, which "reflects the translation of what nurses know into what they do" (Dang & Dearholt, 2017, p. 37). Embedded in the practice component is the 19-step JHNEBP process, which is comprised of three phases—practice, evidence, and translation (PET). The PET process informs practice and learning by creating an "ongoing cycle of inquiry, practice, and learning and identifying best evidence and implementing practice improvements" (Dang & Dearholt, 2017, p. 44). The third interrelated component is learning. The individual clinician and the team learn as they review new evidence for application to practice.

There are discrete steps within each phase of the PET process. For example, the steps that occur in the first phase of the PET process (practice) are: forming an interprofessional team and selecting team leadership, defining the problem and refining the clinical or EBP question, and identifying stakeholders in the EBP project. During the second phase of the PET process (evidence), the team searches for, appraises, and summarizes evidence and makes recommendations for change based on the evidence. During the final phase of the PET process (translation), the team determines if the practice change is appropriate and feasible, develops and implements an action plan, evaluates the outcomes, and shares the outcomes with stakeholders. Tools are available to help guide teams through the different steps in the PET process. The model may be used by individuals or teams of interprofessional clinicians. Advanced practice nurses frequently serve as teachers, role models, and team leaders for implementing the model, whereas BSN-prepared nurses may serve as unit-based EBP champions or be part of an EBP team.

Knowledge to Action Framework

The aim of the Knowledge to Action (KTA) framework, created by Graham and Tetroe, is to improve health and health care by facilitating the translation of knowledge to practice (Graham & Tetroe, 2010). The framework uses a systems perspective and cyclical model to integrate the creation of knowledge with its application. The framework views knowledge as empirical (research-based), contextual, and experiential. The application of knowledge takes into account the context and culture, thus allowing customized application of knowledge to the end user. A central premise of the framework is that, for knowledge translation to occur, there needs to be collaboration between the creators of knowledge and the users of knowledge. Some of the key features of this framework include

that it allows for the adaptation of evidence-informed interventions based on unique variables, and that knowledge users participate in the production of knowledge and its adaptation for use (Graham & Tetroe, 2010, p. 217). This framework may be used with individuals, teams, or organizations to facilitate the translation of knowledge to practice.

Model for Evidence-Based Practice Change

Rosswurm and Larrabee (1999) proposed the Model for Change to EBP, which was renamed in 2009 the Model for EBP Change to reflect that the change is due to EBP (Larrabee, 2009). This is a systematic, six-step model that integrates EBP, research utilization, and change theory. The model uses a team-based approach that may be interprofessional, and includes relevant stakeholders for the problem. The first step in the model is to assess the need for change in practice, which is accomplished by collecting internal data about current practice, such as patient preferences, QI data, or outcome evaluation data. The EBP team then compares this internal data to external data or benchmarks to identify the practice problem, and links the problem to interventions and outcomes. In the second step, the team searches for the best evidence. In the third step, the team will critique and synthesize the evidence, then assess the evidence for feasibility, benefits, and risks. During the fourth step, the team designs the practice change, including defining the change, identifying the resources needed, planning the implementation process, and defining the outcomes. The team will use change management strategies, such as change champions, education, and audit feedback systems. The team will also collect the baseline data during this step. In the fifth step, the team will implement and evaluate the change in practice. This step is usually accomplished by conducting a pilot study to implement the change, then evaluating the process for implementing the change, and the outcomes. The team uses data to decide whether to adapt, adopt, or reject the practice change. In the sixth step, the team will integrate and maintain the change in practice. During this step, the team will share the recommended change with stakeholders, incorporate the change into the standards of practice, and monitor the process for implementing the change and the outcomes associated with the change. Lastly, the team will disseminate the results of the project. Key features of this model are that it is systematic, uses a step-wise approach, uses interprofessional or discipline-specific teams, includes stakeholders and patients, integrates change theory, and uses internal data to identify clinical problems (i.e., patient preferences, QI data).

Promoting Action on Research Implementation in Health Services

The Promoting Action on Research Implementation in Health Services (PARIHS) framework was initially developed in 1998 to understand the complexities associated with the "successful implementation of evidence into practice" (Rycroft-Malone, 2010, p. 110). The nature of evidence, the context or organizational environment, and the approach to facilitating change are factors that affect the successful implementation of evidence into practice. The first factor is evidence. There are four types of evidence, including research evidence, clinical experience, client or caregiver experience, and local data/information, such as audit, performance, or QI data. The second factor is context, which includes environmental elements such as the organizational culture, how the organization's leaders lead, and how practice changes are evaluated (Rycroft-Malone, 2004). The third factor is facilitation which refers to the person or actions that help implement change within an organization. Each of these factors is rated using a high-low continuum. The greatest chance for facilitating successful implementation of EBP occurs when all factors are high (evidence, context, and facilitation). Research evidence is considered high when "it is well-conceived and conducted, that is, robust and judged credible" (Rycroft-Malone, 2010, p. 114). Clinical experience is considered high when it is "explicit and verified through critical reflection, critique, and debate within the wider community of practice" (Rycroft-Malone, 2010, p. 118). Client or caregiver experience is considered high when they are part of the decision-making process. Local data or information may be considered high if it was "systematically collected, evaluated, and reflected upon" (Rycroft-Malone, 2010, p. 118). The context is considered high when the organization encourages change and learning and has empowering leadership. Facilitation is considered high when the facilitator is able to adapt to the context to promote implementation of EBP. This model may be used by individuals or organizations.

Stetler Model of Evidence-Based Practice

The Stetler Model of EBP began as a model for research utilization in the 1970s, and has evolved over time to become a decision-making model that uses critical thinking to determine if research and other evidence is applicable to the clinical issue, as well as how to implement and evaluate the best evidence for practice (Stetler, 2010). The model is viewed as a practitioner-oriented model that may be used by individuals or groups to facilitate the decision-making process as it relates to EBP. The model has five phases. In phase I—preparation, the team will

identify and validate the existence of the problem and search for evidence. Then, the team will validate evidence, critique evidence, assess the level of evidence and the fit of the evidence to the problem in phase II—validation. During phase III—comparative evaluation/decision-making, the team will assess the fit of the evidence to the problem, the feasibility of implementing the evidence, substantiate the evidence, examine current practice, synthesize the evidence, and decide to use or not use evidence. In phase IV—translation/application, the team will apply the evidence to practice, either informally or formally and apply evidence at the individual, group, or department/organization level. Evaluation of the practice change occurs in phase V. During this phase, the team evaluates dynamically based on implementation experiences and outcomes, and determines to continue/sustain EBP or to stop it (Stetler, 2010). This model is designed for use by baccalaureate-prepared nurses with support from advanced practice nurses to assist with evaluation, or by advanced practice nurses.

CONTRAST EVIDENCE-BASED PRACTICE MODELS

EBP models were developed to address a common aim, which is to use the best evidence to improve health outcomes. Most of the models strive to achieve organizational change, and use similar processes to search, appraise, and synthesize evidence for application to practice. The Iowa Model, JHNEBP, Model for EBP change, and the Stetler model use a prescriptive, step-wise approach to implementing EBP; the ARCC© model, KTA framework, and the PARIHS framework provide a conceptual approach to EBP implementation. All of the models, except the Iowa model, use individual or team-based approaches for implementing EBP. The Model for EBP change uses change champions to implement EBP projects, whereas the ARCC© model uses EBP mentors and mentorship to facilitate EBP.

APPLICATION OF EVIDENCE-BASED PRACTICE

Here is an example to illustrate how EBP can be applied to answer a clinical question.

Identify a Problem and Write a Clinical Question

- The nurse manager identifies a trend in the clinical unit's incidence rate of falls with injury in postoperative clients greater than 65 years of age.

- The incidence rate of falls for this population during the first 6 months of the year was 10%, whereas the incident rate for the last 6 months of the year was 20%.
- The clinical question is written using PICO format. What is the effect of hourly rounding (I—intervention) as compared to not rounding hourly (C—comparison) on the incidence of falls with injury (O—outcome) in postoperative clients greater than 65 years of age (P—population)?
- The nurse manager forms an interprofessional team to answer this clinical question.

Search for the Evidence

- The team decides to use the CINAHL and MEDLINE databases to search for evidence.
- Then, they identify the controlled vocabulary terms (hourly rounding, falls with injury, postoperative patients age 65 or older); the Boolean operator (and) to connect the terms, and limitation parameters, such as publication year.
- Lastly, the team reviews the evidence found to ensure that it addresses the clinical question, including the population, intervention, and outcome.

Appraise the Evidence

- The team appraises the level of evidence and the quality of evidence.

Implement the Evidence

- The team gathers information from the clinical experts and the clients/caregivers and uses this information to guide project implementation.
- Then, the team develops and implements a plan to use the intervention in practice.
- Next, the team develops an evaluation plan identifying what data will be collected, by whom, and when.

Evaluate the Outcomes

- The team collects data according to the evaluation plan.
- The team analyzes the data to determine if the outcome was met.
- If the outcome was met, then the team will develop plans to sustain the practice change and to share findings with others.
- If the outcome was not met, then the team will develop plans to phase out (stop) the practice change.

SUMMARY

EBP is a problem-solving approach to clinical decision-making that involves the use of the best available evidence, clinical expertise, and patient preferences and values to improve outcomes. The use of evidence from research, EBP, and QI studies provides the foundations to achieve the Quintuple Aim (improved population health, reduced cost, improved patient experience, enhanced clinician well-being, and improved health equity). All levels of nurses are expected to use EBP to deliver optimal care to our clients. In order to do this, nurses must know how to search for relevant evidence, appraise the evidence, and apply it to nursing practice. Challenges associated with implementing EBP include fast-paced information overload that makes it hard for clinicians to determine what research is valid and reliable versus invalid and unreliable research.

SALIENT POINTS

- Nurses can foster the development of a spirit of inquiry by being inquisitive, asking clinical questions, being open to change, and staying current with the research literature.
- Health care organizations can promote a culture that supports a spirit of inquiry by providing education, mentoring, resources, and time for clinicians to engage in EBP, while recognizing and valuing the contributions of EBP in improving outcomes.
- EBP uses the best, current, relevant evidence coupled with clinician expertise and patient preferences and values to inform the clinical decision-making process.
- EBP has been shown to have a positive effect on patient outcomes, health care quality, and reducing costs.
- All nurses should use EBP to guide their nursing practice.
- EBP is a process, not an event.
- On average, it takes 15 years to implement a practice change.

CRITICAL REFLECTION EXERCISES

1. Identify a clinical question. Select one of the EBP models and describe how you will use it to guide your inquiry into the clinical question.
2. Think about how you can implement EBP in your nursing practice. Discuss four activities that you will use to demonstrate application of EBP to your nursing practice.
3. Identify four activities that you can routinely engage in to develop a "spirit of inquiry."
4. Discuss the criteria you will use to determine if a health care organization facilitates a culture that supports EBP and facilitates a spirit of inquiry.

ⓔ EVOLVE WEBSITE/RESOURCES LIST

American Nurses Association. View this website to learn more about the *Code of Ethics for Nursing with Interpretative Statements* and the *Magnet Recognition Program* for Nursing Excellence. https://www.nursingworld.org/ana/

Institute for Healthcare Improvement. Search this website to learn about the Triple Aim and other initiatives to improve care. http://www.ihi.org/Engage/Initiatives/TripleAim/Pages/default.aspx

National Collaborating Centers for Methods and Tools. Access this website for free educational modules and resources that promote evidence-informed practice. https://www.nccmt.ca/

REFERENCES

Alves, S. L. (2021). Improvements in clinician, organization, and patient outcomes make a compelling case for evidence-based practice mentor development programs: An integrative review. *Worldviews on Evidence-Based Nursing, 18*(5), 283–289. https://doi.org/10.1111/wvn.12533

American Nurses Association. (2015). *Code of ethics for nurses with interpretive statements.* https://www.nursingworld.org/practice-policy/nursing-excellence/ethics/code-of-ethics-for-nurses/coe-view-only/

Carter, E. J., Mastro, K., Vose, C., Rivera, R., & Larson, E. L. (2017). Clarifying the conundrum: Evidence-based practice, quality improvement, or research? The clinical scholarship continuum. *The Journal of Nursing Administration, 47*(5), 266–270. https://doi.org/10.1097/NNA.0000000000000477

Cullen, L., Hanrahan, K., Farrington, M., Anderson, R., Dimmer, E., Miner, R., Suchan, T., & Rod, E. (2020). Evidence-based practice change champion program improves quality care. *The Journal of Nursing Administration, 50*(3), 128–134. https://doi.org/10.1097/NNA.0000000000000856

Dang, D., & Dearholt, S. L. (2017). *Johns Hopkins nursing evidence-based practice: Model and guidelines* (3rd ed.). Sigma Theta Tau International.

Graham, I., & Tetroe, J. (2010). The knowledge to action framework. In J. O. Rycroft-Malone & T. Bucknall (Eds.), *Models and frameworks for implementing evidence-based practice: Linking evidence to action* (pp. 207–221). Wiley-Blackwell.

Iowa Model Collaborative, Buckwalter, K. C., Cullen, L., Hanrahan, K., McCarthy, A. M., Rakel, B., Steelman, V., Tripp-Reimer, T., & Tucker, S. (2017). Iowa model of evidence-based practice: Revisions and validation. *Worldviews on Evidence Based Nursing, 14*(3), 175–182. https://doi.org/10.1111/wvn.12223

Khan, S., Chambers, D., & Neta, G. (2021). Revisiting time to translation: Implementation of evidence-based practices (EBPs) in cancer control. *Cancer Causes and Control, 32*(3), 221–230. https://doi.org/10.1007/s10552-020-01376-z

Larrabee, J. H. (2009). *Nurse to nurse: Evidence-based practice.* McGraw-Hill.

Melnyk, B. M., & Fineout-Overholt, E. (2002). Putting research into practice. *Reflections on Nursing Leadership, 28*(2), 22–25.

Melnyk, B. M., & Fineout-Overholt, E. (2019). Making the case for evidence-based practice and cultivating a spirit of inquiry. In B. M. Melnyk & E. Fineout-Overholt (Eds.), *Evidence-based practice in nursing and healthcare: A guide to best practice* (4th ed., pp. 7–30). Wolters Kluwer.

Melnyk, B. M., Fineout-Overholt, E., Giggleman, M., & Choy, K. (2017). A test of the ARCC© model improves implementation of evidence-based practice, healthcare culture, and patient outcomes. *Worldviews on Evidence-Based Nursing, 14*(1), 5–9. https://doi.org/10.1111/wvn.12188

Melnyk, B. M., Tan, A., Hsieh, A. P., & Gallagher-Ford, L. (2021). Evidence-based practice culture and mentorship predict EBP implementation, nurse job satisfaction, and intent to stay: Support for the ARCC© model. *Worldviews on Evidence-Based Nursing, 18*(4), 272–281. https://doi.org/10.1111/wvn.12524

Nundy, S., Cooper, L. A., & Mate, K. S. (2022). The Quintuple Aim for health care improvement: A new imperative to advance health equity. *JAMA, 327*(8), 521–522. https://doi.org/10.1001/jama.2021.25181

Polit, D., & Beck, C. (2022). *Essentials of nursing research: Appraising evidence for nursing practice* (10th ed.). Wolters Kluwer.

Rosswurm, M. A., & Larrabee, J. H. (1999). A model for change to evidence-based practice. *Image Journal of Nursing Scholarship, 31*(4), 317–322. https://doi.org/10.1111/j.1547-5069.1999.tb00510.x

Rycroft-Malone, J. (2004). The PARIHS framework: A framework for guiding the implementation of evidence-based practice. *Journal of Nursing Care Quality, 19*(4), 297–304. https://doi.org/10.1097/00001786-200410000-00002

Rycroft-Malone, J. (2010). Promoting action on research implementation in health services. In J. Rycroft-Malone & T. Surname

(Eds.), *Models and frameworks for implementing evidence-based practice: Linking evidence to action* (pp. 109–135). Wiley-Blackwell.

Rycroft-Malone, J., & Bucknall, T. (2010). Theory, frameworks, and models laying down the groundwork. In J. Rycroft-Maloner & T. Bucknall (Eds.), *Models and frameworks for implementing evidence-based practice: Linking evidence to action* (pp. 23–50). Wiley-Blackwell.

Speroni, K. G., McLaughlin, M. K., & Friesen, M. A. (2020). Use of evidence-based practice models and research findings in magnet-designated hospitals across the United States: National survey results. *Worldviews on Evidence-Based Nursing, 17*(2), 98–107.

Stetler, C. (2010). Stetler model. In J. Rycroft-Malone & T. Bucknall (Eds.), *Models and frameworks for implementing evidence-based practice: Linking evidence to action* (pp. 51–81). Wiley-Blackwell.

Theories and Frameworks for Professional Nursing Practice

Elizabeth E. Friberg, DNP, RN

 http://evolve.elsevier.com/Friberg/bridge/

INTRODUCTION

Nursing is both a science and an art. The **empirical science** of nursing (relying on or derived from observation, experiment, or practical experience) includes both the natural sciences (e.g., biology, chemistry) and the human sciences (e.g., sociology, psychology). The **art of nursing** is the **ability to use** basic scientific knowledge **to improve the well-being of people** (Phillips, 2016). Nursing is a **knowledge-based, evidence-based discipline** significantly different from medicine. Medicine focuses on the identification and treatment of disease, whereas nursing focuses on the wholeness of human beings (Fawcett, 1993). Nursing claims the health of human beings in interaction with the environment as its domain. Domains define the discipline and set its boundaries. *Knowledge* is commonly defined as the sum of what is known: the body of truth, information, and principles acquired by humankind (Merriam-Webster, n.d.).

Nursing knowledge is the organization of the *discipline-specific concepts, theories, and ideas* published in the literature (both print and electronic media) and demonstrated in professional practice. Nursing's objective to be regarded as a profession (e.g., law, medicine) was the impetus for building a substantial body of discipline-specific knowledge. Many of the existing theories emerged from the response to the simple question, "What is nursing?"

Theories and conceptual frameworks consist of the theorist's words brought together to form a meaningful whole. Theories are not discovered; they are invented by the nurse theorists at a point in time. Therefore they evolve over time yet still have value. Theories are abstractions (Polit & Beck, 2021, p. 112). According to Polit and Beck (2021) theories, conceptual models, and frameworks *provide direction and guidance for structuring professional nursing practice, education, administration,* and *research*. In practice, theories, models, and frameworks help nurses to *describe, explain,* and *predict* everyday experiences. They also assist in *organizing* assessment data, *making* diagnoses, *choosing* interventions, *evaluating* nursing care outcomes, and sometimes *generating* ideas for new research. In education, a conceptual framework provides the general focus for curriculum design. In research, a framework offers a systematic approach to identifying questions for study, selecting appropriate variables, and interpreting findings. The research findings may trigger revision and refinement of the existing theory.

Many nurse theorists have made substantial contributions to the development of a *body of nursing knowledge* and continue to do so today. This richness of the nursing literature reflects that body of knowledge, offering an assortment of perspectives or lenses to view nursing practice. The theories vary in their level of abstraction and their conceptualization of the areas of focus for the nursing discipline. From a historical perspective, nursing theories reflect the influence of the larger society and illustrate increased sophistication in the development of nursing ideas. Continued acquisition of "new knowledge within the discipline of nursing occurs through development of its theories" (Yancey, 2015, p. 275). The intent of this chapter is to provide a comprehensive overview of *select* nursing theories to serve as a foundation for understanding how specific nursing theories relate to individual topics in subsequent chapters.

TERMINOLOGY ASSOCIATED WITH NURSING THEORY

According to Polit and Beck (2021), the term *theory* is used in many ways. *Classic theory* is an abstract generalized representation of observed phenomena and how they are interrelated. The purpose of classic theories is to explain and predict the relationships. *Concepts* (or ideas) are the building blocks of theory propositions (or theory statements) and the relationships between those concepts taken together generate the nature of the theoretical framework. There are *levels of theories*: *grand*, *middle range*, and *practice* theories. The levels of theories are explained later in the chapter. A theory, then, is "defined as propositions that specify the relationships between concepts, which are expected to explain and/or predict the world" (Bender, 2018, p. 2).

A nursing theory is composed of a set of concepts and propositions that claims to account for or characterize the central phenomena of interest to the discipline, in this case nursing. The discipline of nursing addresses human beings, environment, health and illness, and nursing. *Human beings* are the recipients of nursing care and include individuals, families, and communities. *Environment* refers to the surroundings of the client, internal factors affecting the client, and the setting in which nursing care is delivered. *Health and illness* describe the client's state of well-being. *Nursing* refers to the actions taken when providing nursing care to a patient. These concepts, taken together, make up what is known as the *metaparadigm*

of nursing, a multifaceted lens for looking at nursin*g*, which we will use to compare the selected theories. Most nursing theories define or describe these central concepts, either explicitly or implicitly. Because a concept is an abstract representation of the real world, concepts embedded in a theory represent the theorist's perspective of reality and may differ from that of the reader without invalidating the theory. Theories are stepping stones.

Because theories represent abstract ideas rather than concrete facts and may be broad or limited in scope, they vary in their ability to describe, explain, or predict. Theories may be categorized by their level of abstraction as grand theories, midrange theories, or practice theories.

Grand theories (also known as *conceptual models* or *frameworks*) are macro-level representations of the broad nature, purpose, and goals of the discipline (Polit & Beck, 2021). Concepts and their relationships are very abstract, not operationally defined, and not empirically testable. According to Polit and Beck (2021), **conceptual models or frameworks or schemes** are less formal ways of organizing phenomena than classic theories. They are less structured and not formally tested as classic theories but serve as springboards. *Models* are often used as a symbolic representation of the conceptualization. **Schematic models** or **conceptual maps** are visual representations using the concepts as building blocks but with minimal words. A *theoretical* or *conceptual framework* provides the overall conceptual underpinnings of a study, and every study has a framework even if it is not explicitly stated because every study has an underlying **conceptual rationale**. Clearly defining a conceptual rationale or framework helps the consumer/reader to better understand the design and findings of a study (best practice). No matter the nature of the grand theory, grand theory is a macro view/lens for describing, explaining, or predicting the relationships between concepts.

Midrange theories, which may be derived from grand theories, are less abstract, with relatively concrete concepts that address specific phenomena across nursing settings and specialties. Relationships between and among concepts can be defined explicitly and measured. Because they are narrower in scope, midrange theories appear more applicable to practice and remain abstract enough to allow a wide range of empirical research. Liehr and Smith (2017) predict that "ongoing use of middle range theory offers potential for testing and shaping to enhance relevance and optimize the contribution to nursing knowledge development over the next decades" (p. 52).

Practice theories (sometimes called **situation-specific** or **micro-level theories**) are limited further to a patient population or type of nursing practice (Polit & Beck, 2021). They may be derived from existing theories, arise from practice, or emerge from research findings. The purpose of these theories is to describe or explain clinical problems or patient needs that nurses encounter daily within the boundaries of their specialty practices or settings. Therefore they may prescribe specific nursing actions or lead to the in-depth analysis of nursing interventions.

Descriptions of the selected theoretical perspectives presented in this chapter include a brief overview; the theory's basic assumptions about human beings and the environment; definitions of health and illness; a description of nursing, including the goal of nursing; and definitions of concepts and subconcepts specific to each theory. Six grand theories and three midrange theories are presented. Theories and frameworks selected for inclusion in this chapter are those that exemplify the different definitions of nursing along varying levels of abstraction.

Ten theories frequently used in nursing from related disciplines are briefly described. Some theories are more amenable than others to the scheme presented earlier, to summarize selected theories because of their degree of specificity or stage of development. When the needed information is not explicitly detailed by the theorist, inferences are made on the basis of what seems to be implicitly stated. *Direct quotes from the theorists are used whenever possible to ensure that such interpretations are valid and reliable.*

Although the reader is encouraged to consult the primary source to gain a full appreciation of the depth, scope, and extent of the relationships put forth, many of these text sources are no longer available in print. However, noting the year of the citation allows the reader to understand how the theory evolved over time in the view of the nurse theorist, reflecting the influence of practices and societal and environmental changes. This chapter provides the reader the opportunity to engage with the theorist's original work through direct quotes. For those wishing to see details of how the models and theories guide nursing practice over the years, a basic search of the literature using a database such as CINAHL will yield multiple examples.

A statement by Myra Levine (1920–1996), a nurse theorist (Four Conservation Principles theory), speaks to the need for having a variety of theories from multiple perspectives to describe nursing.

> *Exploring a variety of nursing theories ought to provide nurses with new insights into patient care, opening nursing options otherwise hidden, and stimulating innovative interventions. But it is imperative that there be variety—for there is no global theory of nursing that fits every situation.*
>
> *(Levine, 1995, p. 13)*

OVERVIEW OF SELECTED NURSING THEORIES

Grand Theory (Macro Level)

Nightingale's Environmental Theory. Florence Nightingale (1820–1910) conceptualized disease as a reparative process and described the nurse's role as manipulating the environment to facilitate and encourage this process. Her directions regarding ventilation, warmth, light, diet, cleanliness, variety, and noise are discussed in her classic nursing textbook *Notes on Nursing*, first published in London in 1859 and in America in 1860.

Brief Overview. The environment is critical to health, and the nurse's role in caring for the sick is to provide a clean, quiet, peaceful environment to promote healing. Nightingale's intent was to describe nursing and provide guidelines for nursing education.

Assumptions About Human Beings. Individuals are responsible, creative, and in control of their lives and health.

Environment. The environment is external to the person but affects the health of both sick and well persons. As a chief source of infection, the environment must include pure air, pure water, efficient drainage, cleanliness, and light.

Health and Illness. Health is described as a state of being well and using one's powers to the fullest. Illness or disease is the reaction of nature against the conditions in which human beings have placed themselves. Disease is a reparative mechanism, an effort of nature to remedy a process of poisoning or of decay.

Nursing. Nursing is a service to humanity intended to relieve pain and suffering. Nursing's role is to promote or provide the proper environment for patients, including fresh air, light, pure water, cleanliness, warmth, quiet, and appropriate diet. The goal of nursing is to promote the reparative process by manipulating the environment.

Key Concepts. *Environment* refers to conditions external to the individual that affect life and development (e.g., ventilation, warmth, light, diet, cleanliness, noise). Nightingale (1860/1946) identified three major relationships: the environment to the patient, the nurse to the environment, and the nurse to the patient. Examples of these are as follows:

- The need for light, particularly sunlight, is second only to the need for ventilation. If necessary, the nurse should move the patient "about after the sun according to the aspects of the rooms, if circumstances permit, [rather] than let him linger in a room when the sun is off" (Nightingale, 1860/1946, p. 48).

- Nursing's role is to manipulate the environment to encourage healing. Nursing "ought to signify the proper use of fresh air, light, warmth, cleanliness, quiet, and the proper selection and administration of diet" (Nightingale, 1860/1946, p. 6).
- The sine qua non of all good nursing is never to allow a patient to be awakened, intentionally or accidentally: "A good nurse will always make sure that no blind or curtains should flap. If you wait till your patient tells you or reminds you of these things, where is the use of their having a nurse?" (Nightingale, 1860/1946, p. 27).
- Variety is important for patients to divert them from dwelling on their pain: "Variety of form and brilliancy of color in the objects presented are actual means of recovery" (Nightingale, 1860/1946, p. 34).

Rogers' Science of Unitary Human Beings

Martha Rogers (1914–1994) first presented her conceptualizations, *An Introduction to the Theoretical Basis for Nursing*, in 1970, dating back to the 1960s. They evolved into the current science of unitary human beings (SUHB). This theory is sometimes referred to as the Rogerian Model, a conceptual model (Polit & Beck, 2021). She posited that human beings are dynamic energy fields who are integral with the environment and who are continuously evolving. She viewed nursing as a science and an art that focus on the nature and direction of human development and human betterment. Rogers' theory supported the development of derived theories and nursing practice changes beyond the scope of this chapter. The Society of Rogerian Scholars (https://www.societyofrogerianscholars.org/) founded in 1988 continues the evolution of the SUHB grand theory to advance nursing science in the 21st century, including *Visions: Journal of Rogerian Scholar Science*.

Brief Overview. The individual is viewed as an irreducible energy field, integral with the environment. The nurse seeks to promote symphonic (harmonious) interactions between human beings and their environments (Rogers, 1970).

Assumptions About Human Beings. The individual is a unified, irreducible whole manifesting characteristics that are more than, and different from, the sum of his or her parts and continuously evolving, irreversibly and unidirectionally along a space-time continuum. Pattern and organization of human beings are directed toward increasing complexity rather than maintaining equilibrium. The individual "is characterized by the capacity for abstraction and imagery, language and thought, sensation and emotion" (Rogers, 1970, p. 73).

Environment. The environment is an irreducible, pandimensional (pertaining to and across all dimensions of reality) energy field identified by pattern and integral with the human energy field (Rogers, 1994). The individual and the environment are continually exchanging matter and energy with one another, resulting in changing patterns in both the individual and the environment.

Health and Illness. Health and illness are value-laden, arbitrarily defined, and culturally infused notions. They are not dichotomous but are part of the same continuum. Health seems to occur when patterns of living are in harmony with environmental change, whereas illness occurs when patterns of living are in conflict with environmental change and are deemed unacceptable (Rogers, 1994).

Nursing. As both a science and an art, nursing is unique in its concern with unitary human beings as synergistic phenomena. The science of nursing should be concerned with studying the nature and direction of unitary human development integral with the environment and with evolving descriptive, explanatory, and predictive principles for use in nursing practice. The "new age of nursing science" is characterized by a synthesis of fact and ideas that generate principles and theories (Rogers, 1994). The art of nursing is the creative use of the science of nursing for human betterment (Rogers, 1990). The combination of art and science enhances the effect (outcomes) of nursing actions. The goal of nursing is the attainment of the best possible state of health for the individual who is continually evolving by promoting symphonic interactions between human beings and environments, strengthening the coherence and integrity of the human field, and directing and redirecting patterning of both fields for maximal health potential.

Key Concepts. The concepts describe the individual and environment as energy fields that are in constant interaction. The nature and direction of human development form the basis for the following principles of nursing science:

- *Energy field:* The fundamental unit of the living and nonliving. Energy fields are dynamic, continuously in motion, and infinite. They are of two types:
  - *Human energy field:* More than the biological, psychological, and sociological fields taken separately

or together; an irreducible, indivisible, pandimensional whole identified by pattern and manifesting characteristics that cannot be predicted from the parts.

- *Environmental energy field:* An irreducible, indivisible, pandimensional energy field identified by pattern and integral with the human field.
- *Openness:* Continuous change and mutual process as manifested in human and environmental fields.
- *Pattern:* The distinguishing characteristic of an energy field perceived as a single wave.
- *Principles of nursing science:* Principles postulating the nature and direction of unitary human development; these principles are also called *principles of homeodynamics.*
  - *Helicy:* According to Rogers (1989), helicy is "the continuous, innovative, probabilistic, increasing diversity of human and environmental field patterns characterized by repeating rhymicities" (p. 186). Change occurs continuously.
  - *Resonancy:* Rogers (1989) describes resonancy as "the continuous change from lower to higher frequency wave patterns in human and environmental fields" (p. 186). Change is increasingly diverse.
  - *Integrality:* Replacing the earlier concept of complementarity, integrality is "the continuous mutual human and environmental field process" (Rogers, 1989, p. 186). Field changes occur simultaneously.

Orem's Self-Care Deficit Nursing Theory

The foundations of Dorothea Orem's (1914–2007) theory, also viewed as a conceptual model, were introduced in the late 1950s, but the first edition of her work, *Nursing: Concepts of Practice,* was not published until 1971. Five subsequent editions (Orem, 1980, 1985, 1991, 1995, 2001) show evidence of continued development and refinement of the theory. Orem focuses on nursing as deliberate human action and notes that all individuals can benefit from nursing when they have health-derived or health-related limitations for engaging in self-care or the care of dependent others. Three theories are subsumed in the self-care deficit theory of nursing: the theory of nursing systems, the theory of self-care deficits, and the theory of self-care (Orem, 2001). Currently, self-care deficit nursing theory (SCDNT) is widely known and used in nursing practice worldwide.

Brief Overview. The individual practices self-care, a set of learned behaviors, to sustain life, maintain or restore functioning, and bring about a condition of well-being. The nurse assists the client with self-care when he or she experiences a deficit in the ability to perform.

Assumptions About Human Beings. The individual is viewed as a unit whose functioning is linked with the environment and who, with the environment, forms an integrated (unified), functional whole. The individual functions biologically, symbolically, and socially.

Environment. The environment is linked to the individual, forming an integrated system. The environment is implied to be external to the individual.

Health and Illness. Health, which has physical, psychological, interpersonal, and social aspects, is a state in which human beings are structurally and functionally whole or sound (Orem, 1995). Illness occurs when an individual is incapable of maintaining self-care as a result of structural or functional limitations.

Nursing. Nursing involves assisting the individual with self-care practices to sustain life and health, recover from disease or injury, and cope with their effects (Orem, 1985). The nurse chooses deliberate actions from nursing systems designed to bring about desirable conditions in persons and their environments. The goal of nursing is to move a patient toward responsible self-care or to meet existing health care needs of those who have health care deficits.

Key Concepts. The concepts focus on self-care in terms of requisites, demands, and deficits and delineate the nurse's role in client care in the following manner:

- *Self-care:* This refers to "activities that individuals initiate and perform on their own behalf to maintain life, health, or well-being" (Orem, 1995, p. 104).
- *Dependent care agent:* A person other than the individual who provides the care; "the provider of infant care, child care, or dependent adult care" (Orem, 1991, p. 117).
- *Self-care requisites:* Actions that are known or hypothesized to be necessary to regulate human functioning. Three types exist:
  - *Universal:* Common to all human beings; concerned with the promotion and maintenance of structural and functional integrity. These include air, water, food, elimination, activity and rest, solitude and social interaction, prevention of hazards, and promotion of human functioning.
  - *Developmental:* Associated with conditions that promote known developmental processes; occurring at various stages of the life cycle.
  - *Health deviation:* Genetic and constitutional defects and deviations that affect integrated human functioning and impair the individual's ability to perform self-care.

- *Therapeutic self-care demand:* Based on the notion that self-care is a human regulatory function; the totality of self-care actions performed by the nurse or self to meet known self-care requisites.
- *Self-care agency:* Acquired ability to know and meet requirements to regulate own functioning and development.
- *Self-care deficits:* Gaps between known therapeutic self-care demands and the capability of the individual to perform self-care.
- *Nursing system:* Systems of concrete actions for persons with limitations in self-care. These actions are of three types (Orem, 1995):
  - *Wholly compensatory:* The nurse compensates for the individual's total inability to perform self-care activities.
  - *Partly compensatory:* The nurse compensates for the individual's inability to perform some (but not all) self-care activities.
  - *Supportive-educative:* With the individual able to perform all self-care activities, the nurse assists the client in decision-making, behavior control, and the acquisition of knowledge and skill.
- Subsystems of each nursing system:
  - *Social:* The complementary and contractual relationship between the nurse and the client.
  - *Interpersonal:* The nurse-client interaction.
  - *Technological:* According to Orem (1985), the "diagnosis, prescription, regulation of treatment, and management of nursing care" (p. 160).

Roy's Adaptation Model

Sister Callista Roy (1939–present) has continuously expanded her conceptual model from its inception in the 1960s to the present, building on the conceptual framework of adaptation (dynamic evolutionary process of change). She focuses on the individual as a biopsychosocial adaptive system and describes nursing as a humanistic discipline that "places emphasis on the person's own coping abilities" (Roy, 1984, p. 32). The individual and the environment are sources of stimuli that require modification to promote adaptation.

Brief Overview. The individual is a biopsychosocial adaptive system, and the nurse promotes adaptation by modifying external stimuli.

Assumptions About Human Beings. The individual is in constant interaction with a changing environment, and to respond positively to environmental change, a person must adapt. The person's adaptation level is determined by the combined effect of three classes of stimuli: focal, contextual, and residual. The individual uses both innate and acquired

biological, psychological, or social adaptive mechanisms and has four modes of adaptation.

Environment. All conditions, circumstances, and influences surrounding and affecting the development and behavior of persons and groups constitute the environment. Having both internal and external components, the environment is constantly changing.

Health and Illness. According to Roy (1989), "health and illness are one inevitable dimension of a person's life" (p. 106). Health is "a state and process of being and becoming integrated and whole" (Roy & Andrews, 1999, p. 31). Conversely, illness is a lack of integration.

Nursing. As an external regulatory force, nursing acts to modify stimuli affecting adaptation by increasing, decreasing, or maintaining stimuli. The goal of nursing is to promote the person's adaptation in the four adaptive modes, thus contributing to health, quality of life, and dying with dignity (Roy, 2009).

Key Concepts. The following concepts describe and define adaptation in terms of the individual's internal control processes, adaptive modes, and adaptive level:
- *Adaptation:* The individual's ability to cope with the constantly changing environment.
- *Adaptive system:* Consists of two major internal control processes (coping mechanisms):
  - *Regulator subsystem:* Receives input from the external environment and from changes in the person's internal state and processes it through neural-chemical-endocrine channels.
  - *Cognator subsystem:* Receives input from external and internal stimuli that involve psychological, social, physical, and physiological factors and processes it through cognitive pathways.
- *Adaptive modes:* The four ways a person adapts:
  - *Physiological:* Determined by the need for physiological integrity derived from the basic physiological needs.
  - *Self-concept:* Determined by the need for interactions with others and psychic integrity regarding the perception of self.
  - *Role function:* Determined by the need for social integrity; refers to the performance of duties based on given positions within society.
  - *Interdependence:* Involves ways of seeking help, affection, and attention.
- *Adaptive level:* Determined by the combined effects of stimuli:
  - *Focal stimulus:* That which immediately confronts the individual.

- *Contextual stimuli:* All other stimuli present in the environment. These stimuli influence how the individual deals with the focal stimulus.
- *Residual stimuli:* Beliefs, attitudes, or traits that have an indeterminate effect on the present situation.

Neuman's Systems Model

Betty Neuman (1924–present) developed her systems model, a conceptual model, in 1970 in response to student requests to focus on breadth rather than depth in understanding human variables in nursing problems. First published in 1972 (Neuman & Young, 1972), the model was refined to its present form in *The Neuman Systems Model* (Neuman, 1982). The Neuman systems model "is an open systems model that views nursing as being primarily concerned with defining appropriate actions in stress-related situations" (Neuman, 1995, p. 11). Neuman believes that nursing encompasses a wholistic (body, mind, and spirit) client systems approach to help individuals, families, communities, and society reach and maintain wellness. Neuman's focus on the *whole* system explains her use of the term *wholistic* rather than holistic (alternative healing practices). Concepts of the Neuman Systems Model are incorporated in Quality and Safety Education for Nurses (QSEN). The Neuman System Model Trustees Group (https://www.neumansystemsmodel.org/) established in 1988 is committed to the development or use of the Neuman's systems model (NSM) in education, practice, administration, or research.

Brief Overview. This theory offers a "wholistic view" of the client system, including the concepts of open system, environment, stressors, prevention, and reconstitution. Nursing is concerned with the whole person.

Assumptions About Human Beings. In this model, the client is a whole person, a dynamic composite of interrelationships among physiological, psychological, sociocultural, developmental, and spiritual variables: "The client is viewed as an open system in interaction with the environment" (Neuman, 1989, p. 68). The client is in "dynamic constant energy exchange with the environment" (Neuman, 1989, p. 22).

Environment. Both internal and external environments exist, and the person maintains varying degrees of harmony between them. The environment includes all internal and external factors affecting and being affected by the system (Neuman, 1995). Emphasis is on all stressors—interpersonal, intrapersonal, extrapersonal—that might disturb the person's normal line of defense.

Health and Illness. Neuman (1995) asserts that "health and wellness is defined as the condition or degree of system stability" (p. 12). Disharmony among parts of the system is considered illness: "The wellness-illness continuum implies that energy flow is continuous between the client system and the environment" (Neuman, 1989, p. 33).

Nursing. Nursing is a "unique profession in that it is concerned with all of the variables affecting the individual's response to stress" (Neuman, 1982, p. 14). The major concern of nursing is in "keeping the client system stable through accuracy in both the assessment of effects and possible effects of environmental stressors and in assisting client adjustments required for an optimal wellness level" (Neuman, 1989, p. 34). Nursing goals are determined by "negotiation with the client for desired prescriptive changes to correct variances from wellness" (Neuman, 1989, p. 73). This means that nursing interventions designed to improve health are accepted and approved by the individual client during communication with the nurse before implementation.

Key Concepts. The nurse is concerned with all the following variables affecting an individual's response to stressors:
- *Stressors:* Tension-producing stimuli that may alter system stability (Neuman, 1995):
  - *Intrapersonal:* Internal stressors (e.g., autoimmune response).
  - *Interpersonal:* External environmental forces in close proximity (e.g., communication patterns).
  - *Extrapersonal:* External environmental forces at distant range (e.g., financial concerns).
- Concepts related to client system stability:
  - *Flexible line of defense:* Outer boundary that ideally prevents stressors from entering the system.
  - *Normal line of defense:* A range of responses to environmental stressors when the flexible line of defense is penetrated; usual state of wellness (Neuman, 1995).
  - *Lines of resistance:* Protect the basic structure of the client and become activated when the normal line of defense is invaded by environmental stressors.
- *Interventions:* Purposeful nursing actions that help clients to retain, attain, and/or maintain system stability. Three levels of intervention exist:
  - *Primary prevention:* Reduces the possibility of encounter with stressors and strengthens the flexible lines of defense.
  - *Secondary prevention:* Relates to appropriate prioritizing of interventions to reduce symptoms resulting from invasion of environmental stressors; protects the basic structure by strengthening the internal lines of resistance.

- *Tertiary prevention:* Focuses on readaptation and stability. A primary goal is to strengthen resistance to stressors by reeducation to help prevent recurrence of reaction or regression: "Tertiary prevention tends to lead back, in a circular fashion, toward primary prevention" (Neuman, 1989, p. 73).

Watson's Philosophy and Theory of Human Caring

Jean Watson's (1940–present) theoretical formulations focus on the philosophy and science of human caring as the core of nursing. With the aim of reducing the dichotomy between nursing theory and practice, Watson's original theory draws from multiple disciplines to derive a *carative factors framework (vs. curative factors)* that are central to nursing and describes concepts as they relate to the pivotal theme of caring: "Caring is acknowledged as the highest form of commitment to self, to others, to society, to environment, and, at this point in human history, even to the universe" (Watson, 1996, p. 146). The Watson Caring Science Institute (WCSI) is a private nonprofit international organization (https://www.watsoncaringscience.org/). In 2018, Watson explained on the WCSI website:

The caring model or theory can also be considered a philosophical and moral/ethical foundation for professional nursing and part of the central focus for nursing at the disciplinary level. A model of caring includes a call for both art and science; it offers a framework that embraces and intersects with art, science, humanities, spirituality, and new dimensions of mind-body-spirit medicine and nursing evolving openly as central to human phenomena of nursing practice (para. 2).

Brief Overview. Caring, which Watson sees as a moral ideal rather than a task-oriented behavior, is central to nursing practice and includes aspects of the actual caring occasion and the transpersonal caring relationship. An interpersonal process, caring results in the satisfaction of human needs. She recently noted that caring science is rapidly becoming an interdisciplinary or transdisciplinary field of study with relevance to all health, education, and human service fields and professions (Watson, 2018).

Assumptions About the Individual. Individuals (i.e., both the nurse and the client) are nonreducible and are interconnected with others and nature (Watson, 1985).

Environment. The client's environment contains both external and internal variables. The nurse promotes a caring environment, one that allows individuals to make choices relative to the best action for themselves at that point in time.

Health and Illness. Health is more than the absence of illness, but because it is subjective, it is an elusive concept: "Health refers to unity and harmony within the mind, body, and soul" (Watson, 1985, p. 48). Conversely, illness is disharmony within the spheres of the person.

Nursing. The practice of nursing is different from curing. From Watson's emerging perspective, she tried to make explicit nursing's values, knowledge, and practices of human caring that are geared toward subjective inner healing processes and the life world of the experiencing person, requiring unique caring healing arts and a framework called "carative factors," which complemented conventional medicine but stood in stark contrast to "curative factors."

Nursing is a transpersonal relationship that includes but is not limited to the 10 carative processes described in the following Key Concepts. The goal of nursing is to help persons attain a higher degree of harmony by offering a relationship that the client can use for personal growth and development.

Key Concepts. The caring relationship forms the core of nursing, and the caritas processes (evolved from the original carative factors) delineate the domain of nursing practice:

- *Transpersonal caring:* An intersubjective human-to-human relationship in which the nurse affects and is affected by the other person (client). Caring is the moral ideal of nursing in which the utmost concern for human dignity and preservation of humanity is present (Watson, 1985).
- *Caritas processes* (Watson Caring Science Institute, n.d.):
  - Sustaining humanistic-altruistic values by practice of loving-kindness, compassion, and equanimity with self/others.
  - Being authentically present, enabling faith/hope/belief system: Honoring subjective inner, life-world of self/others.
  - Being sensitive to self and others by cultivating own spiritual practices; beyond ego-self to transpersonal presence.
  - Developing and sustaining loving, trusting-caring relationships.
    - Allowing for expression of positive and negative feelings; authentically listening to another person's story.
    - Creatively problem-solving and "solution seeking" through caring process; full use of self and artistry of caring-healing practices via use of all ways of knowing/being/doing/becoming.
    - Engaging in transpersonal teaching and learning within context of caring relationship; staying

within other's framework of reference; shift toward coaching model for expanded health/wellness.

- Creating a healing environment at all levels; subtle environment for energetic authentic caring presence.
- Reverentially assisting with basic needs as sacred acts, touching mind-body-spirit of other; sustaining human dignity.
- Opening to spiritual, mystery, unknowns; allowing for miracles.

MIDRANGE THEORY

Peplau's Interpersonal Relational Theory

Hildegard Peplau (1909–1999) published *Interpersonal Relations in Nursing* in 1952, describing the phases of the interpersonal process in nursing, roles for nurses, and methods for studying nursing as an interpersonal process. Over the years the theory evolved, and in 1991 she published *Interpersonal Relations in Nursing: A Conceptual Framework of Reference for Psychodynamic Nursing* (Peplau, 1991).

Brief Overview. The focus of Peplau's model is the goal-directed interpersonal process: "Psychodynamic nursing is being able to understand one's own behavior to help others identify felt difficulties and to apply principles of human relations to the problems that arise at all levels of experience" (Peplau, 1952, p. xiii). The interpersonal relationship "has a starting point, proceeds through definable phases, and, being time-limited, has an end point" (Peplau, 1992, p. 4). Peplau believed that once the problem that prompts the client to ask for nursing help has been resolved, the relationship ends.

Assumptions About Human Beings. The individual is an organism that lives in an unstable equilibrium and "strives in its own way to reduce tension generated by needs" (Peplau, 1952, p. 82).

Environment. Although the environment is not explicitly defined, it can be inferred that the environment consists of "existing forces outside the organism and in the context of culture" (Peplau, 1952, p. 163).

Health and Illness. *Health* is a "word symbol that implies forward movement of personality and other ongoing human processes in the direction of creative, constructive, productive, personal, and community living" (Peplau, 1952, p. 12). By implication, illness is a condition that is marked by no movement or by backward movement in these human processes.

Nursing. Nursing is a therapeutic interpersonal process because it involves the interaction between two or more individuals who have a common goal. For individuals who are sick and in need of health care, it is a healing art. Six nursing roles emerge in the various phases of the nurse-patient relationship: stranger, resource person, teacher, leader, surrogate, and counselor.

Key Concepts. The nurse-patient relationship consists of four phases:
- *Orientation:* The patient seeks professional assistance with a problem. The nurse and patient meet as strangers and recognize, clarify, and define the existing problem.
- *Identification:* The patient learns how to make use of the nurse-patient relationship and responds selectively to people who can meet his or her needs; the patient and nurse clarify each other's expectations.
- *Exploitation:* The patient takes advantage of all available services. The nurse helps the patient in maintaining a balance between dependence and independence and using the services to help solve the current problem and work toward optimal health.
- *Resolution:* The patient is free to move on with his or her life as old goals are put aside and new goals are adopted. The patient becomes independent of the nurse, and the relationship is terminated.

King's Theory of Goal Attainment

Although the foundation for Imogene King's (1923–2007) theory was developed in 1964, she did not present her entire conceptual framework until the 1971 publication of her book *Toward a Theory for Nursing*. In it she identified the concepts of social systems, health, perception, and interpersonal relations. The midrange theory of goal attainment was refined in *A Theory for Nursing: Systems, Concepts, Process* (King, 1981), in which King asserted that nursing is focused on people interacting with their environments. The goal of this interaction is a state of health, which King defines as the ability of people to function in their roles. The theory is derived from a systems framework and is concerned with human transactions in different types of environments (King, 1995a).

Brief Overview. The individual is viewed as an open system and as one component of a nurse-client interpersonal system whose interactions lead to the attainment of mutually agreed-upon goals.

Assumptions About Human Beings. Human beings are open systems in transaction with the environment and are conceptualized as social, sentient, rational, perceiving, controlling, purposeful, action-oriented beings.

Environment. The theory implies that the open systems of the individual and the environment interact and that both the internal and external environments generate stressors.

Health and Illness. Health is described as an individual's ability to function in social roles. This implies optimal use of a person's resources to achieve continuous adjustment to internal and external environmental stressors. Illness is a deviation from normal, an imbalance in a person's biological structure, psychological makeup, or social relationships.

Nursing. In an interpersonal process of action, reaction, and interaction, the nurse and client communicate, set goals, and explore means to achieve those goals. According to King (1981), "the domain of nursing includes promoting, maintaining and restoring health, caring for the sick and injured and caring for the dying" (p. 4). Nursing's central goal is to help individuals maintain their health so they can function in their roles. As King asserted, "The goal of the nursing system, as a whole, is health for individuals, health for groups, such as the family, and health for communities within a society" (King, 1995b, p. 24).

Key Concepts. Two sets of concepts are included in the theory, one relating to the parties involved in the nurse-client relationship and the other pertaining to the process of goal attainment, as follows:
- Concepts related to the nurse-client relationship:
  - *Personal system:* An individual.
  - *Interpersonal system:* Two or more interacting individuals.
  - *Social system:* Communities and societies.
- Concepts related to goal attainment:
  - *Communication:* The process of giving information from one person to another.
  - *Interaction:* The process of perception between the person and environment or one or more persons, represented by verbal and nonverbal behaviors that are goal directed.
  - *Perception:* An individual's representation of reality.
  - *Transaction:* Identification of mutual goals valued by persons interacting with each other.
  - *Role:* A set of behaviors displayed by the individual, who occupies a given position in a social system.
  - *Stress:* A dynamic state of interaction with the environment to maintain balance for growth, development, and performance.
  - *Growth and development:* According to King (1981), these are "continuous changes in individuals occurring at molecular, cellular, and behavioral levels" (p. 148).

- *Time:* A duration between one event and another.
- *Space:* Defined by "gestures, postures, and visible boundaries erected to mark off personal space" (King, 1981, p. 148).

Leininger's Cultural Care Diversity and Universality Theory (a.k.a. Transcultural Nursing)

Drawing from a background in cultural and social anthropology, Madeleine Leininger's contribution to nursing knowledge is related to transcultural nursing and caring. Her book *Transcultural Nursing: Concepts, Theories, and Practice* (Leininger, 1978) presented her conceptual framework for cultural care and health. She explicated the linkages between nursing and anthropology as she identified and defined concepts such as care, caring, culture, cultural values, and cultural variations.

Brief Overview. Transcultural nursing focuses on a comparative study and analysis of different cultures and subcultures in the world regarding their caring behavior, nursing care, health-illness values, and patterns of behavior, with the goal of developing a scientific and humanistic body of knowledge from which to derive culture-specific and culture-universal nursing care practices (Leininger, 1978).

Assumptions About Human Beings. Clients are caring and cultural beings who perceive health, illness, caring, curing, dependence, and independence differently. The social structure, worldview, and values of people vary transculturally.

Environment. The environment is a social structure, the "interrelated and interdependent systems of a society which determine how it functions with respect to certain major elements, namely: the political (including legal), economic, social (including kinship), educational, technical, religious, and cultural systems" (Leininger, 1978, p. 61). The environment is the totality of an event, situation, or particular experience that gives meaning to human expression and interaction.

Health and Illness. Perceptions of health and illness are culturally infused and therefore cannot be universally defined: "Health refers to a state of well-being that is culturally defined, valued, and practiced, and which reflects the ability of individuals (or groups) to perform their daily role activities in culturally expressed, beneficial, and patterned lifeways" (Leininger, 1991, p. 48). Worldviews, social structure, and cultural beliefs influence perceptions of health and illness and cannot be separated from them. For example, some cultures perceive illness to be largely a personal and internal body experience, whereas others view illness as an extrapersonal or cultural experience. Another example is that many clients of Asian descent believe that health is a personal responsibility, a result of the individual maintaining balance. In Western society, health may be defined by the medical profession.

Nursing. Nursing is a learned humanistic and scientific profession that focuses on personalized (individual and group) care behaviors, functions, and processes that have physical, psychocultural, and social significance or meaning. The goal of nursing is to assist, support, facilitate, or enable individuals or groups to regain or maintain their health in a way that is culturally congruent or to help people face handicaps or death (Leininger, 1991).

Key Concepts. Among the core concepts of transcultural nursing theory are the following:
- *Care:* Phenomena related to assistive, supportive, or enabling behavior toward or for another individual with evident or anticipated needs to ease or improve a human condition.
- *Caring:* Actions directed toward assisting, supporting, or enabling an individual (or group) to ameliorate or improve the human condition or "lifeway" (Leininger, 1991, p. 48).
- *Culture:* Values, beliefs, norms, and lifeway practices of a particular group that guides thinking, decisions, and actions in patterned ways.
- *Cultural care:* The cognitively known values, beliefs, and patterned lifeways that assist, support, or enable another individual or group to maintain well-being; improve a human condition or lifeway; or deal with illness, handicaps, or death.
  - *Cultural care diversity:* The variability of meaning, patterns, values, lifeways, or symbols of care that are culturally derived for health or to improve a human condition.
  - *Cultural care universality:* Common, similar, or uniform care meanings, patterns, values, lifeways, or symbols that are culturally derived for health or to improve a human condition.
  - *Cultural-congruent care:* Assistive, supportive, facilitative, or enabling acts or decisions that fit individual, group, or institutional cultural values, beliefs, and lifeways (Leininger, 1995).
  - *Care preservation or maintenance:* Professional actions and decisions that help people of a particular culture to retain and preserve relevant care values.
  - *Cultural care accommodation or negotiation:* Professional actions and decisions that help people of a

designated culture adapt to or negotiate with others for a beneficial or satisfying health outcome.
- *Cultural care repatterning or restructuring:* Professional actions and decisions that help a client change or modify his or her lifeway to improve health while still respecting the client's cultural values and beliefs.

APPLICATION TO NURSING PRACTICE

The nursing theories and frameworks discussed here offer a variety of perspectives for application to clinical practice. For example, some are process oriented and dynamic, such as Peplau's interpersonal process, King's theory of goal attainment, and Rogers' SUHB. Others are more outcome oriented, such as Roy's adaptation model and Orem's self-care deficit theory. The models of Rogers and Neuman focus on the wholeness of the individual and conceptualize nursing as one component of the individual's life process. King's theory is directed toward the interaction between the nurse and the client, who are inseparable (meaning that the roles are interdependent and undividable). Nightingale and Leininger developed humanistic perspectives, focusing on personalized, individualized care for all, and Roy conceptualizes the nurse as an external regulator whose function is to promote system balance or adaptation. Orem views the nurse as a person who assists the individual with self-care practices when the individual is unable to effectively care for himself or herself. A comparison of the theoretical perspectives discussed in this chapter is presented in Table 5.1.

Many (if not all) of the nursing theories and frameworks presented in this chapter are too broad and abstract to be used in their entirety in any one nursing care situation. For example, Orem describes three types of nursing systems, but for a client who is in the intensive care unit and on life support, only the wholly compensatory nursing system is relevant. Similarly, with Neuman's three levels of prevention, only clients with symptoms resulting from invasion of environmental stressors are appropriate recipients of secondary prevention. Despite these limitations, the theories can guide nursing assessment in terms of what questions to ask and what areas to assess. The type of client, the setting in which care is delivered, and the goal of nursing are what influence the selection of an appropriate theoretical framework for practice. The more specific theories can be readily adapted for use in a practice setting. The more global theories may better serve as frameworks for research, the findings of which can then be applied to practice.

Practice theories, or micro-level theories, may best serve in the development of evidence-based nursing practice (EBP) by providing valid and reliable substantiation of clinical guidelines. Furthermore, use of specific theories to

TABLE 5.1 Comparison of Theoretical Perspectives

Theory/Model	Nursing	Environment	Health	Human Being(s)
Nightingale's environmental theory	Intended to relieve pain and suffering and restore health by manipulating the environment	Conditions external to the person that affect both sick and well persons	State of well-being; using an individual's power to the fullest	An individual who is in control of his or her own life and health and desires good health
Peplau's interpersonal process	Therapeutic interpersonal process	Existing forces outside the organism	Forward movement of ongoing human processes and personality	An organism that lives in an unstable equilibrium and strives to reduce tension generated by needs
Rogers' science of unitary human beings	Science and art; the art of nursing is the creative use of science for human betterment	Pandimensional energy field integral with the human energy field	Patterns of living in harmony with the environment	A unified irreducible whole; more than and different from the sum of parts
Orem's self-care deficit theory	Involves assisting individuals with self-care practices	Linked to the individual, forming an integrated system	State in which human beings are structurally and functionally whole	A unity who functions biologically, symbolically, and socially and whose functioning is linked to the environment
King's theory of goal attainment	Process of action, reaction, and interaction	Interactive with the individual	Ability to function in social roles	An open system in transaction with the environment who is social, sentient, rational, perceiving, controlling, purposeful, and action oriented
Roy's adaptation model	An external regulatory force that modifies stimuli affecting adaptation	Internal and external conditions that surround and affect individuals	State and process of being and becoming an integrated and whole person	A biopsychosocial adaptive system that is in constant interaction with a changing environment
Neuman's systems model	Concerned with variables affecting the individual's response to stress	Internal and external factors affecting and affected by the individual	Optimal system stability	A whole person; a dynamic composite of physiological, psychological, sociocultural, developmental, and spiritual variables
Leininger's cultural care theory	Culturally congruent care behaviors, functions, and processes that have physical, psychocultural, or social significance	The interrelated, interdependent systems of a society	State of well-being that is culturally defined	Caring, cultural beings who perceive health, illness, caring, curing, dependence, and independence differently
Watson's philosophy and science of caring	Transpersonal caring relationship that includes use of 10 caritas processes	Internal and external variables	Unity and harmony within mind, body, and soul	An entity that is nonreducible and is interconnected with others and nature

guide nursing practice facilitates the development of core competencies identified by the Institute of Medicine (2003) as necessary in the provision of quality care by interdisciplinary teams working to ensure patient safety. Chapter 4 provides further content on EBP.

Evaluating the Utility of Nursing Theories: Research Utilization

Not all theories and frameworks are equally comprehensive or equally useful in every situation, and they are not meant to be. The definition of the client and the setting in which care is delivered limit the usefulness of some of the theories and frameworks presented. To be useful in practice, a theory must work in a specific setting: "A nursing theory should *structure* the work, giving the practicing nurse a *frame of reference* (lens) from which to view patients and from which to *make patient care decisions* (emphasis added)" (Barnum, 1998, p. 80). Its concepts must be *operationalized* in ways that promote application of and facilitate nursing activities in that setting. Examination of a theory's usefulness for its intended purpose and the consistency of its internal structure is important. The value and logical structure of a theory can be evaluated by asking questions proposed by Fawcett and DeSanto-Madeya (2013) and Barnum (1998), such as the following:

1. Are the assumptions inherent in the theory clearly stated?
2. Does the model provide adequate descriptions of all four concepts (human beings, environment, health, nursing) of nursing's *metaparadigm* (i.e., multiple philosophical and theoretical frameworks of a scientific school or discipline that support practice, such as nursing practice)?
3. Are the relationships among the concepts of nursing's metaparadigm clearly explained?
4. Is the theory stated clearly and concisely?
5. Does the structure of the theory contain conflicting views?
6. Can relationships between concepts be tested in research (i.e., observed and measured) and applied to practice?
7. Does the theory lead to nursing activities that meet societal expectations (social congruence)?
8. Does the theory lead to nursing activities that are likely to result in favorable client outcomes (social significance)?
9. Does the theory include explicit rules for use in practice, education, or research (social usefulness)?

Polit and Beck (2021) define *research utilization* as the *use* of findings from a study in a practical situation, translating new knowledge into real-world applications. This is different than the broader concept of EBP, which *integrates* research finding (evidence) with other factors (patient values and preferences; clinical expertise; and experiential evidence). *Knowledge translation* (KT) is the term associated with efforts to enhance systematic change in clinical practice (Polit & Beck, 2021). *Translational research* emerged as a discipline devoted to KT and the use of evidence; and study of interventions (practice inquiry), implementation processes (implementation science), and contextual factors that affect uptake of new practices (change theory) in health care. In nursing, this gave rise to the development of the Doctor of Nursing Practice degree. Theories, especially midrange theories, can support continuous quality improvement (CQI) initiatives in health care delivery systems.

The term *nursology* has emerged to capture the crucial role of *nursologists* (a.k.a. nurses) in recent decades to describe nursing's discipline-specific knowledge and is promoted by Jacqueline Fawcett, a nursing theorist (Fawcett, 2021a, 2021b) and her colleagues, stating nurses must know and use the knowledge developed by other nursologists. If we continue to "borrow" knowledge from other disciplines, identifying the rationale for doing so and placing that use within the context of nursing are critical to the future of nursing profession. Fawcett prefers to call practice multidisciplinary instead of interprofessional practice to make a distinction of the various disciplinary perspectives to improve health care outcomes. Interprofessional practice removes the professional boundaries from each discipline which impedes the identification of the "value" each discipline brings to improving health outcomes.

Theories From Related Disciplines

Many nursing theories *derived* their conceptual basis from theories and frameworks developed by scholars from related disciplines and adapted to specific situations. Many of these theories are useful and relevant to nursing in their original form. A brief synopsis of selected theories from related disciplines follows.

One of the theories with wide applicability, *general system theory*, proposes that a system is a set of interrelated parts or subsystems that are in constant interaction with the environment working together toward a common goal (Von Bertalanffy, 1968). Systems take in matter, information, and energy from the environment (input), process it (throughput), and release it back to the environment (output). Some of the output returns to the system as feedback in an attempt to return the system to a steady state (equilibrium) or, in the case of living systems, a condition of balance within the range of normal (homeostasis). A system is more than and different from the sum of its parts and, over time, becomes increasingly complex. The nurse who uses systems theory as the foundation to assess the individual, family, or community as an aggregate, simultaneously considers the relationships among the subsystems, and keeps in mind that a change in one part of the system changes the system as a whole.

Theories of change have been proposed by Lewin (1951) and expanded by Lippitt (1973) that view change as a goal-directed process. Lewin's theory includes three concepts: *force field* (driving and restraining forces for or against change), *motivators* (stimuli indicating the need for change), and *stages of change* (unfreezing, moving, refreezing). Lippitt focuses on the activities of the change agent to bring about the change. These theories provide the foundation for a systematic method of *planning, implementing,* and *evaluating* change in individuals, organizations, and social systems.

Among the several *theories of coping* is one developed by Lazarus (1976) that views coping as a process that leads to adaptation. The major concepts in Lazarus' theory are stress caused by a lack of resources to cope with an environmental event, cognitive appraisal of the stressor to determine the *perceived level of threat*, and *problem-focused coping* (management of the stressor) or *emotional-focused coping* (management of the response) (Lazarus & Folkman, 1984). For clients experiencing an intense level of stress, nursing interventions can use this theory as a foundation designed to alter the perception of the threat level and promote and support the coping process can be derived from the relationships specified by this theory.

Aguilera (1998) provides a theory and framework for successful resolution of a *crisis situation*. She identifies three balancing factors (the perception of the event, the availability of situational supports, and usual coping mechanisms) that prevent an adverse reaction to a stressful situation. When a crisis or psychological disequilibrium occurs, the nurse can use this theory as a foundation to assess the balancing factors to establish a nursing diagnosis. Nursing interventions can then be designed to facilitate the return to equilibrium by assisting the client to establish a realistic perception of the event, providing situational supports, and identifying coping mechanisms.

Both coping and adjustment are embedded in Duvall's (1977) *stages of family life and developmental tasks*, which can serve as the framework for delivering age-specific or situation-specific nursing interventions to the family. Developmental stages encompass three major concepts: *sequential developmental stages, developmental conflicts,* and *identity formation*. Developmental tasks are associated with each stage, and a developmental conflict occurs if the tasks cannot be successfully accomplished. Identity formation is viewed as an ongoing process throughout the life span. Erikson's theory is useful as a framework for assessing an *individual's psychosocial development* and intervening when developmental conflicts are identified (Erikson, 1963, 1982).

Selye's *general adaptation syndrome*, a theory of adaptation to stress, describes three phases of reaction to stress: *stage of alarm*, or immediate reaction to the stressor; *stage of resistance*, or adaptation to the stressor over time; and *stage of exhaustion*, or inability to adapt to the stressor (Selye, 1974). This theory can be applied to clients who are suffering not only psychological or social stress but physiological stress as well.

Maslow's theory of the *hierarchy of needs* is illustrated as a pyramid containing five broad layers of needs on which human functioning is based. The bottom or first-level needs are physiological, followed by safety and security, love and belonging, self-esteem, and self-actualization (Maslow, 1970). The theory contends that basic needs, such as air, water, food, and safety, must be met before meeting higher-level needs such as self-esteem or self-actualization. The application of this theory to nursing practice can provide a framework for client assessment and assist in identifying nursing care priorities.

These theories are only a sample of those developed by related disciplines that have uses in nursing. Indeed, with the drive toward teamwork and collaboration in health care, these theories are relevant to all disciplines. However, as noted before, nurses should explain the use of theories from other disciplines with the context of nursing care when applying these theories, to frame the nursing application of the concepts with nursing practice.

Others, such as Rotter's (1954) locus of control and Bandura's self-efficacy theory (1986), can be found in various chapters in this text. One or more of these theories can serve as a framework for designing interventions for clients throughout the life cycle, developing and implementing research studies, and framing educational curricula. In combination with nursing theories, a wide array of theoretical perspectives in various stages of development is available from which to choose.

SUMMARY

Nursing is a knowledge-based discipline that is significantly different from medicine and focused on the wholeness of human beings. Nursing knowledge is the organization of discipline-specific concepts, theories, and ideas published in both print and electronic media and demonstrated in professional practice. Theories and frameworks provide direction and guidance for structuring professional nursing practice, education, administration, and research.

They provide a way to educate nurses; describe, explain, predict, organize, assess, diagnose, intervene, evaluate nursing practice, and deliver nursing care; and question, study, and interpret research. This chapter provides a historical perspective and a comprehensive overview of some of the many nursing theorists who have made substantial contributions to the development of a body of nursing knowledge. The remainder of this text will introduce additional nursing theories that also contribute to the body of nursing knowledge.

SALIENT POINTS

- A theory is a group of statements that describe the relationship between two or more concepts.
- The main components of nursing theories are person, environment, health/illness, and nursing (nursing's metaparadigm).
- Nightingale's theory focuses on nursing's role in manipulating the environment.
- Peplau's theory centers on the interpersonal process in nursing.
- According to Rogers, the nurse seeks to promote coherence between individuals and their environments.
- As specified by Orem, when a client has a deficit in his or her ability for self-care, the nurse assists the individual with self-care practices.
- King conceptualizes the nurse and the client as components of an interpersonal system who seek to attain mutually agreed-upon goals.
- Roy's theory describes the client as a biopsychosocial adaptive system and the nurse as one who modifies stimuli to promote adaptation.
- Three levels of nursing intervention—primary, secondary, and tertiary prevention—are specified in Neuman's systems model.
- Leininger's theory centers on providing culturally congruent nursing care.
- Watson identifies the caring relationship and *caritas* processes that form the core of nursing.
- The more specific theories, in whole or in part, can be readily adapted for use in any practice setting.
- The more global theories may better serve as frameworks for research, the findings of which can then be applied to practice.
- Theories from related disciplines also have relevance to nursing practice, education, and research.
- All theories have the potential to make substantial contributions to the nursing profession by enhancing the development of a unique body of nursing knowledge.

CRITICAL REFLECTION EXERCISES

1. What is your personal philosophy of nursing? Which of the theoretical perspectives of nursing presented in this chapter is most closely aligned with your philosophy of nursing? Reflect on your most recent patient encounter, and discuss how the chosen theory would guide your care of the patient.
2. How do Florence Nightingale's ideas apply to nursing practice in the current culture of patient safety and quality?
3. Identify the nursing theory or model that would be most useful to you in your practice, and explain why.
4. Compare the definitions of health and illness in two nursing theories, citing similarities and differences. Which one is the most reflective of your own definitions of health and illness? Why?
5. Defend or refute the following statement: "We should have only one nursing theory, rather than several, to guide education, practice, and research."

REFERENCES

Aguilera, D. C. (1998). *Crisis intervention: Theory and methodology* (8th ed.). Mosby.
Bandura, A. (1986). *Social foundations of thought and action: A social cognitive theory*. Prentice Hall.
Barnum, A. (1998). *Nursing theory analysis, application, evaluation*. Lippincott.
Bender, M. (2018). Models versus theories as a primary carrier of nursing knowledge: A philosophical argument. *Nursing Philosophy: An International Journal for Healthcare Professionals, 19*(1). https://doi.org/10.1111/nup.12198
Duvall, E. M. (1977). *Marriage and family development* (5th ed.). Lippincott.
Erikson, E. H. (1963). *Childhood and society* (2nd ed.). Norton.
Erikson, E. H. (1982). *The life cycle completed: A review*. Norton.
Fawcett, J. (1993). *Analysis and evaluation of nursing theories*. Davis.
Fawcett, J. (2021a). Thoughts about models of nursing practice delivery. *Nursing Science Quarterly, 34*(3), 328–330. https://doi.org/10.1177/08943184211010460

Fawcett, J. (2021b). More thoughts about models of nursing practice delivery. *Nursing Science Quarterly, 34*(4), 458–461. https://doi.org/10.1177/08943184211031584

Fawcett, J., & DeSanto-Madeya, S. (2013). *Contemporary nursing knowledge: Analysis and evaluation of nursing models and theories* (2nd ed.). Davis.

Institute of Medicine (IOM). (2003). *Health professions education: A bridge to quality.* The National Academies Press. https://doi.org/10.17226/10681

King, I. M. (1981). *A theory for nursing: Systems, concepts, process.* Wiley.

King, I. M. (1995a). A systems framework for nursing. In M. A. Frey & C. L. Sieloff (Eds.), *Advancing King's systems framework and theory of nursing.* Sage.

King, I. M. (1995b). The theory of goal attainment. In M. A. Frey & C. L. Sieloff (Eds.), *Advancing King's systems framework and theory of nursing.* Sage.

Lazarus, R. S. (1976). *Patterns of adjustment* (3rd ed.). McGraw-Hill.

Lazarus, R. S., & Folkman, S. (1984). *Stress appraisal and coping.* Springer.

Leininger, M. (1978). *Transcultural nursing: Concepts, theories, and practice.* Wiley.

Leininger, M. (1991). *Culture care diversity and universality: A theory of nursing.* National League for Nursing.

Leininger, M. (1995). *Transcultural nursing: Concepts, theories, research, and practice.* McGraw-Hill.

Levine, M. E. (1995). The rhetoric of nursing theory. *Image Journal of Nursing Scholarship, 27,* 11–14. https://doi.org/10.1111/j.1547-5069.1995.tb00807.x

Lewin, K. (1951). Defining the field at a given time. In D. Cartwright (Ed.), *Field theory in social science: Selected papers by Kurt Lewin.* Harper and Brothers.

Liehr, P., & Smith, M. J. (2017). Middle range theory: A perspective on development and use. *Advances in Nursing Science, 40*(1), 51–63. https://doi.org/10.1097/ANS.0000000000000162

Lippitt, G. L. (1973). *Visualizing change.* University Associates.

Maslow, A. (1970). *Motivation and personality* (2nd ed.). Harper & Row.

Merriam-Webster. (n.d.). *Merriam-Webster.com dictionary.* May 31, 2022. https://www.merriam-webster.com/dictionary/knowledge

Neuman, B. (1982). *The Neuman systems model: Application to nursing theory and practice.* Appleton-Century-Crofts.

Neuman, B. (1989). *The Neuman systems model* (2nd ed.). Appleton-Century-Crofts.

Neuman, B. (1995). *The Neuman systems model* (3rd ed.). Appleton-Century-Crofts.

Neuman, B. M., & Young, R. J. (1972). A model for teaching total person approach to patient problems. *Nursing Research, 21*(3), 264–269. https://doi.org/10.1097/00006199-197205000-00015

Nightingale, F. (1860/1946). *Notes on nursing: What it is and what it is not.* Appleton Century.

Orem, D. E. (1980). *Nursing: Concepts of practice* (2nd ed.). McGraw-Hill.

Orem, D. E. (1985). *Nursing: Concepts of practice* (3rd ed.). McGraw-Hill.

Orem, D. E. (1991). *Nursing: Concepts of practice* (4th ed.). Mosby.

Orem, D. E. (1995). *Nursing: Concepts of practice* (5th ed.). Mosby.

Orem, D. E. (2001). *Nursing: Concepts of practice* (6th ed.). Mosby.

Peplau, H. (1952). *Interpersonal relations in nursing: A conceptual framework of reference for psychodynamic nursing.* Putnam.

Peplau, H. (1991). *Interpersonal relations in nursing: A conceptual framework of reference for psychodynamic nursing.* Springer.

Peplau, H. (1992). Interpersonal relations: A theoretical framework for application in nursing practice. *Nursing Science Quarterly, 5,* 13–18. https://doi.org/10.1177%2F089431849200500106

Phillips, J. R. (2016). *Rogers' science of unitary human beings: Beyond the Frontier of Science. Nursing Science Quarterly, 29*(1), 38–46. https://doi.org/10.1177/0894318415615112

Polit, D., & Beck, C. (2021). *Nursing research: Generating and assessing evidence for nursing practice* (11th ed.). Wolters-Kluwer.

Rogers, M. E. (1970). *An introduction to the theoretical basis of nursing.* Davis.

Rogers, M. E. (1989). Nursing: A science of unitary man. In J. P. Riehl-Sisca (Ed.), *Conceptual models for nursing practice* (2nd ed.). Appleton & Lange.

Rogers, M. E. (1990). Nursing science of unitary, irreducible, human beings: Update 1990. In E. A. Barrett (Ed.), *Visions of Rogers' science-based nursing.* National League for Nursing.

Rogers, M. E. (1994). Nursing science evolves. In M. A. Madrid & E. A. Barrett (Eds.), *Rogers' scientific art of nursing practice.* National League for Nursing.

Rotter, J. B. (1954). *Social learning and clinical psychology.* Prentice Hall.

Roy, C. (1984). *Introduction to nursing: An adaptation model* (2nd ed.). Prentice Hall.

Roy, C. (1989). The Roy adaptation model. In J. P. Riehl-Sisca (Ed.), *Conceptual models for nursing practice* (2nd ed.). Appleton & Lange.

Roy, C. (2009). *The Roy adaptation model* (3rd ed.). Prentice Hall.

Roy, C., & Andrews, H. A. (1999). *The Roy adaptation model* (2nd ed.). Prentice Hall.

Selye, H. (1974). *Stress without distress.* Lippincott.

Von Bertalanffy, L. (1968). *General system theory.* Braziller.

Watson, J. (1985). *Nursing: Human science and health care.* Appleton-Century-Croft.

Watson, J. (1996). Watson's theory of transpersonal caring. In P. Hinton Walker & B. Neuman (Eds.), *Blueprint for use of nursing models.* National League for Nursing.

Watson, J. (2018). *Unitary caring science: Philosophy and praxis of nursing.* University Press of Colorado.

Watson Caring Science Institute (WCSI). (n.d.). *Ten carative processes.* May 31, 2022. https://www.watsoncaringscience.org/jean-bio/caring-science-theory/10-caritas-processes/

Yancey, N. R. (2015). Why teach nursing theory? *Nursing Science Quarterly, 28*(4), 274–278. https://doi.org/10.1177%2F0894318415599234

Health Policy and Planning and the Nursing Practice Environment

Debra C. Wallace, PhD, RN, FAAN

ⓔ http://evolve.elsevier.com/Friberg/bridge/

OBJECTIVES

At the completion of this chapter, the reader will be able to:

- Identify selected factors affecting health policy and nursing.
- Describe the processes for developing, implementing, and evaluating policy.
- Discuss selected health programs mandated by federal health policy and how these impact health equity.

- Evaluate health policies for their effect on nursing practice, education, research, quality of care, and the practice environment.
- Discuss strategies for nurse participation in health policy.

INTRODUCTION

The news and media are filled with hot topics related to health care that is influenced by health policy, be it abortion provision, veterans waiting months for clinic visits, how persons survive trauma, medication costs, and more recently, COVID-19 health care. Health policy affects nursing at all levels of preparation, in all settings and specialties, and across all client and population groups. Often, policy decisions, allocations, and regulations dictate where care is delivered, to whom care is delivered, what type of care is delivered, who delivers care, how care is delivered, who pays for care, and what is expected from the care provided. Additionally, practice environment, workplace safety, licensure, certification, accreditation, and educational funding are influenced by health policy and related regulations. Thus, it is important for each nurse to have a working knowledge of health policy, to understand how members of the largest and most trusted health care profession can use and influence policy to improve the health and well-being of society.

Before the 20th century, health care was typically an individual or private sector responsibility in most countries. Many health care facilities were affiliated with religious and civic organizations and groups or educational institutions. Physicians had private office practices with direct fee for service and out-of-pocket payments. The federal government in the United States became involved in the regulation, provision, and financing of health care primarily during the early 1900s. Government involvement, scientific developments, technology, social pressure, and increased costs associated with health care have resulted in the development of a health care industry that exceeds the revenues of manufacturing and agriculture industries. The health care industry is often divided into subsystems that serve populations based on payment decisions and condition specialties.

In industrialized countries in many parts of the world, such as the United Kingdom and Canada, centralized systems of care have been developed through socialized medicine models. In these countries, the infrastructure controls the number and location of health care delivery sites and the training, distribution, and reimbursement of both physician and nurse providers. The nursing practice environment is hospital and community-based and is regulated by the types of services offered, payment decisions, and access points. Regardless of the nation, multiple factors affect the development, implementation, and evaluation of health policy, as well as its influence on nursing and health care. Chapter 1 discusses the effect of these health industry shifts on the profession of nursing.

POLITICS

One of the major factors influencing health policy is politics. Individuals, organizations, agencies, state, and federal processes are involved in developing health policy, the regulations for implementation, and the evaluation of outcomes. For example, a citizen writes a member of Congress and argues that certain needs are not being met for technology-dependent or asthmatic children. An organization such as the American Nurses Association (ANA) may be involved by writing, visiting, and lobbying state and congressional representatives for new and continuing needs of nurses and patients. The need for educational and program grants in the Nurse Reinvestment Act is one example of a law that was passed to support nurses. Federal agencies such as the National Institutes of Health (NIH), the U.S. Food and Drug Administration (FDA), and the Health Resources and Services Administration (HRSA) invite members of Congress to attend administrative hearings and provide input on priority setting, program development, budgetary needs, and evaluation reports. For example, the Veterans Administration (VA) sought additional funding for care and research to improve care, resulting in the Department of Veterans Affairs (DVA) Expiring Authorities Act of 2013, which extended veterans' services to veterans hospitals and clinics, including homeless and disabled veterans, and the Veterans Health Care Choice Improvements Act of 2015 (PL 114-41) which provided for non-VA medical facilities to provide primary care and dialysis, and clarified contract status, funding levels, and required distance from veteran's home to VA facilities.

In addition, political leaders and legislators bring health-related agendas to congressional committees based on their constituents' values, social urgency, and priorities of their own.

Organizations

Nurses are members of many organizations involved in and influencing the development of health policy and health care–related legislation. Nonlegislative citizens also play a political role in health policy development and implementation through participation in and support of civic organizations and activities, such as the American Association of Retired Persons (AARP), Mothers Against Drunk Driving (MADD), American Diabetes Association (ADA),

the March of Dimes, the National Organization of Women (NOW), and the National Rifle Association (NRA). Most professional organizations (e.g., American Medical Association [AMA], American Hospital Association [AHA], American Academy of Nursing [AAN], Coalition for Patients' Rights [CPR]) develop legislative agendas, support political candidates, and employ lobbyists at state and federal levels. The ANA headquarters is in Washington, DC, and allows visibility and access to federal agencies and Congress. State nursing associations often have lobbyists to ensure state laws for advanced practice licensure, Medicaid benefits and coverage, and work environment protections. Lay, civic, and professional organizations, whether associated or not with a political party—such as the AARP, the National Association for the Advancement of Colored People (NAACP), the NRA, the ANA, the National Home Care Association (NHCA), and America's Health Insurance Plans (AHIP)—use grassroots activity, paid lobbyists, campaign support, advertisements, and organized rallies to make an effect on health policies affecting their members and special interest groups. Most health care professional organizations, including the ANA, have a paid lobbyist in each state capital and at least one in Washington, DC. Because these organizations fund political and lobbying activity, a proportion of membership dues to these organizations are not tax-deductible. For example, the ANA uses approximately 25% of its dues for lobbying activities and has a full-time lobbyist in Washington, DC. Many state nursing associations and specialty organizations have their own lobbyist or contract for this work in their state legislature.

Political Parties

Three major political parties are involved in most legislation: the Republican National Committee (RNC), the Democratic National Committee (DNC), and the Independent Reform Party (IRP). More recently, the Libertarian Party (LP) and Green Party (GP) have become more involved and had candidates on presidential and governorship ballots. Political parties set forth the major issues of concern through party platforms during presidential conventions, website postings, and paid media advertisements. The party platforms consist of "planks" that delineate the party's philosophy and stand on issues of the day. Platforms are a consensus of the convention delegates, but they also mirror the presidential candidate's stand and arguments to be used during the campaign. Platform issues, then, often become the agendas of state legislatures and the U.S. Congress. Major issues during the 20th century were health-related, such as gun control, abortion, and Medicare. In the early part of the 21st century, issues surrounding stem cell research and genetics, prescription drug coverage, bioterrorism, universal health coverage, and electronic health records have emerged. The most recent platforms and priority issues can be reviewed on party websites or received from each party's national or state offices. The ANA traditionally has supported more of the Democratic Party's health issue planks.

Political Action and 527 Committees

In addition to the traditional parties, registered *political action committees* (PACs) have been established independently or as a part of a formal organization to (1) raise, spend, and contribute money; (2) assist with campaigns; and (3) lobby on behalf of special interest groups, industries, or segments of society. PACs initiate and influence much of the legislative activity or inactivity on both the state and federal levels. PACs pay for television advertisements, hold public rallies and demonstrations, distribute literature, and invite political and other famous figures to events supporting their positions. Originally PACs represented persons with specific needs who had been overlooked or not protected by society (e.g., those with AIDS, older adults, the homeless, and poor children). Now, PACs have become more commonly representative of particular groups of persons who banded political, human, and financial resources to ensure policies are initiated, funded, extended, or terminated for social and corporate agendas. For example, the ANA has a PAC to address issues related to the health and nursing workforce, including staffing, mandatory overtime, supervision, delegation, and expanded roles. The pharmaceutical industry has multiple PACs to lobby Congress to reduce regulation for drug approvals and to defeat efforts for Medicare fixed price negotiation for medications. The effect of PACs on legislation in the past four presidential elections has been highlighted by the financial support for and against politicians who have voted or will vote on bills relating to an issue. These activities make PACs some of the most powerful entities influencing health policy decisions, especially those related to regulation and allocation of funds. The large amount of funding used for and against campaigns has changed how legislation is formed, what is passed, and the amount and type of appropriations approved. Legislators are finding it more difficult to meet the needs of one special interest group and not offend another group. For example, when political power shifts in state and federal legislatures, the influence of PACs changes. The passage or failure of bills to protect the environment, reauthorize labor unions and workers' rights and safety, change gun control, revise tort reform, cut or raise taxes, or increase the minimum wage may depend on which party is in power. Remaining loyal and supportive of campaign funding sources is important for reelection. The effect is that senators and congressmen

(or state legislators) pass a higher number of bills that require additional federal monies or require states to increase dollars allocated to priority programs or allow elected officials to vote for or against an issue with no simultaneous action. The No Child Left Behind legislation is an example of one *unfunded mandate* in which federal legislation required action but did not result in federal funding to states. The passage of these bills pleases some campaign funders, so they continue to support the candidates in subsequent elections. Another legislative strategy, used to initially please some supporters, is *sunset laws*, which quietly die after a specific time as stated in the law.

Financing

A major discussion is the influence of money on campaigns, resulting in increased access to legislators and greater influence on legislation by PACs and financial contributors. By federal law, the Federal Elections Commission (FEC) regulates the type, amount, and reporting of campaign contributions and expenditures. State commissions handle funds within state, county, and municipal governments. Each candidate, political party, and PAC is required to register and submit regular reports. This is traditionally referred to as *hard money*. *Soft money* is less regulated and refers to funds given to the party but for no specific purpose. Soft money is often used to support campaign activities but under a different guise. For example, instead of giving money to a senatorial campaign for travel to a state capital, the party supports a high school student workshop on a topic that invokes the candidate's position, thus averting the campaign finance rules constraining usage. Campaign finance reports and documentation of PACs, corporate, and other large contributors to each party and candidate are required by the FEC and are available to the public (http://www.fec.gov). Monies spent on media, travel, and food by campaigns have increased tremendously in the past decade. Many of the organizations noted in the preceding section and many nurses, doctors, physical therapists, and patients, donated to these campaigns and the PACs. In federal campaigns from 2021 to 2022, individual contributions are limited to $2900 per candidate, $36,500 per national party, and a total of $109,500 to all candidates, parties, and PACs combined. In contrast, national, state, or local party committee contributions were limited to $5000 per candidate per election and unlimited funds by political parties yearly (FEC, 2022a). These limits had changed from previous elections because of a January 2010 U.S. Supreme Court ruling in *Citizens United v. Federal Election Commission* (559 U.S. 310) that certain limits on campaign contributions were an unconstitutional denial of free speech and inflationary adjustments. Lawsuits to limit or prevent limiting campaign financing continue to be filed in state and federal courts and debated in Congress.

Many state-political contribution limits are similar to national levels or are based on population and candidate numbers each election cycle. In addition to funds raised by candidates, the government provides funds from the taxpayer-supported Presidential Election Campaign Fund (PECF). These monies are designated on federal income tax forms at $3 per taxpayer and then distributed to candidates after they raise a specified amount. For the first time, neither major party presidential candidate chose to receive PECF funds in the 2012 election. The candidates benefited greatly from the amounts the parties or PACs spent on advertisements and other media to support them and by not taking PECF dollars they were not limited in other types of contributions or expenditures. During the 2016 election cycle, more than $4.6 billion was raised by PACs, accounting for more than half of the funds raised. In the 2020 cycle, more than $25 billion was raised, and more than half was PAC money (FEC, 2022b), though final amended reports for some candidates remain pending.

Two modes of funding appeared during the past decades, the first of which was using the Internet to solicit and receive contributions. The second mode of funding is committees, called *527 political groups,* that altered political fundraising and campaign activities. These groups can engage in voter mobilization efforts, issue advocacy, and other activity short of expressly advocating the election or defeat of a federal candidate. There are no limits to how much money they can raise. These organizations are regulated by the Internal Revenue Service (IRS), but not necessarily the FEC if they do not explicitly advocate for an individual's election or defeat or do not directly subsidize federal elections. Thus, this is a major loophole in raising and using soft money. In the past four presidential elections, organizations ran advertisements that showed candidates' positions in a very demonstrative and stark manner. For example, Clinton was portrayed as an untrustworthy crook, Trump as a bigot and a womanizer, and Biden as old and slow.

Understanding the Legislative Process

An important process to understand is illustrated in *How Our Laws Are Made* (U.S. House of Representatives, 2007), which explains how a bill proceeds through the U.S. Congress. Steps, processes, facilitators, and barriers to enacting legislation at the federal level from the introduction of a bill through its enrollment to the president are detailed (Fig. 6.1). This illustration also identifies the House and Senate procedures, including leadership roles and responsibilities, committee assignment, readings on the chamber floor, and resolution between the two chambers. Many of the steps and processes originated in the late 19th century. A system of bells and lights is in place throughout the Capitol building to notify senators and representatives of pending votes and other actions. E-mail and text alerts are also used for notifications. This document also discusses how to "bury" or "kill" a bill and how the majority party ideas often prevail even in the most sacred workings of our democracy. Many state legislatures follow similar protocols and procedures. It is incumbent upon nurses to identify the major committees and legislators that deal with health and nursing issues in their own state and the major pitfalls or bridges where nurse and health-focused legislation may be delayed or strengthened. The state nursing association can assist with identifying those persons, committees, barriers, and facilitators.

Administration and Committees

In addition to the constitutionally mandated process and structure, each Congress or state legislature establishes its own rules for administration and governance that affect how policies are made and which issues are considered. Rules include the number, type, and focus of committees where most of the legislative work takes place. In fact, committee chairpersons, assigned because of seniority, develop the calendar of issues and legislation to be discussed. In the past, and likely continuing, bills that are brought forth for discussion and passage are not necessarily the purview of the particular committee. Rather, these issues may be germane to the constituents of the ranking majority or minority leader, based on the leader's personal beliefs and experience, or related to financial support received from individuals, organizations, and corporations.

Committee structure is determined for each Congress, except for several mandated committees by U.S. or state constitution. In Congress, committee structure was stable from the 1960s through the early 1990s, years during which the Democrats controlled the House of Representatives and often the Senate. During that time, the Committee on Labor and Human Resources had primary responsibility for health care legislation and issues. With a new Republican majority in the House of Representatives and that party's control over the Senate and White House from 2001 to 2008, the committee structure was altered and updated. Similar changes occur each time a national party controls two or three of the legislative houses and the White House. Committees are terminated, and the committee names and jurisdictions are changed. A new Health, Education, Labor, and Pensions Committee in the Senate was charged with primary health policy jurisdiction. However, many committees develop health-related bills and send forth authorizations and appropriations for those bills, such as the Senate Agriculture, Nutrition, and Forestry Committee

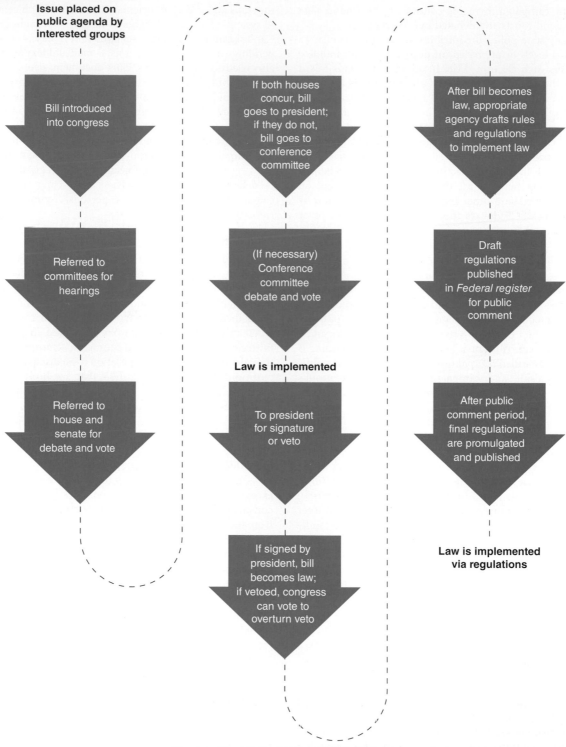

Fig. 6.1 Formal Health Care Policy Process.

(nutrition bill) and the House International Relations Committee (American Red Cross bill). In addition to the committee changes, parties often change the rules of voting, procedures, and how budget decisions are approved. For example, the "nuclear option" of majority voting levels was introduced by Democrats but first used by Republicans. Often these types of change cause mistrust and decrease bipartisanship, resulting in "do nothing" congressional sessions, decreased public understanding of processes, and lowered favorability of congress and leaders.

Congressional Sessions

Congress has two sessions for developing legislation. The 117th Congress began in January 2021 with the first session; the second session began in January 2022. Legislation that has passed both Houses, been resolved in conference committee, been enrolled to the president, and is signed, becomes public law. Laws are signified by the Congress in which they are passed and their chronological order of passage (e.g., Public Law [PL] 114-361: law number 361 passed the 114th Congress). Financial allocations—more precisely, appropriations—are included in bills and usually include funding for 3 to 5 years. However, appropriations depend on the budget bills passed for each calendar year and thus can be revised, reauthorized, repealed, or not funded by subsequent congressional action. In addition, there are unofficial "lame duck" congresses, whereby little is accomplished because everyone is waiting for the election result turnover of political parties in control of congressional houses or majorities.

Chamber Responsibilities

A constitutional directive mandates that all bills raising revenue (what we now call budget bills), including an increase in federal income taxes, originate in the U.S. House of Representatives. Thus, the Senate cannot initiate an income tax increase, but it can increase spending limits and develop new programs that may result in the need for increased taxes and add amendments to bills. Either chamber can be the origin of bills that establish or increase funds through other means, such as airport, gasoline, or Medicare fees and taxes. The Ways and Means, Appropriations, and Finance committees have input on the budget and review legislation originating in other committees that require new or continuing appropriations. Any legislation that includes appropriations, whether continuing or new, are required to be submitted by committees and subcommittees to the chamber budget committees and the congressional Office of Management and Budget (OMB) for calculation, inclusion in the fiscal year appropriations bills, and estimations of spending in the outlying years. On most occasions, the budget committees change or alter the recommended allocations and refer these changes to the committee charged with a specific piece of legislation and to the committee with primary responsibility for that specific area (e.g., health care, education, transportation). Constitutionally, the Senate has primary responsibility for the approval of political appointments, such as judges, ambassadors, the surgeon general, cabinet members, and federal agency directors. In early and recent U.S. history, approval hearings have been contentiously political and philosophical. Health-related issues such as sexual harassment, sex education, government role in health care, constitutional interpretation versus literalist reading, and immigration laws served as litmus tests for appointee approval. Three health issues, abortion, gun control, and the death penalty, continue to be major points for discussion that affect health policy and the appointment of judges to state, appellate, and federal courts, and the U.S. Supreme Court. Universal health care, terrorism, privacy, and environmental issues have resulted in enthusiastic legislative discussions and often a lack of legislative agreement and passage or denial of judicial appointments. Most recently, the COVID-19 vaccine mandates and election regulations have caused disagreement in Congress and the courts.

State Activities

In 2022, all state legislatures (except Nebraska) have two chambers, and their leadership is similar to that of the national Congress in that a speaker of the house, a senate majority leader, and party leaders provide day-to-day administration of the legislative body. In most states, chamber and committee leadership is determined by seniority, past party leadership, respective party caucuses, and persons who aspire to the party ideology and philosophy in setting legislative agendas, just like at the federal level. State legislatures play a large role in the budgetary decisions and health policy and nursing practice, including Medicaid services, health department auspices, certification of hospitals and nursing homes, and nursing licensure and scope of practice and prescriptive privileges within the state. Many state constitutions require a balanced budget submitted by the governor and approved by the legislature. Thus, even in states, health programs and nursing services can be advanced or be in jeopardy depending on annual budgetary decisions. Several states have instituted lotteries or video gambling to increase revenues directly tied to education or specific health programs. Public health initiatives, such as adolescent tobacco use reduction, drunk driving prevention, and school health programs, may be funded with these nonrecurring funds. Public education also may be supported by this type of fund or by recurring income tax funds. In that case, state-supported community colleges, universities, and public schools (e.g., medical, nursing, pharmacy) can increase enrollment and faculty or offer more online and alternative-schedule courses. Similarly, hospitals and health departments are supported by state and local allocations that affect bed capacity, working environment, salaries, construction funds, certificate of need, and services provided.

State legislation also may include mandated overtime or nurse staffing levels in health care facilities. States have passed bills that do not allow mandatory overtime for nurses. Another route to the same result is for nursing boards or other licensing boards to develop regulations concerning appropriate and safe working hours or limitations on overtime. Approximately one-third of states have such statutes. This is an example of just one area among many where nurses can actively participate in the policy decisions to ensure a quality working situation and maximal patient safety and care, as well as expanded roles for registered nurses and advanced practice nurses. The ANA National Database of Nursing Quality Indicators (NDNQI) and Safe Staffing Saves Lives (SSSL) Initiatives, as well as research by Peter Buerhaus, Linda Aiken, Barbara Mark, and Susan Letvak and their colleagues, provide a foundation for those efforts. Press Ganey now owns the NDNQI.

BUDGET PROCESS
Appropriation of Funds

Appropriation bills are required to approve funding for running the federal government each fiscal year (October 1– September 30). Bills, which represent spending by each cabinet department (e.g., Treasury, Labor, Commerce, Health and Human Services, Defense), require congressional approval and presidential signature no later than the beginning of each fiscal year. Near the end of each congressional session, appropriation bills often are combined into one general appropriation bill, which prior to 1997 was called the Omnibus Budget Reconciliation Act (OBRA) and is now known as the Consolidated Budget Resolution (CBR). In the early 2000s, legislation titles began to be focused on social or financial priorities, such as the Taxpayer Relief Act. Specific bills for the cabinet-level governmental agencies are titled, for instance, the Homeland Security Act.

Through the president's proposed budget, with input from the Administration's OMB, this process begins in Congress. After consideration of the proposed budget submitted by the White House, each chamber develops a budget resolution bill by April of each year. Additionally, all legislation under consideration that includes funding recommendations or appropriations is required to be submitted by committees to the Congressional Budget Office (CBO). The CBO reviews and calculates the actual costs to the federal government and considers how a particular

appropriation fits into the proposed budget or *reconciliation bill.* One important issue at both state and federal levels is that revenue and expenditure estimates by varying interested parties are calculated with similar factors such as inflation, economic growth, gross domestic product (GDP), and consumer price index.

In recent decades, state and federal budgets often are achieved through crisis management. This may have been because of a lack of clarity about legislation, large amounts of legislation to consider and act on, political strife, or budget shortfalls or surpluses. Disagreements and animosity have caused a delay in the mandated federal budget approval in Congress. The lack of approval for a reconciliation or consolidation bill has caused the federal government to shut down on more than one occasion. This type of crisis management resulted in special amendments being added to bills at the "11th hour" to convince certain representatives and senators to agree to vote for the final bill. This deal-making and "pork barrel" special interest spending added to what may have been appropriate legislation and allocations in an earlier version of a bill. Many bills were delayed in the early 2000s primarily because of discussions regarding terrorism funding or major disagreements on appropriations. In the most recent decade, multiple continuing budget resolutions were required to keep the government open. In December 2013 a continuing budget resolution bill titled the Bipartisan Budget Act of 2013 was passed by the House and Senate. In addition, this bill contained the Pathway for SGR Reform Act of 2013, which addressed Medicare payments to physicians and hospitals, special needs populations, and long-term care and repeals the Patient Protection and Affordable Care Act (ACA) changes to hospital disproportionate care (Medicaid). The fall 2017 continuing resolutions ranged from 2 days to 2 months because of the lack of agreement on budget priorities and allocations. A similar pattern occurred in subsequent years.

Another type of spending, *emergency spending,* may not be included in the fiscal year reconciliation bill but can be approved through supplemental appropriation bills. For example, after the September 11, 2001, terrorist attacks, Super Storm Sandy in 2012, the Texas floods and California wildfires in 2017, and 2020 and 2021 COVID-19 pandemic special funds and Federal Emergency Management Agency and Centers for Disease Control and Prevention (CDC) increases were approved to provide disaster relief and emergency actions. Multiple *supplemental bills* have been passed to increase homeland security (Transportation Safety Administration), defense spending (the war in Iraq), health crises at home and internationally (Ebola crisis), or to deal with other expenses not approved through the traditional congressional budget processes. This is less likely at the state level because of balanced budget statutes. Also, many states have "rainy day" funds.

Authorization of Programs

Authorization and reauthorization bills (with funding requests) are required to establish or continue programs and to fund those mandates. The initial authorization is usually a separate bill named for the issue or program being established, for example, the Older Americans Act, the Ryan White AIDS Act, and the Public Health Service Act. New governmental agencies may be initiated or established, as was the case with the Administration on Aging (AOA) in 1965 and the Department of Homeland Security in 2002. Future authorization and reauthorization bills are required to make changes in governmental agencies, expand programs, and continue or alter funding levels. However, some authorization bills that are passed do not contain any funding levels. Rather, these bills are used to establish programs that are to be funded by governmental departments within present allocations or by individual states, or they are *unfunded mandates.* For example, the Brady Bill gun control legislation requires background checks on gun purchasers before a license is issued. The federal law contained no continuing funds; thus, states must provide funds or be in violation of the law, and as a result, often suffer a loss of government monies for law enforcement. The Patient Self Determination Act and the No Child Left Behind bill are similar federal mandates with no state funding allocated. Several bills, like the Family and Medical Leave Act, contained only federal regulatory allocations. Some authorization bills purposely contain no funding recommendations so that members of Congress can support the issue without providing funding. The regulatory body may not be provided funding to oversee state implementation of the act. Mandating the Culturally and Linguistically Appropriate Services (CLAS) standards for health providers and agencies is another example in which a federal law required states to implement statutes and services, but little or no funding was provided.

Fiscal Responsibility

Several efforts were made in previous decades to mandate a balanced budget at the federal level. The Gramm-Rudman-Hollings law was passed in 1985 (PL 99-177), but the U.S. Supreme Court subsequently found this law to be unconstitutional. Other attempts were made over the next two decades, but no bill reached final approval in Congress or presidents vetoed them. Thus, no bill passed that would have allowed the public to vote on a constitutional amendment. Rules within Congress have been passed to constrain budgets. The Senate has the Byrd rule, named after the long-serving senator from West Virginia so

that any senator can raise an objection to any budget reconciliation bills, amendments thereto, and reconciliation conference reports and it will be stricken. The house has no such rule but understands how the Senate must abide by the rule unless 3/5 of the Senate (60 votes) votes to suspend the rule. With closely divided chambers, reaching that level of vote is difficult. In December of 2017, PL 115-97, the Tax Cuts and Jobs Act that changed income taxes was passed even though it may have violated the Byrd rule. The strategy used by the majority party was that tax changes were attached to a previously approved bill that was not a reconciliation bill (H.R.1) and was not actually part of the budget reconciliation process. Thus, a simple majority of senators could pass the bill. In addition, the bill wording and calculations were such that the bill added only $1.4 trillion to the federal debt, thus following the self-imposed congressional rule. In December 2021, Public Law 117-73 was signed by President Biden to increase the federal debt limit by $2.5 trillion, passed in the Senate with only Democratic support in a simple majority rule.

Appropriation or budget bills are required for the functioning of the federal government or other legislation, and thus specialized "pet" programs are often attached to the budget bills to get them enacted. For example, several times the Nurse Education Act's appropriation bills were tacked on to the budget to ensure they were passed during that fiscal year before Congress adjourned. Much of the time, pork-barrel amendments are approved to gain the votes of specific members of Congress. Even though the spending will benefit constituencies, the programs often are not federal mandates or related to the responsibilities of the government. Because many of these amendments are added at the 11th hour and at times in conference committees to resolve the House and Senate differences, the public and some legislators are often not aware of these expenditures until they have been approved. The president does not have *line-item veto authority* and therefore must accept or veto each appropriation bill in its entirety to enact the fiscal year budget. Similar actions occur in state legislatures for appropriation bills for services such as museums, bypass highways, and new post offices, though some governors have a line-item veto and can delete specific budget items from the budget. A legislative veto override would be required to reinstate that item.

Economics

A majority of the budget for the U.S. Department of Health and Human Services (DHHS) is for *entitlement programs,* which means that only one-third or less of the amount appropriated by Congress for this department can be controlled or used in discretionary ways. The NIH, the Centers for Medicare and Medicaid Services (CMS), and the Bureau of Health Professions (BHPr) are included in the DHHS budget. Nursing leaders and others have continually worked to increase these budgets, and these efforts resulted in budget increases. In calendar year 2020, CMS expenditures for federal Medicaid obligations totaling $671.2 billion and federal Medicare obligations totaling $829.5 billion were expended (CMS, 2022a).

Overall U.S. national health care spending grew 9.7% in 2020, averaging $12,530 per person and more than $4.1 trillion. The health care portion of the GDP was 19.7% (CMS, 2022a). However, some of the rise was attributed to COVID care. Regardless, hospital care is still provided for one-third of all private and public expenditures. In addition to providing health care coverage, agencies fund many health-related activities, such as food inspections, drug approvals, and research. For example, the NIH fiscal year 2021 budget was $42.93 billion, with the National Cancer Institute receiving $6.56 billion and the National Institute of Nursing Research (NINR) receiving $175 million (NIH, 2022). Various federal agency heads and deputies submit budget requests to congressional committees each year through letters, hearings, and routine budgetary processes.

Congress has been borrowing from the Social Security Trust Fund since the early 1980s to meet annual operating costs and appropriations across the government. Social Security (SS) includes Medicare and Medicaid health coverage programs, Supplemental Security Income (SSI), retirement pension income, and disability income. More than 65 million persons in 2020 were covered using SS pension or income payment programs; the retirement income and Medicare programs that are funded by current worker payroll taxes do not contain enough money to fund those same workers when they reach 65 years of age or full SS retirement age. The General Accounting Office (GAO) estimates that the SS Trust Fund will be unable to meet its full obligations starting in the year 2034. Debate continues over how a government with a large national debt and a large tax base can best serve its citizens, given the promises made to citizens regarding retirement and health insurance in old age. Several of the major proposals to change SS through decreased benefits to younger workers, change in the age of eligibility for SS, initiation of private health savings accounts, gradually increasing the salary cap for paying SS taxes, and a means-tested eligibility for full benefits have been enacted. Others remain under debate annually. The ACA passage revised Medicare, Medicaid, and access to care, but the implementation of all titles was delayed because of political and budgetary decisions during the 112th and 113th Congresses. The 115th Congress removed the ACA individual mandate and Presidential Executive Order decreased or terminated the exchange subsidies, which would save the federal government money. Court

actions continue regarding the latter order, while the 11 million persons covered under these plans continue to enroll annually. The ACA exchanges were largely subsidized by the federal government, though presidential orders have left states in limbo with respect to funding. Local agencies and school boards are often the most successful in dealing with budget shortfalls because they have not had—or have not chosen to use—the ability to borrow funds, incur long-term debt, or move costs from one budget year to another. This was true until the COVID-19 pandemic, which has caused many costs to local governments and schools related to cleaning, loss of staff, and personal protective equipment purchase requirement. More discussion on health-related economics can be found in Chapter 7.

HEALTH PROGRAMS

Two main types of federal health care programs exist, discretionary and entitlement. *Discretionary programs* are subject to annual appropriations by Congress and are considered controllable budgetary items. For this discussion, these programs primarily consist of categorical health services, training, and research programs. Categorical health services are services for somewhat narrowly defined categories of problems, such as programs for communicable diseases and family planning services. An example of a training program is the Nurse Reinvestment Act (PL 107-205), and an example of a research program is the NINR at the NIH.

Entitlements are those health care programs in which budgetary expenses are more difficult to control. Citizens who benefit from these programs are "entitled" to the benefits by law because of a specified age, disability, economic status, or prepayment. The federal government is obligated to pay these benefits regardless of the number of enrollees or the costs. The only major avenue to cut costs is by changing either the authorization or eligibility criteria through legislation. Costs cannot be limited by appropriating less money for expenditures. SS, veterans' compensation and pensions are examples of income entitlement programs. Health care entitlement programs are Medicare, Medicaid, and State Children's Health Insurance Programs.

The enactment of the Social Security Act (SSA) in 1935 marked the first major act of government involvement in health. The Act provides federal grants to the states for public health; maternal and child health; services for disabled children; and public assistance for the aged, blind, and families with dependent children. The role of the federal government in the provision of health care was expanded with the 1965 passage of Title XVIII and XIX amendments to the SSA, creating Medicare and Medicaid. These two programs have changed the face of health care and continue to have a large role in the provision of health care services. The addition of disabled persons and those with end-stage renal disease to Medicare in the 1970s increased costs and care. In 1997 Title XXI, the State Children's Health Insurance Program was added, which dramatically increased the number of children now covered by federal and state legislations and budgets. Much of the discussion in the 105th through the 115th Congresses was related to how to deal with the increasing costs of these entitlement programs and to propose strategies for reforming the programs. The ACA of 2010, the Bipartisan Budget Bill of 2013, the Pathway for Sustainable Growth Rate Reform Act of 2013, Medicare Access and CHIP Reauthorization Act (MACRA) of 2015, and the Tax Cut and Jobs Act of 2017 legislate access to care, entitlement payment changes, and national budget cuts. Medicare and SS are major entitlements for budgetary expenses, but because they affect more than half of Americans, cutbacks and revisions are difficult politically and socially.

Implementation and Regulation

Multiple governmental agencies plan, implement, and evaluate health policy in the United States. The major agencies are headed by political appointment cabinet officials, directors, and administrators but are staffed by career civil servants. For example, the U.S. House of Representatives has 435 elected members, but 10,000 staff members are employed for duties such as cleaning, moving, painting, preparing and serving food, providing mail and phone services, and staffing the infirmary. Congressional legislation and presidential executive orders and mandates can alter workings across staff divisions of the executive, judicial, and legislative branches of government. The Balanced Budget Act of 1997 mandated changes in the administration and implementation of federal programs. Before the 1990s most federal departments or regulatory oversight had changed very little. The Government Performance and Results Act of 1993 was a major effort to enhance the accountability of agencies. The Federal Funding Accountability and Transparency Act of 2006, signed by President Bush, was another attempt to clarify governmental action and spending to the public. In the 110th Congress, Senator Obama introduced a revision titled the Strengthening Transparency and Accountability in Federal Spending Act of 2008, but the bill died when that congressional session ended. Similar bills were introduced in 2013 (S. 1217: Housing Finance Reform and Taxpayer Protection Act) but remained in committee. However, several states have passed laws to increase transparency, access to government spending documents, and streamlined governmental structure.

The DHHS is charged with protecting and ensuring the health of the nation and is headed by the Secretary of Health. Multiple agencies and divisions are included in the DHHS, and several assistant secretaries are responsible for administrative aspects. The Surgeon General is an Assistant Secretary of Health and heads the Office of Public Health and Science (OPHS). An Assistant Secretary for Aging heads the AOA and the Administration for Children and Families (ACF). Other agencies are headed by a commissioner (e.g., FDA) or director (e.g., NIH). Agencies include several sections or divisions. For example, the NIH has 27 institutes and centers, including the NINR, the Eunice Kennedy Shriver National Institute for Child Health and Human Development (NICHD), and the National Institute on Mental Health (NIMH). In Atlanta and other regional offices, CDC houses 17 centers, institutes, and offices that conduct research, including the National Center for Chronic Disease Prevention and Health Promotion (NCCDPHP); the National Center for HIV/AIDS, Viral Hepatitis, STD, and TB Prevention; the National Center for Health Statistics (NCHS); and the Office of Public Health Preparedness and Response (PHPR). Most federal government agencies and state agencies have civil rights, legal, public relations, and budget sections staffed by career employees. These agencies have public Internet sites for consumers and professionals to obtain program and contact information. Many political, professional, and health-related agencies and organizations also house websites and social media account for rapid and wide public access and dissemination of information.

Each federal agency has specific auspices or sponsorship, although these are not always consistent with the appropriation focus. The Department of Agriculture directs the commodity distribution program (e.g., nonfat dry milk, cheese products), the National School Lunch Program (NSLP), farm programs, and food inspection. The CMS directs Medicare, Medicaid, and Children's Health Insurance Programs; the Department of Labor houses the Occupational Safety and Health Administration (OSHA); the CDC houses the National Institute of Occupational Safety and Health (NIOSH). Most states have similar agencies and auspices to manage public programs. Some have separate offices for health care. For example, the Division of TennCare administers the Medicaid program in Tennessee, and the KanCare Medicaid program is in the Division of Health Care Finance under the Kansas Department of Health and Environment.

Whereas laws are written in broad language, the *rules and regulations* to implement these laws are very specific and often can be revised without changing the original law. Agencies are charged with implementation, financial oversight, legislative interpretation, and the development of regulations and rules governing their respective programs.

Often agencies are required to interpret the purpose and intent of congressional or state legislation to implement such laws. The perceptions, political savvy, and experiences of the agency's director, staff, and proponents effect this interpretation of the issue under consideration. For example, former DHHS Secretary Tommy Thompson reworded family planning regulations to include abstinence-only programs, President Clinton used presidential directives for regulations to allow stem cell research on embryos not used by couples who went through in vitro fertilization procedures, and President Bush wrote executive orders to allow only currently available stem cell lines to be used rather than new embryonic lines and vetoed bills to allow federal funding for certain research. In 2009, President Obama used executive orders to lift the ban on federal funding for "promising" embryonic stem cell research. According to multiple media outlets and not disputed by officials, President Trump's administration recommended that five terms should not be used in federal budget request documents for FY 2019 (e.g., evidence-based, entitlement, diversity). It is unclear how this will affect the actual practices, structure, and research of the CDC. Thus, interpretations and changes in regulations can be related to the number and types of citizens served in a particular program, the increase or decrease in appropriations, the social or ethical values of directors and department heads, the political climate, and societal crises.

In some instances, the auspices and appropriations are not consistent. The Department of Agriculture receives appropriations for elder nutrition programs, but these are administered under the Area Agencies on Aging (AAOA) through state, regional, and local agencies. The Department of Labor has administrative responsibility for the Senior Community Service Employment Program (SCSEP), which is under the auspices of the AAOA. The Bureau of Census collects vital data, but the NCHS and Department of Labor analyze those data for developing policy and allocation decisions. Thus, some health-related policy legislation and appropriations require extra effort to determine the auspices, regulation, and implementation and whether duplication or omission occurs, and thus where influence can be used.

Evaluation of specific policies and their implementation is often limited at the federal level. This evaluation of process, structure, and outcomes has become an emphasis and accountability, especially for the SS, Medicare, and Medicaid programs and costs. Process and structure are often difficult to change in large, bureaucratic organizations of state and federal government. Annual performance plans now required of agencies should assist in more clearly evaluating program effectiveness and efficiency and revising structure and process to meet the outcomes.

Two such health-related efforts are the *Healthy People* national objectives and the initiatives to eliminate racial and ethnic disparities at the DHHS. Because these two efforts reflect new targets and new census health data, new populations and new social determinants of health have emerged as areas of focus. The initiatives are integrated into policies, regulations, and even research requirements. Thus, policy at the federal, state, and local levels is affected by efforts to improve the health of our community through system, policy, and funding decisions. Nursing has been involved in both efforts at multiple levels and across the education, practice, and research arenas.

LEADERSHIP

Several persons and organizations have provided leadership to ensure the passage of major health policies and regulations. Surgeon Generals Koop, Elders, and Satcher supported efforts to deal with chronic diseases, prevent and reduce health risks through education, and target efforts based on *Healthy People* initiatives. Dr. Richard H. Carmona (formerly a nurse), who served as Surgeon General, was a less visible leader partially because of the focus on bioterrorism and the overshadowing of the White House leadership related to stem cell research and abstinence education. David Kessler, Commissioner of the FDA, worked to protect consumers through the regulation of nutritional and dietary supplements. He also argued for the regulation of tobacco. The Tobacco Master Settlement Agreement was reached between the four largest tobacco companies and 46 state attorneys general, but not under the purview of the FDA. The lawsuit was brought by state departments of justice suing for repayment of public dollars (Medicare and Medicaid) spent on providing health care to those with tobacco-related illnesses. The $360 billion settlement agreed to by the tobacco industry is being paid over a 25-year period. The termination of soliciting adolescent smokers, bans on tobacco advertisements within specific distances of schools, and supplementation of education and prevention programs were required. However, money in most states is not being used for the purposes noted. This is an example of the judicial branch of government playing a role in health policy and planning. Another highly visible leader in health care regulation, Dr. Julie Gerberding served as director of the CDC, and her tenure was marked by multiple national occurrences of food-borne illnesses (e.g., *Escherichia coli*, salmonella). The CDC, under Dr. Tom Friedman's leadership, was faced with H1N1 flu, Ebola, and Zika outbreaks. Dr. Kathleen Sebelius, the former Secretary of the DHHS, was active in the implementation of the ACA. Dr. Anthony Fauci, director of the National Institute of Allergy and

Infectious Disease, and Dr. Rochelle Walensky, director of the CDC, have led COVID-19 pandemic efforts. Executive orders and congressional actions guided this pandemic response.

Legislators

Senators Edward Kennedy (D-MA), Barbara Mikulski (D-MD), Paul Simon (D-IL), and Nancy Kassebaum (R-KS) led health-related legislative efforts during the 1980s, 1990s, and early 2000s in the U.S. Senate. In the House of Representatives, efforts were led by Henry Waxman (D-WI), John Lewis (D-GA), Joseph Kennedy (D-MA), and nurse Lois Capps (D-CA). Legislative efforts during this time focused on programs for vulnerable populations such as children, the elderly, and low-income persons, as well as appropriations for new and continuing programs. Health policy efforts in the early 2000s were related to managed care (both private and public sector) and consumer rights regarding their health care coverage, use of personal information, the Health Insurance Portability and Accountability Act (HIPAA), and competency of providers. Representative Lois Capps led the initial Nurse Reinvestment Act effort in 2002. In 2007 Senator Brownback led efforts to develop electronic medical records (EMR) and Senator Akaka worked to block the establishment of electronic records unless privacy could be ensured. In 2008, Medicare, Medicaid, and the Children's Health Insurance Program (CHIP) were a major focus by both parties, with Senators Edward Kennedy and Hillary Clinton and James Clyburn in the House leading the efforts. In January 2009 the 111th Congress passed new State Children's Health Insurance Program (SCHIP) legislation that expanded coverage. During the 110th Congress, Senators Brownback (R-KS), Casey (D-PA), Inhofe (R-OK), Spector (R-PA), and Coleman (R-MA), along with Representative Watson (D-CA), introduced the compassionate care ACCESS Act to provide for physician and patient FDA options for experimental treatments. Most recently, Senators Mikulski and Collins (R-ME) and Representative Capps (D-CA) were leading supporters of increasing Nursing Workforce Development funds, HRSA nursing education funds, and extension of the Health Care and Education Reconciliation Act (PL 111-152). Representatives Walden (R-OR), Schwartz (D-PA), Bonamici (D-OR), Noem (R-SD), Peterson (D-MN), Cramer (R-ND), and Daines (R-MT) and Senators Moran (R-KS), Thune (R-SD), and Tester (D-MT) sponsored legislation that allows nurse practitioners, clinical specialists, and midwives to receive federal payments (Medicare) for home health, primary care, and rural services. Representatives Rohrbacher (R-CA), Johnson (a nurse; D-TX), Smith (R-TX), and Sablan (D-MP at large) cosponsored PL 114-255, the 21st Century Cures Act that provides funding for the opioid crisis and research, the BRAIN Initiative, adding patient experiences to drug side-effect information, and establishing a Task Force on Research Specific to Pregnant Women and Lactating Women. In addition, congresswoman Johnson called for and coauthored the Helping Families in Mental Health Crisis Act of 2015, which was included in PL 114-255. In 2013, six nurses served in the U.S. House of Representatives (Bass, D-CA; Black, R-TN; Capps, D-CA; Ellmers, R-NC; Johnson, D-TX; McCarthy, D-NY), and in 2018 three nurses served (Bass, Black, Johnson). Ms. Capps served for 20 years, and Ms. Johnson was the first RN elected to Congress in 1993. In 2022, Lauren Underwood (D-IL) and Cori Bush (D-MO) are nurses that serve in the U.S. House. No nurse has been elected to the U.S. Senate; however, physicians, pharmacists, and opticians have served as senators.

Many nurses have provided leadership at the national level to contribute to health policy and ensure that its influence on nursing is positive. ANA presidents have long been visible and active proponents of nursing and health. Virginia Trotter Betts and Beverly Malone were instrumental in setting the original Nursing's Agenda for Health Care Reform (NAHCR) to promote the passage of third-party reimbursement changes for advanced practice nurses, accreditation of home health agencies, and provision of childhood immunizations. Betts and Malone later were appointed Assistant Secretaries of Health at the DHHS. Debbie Gettis, a registered professional nurse, served as the AIDS advisor to President Clinton. Nurses have been elected to the National Academy of Sciences Institute of Medicine (e.g., Dorothy Brooten, Martha Hill, Peter Buerhaus), which advises Congress on health matters. Ada Sue Hinshaw and Patricia Grady served as the initial directors of the National Center for Nursing Research (NCNR), which became the NINR. In 2022, Dr. Sharon Zenk serves as NINR director.

Nancy Bergstrom and Thelma Wells have provided leadership in the development of guidelines for practice for the Agency for Healthcare Research and Quality (AHRQ, formerly the AHCPR), and Nancy Fugate-Woods and Ora Lea Strickland spearheaded a national focus on women's health. Peter Buerhaus (an economist), Cheryl Jones, and Linda Moody have served as scientists at the national level to develop recommendations and projections for the nursing workforce, staffing, and economic needs. Janet Allan, Lucy Marion, and Carol Loveland-Cherry have served on the U.S. Preventive Services Task Force, and Audrey Nelson led patient safety and quality of care efforts at the DVA. Martha Hill served as President of the AHA and Terry Fulmer served as President of the Gerontological Society of America (GSA). Nurses have been appointed to formal policy-level impact positions. Dr. Debra Barksdale was an original member of the Board of Governors for the Patient-Centered Outcomes Research Initiative (PCORI). Drs. Beth Collins Sharp and Cheryl Jones served as senior advisors and scientists at the AHRQ. Dr. Clair Caruso served as Research Scientist at NIOSH. At higher levels, Dr. Mary Wakefield served as the Administrator of the HRSA and Marilyn Tavenner was the Director of the CMS. Internationally, Stephanie Ferguson served as director of the International Council of Nurses (ICN) Leadership for Change Program and its ICN-Burdett Global Nursing Leadership Institute, as well as being a White House Fellow earlier in her career.

Think Tanks, Foundations, and Organizations

Other sources of health policy and planning encompass private or public "think tanks," philanthropic foundations, and policy centers that directly affect nursing. One example is the Pew Health Professions Commission (PHPC), formed to study the future needs of the health care system in the United States. Multiple reports have been issued by this commission over the past three decades. The reports delineate the nature of health care work, the restructuring of health care professional regulation, the number and types of professionals needed, and the training and education of professionals. Much of the discussion is, by necessity, in the context of an evolving health care system with dynamics not yet known. Although widely heralded, the commission's *Reforming Healthcare Workforce Regulation Policy: Considerations for the 21st Century* and the recommended competencies for the 21st-century health professional are slowly being enacted. The Robert Wood Johnson Foundation (RWJF) funds large demonstration projects to address varying health issues and populations. In addition, the RWJF established the Initiative on the Future of Nursing, Nurse Faculty Scholars, New Careers in Nursing Scholarship Program, the Interdisciplinary Nursing Quality Research Initiative (INQRI), Disparities Research for Change, and Public Health Law Research. The John A. Hartford Foundation partners with universities to improve nursing education for elder care through centers, student fellowships, and the development of best practice guidelines. The National Academy of Medicine (NAM), formerly known as the Institute of Medicine (IOM), is one of the three independent peer professional academies that include the National Academies of Science (NAS) and the National Academy of Engineers (NAE), which advise Congress on health matters through position papers, expert witnesses, and recommendations for legislative initiation, approval, and funding. The IOM report *The Future of Nursing: Leading Change, Advancing Health* (targeting 2020 achievements) continues to lend support for HRSA funding, Department of Education (DOE), accreditation approvals,

The Joint Commission activities, and the nursing-led Magnet Hospital accreditation program. A new Future of Nursing 2030 report has been released and includes initiatives for health equity, new models of education, care delivery changes, and control costs (NAM, 2021).

NURSING

Nursing currently has several issues that are affected by and affect health policy. First, there are workforce needs; that is, the qualifications and types of roles nurses will be required to fill. The American Association of Colleges of Nursing (AACN), the PHPC, and the IOM, now the National Academy of Medicine, recommended an increase in the number of registered nurses at the baccalaureate level and advanced practice nurses with master's and doctoral-level preparation (AACN, 2020; National Academy of Medicine [NAM], 2021), though the need for registered nurses is lagging behind projected needs (U.S. Bureau of Labor, 2022). This shortage has resulted in expanded online education, RN to BSN and RN to MSN options, training of medics and corpsmen in associate degree and bachelor's degree nursing, innovative models for second-career students, and new articulation agreements. A second issue is that of programs for nurse educators at the doctoral level to prepare nurses for the workforce needs. Although many doctoral programs have opened in the past three decades, the number of doctoral-prepared nurse educators available for appropriate training and education of the projected workforce has not kept pace with market need (AACN, 2020, 2021). A third nursing issue is that of competency-based education and practice, in which nurses demonstrate critical thinking, judgment, and decision-making skills, cultural competence, and engage in collaborative interprofessional practice. Curricular, regulation, and certification changes have been implemented. In the mid-1990s the National League for Nursing Accreditation Commission (NLNAC) for baccalaureate and master's degree programs began an increased emphasis on critical thinking and community-based care. Additional essentials were distributed through 2010. The AACN-East, in 2021, released new Essentials of Nursing Education that focus on competencies needed at two levels of practice (entry-level and advanced-level nursing practice) rather than specific BSN, MSN, or DNP academic programs. Ten domains and the associated competencies are identified and focus on four spheres of care (disease prevention, promotion of health and wellbeing, chronic disease care, regenerative or restorative care, and hospice/palliative/supportive care). In addition, several position statements regarding diversity, inclusion and equity, genetics education, opioid crisis management, and enhancing veterans care have been published as new priorities occur. The Commission on Collegiate Nursing Education (CCNE) and Accreditation Commission for Education in Nursing (ACEN), the professional accreditation bodies, require that undergraduate programs target their mission to local and regional health rather than taking a "cookie-cutter" approach to curriculum. The American Association of Critical-Care Nurses (AACN-West), the Association for Women's Health (AWH), Obstetrical and Neonatal Nurses (ONN), and the Oncology Nursing Society (ONS) offer certification for nurses. The American Nurses Credentialing Center (ANCC) provides both specialty roles (e.g., case management, nurse practitioner, clinical specialist) and population (e.g., mental health, adult, pediatric) certifications. Recent changes that may influence the workforce include changes to certification for advanced practice nurses in both education and practice requirements. These changes eliminated the stand-alone gerontological nurse practitioner certification; added requirements for pharmacology, physical assessment, and pathophysiology for nurse educators at the master's level; and increased the emphasis on DNP for advanced practice level nurses. The Department of Labor projects that the largest job growth through 2030 will be in the health care sector, with nurse practitioners a high growth area (U.S. Bureau of Labor, 2022). For this to occur, the shortage of nursing faculty will need to be alleviated and new models of education will be required to meet future student needs.

Several organizations have a major effect on health policy and nursing. The NAS is often involved in discussions of, and decisions for, auspices and allocations for the HRSA branches and nurse education acts in Congress. In fact, the Higher Education Opportunity Act of 2008 (PL 110-803) required the DHHS secretary to negotiate with the IOM to conduct a study on the capacity of nursing schools to meet the needs of the nation. More importantly, *The Future of Nursing* landmark report and recent update (NAM, 2021) detail multiple strategies to ensure a competent and adequate nursing workforce to meet future health needs. One such policy change in late 2016 was that the U.S. DVA amended provider regulations to permit full authority to VA advanced practice registered nurses (APRNs) to practice to the full extent of their education, training, and certification. This includes clinical specialists, nurse practitioners, and nurse midwives who meet specific education and certification requirements. Nurse anesthetists have not been fully approved, and APRNs may have limited scope for writing prescriptions based on state practice acts and VA regulations. Another policy effort is the HRSA effort to expand RN roles in primary care settings through innovative models of training, including the use of mobile health and telehealth. Both

of these two efforts are strategies to improve access and health outcomes. In addition, efforts can increase the visibility of a well-prepared, trusted, and large nursing profession.

The ANA, American Public Health Association (APHA), AMA, GSA, and American Dental Association (ADA) provide expert testimony to state and federal agencies and decision-making bodies on topics from product development and liability to school lunch programs; immunizations; disaster relief; bioterrorism; domestic violence; and lesbian, gay, bisexual, transgender, queer or questioning, intersex and allies (LGBTQQIA) health. Also, a national coalition effort (Nurses on Boards Coalition [NOBC]) has been to place 10,000 nurses in leadership, legislative, and other governing board-type positions by 2020 and beyond to influence priorities, allocations, and policies so that when health needs arise, such as the current opioid crisis, nurses activate (http://www.nursesonboardscoalition.org). Through activities noted in this section, nurses can lend a voice to the health needs of the vulnerable and underserved.

HEALTH POLICIES

Health policies, or decisions regarding the health care system, are developed and implemented through several avenues. Congressional and state legislation; federal, state, and local rules and regulations for agencies; and appropriation decisions are methods to develop health policy. Some health policies are reached only through legislation, whereas others are developed by multiple avenues. All these avenues are affected by public opinion, the economy, societal demographics, professional expertise, technology, and knowledge about health.

Health Policies Before 1990

Three of the most influential health policies have been the SSA of 1935 and the amendments that established Medicare and Medicaid in 1965. Many of our national concerns with health and welfare have been addressed by amendments to these policies. Issues such as abortion, family planning, nutrition, and disability and those related to *vulnerable populations* (the chronically ill, mentally ill, elderly, poor, and minorities) are included as major concerns and foci of programs and payments. These are also the largest programs in terms of population covered and dollars spent. With the aging of the population, technological and pharmaceutical advances, and changes in the racial/ethnic face of society, the original intent and expected costs of these programs have been far exceeded. A major issue today is how to continue these programs as a *safety net* for society. Many bills and acts have been passed that directly and indirectly affect the health of society. In the 1960s the Hill-Burton Act was funded for hospital construction and some nursing schools. Legislation for payment to nurses was included in the Rural Health Clinics Act of 1977 and extended with OBRA of 1989. In the 1970s and 1980s, increased emphasis was placed on disease prevention, risk reduction, and research on the leading causes of death (cardiovascular disease, cancer). A landmark change was the OBRA of 1982 established the diagnostic-related groups (DRGs), which resulted in a prospective payment system (PPS) for Medicare hospitalization. Legislation regarding mental health, school lunch programs, disease research, rural manpower, and end-stage renal disease and disability were added to Medicare eligibility. The 1987 OBRA (PL 101-203) changed Medicare payments to hospitals, altered health maintenance organization (HMO) requirements, and authorized nurse practitioners (NPs) and clinical nurse specialists (CNSs) to certify patient needs for nursing home care.

Health Policies 1990 to 2000

The 1990s were perhaps the most prolific decades for health policy reform and regulation for specific diseases, conditions, and vulnerable groups (Table 6.1). The Patient Self-Determination Act allowed persons to make decisions regarding their own health care. The Ryan White Act was passed to deal with issues related to HIV and AIDS. New NIH guidelines for the inclusion of women and children in research altered past trends, the use of past findings, and subsequent health policies. As the number of homeless persons increased, private and public sectors had difficulty dealing with the costs and spectrum of services, and the McKinney Homelessness Act was passed with both funded and unfunded mandates. The Americans with Disabilities Act has affected health care and work and practice environments and the justice system.

Major changes in Medicaid occurred in 1996 with the passage of the Personal Responsibility and Work Opportunities Act (Welfare) and Temporary Assistance to Needy Families, which replaced Aid to Families with Dependent Children. The 1997 Balanced Budget Act included SCHIP in the form of block grants to states to provide health care coverage to more low-income children. However, reports indicated that many children remained uncovered, resulting in the passage of the Children's Health Insurance Program Reauthorization Act (CHIPRA) in 2009, which provided appropriations through 2013. Additional congressional actions have extended funds.

Policies and new regulations in the 1990s also affected nurses and other health care workers. Parenting and caregiving concerns resulted in the Family and Medical Leave Act, and OSHA guidelines were developed regarding work-at-home employees. Reauthorization of programs and allocations for older Americans, children, and indigent care each year has an effect on nursing and health care. The Health Professions Education Partnerships Act included the Nursing Education and Practice Improvement Act, which established the National Advisory Council on Nurse Education and Practice (NACNEP) workforce needs. A major purpose of the Health Professions Education Partnerships Act was to consolidate health profession education, training, recruitment of minorities, and rural placements. Additionally, Health Care Financing Administration (HCFA)/CMS regulations were revised during the latter part of 1998 and 1999, which changed payment, diagnostic capabilities, and reimbursement for advanced practice nurses. In 2000, the National Center on Minority Health and Health Disparities (NCMHD) was established as part of the NIH that focused on health concerns across the federal agencies.

Health Policies 2001 to Present

Many new policies initiate, establish, or reauthorize nursing and health issues. The Nurse Reinvestment Act, the Medicare Prescription Drug Improvement and Modernization Act, and the Veterans' Health Care Authorization Act (Table 6.2) are such policies. The Medicare Modernization Act was an attempt to provide relief from high-cost prescriptions for the elderly and disabled. Drug discount cards were distributed to qualified elderly and disabled persons to be used beginning in January 2006. As of August 2022, almost 50 million Medicare beneficiaries received Part D coverage and 2019 expenditures were $183 billion (Cubanski & Damico, 2022; Cubanski & Neuman, 2021), far greater than the $750 million per year estimated when Part D passed Congress. Consumers and vendors can update or change plans each year. The cost of this law is continually being updated. Medicare Part A is the traditional fee-for-service hospital insurance coverage, and Part B is coverage for office visits and preventive care. Part C is an option to Part A and allows persons to be in a managed care plan that may be less expensive, include wellness programs, and not require prepayment, and it may offset or cover Parts B and D premiums.

Mental health coverage has grown steadily over the past 20 years, culminating in the Paul Wellstone Mental Health and Addiction Equity Act of 2007 (PL 110-343). Politics was a factor even with this legislation because it was tacked on to the Emergency Economic Stabilization Act of 2008 (which provided for the Troubled Asset Relief Program [TARP]) that was sure to pass after the housing and banking crash. The Comprehensive Addiction and Recovery Act of 2016 began a major effort to address pain management and reduce opioid abuse. Many states also have begun efforts that include provider and prescription tracking databases and limits on opioid medication prescriptions.

TABLE 6.1 Selected Policies Affecting Health and Nursing Passed From 1990–2000

Year	Title	Content/Purpose
1990	Patient Self-Determination Act (PL 101-508)	Required all Medicare/Medicaid-paid health care institutions to provide or ask for advance directives
1990	Occupational Safety and Health Act, amended (PL 101-552)	Describes general working conditions, guidelines for handling blood and body fluids, prevention of infectious disease, and biohazard waste disposal
1990	Trauma Care Systems Planning and Development Act (PL 101-590)	Established guidelines for trauma care services; replaced 1973 Emergency Medical Services Act
1990	Americans With Disabilities Act (PL 101-336)	Prohibits discrimination against persons with disabilities in five specific areas
1992	Breast and Cervical Cancer Mortality Prevention Act (PL 101-354)	Provides grants to states for screening, referrals, educational programs, training, quality assurance programs, and research
1992	Mammography Quality Standards Act (PL 102-539)	Requires certification, accreditation, and inspection of centers, including equipment, technicians, and records
1993	Family and Medical Leave Act (PL 103-3)	Establishes leave (job security) for employees caring for an ill child or family member, experiencing childbirth or adoption, or experiencing own illness
1996	Welfare Reform Act (PL 104-93)	Limits adults to 5 years on welfare; must work within 2 years
1996	Health Insurance Portability and Accountability Act (PL 104-191)	Provides for portability when changing jobs, limits preexisting conditions, requires congressional reports to evaluate the effect
1996	Newborn's and Mother's Health Protection Act (PL 104-326)	Mandates medical decision for minimum 48-hour stay after delivery; *provider* includes midwife and nurse practitioner
1997	Balanced Budget Act (PL 105-33)	Medicare direct payment to advanced practice nurses; Children's Health Insurance Program; welfare-to-work
1998	Health Professions Education and Partnership Act (PL 105-392)	Consolidated health professions education and training and minority health education and training; nursing education funding
1999	Healthcare Research and Quality Act (PL 106-129)	Changed name of Agency for Health Care Policy and Research (AHCPR) to Agency for Healthcare Research and Quality (AHRQ); mandates and funds quality and outcomes research
2000	Minority Health and Health Disparities Research and Education Act (PL 106–525)	Established the National Center on Minority Health and Health Disparities at National Institutes of Health

The growth of genomic medicine and the privacy issues regarding genetic information resulted in the Genetic Information Nondiscrimination Act of 2008 or GINA (PL 110-233), which prohibits discrimination or categorization of applicants or employees based on that information and mandates that genetic information be treated as confidential medical information. Many states have implemented similar laws for genetic protection. (Further discussion of the genetic and genomics topic occurs in Chapter 16.) Other laws passed addressed veterans' health, domestic violence, premature birth, and nursing education with reauthorizations, changes to regulations and programs, and renewed allocations. The ACA addressing health reform in 2010 and later actions are addressed in a separate section that follows.

Managed Care

The rise in health care costs has contributed to the rise of managed care organizations and more policy focused on health care costs over the past three decades. Care provided

TABLE 6.2   Selected Policies Affecting Health and Nursing Passed From 2001–Present

Year	Title	Content/Purpose
2003	Nurse Reinvestment Act (PL 107-205)	Provides funding for nurse recruitment, retention, education, and care for special populations and underserved areas
2003	Medicare Modernization Act (PL 108-173)	Provides prescription drug benefit (Part D); enhances new Medicare Advantage regional health plan choices (Part C)
2004	Asthmatic Schoolchildren's Treatment and Health Management Act (PL 108-377)	Rewards states that require schools to allow students to self-administer medications for asthma or anaphylaxis
2007	Paul Wellstone Mental Health and Addiction Equity Act (PL 110-343)	Requires equity in the provision of mental health and sub-stance-related disorder benefits under group health
2007	Conquer Childhood Cancer Act (PL 110-285)	Amends the Public Health Service Act to advance medical research and treatments into pediatric cancers; ensures patients and families have access to the current treatments and information regarding pediatric cancers
2007	National Breast and Cervical Cancer Early Detection Program Reauthori-zation Act (PL 110-18)	Established to provide waivers relating to grants for preventive health measures with respect to breast and cervical cancers
2007	Trauma Care Systems Planning and Development Act (PL 110-23)	Established to amend the Public Health Service Act to add requirements regarding trauma care and for other purposes
2007	Joshua Omvig Veterans Suicide Prevention Act (PL 110-110)	Developed to direct the Secretary of Veterans Affairs to develop and implement a comprehensive program designed to reduce the incidence of suicide among veterans
2007	Charlie W. Norwood Living Organ Donation Act (PL 110-144)	Established to amend the National Organ Transplant Act to provide that criminal penalties do not apply to human organ paired donation
2008	Genetic Information Nondiscrimina-tion Act (PL 110-233)	Established to prohibit discrimination of applicants and employees based on genetic information
2009	Children's Health Insurance Program Reauthorization Act (PL 111-3)	Established to amend Social Security Act Title XXI to reautho-rize the CHIP program through year 2013 at increased levels
2012	Child Protection Act (PL 112-206)	Penalties for child pornography, defines child witness protec-tion, and establishes task force
2013	Violence Against Women Reauthoriza-tion Act	Reauthorizes funds and enforcements
2013	Prematurity Research Expansion and Education for Mothers who deliver Infants Early (PL 113-55)	Authorizes the PREEMIE act through 2017, includes priority for telehealth services, prenatal and postnatal care, and establishes the Advisory Committee on Infant Mortality
2015	Medicare Access and CHIP Reautho-rization Act (MARCA) (PL 114-10)	Revised physician rates, changed to merit-based incentive program (including NP, CNS, CRNA); established metrics for HER; study telehealth; revised Medicare Advantage payment; extends CHIP, SSA titles V, XX, etc.
2016	Comprehensive Addition and Recovery Act (PL 114-198)	Pain management best practices; opioid abuse reduction
2017	Tax Cut and Jobs Act (PL 115-97)	Removed the individual mandate and penalties
2021	American Rescue Plan Act (PL 117-2)	Funds for COVID-19 vaccine Funds for health-care workforce Funds to agencies to assist persons with social determinants of health risks

under cost agreements has become the primary substructure for health care. Capitated costs under Medicare started in 1983 with DRGs. Formal Medicare Choice and Medicare Advantage managed care plans were established through care choice options in the mid- to late-1990s. The number of Americans participating in managed care plans increased steadily between the 1990s and 2005. In 1998, approximately 80% of Americans with employer-sponsored health insurance had managed care plans. Medicare included options for Part C Medicare Advantage Plans that could be chosen by Medicare-eligible persons. In 2021, almost 30% of Medicare beneficiaries (20 million) were enrolled in managed care plans called Medicare Advantage programs or Part C. Initial Medicaid managed care plans were established through HCFA 1915(b) and 1115 waivers to states in the early 1990s and have continued through 2021. In addition, CHIP and ACA allowed states to expand Medicaid programs and enrollment in managed care. By 2022, Medicaid-eligible persons numbered more than 70 million, the great majority of whom are covered under managed care.

A presidential order required the DHHS to enact regulations of consumer rights for Medicare and Medicaid beneficiaries with managed care options. However, the bipartisan debate continues over accountability and liability with managed care. State courts, and now the U.S. Supreme Court, deal with the issue of whether a patient has the right to sue a managed care organization for services provided or withheld based on economic rationale rather than clinical decision-making. Individuals have the right to notification of denial, changes in benefits, provider networks, and network institutions such as hospitals and pharmacies. In addition, most states provide the right to information—written and verbal—concerning the appeal or grievance processes, including a mechanism for arbitration over disputed denial of care. National- and state-level patient "bills of rights" have been enacted that require these issues and ensure equitable care. The Employment Retirement Income Security Act (ERISA) of 1974 and its reauthorizations also ensure certain worker rights regarding health care coverage as part of retirement benefits.

The most recent federal managed care activity is the addition of Accountable Care Organizations (ACOs) under Medicare as required by the ACA. This type of managed care organization is different from the original managed care that was started in the 1980s. The original managed care was directed at controlling or capitating costs as the primary goal and was often a business organization that may or may not have medical or other health professionals in charge. The ACOs are groups of physicians, providers, hospitals, and clinical and other health services that organize together to provide comprehensive services and coordinate health care. The purpose was to improve the quality of care, which is assumed to be cost-effective and improve health. Based on effectiveness and enrollment, ACOs can earn rewards or deficits from CMS in the Shared Savings Program. There are many allowances for confidential and proprietary information not shared with patients from ACOs. The CMS quality metrics are just being fully implemented in 2018. As of 2022, there are 483 ACOs with 1353 hospitals and 528,996 physicians, physician assistants (PA), NP, and CNS providers covering more than 11 million beneficiaries (CMS, 2022b).

State Nurse Practice Acts

Legislation and related policies that directly affect nurses are addressed in state practice acts, or other legislation governing health care professionals. The nurse practice acts, other legislation, and corresponding rules and regulations define educational preparation and programs, eligibility for licensure, and the scope of practice. All states require eligible nurses to pass the National Council Licensure Examination (NCLEX-RN) for initial registered nurse licensure. Candidates for licensure must have graduated from a program approved by the state board of nursing, but the requirements for graduation from a nationally accredited school vary among states. Nursing practice in most states includes research, education, administration, counseling, and clinical practice or direct patient care. The interstate RN and licensed practical nurse/licensed vocational nurse (LPN/LVN) licensure compact was initially developed through the National Council of State Boards of Nursing (NCSBN) in 1998, and the first states joined in 2000. In 2013, the compact had 24 member states and in 2022, 39 states and territories were members. This compact allowed RNs to practice in member states without having a separate license, especially for persons living near state borders. In July 2017, the Enhanced Licensure Compact (eNLC) was enacted when the North Carolina governor signed legislation that provided the 26th and final required state membership. January 19, 2018 is the initial date that member states can issue the new compact RN or LPN/LVN licenses. This initiative provides for new telehealth care provisions and other nonlocation-based practices. Nursing has found that it often can best manage its practice through rules and regulations that require only a state-recognized licensing board or committee to approve changes rather than null legislative action. Nursing licensure and the compact and state nurse practice acts are discussed further in Chapter 11.

In addition to state boards of nursing, many national organizations play a role in defining practice. The NCSBN develops the licensure examination for nurses. The ANCC and various national specialty organizations determine eligibility, educational qualifications, experience, and examinations for national certification required in many states. This is especially true for advanced practice nursing. In some states, an advanced practice nurse can practice without certification but cannot have prescriptive privileges unless national certification is obtained. In other states, certification either is not required or is required for both.

State practice acts are statutes requiring legislative approval for establishment and amendment. In the past, most changes occurred in the legislative arena. More recently, state boards of nursing have developed specific rules and regulations concerning practice that can be changed without legislative activity. This avoids the possibility of undesirable statute revisions that might occur when "opening" the practice act for legislative revision. Additionally, the rules and regulations allow the nursing profession to articulate the practice, roles, and responsibilities of nurses rather than having other entities define nursing. One example is that of anesthesia assistants or unlicensed personnel. For example, there is a national movement to allow anesthesia assistants and other unlicensed personnel to accept responsibilities and use titles traditionally reserved for RNs, LPNs, and certified registered nurse anesthetists (CRNAs). In addition, nurse practitioners are actively collaborating with state nursing associations and national nursing, lay, and professional organizations to achieve prescriptive privilege and independent practice.

NURSING AND HEALTH POLICY

Health policy, regulations, allocations, and care affect nursing and the practice environment and are in turn affected by nursing in several ways. The following sections focus on nursing practice, education, research, and the nursing discipline. The discipline requires professional nurses to conduct scholarly inquiry and participate in social and public policy through multiple avenues.

Practice

Today the health care arena requires nursing administrators and staff to be aware of economic, communication, transparency, and ethical issues to a greater extent than previously encountered. This entails knowledge of budgets and health payment, the use of community resources, product evaluation, technology, benchmarking, patient safety, quality, and outcomes accountability. Consumers are more educated and aware of their health needs and rights in today's world. Although the types of services may be different according to a particular agency, setting, or location, a standard level of competency, transparency, and accountability is required in all practice environments.

One effort to indicate quality and accountability by health care institutions is the Magnet hospital program. The ANA, through the ANCC, developed the Magnet Nursing Services Recognition Program (MNSRP) in the late 1990s. This program is a voluntary external professional nurse peer review of the nursing practice and care environment of any hospital that wishes to participate. The review includes an examination of the extent to which a hospital meets specific standards of care, which are incorporated within the model of professional practice at each site. The process of applying for Magnet status involves both a written application and a site visit by a board of experts. Applicants are required to demonstrate nurse-sensitive quality at the unit or system level and to meet established state, regional, or national benchmarks. Governance, research, patient safety, and feedback processes are all part of Magnet criteria. If a facility is designated as a Magnet hospital, the effective practice environment and the resulting quality of nursing care should be evident.

For individual nurses, standards are provided by professional organizations, including the ANA's *Standards of Clinical Nursing Practice, Scope and Standards of Advanced Practice Registered Nurses,* and other specialty standards for practice, in response to both societal and professional requests for clarification of nursing. Identification of competencies, such as those for wound and ostomy care, cultural competence, and genetics, may be required for nurses across practice settings. Studies examining nurse competence also are needed. Effectiveness studies that support competent and quality practice also influence legislation. The RWJF established the INQRI in 2005. Nurses Dunston, Boyle, and colleagues at the University of Kansas led those efforts to develop measures of acute care nursing through the ANA-supported National Database for Nursing Quality Indicators (NDNQI), now owned by Press Ganey. Dr. Linda Cronenwett led the phased Quality and Safety in Education for Nursing (QSEN) initiative that developed content and competencies to improve quality and safety in the nursing curriculum. These guidelines and activities indicate to legislators and the public that nursing contributes to better health outcomes, quality care, and cost-appropriate care.

Self-development, continuing education, certification, and learning new skill sets (retooling) will be required as the health care delivery system continues to evolve. This learning must be of an interprofessional nature, including terminology and new taxonomy languages, client needs, treatment, and evaluation of outcomes, quality, and access. Hospitals and clinics will continue as settings, but the move to community-based settings, long-term care, alternative care settings, and delivery methods that assist clients to achieve health must be initiated and embraced. Care coordination, quality improvement, leadership, and chronic care management can assist in meeting the needs of specific populations. Homeless clinics, parish nursing, mobile health, and collaborative efforts with physician practices and school systems are additional delivery methods that provide community-based care to vulnerable populations. Expanding roles for APNs and RNs in settings such as primary care, health departments, telehealth, and outpatient clinics can improve access to care, and the quality of care provided.

Education

Authorization for nursing education originated with the Nurse Training Act of 1964. Between 1965 and 1971, more than $380 million was spent on nursing education for both students and institutions. In the 1990s, with the onset of managed care and increased competition for health care dollars, the nursing education legislation was twice not enacted. Passage of the Health Professions Education Partnership Act in 1998 changed the tradition by which nursing was the only health profession to retain a separate funding law. Congressional funding for nursing education has increased and expanded to include baccalaureate, master's, and doctoral levels, but enrollments have not increased to meet the projected needs in most areas of the country as of 2022.

To address the major shortages specific to nursing, the Nurse Reinvestment Act and subsequent legislative versions have been passed. The focus of these efforts was on funding and implementing strategies for nurse recruitment and nurse retention. Scholarships (Nursing Loan Repayment and Scholarships) are available to those nurses willing to work in health care facilities with a critical nursing shortage. HRSA has revised priority from primarily funding master's nursing programs to increased funding for nursing doctoral programs, especially Doctor of Nursing Practice programs. The funding is in multiple areas, including traineeships to students, the Nurse Faculty Loan Program, and DNP program grants with clinical partners. In addition, the Jonas Center for Nursing Excellence established the Jonas Nurse Leaders Scholar Program, which provides funding for doctoral education for aspiring nurse leaders and veterans, funding multiple schools and scholars each year. Shortages in practice settings will become greater as baby boomers retire, and nursing faculty will continue to be recruited to prepare the nurses necessary for health care in the next few decades. Grants and contracts are awarded to schools of nursing that expand their programs by increasing enrollment in 4-year programs, providing internships and residency programs for nursing students, and providing new programs such as distance learning using new technologies. This Nurse Education, Practice, Quality, and Retention

(NEPRQ) program fosters the area of practice by providing funding for nurses caring for underserved populations and populations in noninstitutional settings, as well as for nurses interested in developing primary care, mobile health, and cultural competencies. Low-interest-rate loans—for instance, through the Nurse Faculty Loan Program (NFLP)—are available to master's and doctoral students who agree to work full-time in a school of nursing or nursing department after graduation or the NURSE CORPS scholarship and loan repayment program for ADN, BSN, or graduate program students. Nursing Workforce Diversity (NWD) grants provide educational funds to persons from disadvantaged backgrounds. The HRSA nursing workforce FY 2020 funding for Title VIII specific to nursing was $264 million, and the Consolidated Appropriations Act of 2021 increased overall for HRSA Title VII and VIII workforce training. Large increases in mental and behavioral health training were included, with nursing-specific priorities less clear.

Federal dollars are the largest source of external funding for nursing education, primarily provided through the DHHS BHP. Most of these federal dollars provide program funding; however, available funding for nursing students themselves is often inadequate. Various foundations provide scholarships for nursing workforce development. The Jonas Foundation has established a center for nursing and veteran's health care that provides leadership training, scholarship funds, and innovative models of nursing education. The John A. Hartford Foundation has funded gerontology centers, training programs, fellowships, and educational innovation for two decades. Partnerships with medical centers, ACOs, and payers, such as the University of Kentucky and the Norton Healthcare Institute for Nursing, to increase the number of advanced practice graduates and the University of North Carolina Hillman Scholars Program in Nursing Innovation to expose BSN-level students to leadership opportunities both provide additional avenues to develop and grow the nursing workforce.

The NLN initiated the accreditation of nursing programs. Policies relative to accreditation came under scrutiny by the U.S. Department of Education in the 1990s, and the NLNAC was established as a freestanding entity. In 1999 the CCNE, which evolved from the AACN, gained recognition from the Department of Education and now accredits most baccalaureate and graduate programs. In 2013 the NLNAC was dissolved, and a new body, the Accreditation Commission for Education in Nursing (ACEN), was created. Subsequently, NLN announced plans for a new accreditation department (NLN) Commission for Nursing Education Accreditation (CNEA) on February 21, 2013, in response to the needs of the nursing education community and the nursing profession. This organization accredits associate, baccalaureate, and graduate degree programs. These accrediting bodies understand the importance of the Pew Commission Report, the Kellogg-sponsored Sullivan Commission DHHS priorities, and congressional requirements, as well as innovation and an evolving health care arena. Schools and staff development departments are encouraged to initiate new curricula, develop creative teaching methods, stimulate lifelong learning, evaluate innovative methods and modes of delivering content, establish competency-based educational programs that may include simulation and e-learning, focus on *Healthy People 2030,* address health disparities and diversity issues across practice, education, and research settings, and evaluate care delivered at all levels across settings. The AACN released new Essentials for professional nursing education, the Consensus Model for APRN Regulation: Licensure, Accreditation, Certification, and Education; and the quality indicators and Pathways to Excellence for research doctoral education are excellent beginning guidelines that will need to be evaluated and revised as the health care industry changes. Clinical doctorate programs, including the DNP, are now funded by the HRSA through Advanced Nursing Education Workforce (ANEW) program grants. In addition, workforce, staffing, and quality of care studies are germane to nurses at the local and state levels as nurses lobby for continued authorization of funding programs and reimbursement and demonstrate quality-of-care benchmarks.

Successful efforts to foster collaboration and improve evidence-based practice and provide effective education are needed. The studies and directions they lead to, based on findings, will influence the practice environments by identifying appropriate staffing, quality, and effective workforce development to improve health.

Research

The establishment of the NINR at the NIH in 1993, and its reauthorizations, have affected nursing research. First established as the NCNR in April 1986, with the purpose of providing a strong scientific base for nursing practice, it became the NINR in 2000 and serves as an integral part of the NIH. The NINR National Advisory Council for Nursing Research (NACNR) participates in setting the NIH agenda, budget priorities, and funding recommendations. The NINR has led the NIH efforts to include the elimination of health disparities in its strategic plan. The program areas at the NINR in the 1990s were consistent with the national priorities set by the NIH and *Healthy People 2020.* The priority focus areas identified by the NINR for the new 2022–2026 strategic plan are Health Equity, Social Determinants of Health, Population and Community Health, Prevention and Health Promotion, and Systems and Models of Care.

The NINR funds investigators who are not nurses; likewise, nurses receive funding from institutes other than the NINR. An interdisciplinary focus of projects is emphasized across program areas shared with many institutes, including the National Institute on Aging (NIA), the NIMH, the NICHD, the NIMHD, NIOSH, and the AHRQ. NIOSH funds studies and interventions for workplace safety, as well as education and research centers (https://www.cdc.gov/niosh/index.htm). The AHRQ supports the efforts to define patient safety indicators, improvement of delivery systems, clinical decision-making, and consumer assessment of health plans (http://www.ahrq.gov). The Eunice Kennedy Shriver NICHD supports studies related to the Best Pharmaceuticals for Children Act, and the NIMHD funds Centers of Excellence (COE) in Health Disparities Research. Nurses serve as nurse principal investigators and directors of these types of centers.

The Substance Abuse and Mental Health Services Administration (SAMHSA) has supported demonstration projects to develop tools for Preadmission Screening and Resident Review (PASRR) for nursing homes (see http://www.samhsa.gov) and training programs for mental health professionals. One of the newest forms of interdisciplinary study the federal government funds is the PCORI. Dr. Debra Moser, a nursing professor, led the team in comparing heart health interventions among the underserved in Appalachia. The Clinical and Translational Science Awards efforts and activities have been led by nurses such as Drs. Catherine Gillis and Teresa Kelechi.

Nurses provide leadership in many ways. For example, Dr. Martha Hill, former dean of The Johns Hopkins University School of Nursing, cochaired the committee to develop the IOM's *Unequal Treatment* report, which guides much of the system and disparities interventions. Dr. Audrey Nelson led efforts to improve patient safety and quality of care through the VA. Dr. Cornelia Beck, a Distinguished Professor at the University of Arkansas Medical Sciences, provided leadership in the national efforts to alleviate suffering from Alzheimer's disease. In addition, HIV/AIDS work has been led by Drs. William Holzemer and Nancy McCain, with an emphasis on biobehavioral interventions. AAN EdgeRunners, Drs. Szanton, Jemmott, Villaruel, Lipman, Hench, Reiss-Brennan, Gerrity, Ortega, and Reed provide innovative and effective models of care for elders, children, rural health, and mental health patients (AAN, 2022).

Research directions have been guided by foundations such as the RWJF and the W. K. Kellogg Foundation, which have funded community and rural health initiatives. Findings from nursing investigations and experience have resulted in input to the development of practice guidelines. The work of Drs. Bergstrom, Wyman, and Wells and their colleagues influenced the AHRQ practice guidelines for decubitus ulcers and incontinence. Nurses identify science agendas through regional and national organizations (Chipps et al., 2021). Also, nurses develop guidelines such as the Report of the American College of Cardiology on Pathways for heart failure patients (Maddox et al., 2021). Nurse researchers have investigated factors related to different health concerns in U.S. and international populations (Melhem et al., 2022), as well as the effectiveness of interventions for vulnerable populations (Amirehsani et al., 2021; Derella et al., 2021). In addition, Elaine Larson, Patricia Stone, and colleagues at Columbia Medical Center have built knowledge to prevent infections in hospitals and provided a cost analysis of those interventions.

The NINR, Sigma Theta Tau International, the four regional nursing research societies (Southern, Midwest, Eastern, and Western), specialty organizations, Friends of NINR, and the National Nursing Research Roundtable meet annually to discuss and plan for the direction, implementation, and funding of nursing research. Regional and national conferences and the Council for the Advancement of Nursing Science (CANS) State of the Science Congress highlight nursing research findings that influence health care delivery, costs, access, and outcomes. Congressional members and persons from local, state, and regional political and legislative arenas are invited to attend these meetings to discuss nursing and health care efforts and needs. Additional research activities include the VA Nursing Research Initiative (NRI), the American Nurses Foundation (ANF) awards, AHRQ nursing fellowships and grants, the RWJF, the W. K. Kellogg Foundation, and the Templeton Foundation. Nurses also fill positions as clinical researchers in medical centers across the country and conduct ongoing studies.

Outcomes and Quality

Outcomes and comparative effectiveness research are now required to determine the effectiveness and accountability of practice. Much effort is directed at defining what constitutes outcomes and how to measure them. Outcome research is a priority in the area of health services research. One policy initiative was the enactment of the Healthcare Research and Quality Act of 1999, which changed the name of the Agency for Health Care Policy and Research (AHCPR) to the AHRQ. This emphasis provides that research on outcomes and quality will provide a foundation for future policy, regulation, and allocation decisions for health care. National health indicators, *Healthy People 2030,* and the DHHS initiative to eliminate racial and ethnic disparities provide another set of outcomes and measures of quality. Examining system outcomes is one avenue of research. System outcomes are those related to direct and indirect material and financial costs, length of stay, manpower, provider qualifications, and provider and payer satisfaction. Delivery system change, nurse workforce issues, and client outcomes such as consumer satisfaction, health status outcomes, adaptation, and function require study. Nurses will lead many of these efforts. For example, Li and Jones (2021) investigated (https://pubmed.ncbi.nlm.nih.gov/33814158/) care provision by Nurse Practitioners and physicians, with findings that NPs were likely to provide more therapeutic or preventive care than physicians. Bacon and colleagues (2021a) report that organizational climate is related to the failure to rescue patients and mortality in acute care. Also, the team found that an organizational safety climate is related to nurse resource management (Bacon et al., 2021b). Another focus in patient outcomes research is the avoidance of missed care opportunities (Campbell et al., 2020) that nurses identify for a variety of reasons including resources and staffing. One such study was in Alabama, where Campbell and colleagues (2020) investigated built environment and care patterns, findings of which suggested that nurses identify opportunities for missed care and reasons for poor care.

In addition, nursing should be involved in the transformation of the health system and the determination of metrics for quality practice and patient outcomes. The use of QSEN, the National Quality Strategy, HP2030, and PCORI offer nurses methods by which to participate and lead outcomes and quality efforts. This will be a specific area for nursing to address in future practice, education, and research efforts. Future nursing efforts will be guided by the ANA's health policy analyses, position statements, and ethics and practice guidelines to set forth priorities for workforce development, quality care, health access, and evolving practice environments, as well as partnerships such as the National Quality Forum. Beyond the health disparities work that has been completed, the new focus on health equity and how structural racism impacts the social determinants of health, built environment and resulting health outcomes is highly important. All the national organizations and the NINR include equity as the lens that must be used across education, practice, research, and delivery arenas. The Code, professional priorities, and societal trust in our profession necessitate a transformation. As noted in the next section, achieving health equity involves active participation in health policy.

NURSE PARTICIPATION IN HEALTH POLICY

Nurses have increasingly become active participants in the health policy arena as advocates and activists and in writing health policies at the state and federal levels. Nursing has progressed through several stages in its political development and involvement in the policy arena. Nursing is currently at the "leadership" stage, where it is recognized as a political entity with a recognizable agenda that guides health policy. The ANA has been consulted for advice and has offered recommendations on health care reform and health policies, such as the Women's Health Initiative (WHI). A prime example occurred during the debate about health care reform in 2010 and subsequent years. The ACA implementation discussions resulted in ANA issuing briefs, position papers, and principal statements on access to care for immigrants, nursing workforce development, use of unlicensed personnel, expanding NP practice, staffing guidelines, and measuring the quality of care. These documents have been developed and shared with leaders of organizations representing health care providers, insurers, policymakers, employers, labor unions, and consumers. However, nursing often misses opportunities for input, such as with the Oral Health Initiative, partially because nurses fail to recognize or champion one another as experts.

Representative Capps (D-NC), a nurse, was instrumental in writing the initial Nurse Reinvestment Act in 2002. The original intent has been accomplished primarily through HRSA funding for graduate programs, nurse scholarships, grants to health care facilities to improve nurse retention and patient safety, faculty loan repayment, and funding for new undergraduate programs. Reauthorizations have been enacted since that time. In addition, the ACA (PL 111-148) and the partnering Health Care and Education Reconciliation Act of 2010 (PL 111-152) established the Graduate Nurse Education Demonstration program to develop a system of payments to hospitals for the costs of clinical training for APNs, reauthorized the Nursing Workforce Development programs, and created a National Health Care Workforce Commission. However, the appropriation of adequate support continues to be a concern.

Nurses have been instrumental in the policy arena, advocating for change in policies that affect nurses and health. Nurses are involved in numerous legislative efforts such as the NLSP and state and local efforts to improve nutrition for children. National efforts are evaluated for impact. In another example, nurses who were members of Virginia's Old Dominion Society of Gastroenterology Nurses and Associates (SGNA) initiated the introduction of legislation to promote insurance payment for colorectal screening. This effort began when a nurse working at a gastroenterology unit in Virginia became concerned about the number of patients who were diagnosed with late-stage colon cancer because they did not get early screening. The President of SGNA contacted Virginia State Senator Emily Couric, sharing the group's concern about the lack of colorectal screening and asking her to

write a legislative mandate for insurance coverage of colonoscopies. Through these efforts, Virginia became the first state to pass legislation mandating insurance coverage for colonoscopies to all individuals, including those covered by Medicaid. In addition, Senator Couric's sister, Katie Couric, and others participate in the Screen for Life: National Colorectal Cancer Action Campaign (CDC, 2022). In the past two decades, there have been more than 678,000 television, 1 million radio, and 628,000 digital public service announcements to inform the public about colorectal cancer screening.

In other areas, NPs have been active in passing state laws dealing with prescription drug rights. Nurse anesthetists have been active in legislation dealing with their practice. The North Carolina Association of Nurse Anesthetists (NCANA) has been active in fighting to preserve the authority of CRNAs in North Carolina and against legislation that would allow licensing of anesthesiologist assistants. Julie Ann Lowery, President of the NCANA, reached out to grassroots groups and North Carolina residents to encourage nurses' involvement in preventing legislation that would jeopardize CRNAs' practice in North Carolina.

These are only a few examples of nurse activism in the policy arena. As nurses become more informed, passionate, and committed in their policy arena leadership role, legislation at the state and federal levels will require input from nurses to advocate for patients, the public, and themselves.

HEALTH CARE REFORM 2010 TO 2021

The historic health care insurance reform law, the ACA of 2010 (PL 111-148), was signed into law by President Obama on March 23, 2010, and its companion Health Care and Education Affordability Reconciliation Act (PL 111-152) was signed into law on March 30, 2010. Bills are typed in a particular format that greatly expands the number of pages, and the complexity of the current health care system required that many interconnections be addressed.

The government website (http://www.healthcare.gov) provides useful information for patients who are enrolled or wish to enroll in ACA exchanges. Table 6.3 provides a summary of the 10 titles included in the ACA, including the elements of the companion Reconciliation Act. The Office of Consumer Information and Insurance Oversight (OCIIO) was created within the DHHS to implement many of the provisions of the legislation that address private health insurance. Some provisions were enacted in 2010, and other provisions were enacted over the past few years. The full Act was anticipated to be implemented by 2014; however, legislative, regulatory, and political issues delayed some provisions until 2018. For example, the individual mandate to purchase health insurance was delayed because

TABLE 6.3 Patient Protection and Affordable Care Act of 2010 (PL 111-148) and Health Care and Education Reconciliation Act of 2010

Summary With Designation of New and Existing Authorities

Title	Description
Title I: Quality Affordable Health Care for All Americans	This Act allows individuals, families, and small business owners to make decisions about their health care. Premium costs are reduced for millions of working families and small businesses by providing hundreds of billions of dollars in tax relief—the largest middle-class tax cut for health care in history. Out-of-pocket expenses are capped, and preventive care must be fully covered without out-of-pocket expense. For many Americans, their insurance coverage is not expected to change. Qualified health plans have been defined, and exchange pools have been established for Americans without insurance coverage so they can choose their insurance coverage. The insurance exchange pools' buying power gives Americans choices of private insurance plans that have to compete for their business based on cost and quality. Small business owners may choose insurance coverage through this exchange and receive a tax credit to help offset the cost of covering their employees.
	The Act bans insurance companies from denying insurance coverage because of preexisting medical conditions and provides consumers new power to appeal insurance company decisions that deny provider-ordered treatments covered by insurance.
	The DHHS Secretary has the authority to implement many of these new provisions to help families and small business owners have the information they need to make the choices that work best for them.
Title II: The Role of Public Programs	The Act extends Medicaid while treating all states equally. It preserves CHIP, the successful children's insurance plan, and simplifies enrollment for individuals and families.
	Community-based care for Americans with disabilities is enhanced, and states will have opportunities to expand home care services to people with long-term care needs.
	The Act gives flexibility to states to adopt innovative strategies to improve care and the coordination of services for Medicare and Medicaid beneficiaries.
	The Secretary has the authority to work with states and other partners to strengthen strategic public programs.
Title III: Improving the Quality and Efficiency of Health Care	The Act closes the Medicare prescription coverage gap called the "donut hole." In addition, the Act provides incentives for providers and hospitals that improve care and reduce errors.
	The Act enhances access to health care services in rural and underserved areas. Funding is provided for school-based and nurse-managed centers to assist in providing this care.
	Another change is the addition of a group of doctors and health care experts, rather than only members of Congress, who identify ideas to improve quality and reduce costs for Medicare beneficiaries.
	The Secretary has the authority to take steps to strengthen the Medicare program and implement reforms to improve the quality and efficiency of health care.
Title IV: Prevention of Chronic Disease and Improving Public Health	The Act directs the creation of a national prevention and health promotion strategy that incorporates the most effective and achievable methods to improve the health status of Americans and reduce the incidence of preventable illness and disability in the United States. Included in this title are the availability of science-based nutrition information and waiving copayments for America's seniors on Medicare for prevention and health screenings.
	The Secretary has the authority to coordinate with other departments, develop and implement a prevention and health promotion strategy, and work to ensure that more Americans have access to critical preventive health services.

Continued

TABLE 6.3   Patient Protection and Affordable Care Act of 2010 (PL 111-148) and Health Care and Education Reconciliation Act of 2010

Summary With Designation of New and Existing Authorities—cont'd

Title	Description
Title V: Health Care Workforce	The Act funds scholarships and loan repayment programs to increase the number of primary care physicians, nurses, physician assistants, mental health providers, and dentists in the areas of the country that need them most. In addition, funds are provided to expand, construct, and operate community health centers, with specific funding for nurse-managed health centers. Expansions are also noted for the advanced education nursing programs, the Nurse Faculty Loan Program, the Nurse Loan Repayment and Scholarship Program, and the Nursing Student Loan Program. The Secretary has the authority to take action to strengthen many existing programs that help support the primary care workforce.
Title VI: Transparency and Program Integrity	The Act includes the Nursing Home Transparency program so that consumers can compare facilities. The Act protects whistleblowers, and it requires staffing accountability and disclosure. Finally, the Act imposes rigorous disclosure requirements to identify high-risk providers who have defrauded the American taxpayer. It gives states new authority to prevent providers who have been penalized in one state from setting up in another and the flexibility to propose and test tort reforms for improving health care. The Secretary has new and improved authority to promote transparency and ensure that every dollar in the Act and in existing programs is spent wisely and well.
Title VII: Improving Access to Innovative Medical Therapies	The Act extends drug discounts to hospitals and communities that serve low-income patients and creates a pathway for the creation of generic versions of biological drugs. The Secretary of Health and Human Services has the authority to implement these provisions to help make medications more affordable.
Title VIII: Community Living Assistance Services and Support Act (CLASS)	The Act provides Americans with a new option to finance long-term services and care in the event of a disability. It is a self-funded and voluntary long-term care insurance option. Workers pay premiums to receive a daily cash benefit if they develop a disability. Need is based on difficulty in performing basic activities such as bathing or dressing. The benefit is flexible—it could be used for a range of community support services, from respite care to home care. Safeguards will be put in place to ensure that its premiums are enough to cover its costs. The Secretary has the authority to establish the CLASS Program.
Title IX: Revenue Provisions	The Act provides new tax credits that will reduce health premium costs for middle-class families and allow them to exchange pools for insurance purchase. Families making less than $250,000 are the primary targets of these provisions. This title will be implemented by the U.S. Department of the Treasury.
Title X: Family Planning Program	The Act reauthorizes the Indian Health Care Improvement Act (IHCIA), which provides health care services to American Indians and Alaskan Natives. The Secretary, in consultation with the Indian Health Service, has the authority to implement the Indian Health Care Improvement Act.

of website access problems, then by legislation in December 2013. The business mandate was delayed allowing time for regulations and consideration of cost levels, mostly by Executive Orders of President Obama in January and February 2014. As of January 2022, 39 states and the District of Columbia regular and expanded Medicaid programs under the ACA covered more than 76 million persons, up from 55 million in 2017 (CMS, 2021). These expansions include a combination of eligibility changes by poverty level, services provided, and CMS-approved waiver programs that are highly subsidized by the federal budget. The remaining 12 states are Alabama, Florida, Georgia, Kansas, Mississippi, North Carolina, South Carolina, South Dakota, Tennessee, Texas, Wisconsin, and Wyoming. The ACA Medicaid expansion was designed to address the high uninsured rates among adults living below the poverty line by providing coverage options for individuals with limited access to employer coverage and/or limited income to purchase coverage in the individual insurance market. Additionally, the expansion was designed to end categorical eligibility for Medicaid. With many states opting for Medicaid expansion, millions of adults have been added to insurance coverage. However, the millions of persons in the nonexpansion states remain outside of this health insurance reform initiative. Within that insurance gap, those persons do not qualify for publicly financed coverage in their state, do not have access to employer-sponsored coverage, or cannot afford to purchase insurance on their own. Most of these people are the "working-poor," employed either part-time or full-time but still living below the poverty line. Based on the state-specific population characteristics, these decisions not to expand disproportionately affect people of color, particularly black Americans in eastern and southern states. This has implications for efforts to address health disparities and health equity in health coverage, access, and outcomes among people of color. The ACA allows persons younger than 26 years of age to remain or return to their parent's insurance coverage if certain conditions are met, removes lifetime limits on health coverage, and removes the use of preexisting conditions as a reason to deny or terminate coverage. An online web portal is used for persons to enroll in the health insurance market through exchanges. States have made decisions regarding developing their own insurance exchanges or allowing the federal government to develop an exchange within the state.

In addition, the ACA allowed an expansion of Medicaid, which many states have enacted, as noted previously. The decisions were logistical, political, and financial. As with any legislation, the ACA titles will be revised, removed, or implemented in future years. In addition, courts will be involved in decisions regarding the ACA in the future, like the 2013 U.S. Supreme Court decisions on the ACA that the individual mandate is required and that Medicaid expansion could not be required by the states. One such change has been the repeal of the individual mandate and associated penalties and tax liabilities in the Tax Cut and Jobs Act of 2017 (PL 115-97). Another change has been the level of federal government subsidies provided for exchanges in 2017. Given the needs, costs, and political discourse, additional changes to ACA titles, regulations, and allocations will occur, as will continued legal challenges to the law and sections of the law.

SUMMARY

As members of the largest group of health professionals and major providers of care, nurses can influence health care policy as individuals and as professionals. Consumers of health care, including nurses, desire affordable, accessible, and high-quality care. Nurses are obligated to ensure that the public has access to quality health care at controlled costs. Identifying and prioritizing client needs with sensitivity to culture and diversity, acquiring and demonstrating a knowledge of treatments and interventions (both nursing and interdisciplinary), maintaining a focus on outcomes (client, system, and provider), and ensuring safe, quality care in multiple environments are basic responsibilities of professional nursing in the 21st century.

Armed with information on how to influence health care policy, nurses serve as advocates for patients and active participants in the formation of effective health care policy. Organizational membership in regional, state, or national organizations and letter writing are two traditional activities for nurses involved in policymaking. More focused involvement can be achieved through collective actions as members of PACs and political parties. Social, civic, professional, and lay organizations with an interest in specific populations and concerns also provide a mechanism by which nurses can influence legislation and allocation decisions. Another avenue is to run for elected office or sit on boards, committees, councils, or commissions, especially those that make policy and funding decisions that affect health care. Opportunities exist and can be developed to share expertise and communicate nursing needs through consultation with elected officials, health agencies, foundations, educational institutions, and funding agencies. Policy decisions regarding financial resources influence the type of nursing staff, the number of nurses, the amount and type of management and support services, and the extent of educational program and research funding, all of which affect the practice environment and quality of nursing and health care. The settings and payment of care affect access and the spectrum of services available to the most vulnerable populations. Through professional and personal knowledge, expertise, and experience, nurses can act in research, practice, and education areas. Politics, legislation, and economics provide ample opportunity and challenge for nursing involvement. Taking advantage of these opportunities and meeting the challenge of ensuring access to high-quality health care for all can be achieved through greater involvement in the health policy arena.

SALIENT POINTS

- Health policy is influenced by many factors, including politics, economics, demographics, and personal and societal priorities.
- Legislation is a complex process that includes multiple players, takes time, and involves political and special interests at local, state, and federal levels.
- A large portion of the federal budget and expenditures is directed at health programs, specifically Medicare, Medicaid, and Social Security entitlements.
- Federal and state legislation, as well as rules and regulations to implement policies, influence the availability, access, and spectrum of nursing practice and health care.

- New demographics, equity concerns, and health needs will require changes in the delivery of health care, to whom it is delivered, and the environment and practices of care.
- Outcomes and quality focus are required to ensure quality and useful nursing practice, education, and research.
- Nurses have a responsibility to participate in health policy and planning to ensure the quality and safety of health care and an effective practice environment.
- Knowledge and involvement are keys to influencing health policy.

CRITICAL REFLECTION EXERCISES

1. What are the major health care issues in your community, state, and region? What are some solutions to these problems? How might you become involved in implementing these solutions?
2. Discuss how a practice, workplace, education, or research situation in your experience was directly affected by health policy decisions or allocations. What are the options for changing that policy? What are the barriers and facilitators to changing the policy?
3. Discuss how entitlements should be addressed with a health care provider, a health care economist or

businessperson, and a client. Develop three strategies and share these with your state or national legislator and your professional organization.
4. Discuss your nursing practice and workplace environment and how these are affected by policy decisions at the local, state, and federal levels.
5. What are your responsibilities to ensure access to health equity, quality, timely, appropriate, and cost-effective care?
6. How does the Patient Protection and Affordable Care Act affect your community, state, or agency?

REFERENCES

American Academy of Nursing (AAN). (2022). *Edge Runner profiles.* American Academy of Nursing. https://www.aannet.org/initiatives/edge-runners/profiles

American Association of Colleges of Nursing (AACN). (2020). *Nursing shortage.* American Association of Colleges of Nursing. https://www.aacnnursing.org/news-information/fact-sheets/nursing-shortage

American Association of Colleges of Nursing (AACN). (2021). *Nursing faculty shortage.* American Association of Colleges of Nursing. https://www.aacnnursing.org/News-Information/News/View/ArticleId/25043/data-spotlight-august-2021-Nursing-Faculty-Shortage

Amirehsani, K. A., Hu, J., Wallace, D. C., & McCoy, T. P. (2021). Herbal/plant remedies and supplements used by Hispanics/Latinxs for diabetes: Source of functional foods? *The Science of Diabetes Self-Management and Care, 47*(1), 94–104. https://doi.org/10.1177/0145721720983221

Bacon, C. T., McCoy, T. P., & Henshaw, D. S. (2021a). Exploring the association between organizational safety climate, failure to rescue, and mortality in inpatient surgical units. *The Journal of Nursing Administration, 51*(1), 12–18. https://doi.org/10.1097/NNA.0000000000000960

Bacon, C. T., McCoy, T. P., Henshaw, D. S., & Stabel, C. L. (2021b). Organizational safety climate and job enjoyment in hospital surgical teams with and without crew resource management training. *The Journal of Nursing Administration, 51*(11), E20–E26. https://doi.org/10.1097/NNA.0000000000001071

Campbell, C. M., Prapanjaroensin, A., Anusiewicz, C. V., Baernholdt, M., Jones, T., & Patrician, P. A. (2020). Variables associated with missed nursing care in Alabama: A cross-sectional analysis. *Journal of Nursing Management, 28*(8), 2174–2184. https://doi.org/10.1111/jonm.12979

Centers for Disease Control and Prevention (CDC). (2022). *Screen for life: National colorectal cancer action campaign.* Centers for Disease Control and Prevention. https://www.cdc.gov/cancer/colorectal/sfl/about.htm

Centers for Medicare and Medicaid Services (CMS). (2021). *Medicaid and CHIP total enrollment chart—July 2021.* Centers for Medicare and Medicaid Services. https://www.medicaid.gov/medicaid/program-information/medicaid-and-chip-enrollment-data/report-highlights/index.html

Centers for Medicare and Medicaid Services (CMS). (2022a). *Medicare shared savings program fast facts January 2022*. Centers for Medicare and Medicaid Services. https://www.cms.gov/files/document/2022-shared-savings-program-fast-facts.pdf

Centers for Medicare and Medicaid Services (CMS). (2022b). *National health expenditures*. Centers for Medicare and Medicaid Services. https://www.cms.gov/Research-Statistics-Data-and-Systems/Statistics-Trends-and-Reports/NationalHealthExpendData/NHE-Fact-Sheet

Chipps, E. M., Joseph, M. L., Alexander, C., Lyman, B., McGinty, L., Nelson-Brantley, H., Parchment, J., Rivera, R. R., Schultz, M. A., Ward, D. M., & Weaver, S. (2021). Setting the research agenda for nursing administration and leadership science: A Delphi study. *The Journal of Nursing Administration*, 51(9), 430–438. https://doi.org/10.1097/NNA.0000000000001042

Cubanski, J., & Damico, A. (2022). *Key facts about Medicare Part D enrollment and costs in 2022*. [Issue Brief]. Kaiser Family Foundation. https://www.kff.org/medicare/issue-brief/key-facts-about-medicare-part-d-enrollment-and-costs-in-2022/

Cubanski, J., & Neuman, T. (2021). *Relatively few drugs account for a large share of Medicare prescription drug spending*. [Issue Brief]. Kaiser Family Foundation. https://www.kff.org/medicare/issue-brief/relatively-few-drugs-account-for-a-large-share-of-medicare-prescription-drug-spending/9

Derella, C. C., Tingen, M. S., Blanks, A., Sojourner, S. J., Tucker, M. A., Thomas, J., & Harris R. A. (2021). Smoking cessation reduces systemic inflammation and circulating endothelin 1. *Scientific Reports*, 11(1), 24122. https://doi.org/10.1038/s41598-021-03476-5

Federal Elections Commission (FEC). (2022a). *Contribution limits for 2021–2022 federal elections*. Federal Elections Commission. https://www.fec.gov/help-candidates-and-committees/candidate-taking-receipts/contribution-limits/

Federal Elections Commission (FEC). (2022b). *Campaign finance disclosure portal*. Federal Elections Commission. https://www.fec.gov/data/browse-data/?tab=raising

Li, Y., & Jones, C. B. (2021). Care received by patients from nurse practitioners and physicians in U.S. primary care settings. *Nursing Outlook*, 69(5), 826–835. https://doi.org/10.1016/j.outlook.2021.02.007

Maddox, T. M., Januzzi, J. L., Jr., Allen, L. A., Breathett, K., Butler, J., Davis, L. L., Fonarow, G. C., Ibrahim, N. E., Lindenfeld, J., Masoudi, F. A., Motiwala, S. R., Oliveros, E., Patterson, J. H., Walsh, M. N., Wasserman, A., Yancy, C. W., & Youmans, Q. R. (2021). 2021 Update to the 2017 ACC Expert Consensus Decision Pathway for Optimization of Heart Failure Treatment: Answers to 10 pivotal issues about heart failure with reduced ejection fraction: A report of the American College of Cardiology Solution Set Oversight Committee. *Journal of the American College of Cardiology*, 77(6), 772–810. https://doi.org/10.1016/j.jacc.2020.11.022

Melhem, B. G., Wallace, D. C., Adams, J., Ross, R., & Shreeniwas, S. (2022). Predictors of advance care planning engagement among Muslim community dwelling adults living in the United States. *Journal of Hospice and Palliative Nursing*, 24(3). https://doi.org/10.1097/NJH.0000000000000842

National Academy of Medicine (NAM). (2021). *The Future of Nursing 2020–2030: Charting a path to achieve health equity*. National Academies of Medicine. https://nam.edu/publications/the-future-of-nursing-2020-2030/

National Institutes of Health (NIH). (2022). *Operating plan for 2021*. National Institutes of Health. https://officeofbudget.od.nih.gov/pdfs/FY21/cy/FY%202021%20NIH%20Operating%20Plan_Web.pdf

U.S. Bureau of Labor. (2022). *Employment projections 2020–2030*. U.S. Bureau of Labor. https://www.bls.gov/news.release/ecopro.nr0.htm

U.S. House of Representatives. (2007). *How our laws are made. Document 110-49*. U.S. House of Representatives. https://www.gpo.gov/fdsys/pkg/CDOC-110hdoc49/pdf/CDOC-110hdoc49.pdf

PART II

Dimensions of Professional Nursing Practice

7

Economic Issues in Nursing and Health Care

Richard Ridge, PhD, MBA, RN, NEA-BC

ⓔ http://evolve.elsevier.com/Friberg/bridge/

OBJECTIVES

At the completion of this chapter, the reader will be able to:

- Describe how the economic concepts of supply, demand, complements and substitutes, competition, and market failure apply to nursing and health care.
- Compare and contrast various methods of cost evaluation applied to health care.
- Differentiate between present and evolving types of insurance and methods of payment and their relation to health care cost, quality, and access.

- Compare and contrast the economic foundations of emerging models for health system reform.
- Assess the economic aspects of the nurse labor market in relation to national health workforce challenges.
- Discuss opportunities for nurses at all levels in the context of the Future of Nursing Report, 2020–2030: Charting a Path to Achieve Health Equity.

INTRODUCTION

With the passage of federal Medicare and Medicaid programs in the mid-1960s; the rise of third-party payment models; emergence of health care employment benefits; health care cost containment initiatives of starting in the mid-1970s; and significant advances in health care technology in recent decades, awareness and consideration of health care decision-making by individuals and professional providers is more critical. The associated increases in insurance rates, employer benefit costs, and taxes placed additional burdens on the economy (Sovie, 1985).

By the mid-1980s, with the pressure mounting to contain rising health care costs and to meet the health needs of the population, interest in applying economic concepts and principles to issues in health care evolved. In the first edition of *Nursing Economics*, Dayani (1983) argues that nurses must adapt to what society "*needs*" and "*wants*" and what society is "*willing to pay*." Understanding basic health care economics is an important aspect of empowering nurses to *define*, *regulate*, and *self-govern* the nursing profession.

Sovie (1985) identified the *value* of managing nursing resources in a constrained economic environment. Historically, managing costs and revenues had been separated from the clinical and management functions within health care organizations. However, the spiraling cost of health care as a portion of the nation's overall economy and the inefficient distribution and use of scarce resources within the health care sector underscore the need to incorporate *economic principles* in clinical and care management decision-making.

According to the National Council of State Boards of Nursing (NCSBN), there are 4,096,607 licensed Registered Nurses (RNs) and 920,655 Licensed Practical Nurses in the United States (NCSBN, 2020). Nurses, as the largest health care workforce sector, are in a unique position to influence the efficient and effective use of scarce health care resources. Nurses involved in clinical practice, administration, education, policy-making, and research can use principles of economics to (Buerhaus et al., 2012):

- Provide nursing care in the most cost-effective manner.

- Protect the scope of nursing practice by demonstrating the quality and value of nursing services in relation to other professionals.
- Develop opportunities to expand settings for nursing practice by demonstrating the cost and quality of nursing interventions.
- Understand what purchasers and consumers want from nursing and take steps to satisfy these needs and demands.
- Promote health system change to expand access, improve the quality, and ensure more equitable distribution of health care resources.

The purpose of this chapter is to introduce the reader to *basic economic concepts* that affect professional nursing practice and, more broadly, the delivery of health care services. The chapter is organized into *eight sections*. The first section introduces *health economics and its value* in understanding the health care system. The next section discusses the context and trajectory of *health care reform* leading up to the origin and launch of The Patient Protection and Affordable Care Act of 2010 (ACA). The third section addresses the *basics of health insurance, reimbursement,* and *payment structures*. The fourth section focuses on *health care delivery redesign and the transition* from fee-for-service to population health incentive systems. The fifth section discusses the *impact* of the ACA on costs, quality, access, and opportunities for nursing. The sixth section introduces *methods for evaluation of health systems* in terms of *cost, quality, value,* and *technology assessment*. The seventh section addresses the *nursing workforce* in terms of the labor market, supply and demand, and its cyclical nature. The final section discusses the *economic impact of the COVID-19 pandemic* on the health care industry and the overall economy.

HEALTH ECONOMICS

Economics is concerned with how scarce resources are allocated among alternative uses to meet and satisfy human wants (Henderson, 2018). Models are based on assumptions. Economic models assume that rational behavior drives human decisions and that consumers behave in a purposeful manner under conditions of scarcity. Resources are generally finite, and individuals, motivated by self-interest, respond to incentives to improve their own situation.

As economists started to work on problems in health care, *health care economics* emerged as a discipline of study (McPake et al., 2020). There are two distinct ways in which society can make decisions about how resources, including those in health care, are produced and distributed to those who want them. *First,* the supply, demand, and prices determine how goods and services are distributed (market-driven

approach). *Second,* resources may be collected by a centralized government, which also takes on the task of supply and demand by allocating resources across the population (universal health care approach). Most societies, including the United States and western countries, have evolved to embody aspects of each type (McPake et al., 2020).

In countries where there is a greater role of markets, as in the United States, health care economics seeks to help us understand markets in terms of how consumers express preferences, their ability and willingness to pay, the supply of labor, goods, and services, and how service providers are organized and interact with each other (McPake et al., 2020). Specifically, health economists seek answers to three basic questions:

- What are the main factors that affect choices?
- How are health care goods and services produced and how do we minimize costs and maximize efficiency?
- How do we address the consumer's needs and responsibilities within a social framework that values societal norms and population health?

Health economics is concerned with the allocation of resources between competing demands. *Demands* are assumed to be infinite with *supply* of resources considered finite. Thus, the concept of *scarcity,* resource availability relative to demand, becomes the fundamental problem of study. Health economics is the study of the *production and distribution* of health care resources and their *effect* on a population. *Health care resources* consist of medical supplies, such as pharmaceutical goods, latex gloves, and bed linens; personnel, including nurses, physicians, and other allied health professionals; and capital inputs, including hospitals and nursing home facilities, diagnostic and therapeutic equipment, and other items used to provide health care.

Economists are interested in how *society* makes important decisions regarding the consumption, production, and distribution of these goods and services within the health care sector and in relation to other societal needs, such as education, housing, and defense.

Although economic theory is complex, it is guided by a relatively small set of principles and concepts. A few of these concepts and associated health care examples are presented in Box 7.1 and provide the foundation for a more detailed explanation of how economic principles underpin current health care issues discussed in this chapter (Henderson, 2018). Typically, economists assume certain "conditions" to understand human behavior in relation to the production and distribution of resources.

A fundamental premise of economics is that in a perfect free market the supply of a good or service will attain an equilibrium with the demand for the respective good or service. The free-market system is grounded by the primacy of the consumer and supply, or production is determined

BOX 7.1 Economic Concepts With Health Care Examples

Concept	General Description	Health Care Examples
Markets	Markets are comprised of buyers (consumers) and sellers (producers) who interact (directly or through intermediaries) to trade goods and services.	Health care has several interdependent markets such as: education, personnel, health insurance, pharmaceutical, and others.
Market Forces	Market forces are mechanisms that determine prices and quantities of the product or service, communicate price information, and distribute the products and services.	The current market forces for health care in the U.S. tend to incentivize delivery of hospital-based in-patient services to the acutely ill, as compared to health promotion and preventive care.
Market Failure	Market failure is a situation in which inefficient distribution of a good or service results from a failure in market forces that leads to excessive costs or too few benefits.	One type of health care market failure is due to information asymmetry between the provider and consumer, such as the maldistribution of services that results when consumers have insufficient information regarding costs, alternatives, and outcomes.
Supply & Demand	The dynamic interplay of supply and demand drives markets. As prices increase, supply rises, while demand declines. As prices decrease, supply generally decreases, and demand increases.	In the nursing labor market, increased wages would lead to an increase in the supply of nurses, and wage controls would likely lead to a decrease.
Opportunity Costs	Opportunity costs represent the value or benefit that is relinquished by not choosing the alternative.	In an economic evaluation of a safe-lift program, the saved wages of noninjured staff would represent an opportunity cost.
Cost & Benefits	Consumers generally behave rationally when trying to maximize their benefits in relation to costs.	Costs and benefits are considered when an individual decides whether to obtain a vaccine.

by what consumers want and can buy. The balance between supply and demand was said by Adam Smith, the founder of modern economics, to be determined by the "invisible hand of the marketplace" (Henderson, 2018). Although some modern economists do not fully agree with the invisible hand notion, most do agree that fully free markets do not really exist, due to governmental price controls and other policies that influence supply and demand. Specifically, some health care sector features violate several economic theory assumptions related to supply, demand, and free markets (Henderson, 2018).

Uncertainty

Historically, the *need* for health care services is *irregular* and *cannot be predicted* by either consumers or providers (Arrow, 1963; Henderson, 2018). Consumers who *demand* health care *cannot predict* when illness or catastrophe will

strike, and health care providers *cannot forecast* the costs of the treatment(s) required. Health care professionals who provide health care interventions also face *uncertainty* regarding when *patients will present themselves* for treatment and the extent to which *patients will respond* to prescribed treatment regimens. The unexpected and often costly nature of illness gives rise to the *purchase of insurance* as a safeguard against the cost of health care treatment in the event of illness (Folland et al., 2017). However, the availability of insurance coverage contributes to overall spending on health care which is discussed later in this chapter (Henderson, 2018). However, on a macro level, models based on big data stored in cloud-enabled platforms are under development to predict health care needs for specific services and segments of the population but are not yet applicable to larger population segments (Ramakrishnudu et al., 2021).

Supply and Demand

Supply and demand in health care economics relates to services and goods that consumers consider for *purchase* and that providers and insurers are willing to *produce*. Goods and services are produced and allocated among competing uses by achieving a balance between consumers and producers. The supply and demand of goods and services are influenced by *consumer preferences*, *choices*, and *prices*. *Price elasticities* provide a good example of the interaction between supply and demand. As prices increase, consumer demand for a particular good or service will tend to decrease (Ellis et al., 2017). In addition to the short-term impact of price on demand, the longer-term impact of price on supply should be considered, because price increases and decreases also influence the extent to which specific goods and services will be produced (McPake et al., 2020).

Insurance and Third-Party Payment

Consumers buy insurance to guard against the risk and uncertainty of illness. Insurance introduces an intermediary between the consumer (person requiring health care) and the providers of care (health care professionals and organizations). Consumers do not pay the full price for their health care and are separated from making decisions about services based on the price of those services. In economic theory, *price* is the key measure used to determine what a consumer is willing to pay for a good or service and enables an organization to gauge its output in relation to consumer desires and buying behaviors (Folland et al., 2017). Insurance also changes the demand for care, and it potentially changes the incentives for providers to offer certain types of treatments that are reimbursed by insurance (Folland et al., 2017). Health insurance in the United States is provided from public and private sources, and with varying levels of cost sharing in terms of premiums, copays, and coinsurance.

Problems With Information

Economic theory assumes buyers and sellers have *equal information* about the *cost, price,* and *quality of goods and services*. However, in health care markets, professionals (the sellers) typically have more information about treatment options than do clients (the buyers). In some instances, information is unknown to both the professional and the individual. For example, when a person has cancer that has not yet been detected by regular screenings, a treatment course cannot be formulated because neither party knows health care services are needed. The lack of symmetrical information is a problem because it distorts the basic mechanism of consumer sovereignty, in which consumers (clients) dictate what goods and services are produced because they know what they want and what they are willing to pay (Folland et al., 2017).

Not-for-Profit, Investor-Owned, and Government Firms

Economists assume that organizations seek to maximize profits and that models of firm behavior explain how businesses allocate resources to increase profits. It is important to note that *all* businesses must take in more money than they spend (make a profit or surplus) for continued operations. Many health care providers—including hospitals, nursing homes, and insurance companies—are operated as not-for-profits. As shown in Fig. 7.1 the three types of *acute care* hospitals represent the majority of hospital types: 2946 nongovernment *acute care* not-for-profit hospitals comprise the largest segment at 48% (American Hospital Association [AHA], 2021). Combined with the 1233 (20%) investor-owned community *acute care* hospitals and the 962 (16%) state and local government-owned hospitals, *acute care* hospitals comprise most hospitals in the United States. The 208 federal hospitals primarily represent the Veterans Health Administration (VHA) hospitals, essentially the largest integrated care delivery system (IDS) in the United States. Nonfederal psychiatric hospitals comprise almost 10% of all hospitals, and the smallest segment represents all others, including nonfederal long-term care hospitals and hospital units within an institution such as a prison or school infirmary. Most hospitals are *community hospitals* by AHA's definition which can be found at the link to Fig. 7.1. Most community hospitals are not-for-profit facilities, which we will discuss next. The specific breakdown of *community hospitals* by ownership type is shown in Fig. 7.2. Of the subset of 5141 community hospitals, 1233 (21%) are investor-owned for-profit hospitals and 2946 (57%) are privately owned not-for-profit organizations. The remaining 962 (20%) are owned by state or local governments (AHA, 2021).

The *nonprofit designation* means the facility does not pay state or local property taxes or federal income taxes because it is considered a charity; instead, it provides *community benefit*, including uncompensated care, in accord with state and federal laws and tax codes (Herring et al., 2018). The ACA now requires nonprofit community hospitals to: (1) conduct regular *community health needs assessments* with an accompanying implementation strategy, (2) establish a *formal financial assistance policy for medically necessary and emergency care*, (3) comply with *specified limitations on hospital charges* for those eligible for financial assistance, and (4) comply with *specified billing and collections requirements*. However, the new ACA requirements do not include a specific minimum value of community benefits that a hospital must provide to qualify for tax-exempt status (Herring et al., 2018). Indeed, in the study using data drawn from the Internal Revenue Service (IRS), AHA, and Centers for Medicare and Medicaid Services (CMS), the

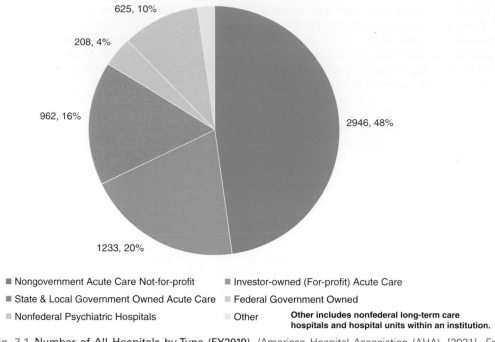

Fig. 7.1 Number of All Hospitals by Type (FY2019). (American Hospital Association (AHA). [2021]. *Fast facts on U.S. hospitals.* https://www.aha.org/statistics/fast-facts-us-hospitals)

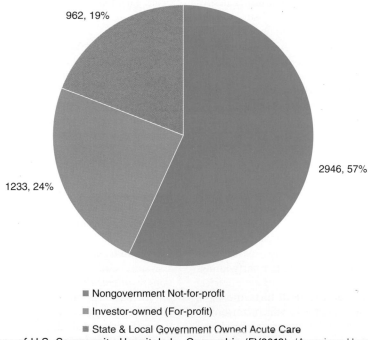

Fig. 7.2 Number of U.S. Community Hospitals by Ownership (FY2019). (American Hospital Association (AHA). [2021]. *Fast facts on U.S. hospitals.* https://www.aha.org/statistics/fast-facts-us-hospitals)

incremental community benefit exceeded the tax exemption for only 62% of not-for-profit hospitals (Lown Institute, 2021). The Lown Institute now includes a community benefit metric in their hospital ranking index and they include a calculation of "fair share spending," which compares not-for-profit hospitals' community spending to the value of their tax exemption (Fair Share Spending). Based on this methodology, 72% of private not-for-profit hospitals were identified as spending less on charity care and community investment than they received in tax exemptions. Several local, state, and federal level challenges to not-for-profit hospitals' tax-exempt status have been made, with at least one hospital losing its tax-exempt status and another being required to pay property taxes after failing to meet its state obligations for a tax exemption.

Investor-owned hospitals are a significant trend in the United States, having increased from 12% of all hospitals to 20% in 2021. Most investor-owned hospitals are part of publicly traded multihospital chains, while others are owned by private investors. As corporations, they are governed by boards of directors and pay local, state, and federal taxes but generally impose strict cost controls, limit investments, and charge higher rates for inpatient services because of their primary commitment to shareholders and financial performance (Bruch et al., 2021).

The trend of community hospitals to merge, form, or join systems has continued, with system-affiliated community hospitals at 67% (up from 51% in 1999) and independent community hospitals at 33% (down from 49% in 1999) (AHA, 2021). Numerous factors drive community hospitals to affiliate with systems, including the ability to fund capital expenditures and achieve greater levels of *economies of scale* (cost advantages achieved by spreading out the fixed costs of services over a larger number of services). For example, a hospital merger or acquisition will likely result in fewer administrative departments and personnel and less duplication of high-cost technology. Evidence of economic benefit and impact of hospital mergers and acquisitions appears to be mixed (AHA, 2020; Beaulieu et al., 2020).

Restrictions on Competition

Competition is a force that produces the most efficient allocation of resources because owners must use their resources to produce the highest satisfaction for society. Economists assume markets are perfectly competitive, consisting of numerous buyers and sellers, with no power over price, who have complete information and can enter and exit the market freely by selling similar goods or services (McPake et al., 2020). Health care markets *violate* several of these assumptions, as discussed previously, such as asymmetrical information; weak pricing mechanisms due to third-party payment (insurance); and blocked market entry by professional practice licensure, advertising restrictions, and provider competition restrictions. In economic terms, health care services can be considered along a continuum of *public good,* which reflect the degree to which nonpayers can be excluded from receiving a service, and the degree to which one person's consumption may limit another person's consumption. For example, state and federal regulations or other outside entities ensuring quality of care and equitable geographic resource distribution may consider health education, mass immunizations, and other public health initiatives as a *public good* while specialized cancer treatments and cosmetic surgery are not (Konar, 2018; McPake et al., 2020).

Role of Equity and Need

Economics is concerned with the distribution of scarce resources so that society receives the highest possible satisfaction from the combination of goods and services produced from these resources. *Distributive justice,* or *equity,* is the extent to which resources are allocated in a fair and equal manner to everyone involved (Konar, 2018). In pure market economies, the price mechanism is used to strike a balance (equilibrium) between the price suppliers charge and the price purchasers are willing to pay. In pure egalitarian systems, governments ensure everyone receives an equal distribution of resources (McPake et al., 2020).

The U.S. health care system is a *mixed system* in which goods and services are distributed both by *markets* and by *government.* This *mixed system* is a factor in the inequitable distribution of health care resources most notably seen in the *lack of universal insurance* or *universal access to health care services* in the United States. Advocates argue that in a *just society* people ought to get the health care they need (universal access), regardless of their ability to pay for these services (universal coverage), promoting fairness, equality, greater transparency, and accountability in health care (Meyer, 2017). This topic is addressed in more detail in the section on health care reform.

Government Subsidies and Public Provision

The health care sector has more government intervention than other sectors of the national economy because of the *uncertainty* in the demand-for and provision-of services. In the United States, state and federal governments play major roles as financiers and payers of health care through the **Medicare**, **Medicaid**, and **State Children's Health Insurance Programs (SCHIPs)**, which will be addressed in more detail in the next section. Publicly owned state and federal hospitals and other facilities, including those of the Veterans' Health Administration, impact health care market dynamics (McPake et al., 2020). Thus, public provision of services and subsidies to providers and consumers through direct care delivery, tax credits, increased federal and state taxes, and differential funding of critical-access and other hospitals influences the health care economy and contributes to some level of *market failure*, discussed later in this chapter (Henderson, 2018).

HEALTH INSURANCE, REIMBURSEMENT, AND PAYMENTS TO PROVIDERS

Because medical care is costly and it is difficult to predict when one might need medical services, insurance functions as a buffer from the financial risks associated with treating illness or disease. People buy insurance to avoid the many *risks* and associated costs of illness and seeking medical treatment such as the risk: (1) to one's health or life associated with illness or disease, (2) a given treatment course will not cure or alleviate the underlying disease, (3) unavoidable harm from the treatment itself or by the lack of skill or negligence on the part of the provider, and (4) incurring substantial costs for treatments. Individuals can take certain personal actions to reduce the risk of illness (e.g., getting vaccinations, avoiding dangerous environments, or leading a healthy lifestyle), but considerable risk remains largely uncertain.

People buy health insurance to avoid the risk of having to pay for expensive medical care. Stated a different way, people are "risk averse" and try to safeguard their wealth or resources by buying insurance as protection from the financial consequences of an unpredictable event. Economists view risk aversion as a characteristic of people's utility functions (McPake et al., 2020). *Marginal utility* is the extra satisfaction, welfare, or well-being (utility) gained from consuming one more unit of a good or service. In the case of insurance, it is believed that people are more likely to buy insurance to cover low-probability events involving large losses than high-probability events associated with small losses (McPake et al., 2020).

Although it is difficult to predict when an individual will become sick or need expensive medical care, the risk for large numbers of people (or the expected value of all losses averaged over all people) is quite predictable. Insurance spreads risk across a group of people and involves a series of trades between people. This practice is known as *risk pooling*. Money is shifted between people who are healthy to people who are sick and in need to pay for expensive medical care. Insurance pools potential losses, but it does not eliminate or reduce the losses (i.e., *pricing* risks, not in *taking* risks). Insurance companies sell policies to large groups of people with predictable or average risks. Members pay a premium, which covers all losses across the group of policy holders and management fees (McPake et al., 2020). Sharing costs across a broader risk pool increases costs for the healthy for the benefit of those who utilize more care. Segmenting the risk pool promotes savings for the healthy users while increasing costs for those with greater health care utilization (Mathauer et al., 2019).

Moral hazard occurs when a person's behavior changes based on their insurance coverage. In the event of an illness or other adverse event, the insured person is offered medical care at a reduced price. Moral hazard in health insurance markets occurs to the extent that insurance increases the quantity of medical care used, as discussed previously under the topic of *uncertainty* (Henderson, 2018). One way insurance companies offset the risk of moral hazard is to require *cost sharing* with consumers. *Deductibles* and *copayments* are two commonly used methods.

Copayment is a sharing relationship between the consumer and the insurance company, as detailed in a specific policy. When consumers seek medical care, the insurance company pays for some of the costs and the consumer pays for the remainder (the copayment). A *deductible* is a fixed amount that the consumer must pay toward a medical bill each year before any insurance payment is made. Deductibles are designed to generate more prudent care decisions on the part of the policy holder because they dissuade consumers from submitting claims to the insurance company for "small" losses or minor services (Henderson, 2018).

Consumers purchase health care (demand) depending on their perceptions of the effect of the care on their desired health (Babalola, 2017; Henderson, 2018). The decision to purchase health care also depends on the cost of care to the consumer. Total consumer costs of health care include *monetary costs* (e.g., copayment, deductibles, insurance premiums, out-of-pocket expenses, lost time from wages and work) and *nonmonetary costs* (e.g., risk, pain, inconvenience).

The demand for health care also depends on the willingness of consumers to purchase services after *weighing the expected benefits of the care against the costs of the care.* If consumers carry insurance, their direct out-of-pocket expenses for the care will be less than if they are uninsured (Henderson, 2018). Therefore, the insurance status of consumers effects the costs of care (to the consumers) and thus their demand for care.

Despite the fact consumers make copayments and pay deductibles, they are generally *insulated* from the high costs of health care because insurance companies typically pay such a large portion of a bill. This separation of consumers from the price of health care resulting from health insurance coverage (either private or public) has dramatically *increased demand* for health care services. However, because demand is based on willingness and ability to purchase, demand for health care does not necessarily correlate with the need for health care. Demand for health care services changes over time as societal demographics and morbidity patterns change. For instance, as baby boomers continue to age, the percentage of the population age 80 years and older will continue to increase proportionately. Their demands for health care will contribute to the already increasing demands of an existing elderly population (Feinberg & Spillman, 2019). As the large baby boomer cohort ages, there is expected to be a smaller number of spouses and children available as caregivers due to women having fewer children, delaying childbearing, and other social and economic trends affecting the availability of family caregivers (Feinberg & Spillman, 2019).

Demand for specific services is also influenced by the recommendations and decisions of health care providers (Henderson, 2018). Because providers of care possess *more knowledge* regarding treatment options than do consumers, the practice styles of providers and how much information they share with consumers can greatly affect the demand and consumption of services. Similarly, fear of litigation can lead to the overuse of (often unnecessary) diagnostic tests or therapeutic interventions and ultimately result in higher health care costs. The so-called *defensive practice style* has been estimated to comprise between 2% and 10% of health care spending (Henderson, 2018).

The demand for health care services is not directly related to the amount or quality of services purchased as in other industries. This, in conjunction with the high levels of *uncertainty* and the *unequal information* among consumers, providers, and payers, leads to a situation called *market failure. Market failure* is characterized by the inability of buyers and sellers to strike a balance in the *supply* and *demand* of goods and services and ultimately fail to produce a socially desirable level of output (McPake et al., 2020). For example, variation in the quality of care is an example of market failure arising from imperfect consumer information about physician practice patterns, implying that some patients are getting too-much and some too-little treatment.

Supply-side drivers leading to market failure include the cost of care for hospital and physician services, access to care because of the prohibitive cost of health insurance, and medical outcomes and population health status in light of invested resources. Demand-side factors of market failure in health care include the third-party insurance mechanism in which the insurance company or government entity under the Medicare and Medicaid programs is the primary purchaser of health care services (Henderson, 2018).

Types of Insurance and Payment Methods

There are generally two approaches to health care financing through insurance: *private insurance* and *social insurance (public). Private insurance* provides reimbursement

for expenditures or direct payments to those in need of care and is based on the premise that premiums reflect medical spending (Henderson, 2018). In principle, those with higher expected spending pay higher premiums or via additional cost-sharing mechanisms. *Public insurance* does not factor higher risk into premiums, but rather those with higher incomes pay more. The U.S. health care system incorporates both approaches.

There are five dominant methods consumers use to pay for their health care in the United States: out-of-pocket payment, private individual insurance, health savings account (HSA), employer-sponsored group insurance, and public or government-sponsored individual or group insurance. Premiums are upfront payments, paid in advance of receiving services, on behalf of an individual or family. Premiums for private plans may be subsidized by an employer, and some government-provided or supported plans require premiums.

Out-of-Pocket Payment

Out-of-pocket payment for health care services is the simplest form of financing because the consumer directly pays the provider for services. This was the dominant model of paying for health care services in the 19th and early 20th centuries when the technology and available interventions to cure disease or alleviate the symptoms of illness were relatively weak. However, out-of-pocket payment is a flawed way to pay for health care, especially because health care services have become more complex and increasingly expensive. Individuals cannot save or borrow enough money to pay for health care services (Henderson, 2018). Out-of-pocket expenses, as previously discussed, include copayments and coinsurance.

Private Individual Insurance

This form of financing adds a third party (the insurance company) to the relationship between the consumer and provider. Payment for health care services is divided into two parts, a *premium* paid by the individual to the insurance company and a *reimbursement payment* to the provider from the insurance company. *Indemnity insurance, a type of private insurance*, added a third payment transaction: a reimbursement to the individual from the insurance company after the individual has paid the provider. Two-thirds of the population is covered by some type of private third-party health insurance plan (Keisler-Starkey & Bunch, 2021).

Health Savings Accounts

HSAs were created by Congress in 2003 to allow individuals to pay for selected health care expenses with pretax dollars such as out-of-pocket expenses not covered by the health plan. Individuals preselect the amount of money they have withheld from their gross income; approved expenses are covered from this account; the individual saves the amount of money they would have incurred in income tax. In 2021, 58% of all firms offered HSAs or a posttax reimbursement program as part of a High-Deductible Health Plan (HDHP) (Kaiser Family Foundation [KFF], 2021).

Employer-Sponsored Group Insurance

Employer-sponsored group insurance came into being during the Great Depression and expanded rapidly after World War II (Starr, 1982). The AHA first established the Blue Cross of California in 1939, offering hospital insurance to groups of workers. The first employer-based insurance plans were initiated by physicians and hospitals seeking a steady source of income, generous reimbursements, and protection from cost controls (Starr, 1982), all of which had declined during the Great Depression because people were not able to pay for their medical and hospital expenses out-of-pocket.

With employer-based insurance, the employer pays a proportion of the premium to purchase health insurance on behalf of their employees (Fronstin et al., 2021). Thus, in the United States, health insurance became a *benefit of employment*. The government treats employee health benefits as a tax-deductible business expense for employers. Because each dollar of employer-sponsored health insurance results in a reduction in taxes collected, the federal government is in essence *subsidizing employer-sponsored insurance*.

Public or Government-Sponsored Insurance

The U.S. government became involved in the financing of health care during the Great Depression (Starr, 1982). Individuals not participating in the labor force, especially the elderly and those with chronic conditions or low incomes, found it increasingly difficult to buy insurance on their own. This led to the creation of the government-sponsored **Medicare** and **Medicaid** programs in the mid-1960s, the **SCHIP** in 1997, the establishment of **HSAs** in 2003, and the more recent **ACA of 2010**. Although many elements of the ACA remain law, key elements were removed in the 2018 Tax Bill, signed into law in January 2018. The ACA penalties related to the *individual mandate* were eliminated, *insurance subsidies* were reduced or eliminated, and *health plans with minimal coverage for prevention and care* were approved (Norris, 2021). However, several states have their own mandates for insurance, and penalties in these states may be imposed for not being insured.

Government health insurance for the poor and elderly adds the taxpayer to the equation as the ultimate payer. Much like private insurance, beneficiaries are required to contribute to receiving benefits. *Taxpayers* need to contribute a certain amount to Social Security taxes to be eligible for Medicare (Henderson, 2018). In comparison, the state-funded Medicaid program is funded by taxpayer contributions, although not all taxpayers are eligible for Medicaid benefits. Because these programs are tax-funded, there is a double subsidy at play for taxpayers. As with private insurance, benefits are shifted from those who are healthy to those who are sick. The government-sponsored programs add an additional distribution of funds between the wealthy and the poor. That is, the healthy middle-income employees generally pay more Social Security taxes than they receive in health services, while unemployed, disabled, and lower-income elderly persons may receive more in health services than they contribute to taxes (Center on Budget and Policy Priorities, 2020b).

The three government-sponsored or provided insurance programs: Medicaid, Medicare, and SCHIP, are differentiated in terms of the target population, funding mechanism, and covered services. **Medicaid** is designed to provide health coverage for low-income people. The Federal government establishes parameters for all states, the District of Columbia, and the U.S. territories, with each state administering its own program, which results in *variation between states*. Differences in eligibility income levels and covered services result from the flexibility in designing and administering their own programs (Center on Budget and Policy Priorities, 2020a). Further flexibility is given to the individual programs through the CMS ***Section 1115 waiver*** process (CMS, n.d.-a). The waiver process allows for experimental, pilot, or demonstration projects deemed likely to assist in promoting the Medicaid program's objectives, through which almost 600 individual waivers are in process as of 2021 (Medicaid.gov, 2021).

Medicare is federally supported and administered for people ages 65 and older, regardless of income, medical history, or health status. The program was expanded in 1972 to include certain people under age 65 with a long-term disability (KFF, 2019). Medicare helps pay for many medical care services, including hospitalizations, physician visits, prescription drugs, preventive services, skilled nursing facility, home health care, and hospice care. *Medicare Part A* requires no premium if the participant has paid Social Security tax for 10 or more years and covers hospital care. Recipients' out-of-pocket costs include deductibles and coinsurance and include limits on hospitalization days per benefit period, and lifetime limits on days more than 90 during a specific benefit period. *Medicare Part B* requires a sliding-scale income-dependent premium and covers physician visits, outpatient services, preventive services, and some home health visits. Deductibles apply, except for annual wellness visits and certain preventive services such as mammography or prostate cancer screenings (KFF, 2019). *Medicare Part C* refers to the Medicare managed care program, Medicare Advantage, through which participants can enroll in a privately offered approved health maintenance organization (HMO) or preferred provider organization (PPO) and receive all Medicare Part A and Part B benefits through this managed program. Premiums, deductibles, copays, and coinsurance out-of-pocket expenses apply, but medication coverage is included. Over one-third of all Medicare recipients are enrolled in a Medicare Advantage plan. *Medicare Part D* covers outpatient prescription drugs through private plans that contract with Medicare. Participation is voluntary and premiums are required, but one in four participants receives some level of low-income subsidy (KFF, 2019).

The SCHIP provides low-cost health coverage to children in families that earn too much to qualify for Medicaid (Healthcare.gov, n.d.). SCHIP is administered by the states but jointly funded by the federal government. States may call these programs something other than CHIP. States may use the funding to expand Medicaid, offer a separate child health insurance program, or offer a combination of these two approaches. SCHIP was planned to be phased out as part of the ACA but since Medicaid expansion was not universally accepted, the program's 23% federal match rate was extended for 6 years, beginning in 2018 (KFF, 2018).

Government-Provided Health Care Services

With 1293 health care facilities, including 171 medical centers, the VHA is the largest integrated health care delivery system in the United States. The VHA serves over 9 million veterans (VHA, 2021). As a centrally administered system, the VHA can implement large-scale innovative changes to improve care, including the single largest implementation of the Clinical Nurse Leader (CNL) role (Veterans Affairs, n.d.) in the United States. Developed by the American Association of Colleges of Nursing (AACN, 2020) in collaboration with academic and practice leaders in response to quality and safety issues identified by The Institute of Medicine (IOM) reports in 2000, the role is designed to address gaps in care delivery related to the growing complexity and fragmentation of health care. By 2013, the VHA had reported that over 70 VHA medical centers were participating in the program.

HEALTH CARE DELIVERY REDESIGN: FROM FEE-FOR-SERVICE TO POPULATION HEALTH

The widely influential report, *Crossing the Quality Chasm* (IOM, 2001), highlighted the need to better align payment methods for health care with quality improvement goals. Indeed, this work built on the managed care principles of

HMO or PPO initiatives and became embedded within the ACA a decade later.

The traditional fee-for-service (FFS) payment system is based on a unit of service, such as a visit or procedure. The financial incentive to the hospitals and providers is to produce more of the unit that is being reimbursed leading to increased intensity of care and treatment of more patients (volume). In addition to the difficulties and expense associated with coordinating payments, this system is not designed to incentivize quality or safety (value), especially regarding the predominance of chronic preventable medical conditions and the emphasis on acute care.

Principles of *managed care* provide the foundation for the shift from fee-for-service to a *population health model* in which lower costs and higher levels of population health are achieved. Key principles include that health care costs can be affected by changing patient utilization, physician practice styles, and the introduction of information technology (Henderson, 2018). Demand-side cost-sharing in the form of co-pays and coinsurance influence *consumer behavior* and reduce spending. On the provider or supply-side, utilization is influenced through *selective contracting* with lower-cost providers, *risk-sharing* arrangements between providers and insurers, and *utilization review* and control and *case management*.

Impact of the Affordable Care Act (2010) on Costs and Quality

The ACA was signed into law in 2010 and is commonly referred to as *Obamacare*. The law addresses all three major aspects of health care policy and economics: *cost*, *quality*, and *access*. The law provides numerous rights and protections for consumers, along with subsidies through tax credits and cost-sharing reductions that make health coverage more affordable. The major provisions of the ACA are organized into two main groups, *Access*, and *Cost* and *Quality*, as organized in Fig. 7.3 and described in detail in the law's summary (https://www.govinfo.gov/content/pkg/PLAW-111publ148/pdf/PLAW-111publ148.pdf). The impact on *access* is addressed in Chapter 6: Health Policy and Planning and the Nursing Practice Environment.

Cost and Quality. In addition to addressing access, the ACA also launched several innovative changes in how health care is paid for and delivered. At the outset, hospitals agreed to across-the-board reductions in Medicare payments, anticipating increased numbers of paying patients and reduced levels of uncompensated care (Blumenthal & Abrams, 2020). Several new programs were introduced to improve the overall *value* of health care, by reducing costs and increasing quality. These value-focused programs are divided into two categories, as shown on the right side of Fig. 7.3. Programs in the first category were enhancements

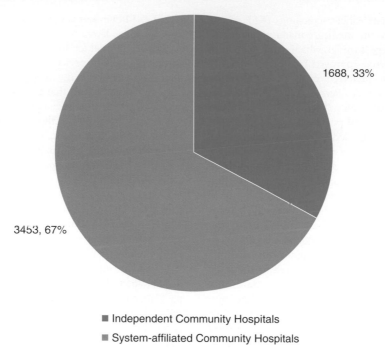

1688, 33%

3453, 67%

■ Independent Community Hospitals
■ System-affiliated Community Hospitals

Fig. 7.3 U.S. Community Hospitals: System Affiliated Versus Independent (FY2019).

to payments made within the *traditional* fee-for-service plans of Medicare and Medicaid. Programs in the second category were entirely *new* (*nontraditional plan related*) and implemented in addition to the enhanced traditional Medicare and Medicaid payment schemes.

Traditional fee-for-service payment plan programs. The category of enhancements to the traditional FFS payment plans, also referred to as pay-for-performance (P4P), includes programs designed to improve quality and decrease costs through various combinations or financial incentives and rewards. This category includes the *Hospital Readmission Reduction Program (HRRP)*, the *Hospital-Acquired Condition Reduction Program (HACRP)*, and the *Hospital Value-Based Purchasing Program (HVBP)*.

Hospital readmission reduction program. Prior to the ACA, there was wide variation in Medicare readmission rates across procedures and diagnoses, with 30-day readmission rates as high as 24.7% among some patient diagnostic groups (Weiss et al., 2010). Under the HRRP rules, hospitals with a higher-than-average risk-adjusted rate of readmissions for patients with one of six clinical conditions would incur a financial penalty. Although initial studies showed some reduction in readmissions by 2015, later studies suggest that changes in risk classification rather than changes in actual rates accounted for the apparent decrease. In response to these findings, adjustments

for socioeconomic factors were added in 2016 but the impact of these changes on readmission rates has yet to be adequately evaluated (Blumenthal & Abrams, 2020).

In fiscal year (FY) 2022, CMS will penalize 2499 (82%) of the 3046 hospitals assessed for excessive Medicare patient readmission rates, similar to FY2021, with 83% of hospitals penalized (CMS, 2021c). The average penalty will be 0.64%, with a maximum penalty of 3%, resulting in an estimated $521 million (Rau, 2021). An additional 2216 hospitals are exempt from the program because they specialize in the care of children, psychiatric patients, or veterans. Rehabilitation, long-term care, and critical access hospitals are also exempt.

Hospital-acquired conditions reduction program. Efforts to reduce the incidence of various hospital-acquired conditions and their associated costs to Medicare predate the ACA. In 2008, CMS identified 10 categories of conditions for which hospitals do not receive payments, including *care for pressure ulcers, surgical site infections, injuries from falls,* and *other hospital-acquired injuries* (CMS, n.d.-b). The HACRP builds on this with additional penalties for hospitals in the worst-performing quartile. The performance measure is tracked annually, and overall Medicare payments to these hospitals are reduced by 1%. In the latest report available through AHRQ, the *overall HAC rate* had decreased by 13% from 2014 to 2017

(Agency on Healthcare Research and Quality [AHRQ], 2019). Initial data show that low-performing hospitals generally do not improve despite being penalized (Sankaran et al., 2019). A retrospective study using Medicare data from 2006 to 2015 showed a 2% to 3% annual decline in falls and injurious falls in acute care patients from 734 hospitals, which coincides with the first 9 years of the introduction of the penalty (Shorr et al., 2019).

Hospital value-based purchasing. The Medicare Prescription Drug, Improvement, and Modernization Act of 2003 and the Deficit Reduction Act of 2005 allowed the CMS to reward acute care hospitals for the quality of care they provide to Medicare patients (pay for quality model). The ACA of 2010 builds on this *incentive* concept by rewarding hospitals with better patient outcomes with funds created by withholding portions of payments from hospitals with lower-quality outcomes.

The HBVP's primary purpose is to improve care through *economic incentives and penalties.* The funds to support VBP incentive payments to hospitals are generated through reductions in diagnosis-related group (DRG) payments (CMS, n.d.-c). Beginning in FY2013, 1% was withheld from hospitals' Medicare payments, with incremental annual increases culminating in 2% being withheld by 2017 and beyond. The CMS calculates payments based on **Total Performance Scores (TPS)** of **Clinical Process of Care (quality measures)** and **Patient Experience of Care (Hospital Consumer Assessment of Healthcare Providers and Systems [HCAHPS] patient satisfaction)**. Beginning in 2013 the quality measures contributed 70% to the overall score and patient satisfaction contributed 30%. As of 2018, the four domains of value and percentages had shifted and remain at 25% each, as shown in Fig. 7.4. A total of 22 measures are distributed among the four domains of Clinical Outcomes, Person & Community Engagement, Safety, and Efficiency & Cost Reduction (CMS, 2021a).

For FY2021, total funds available for value-based incentive payments were approximately $1.9 billion (CMS, 2021b). In approximately 55% of participating hospitals, 1450 received Medicare payments higher than the amount that was withheld. The average net increase in adjustments was 0.69% and the average decrease in payment adjustments was –0.45%. The highest-performing hospital received a net increase of 3.94%, and the lowest-performing hospital incurred a net decrease of –1.62% (CMS, 2021a).

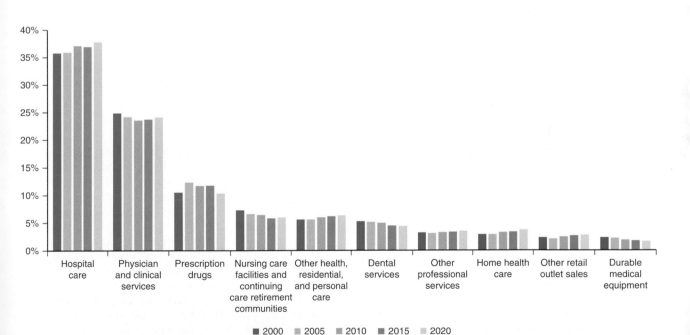

Fig. 7.4 Distribution of Personal Health Care Spending by Types of Service (Excludes Administrative Costs, Research, and Investments) Total Personal Spending = $3.93 trillion (Centers for Medicare and Medicaid Services [CMS], 2021a). (National Health Expenditure Data [Data set], Table 06, Personal Health C are Expenditures. https://www.cms.gov/research-statistics-data-and-systems/statistics-trends-and-reports/nationalhealthexpenddata/nhe-fact-sheet)

Quality measures include specific criteria for a set of common medical and surgical conditions such as anterior myocardial infarction, heart failure, pneumonia, and patients undergoing surgeries. Examples include patients receiving fibrinolytic therapy within 30 minutes of hospital arrival and receiving primary percutaneous coronary intervention within 90 minutes of hospital arrival. Other measures relate to discharge instructions for patients with heart failure and prophylactic antibiotics before surgery. The patient experience domain relates directly to the **HCAHPS Survey**.

The HCAHPS is a national standardized survey used to measure CMS patients' perceptions of care. The survey asks questions about critical aspects of the patients' hospital experiences, including communication with nurses and doctors, the responsiveness of hospital staff, the cleanliness and quietness of the hospital environment, pain management, communication about medicines, discharge information, overall rating of the hospital, and whether they would recommend the hospital to others. Most measures are directly or indirectly related to nursing practice, nurses' work environment, and workload.

To understand the financial effect at the hospital level, it is helpful to look at a contrived example of how Medicare dollars are withheld and divided. Using the FY2020 CMS HVBP withheld amount of $1.9 billion, each of the 2677 participating hospitals would have had an average of $709,750 or 2% withheld and would have either forfeited this amount as a penalty for performing below the mean or could have received a financial incentive for performing above the mean. The average hospital will initially have $727,272 withheld, and half of the hospitals could receive up to two times $727,272, or $1.45 million (CMS, 2021a).

Nursing continues to be at the forefront of the positive effect on improving HVBP measures. Several studies have examined the impact of *Magnet* hospital designation on HBVP and associated measures. *Magnet* hospitals serve as a suitable indicator of nursing excellence, as embodied within the *Magnet* model domains. Elements of the model include transformational leadership, structural empowerment, exemplary professional practice, new knowledge, innovations, improvements, and empirical outcomes. Early in the implementation of the program, *Magnet* hospitals outperformed non-Magnet hospitals regarding patient experience, clinical processes, and total score (Lasater et al., 2016). In a more recent study, *Magnet* hospitals were 38% less likely to receive penalties as compared to nondesignated hospitals (Dierkes et al., 2021). In another cross-sectional study using CMS data, *Magnet*-designated hospitals were again found to outperform nondesignated hospitals in terms of patient experience, care processes, and total

performance (Spaulding et al., 2020). Thus, the **value of nursing**, as represented by the Magnet Model, can be directly tied to financial performance.

In November 2021, CMS determined that circumstances caused by the COVID-19 public health emergency significantly affected hospital performance and reporting and CMS's ability to accurately collect the data required to calculate total scores and assign penalties and rewards. Thus, payment adjustments under the HVBP were *suspended* by CMS for FY2022 due to the COVID-19 pandemic (CMS, 2021b). As a result, CMS does not plan to calculate scores nor determine penalties or incentives until a decision is made for FY2023.

Nontraditional plan-related programs. Under the ACA, the nontraditional plan-related category programs (see Fig. 7.3) were established beyond the boundaries of the traditional payment mechanisms of Medicare and Medicaid and include four programs to reduce costs and improve quality and safety.

Accountable care organizations. The contemporary concept of Accountable Care Organizations (ACOs) is generally believed to have been created at a public meeting of the Medicare Payment Advisory Commission (MedPAC) in 2006 (Fisher et al., 2006). In their follow-up policy paper, the authors argued that cost-containment, payment reform, and quality improvement approaches that focus on individual physician's risk reinforce fragmentation of care and lack of coordination experienced by patients with serious illness. Instead, they proposed an approach that would be led by physicians and hospitals within relatively coherent systems, where patients received their care. ACOs should be created with a virtual "extended hospital medical staff" that "work within and around" local hospitals.

The Medicare shared savings program. Instituted by the ACA creates financial incentives for hospitals, physicians, and other health care providers to limit growth in health care costs through improved coordination of care (CMS, n.d.-d). The SSP is operationalized through the ACOs, who contract with CMS and agree to be held *accountable* for the *quality*, *cost*, and *experience* of an assigned traditional Medicare fee-for-service population. Before the Shared Savings Program (SSP) and ACOs, financial incentives for combined physician and hospital entities were limited to a few pilot programs created to establish feasibility. Hospitals are now allowed to formally partner with physicians and other providers through the legal and financial entity of the ACO. The ACO is held accountable for improving the outcomes and experience for individuals and populations. Better coordinated care helps ensure that patients receive the right care at the right time, with less duplication and fewer errors.

ACOs are like HMOs, yet there are key differences. HMOs are primarily insurance providers who assume the risk for a population of members within their service programs. *First*, ACOs generally comprise fewer enrollees; current regulations require a minimum of 5000 Medicare beneficiaries. *Second*, ACOs, at least as currently defined, bear less financial risk. ACOs are rewarded for high performance but not accountable for 100% of the costs as in the HMO model. The ACOs' enrollees are tracked and monitored by the ACO and CMS. The ACO selects one of two options at the outset: operate on a shared savings agreement *or* elect a higher-risk option that allows the ACO to share savings and losses, thus attaining a higher share of any savings generated.

Since 2010, over 900 ACOs have formed over 1300 payment contracts with public and commercial payers, managing care for approximately 10% of the U.S. population (Muhlstein et al., 2019). As of 2019, there were more than 1500 public and private ACOs covering 44 million patients or nearly two-thirds of all Medicare recipients. Kaufman et al. (2019) identified 42 studies of ACOs and their impact on costs, utilization, and outcomes. The most consistent findings across all studies were reduced inpatient use, reduced emergency department visits, and some improvement in measures related to preventive care and chronic disease management. Several studies have shown a net savings of approximately 2% while maintaining or improving quality (Muhlstein et al., 2019). Some recent studies suggest that physician-led ACOs may outperform non-physician-led ACOs (McWilliams et al., 2018; Sullivan & Feore, 2019).

Bundled payments for care improvement. Several Bundled Payments for Care Improvement (BPCI) initiatives were implemented to test whether linking payments for all providers that deliver care during an episode of inpatient hospitalization and subsequent care could reduce Medicare expenditures while maintaining or improving the quality of care (CMS, 2021a). Several variations of the model were designed to give multiple providers a single, prospective payment for the treatment of a surgical or medical condition. As of 2021, more than 125 hospitals, physician groups, and post–acute care organizations have participated. Hip and knee surgery were the most common surgical procedures and congestive heart failure was the most common medical condition (Blumenthal & Abrams, 2020). BPCI appears to have reduced expenditures for surgical procedures such as hip and knee replacement, but the savings may not exceed the administration costs of the program (Dummit et al., 2016). The results for the medical conditions were less promising, and although the original program was suspended in 2018, a new iteration has been launched, which will run until at least 2023. Evaluation evidence is limited due to the small number of programs (Joynt Maddox et al., 2018).

Primary care enhancements. Three programs were launched to strengthen the primary care infrastructure, with mixed results (Blumenthal & Abrams, 2020).

The comprehensive primary care initiative. Attempted to coordinate increased payment from private and public sources to promote improved primary care outcomes. Comprehensive Primary Care Initiative (CPCI) was associated with a 2% reduction in costs because of decreased emergency room visits, but no net savings were realized. A considerably larger scale program, **Comprehensive Primary Care Initiative Plus**, was launched in 2018, which involves 14,810 primary care practitioners in 2851 practices serving 15 million patients in 18 different markets across the United States. As the program is in the implementation phase, evaluation data are unavailable. Interestingly, Nurse Practitioners and Clinical Nurse Specialists are identified as eligible participants for the program (CMS, n.d.-b). Nurse practitioners are also eligible to participate in the **Independence at Home Demonstration Program,** a pilot program renewed in 2018, that provides intensive home-based primary care for homebound patients. Initial results have shown a significant decrease in emergency department visits and hospitalizations, as well as increased consumer and caregiver satisfaction (U.S. Department of Health and Human Services [USDHHS], 2018).

Center for Medicare and Medicaid innovation. The Center for Medicare and Medicaid Innovation (CMMI) was created to *test innovative payment and delivery models* to reduce costs while preserving or enhancing the quality of care for populations served by Medicare, Medicaid, and CHIP. Two other nongovernmental entities were established to effect innovation and change in care delivery and payment systems.

First, **the independent payment advisory board.** Was created and empowered to make changes to Medicare payment rates and program rules. Previously, congressional approval was required to make any changes in payments, and the intent was to shift payment decision-making to "experts using evidence" rather than the highly politicized Congress (Spatz, 2018). Designed to set rates if Medicare spending exceeded the targets established by the ACA, the program stalled when published targets were never exceeded up to 2018. Board members were never appointed, and the program was phased out in 2018.

Second, **the patient-centered outcomes research institute (PCORI, 2020).** Was established as a nongovernment advisory entity comprising patients, physicians, nurses, hospitals, drug makers, device manufacturers, insurers, payers, government officials, and health experts. PCORI examines the relative health outcomes, clinical effectiveness, and appropriateness of different medical treatments by evaluating existing studies and conducting their own (PCORI, 2020). Reauthorized by Congress in 2019, PCORI awarded $158 million to fund 36 comparative clinical research studies.

Additional reform.

2021 No surprises act. The No Surprises Act (NSA) of 2021 establishes federal protections for consumers who unexpectedly and often unknowingly receive care from out-of-network providers. Examples include receiving additional bills from nonnetwork anesthesiologists, laboratories, and specialists. These surprise medical bills pose financial burdens on consumers when health plans deny these out-of-network services when the consumer had originally sought in-network care (Pollitz, 2022). The NSA will establish a process for determining the payment amount for surprise, out-of-network medical bills to include negotiations between plans and providers, and if negotiations are unsuccessful, an independent dispute resolution will be used.

2021 promoting competition in U.S. health care. An executive order on promoting competition in the American Economy was issued by the President in 2021 (The White House, 2021). The order includes over 70 executive branch and agency initiatives aimed at promoting competition within and across many economic segments, including health care. Four focus areas are identified in which lack of competition in health care increases prices and potentially reduces access: *prescription drugs*, *hearing aids*, *hospitals*, and *health insurance*. Specific direction includes importing pharmaceuticals from Canada, removing barriers to making generic drugs available, proposing rules to allow hearing aids to be sold over the counter, reviewing and revising merger guidelines to ensure consumers are not unfairly financially harmed, accelerating the enforcement of hospital price transparency rules, and standardizing options on the health insurance exchanges. In August of 2022, Medicare was authorized to negotiate pharmaceutical drug prices for a limited set of drugs annually under the **Inflation Reduction Act of 2022** (effective in 2023) and the Food and Drug Administration (FDA) issued a new rule authorizing the purchase of over-the-counter hearing aids for mild-to-moderate hearing loss without a medical exam or fitting.

Opportunities for Nursing

Specifically, ongoing health care reform provides numerous opportunities for nursing at the general and advanced practice levels, within the care delivery and academic domains, to address issues and challenges related to health care cost, access, and quality. Nurses are a "pivotal component" in leading change across various health care delivery sites and organizations (National Advisory Council on Nurse Education and Practice [NACNEP], 2019). In their report to Congress and the DHHS Secretary, NACNEP emphasizes changes in policy, legislation, and research to strengthen nursing's ability to lead and practice in the **Value-Based Care** (VBC) environment. Advocating for investment through **Title VIII** to advance nursing education and practice, the Council identified four major recommendations:

1. Fund demonstration projects that study costs, access, and quality outcomes of nurse-led interdisciplinary teams.
2. Support partnerships between community health centers and academia through which the value of advanced practice registered nurses (APRNs), with and without full practice authority, can be studied and compared in terms of patient, cost, and quality outcomes.
3. Fund academic and practice initiatives that advance the development of undergraduate and graduate nurse competencies associated with improved population health outcomes (e.g., case management, care coordination, utilization management, team-based care, and understanding of health care finance).
4. Fund educational and training initiatives in the areas of population health, data analytics, informatics, and connected care (e.g., telehealth) to address the needs of rural and underserved communities.

As financial incentives shift the focus of care from hospitals to less expensive venues in the community, APRNs and nurses in home and community nursing practice settings will likely be afforded significant opportunities to lead and implement change. APRNs will likely assume greater responsibility in primary care as state nurse practice acts and related legislation at the federal and state levels loosen restrictions on nursing practice and promote higher levels of fee equity between primary care providers of all disciplines.

The Future of Nursing Report, 2020–2031 (2021). The National Academies of Science, Engineering, and Medicine's (NASEM), **2021 Future of Nursing Report** presents a comprehensive and inspiring vision of how nurses in different roles can develop, provide, and facilitate individualized evidenced-based care that optimizes outcomes for diverse patients and communities (NASEM, 2021). An overview of the Future of Nursing reports (2010 & 2020) can be found in the Appendices.

An important aspect of the vision is to restructure and redesign payment models for nursing that recognize and reward the value that nurses contribute to direct care and supporting team-based care. The essential contributions to care include coordinating and managing care, helping patients and families navigate the health system, and providing patient education. Thus, one of the key conclusions in the Report is that "payment mechanisms need to be designed to support the nursing workforce and nursing education in addressing social needs and social determinants of health to improve population health and advance health equity" (NASEM, 2021, p. 8).

Nursing is considered a "cost" in hospital services, and something that should be minimized and contained. Since hospitals are not directly compensated for providing nursing care, unlike physician service, there is little financial incentive to match the right amount and skill sets to patients, aside from the indirect efforts through various nurse-sensitive value-based-purchasing initiatives previously mentioned (Aiken, 2008). Since at least the initial 2001 IOM report, the argument has been offered that direct reimbursement for nursing care would have a positive impact on the quality of care by reducing incentives to inappropriately ration care (Aiken, 2008; Welton, 2006; Welton et al., 2006). A summary of the key IOM reports can be found in the Appendices.

The 2020 *Future of Nursing Report* extends the vision to beyond hospitals, to all settings. The new payment models, ACOs, and VBP provide an opportunity for payment reform that recognizes and rewards the **value of nursing care**. The FFS model that underlies payment approaches provides a fundamental economic function in the supply and demand of health care and is how care has been billed and compensated. All types of insurance require **two components for a bill**: the **service** that was provided, represented by **Current Procedure Terminology (CPT) codes**, and the **condition** that was addressed, represented by an **International Classification of Diseases, 10th Revision (ICD-10) code**. Each payor has a fee schedule based on these codes, which are generally negotiated as a percentage of the Medicare fee schedule, which is updated annually by CMS. The proprietary CPT codes are owned, managed, and licensed by the American Medical Association (AMA), and have long been criticized for undervaluing cognitive work and overvaluing procedural work. The creation and valuation of codes for *care coordination*, *patient assessment*, *end-of-life counseling*, *health education*, and *preventive services* have not been prioritized. The Report advocates for a reform of the FFS that supports key nursing roles, through a *payment redesign* that allows nurses and organizations to bill and receive payment for nursing care.

Aside from payment reform, within the current payment system, there are many opportunities for nurses to drive health care transformation (Salmond & Echevarria, 2017). Regardless of the specific legislation or administrative rules enacted, drivers of change will likely persist. *Drivers of health care change* include: (1) cost, (2) waste, (3) lack of standardization, (4) quality, (5) health systems infrastructures, (6) reimbursement incentives, (7) aging demographics and increased longevity, (8) chronic illness, and (9) health care disparities. In this model, nurses can leverage their skill sets in four major areas: (1) focus on wellness, (2) patient- and family-centered care, (3) care coordination, and (4) data analytics with a focus on outcomes and improvement. In this model of the future, nurses will continue to assume roles to advance health, improve care, and increase value for all stakeholders in health care (Salmond & Echevarria, 2017).

HEALTH SYSTEMS EVALUATION: COST, QUALITY, VALUE, AND TECHNOLOGY

The existence of trade-offs is an inevitable consequence of scarcity and a fundamental premise underlying the need for economic-based evaluation methods in health care (Henderson, 2018). Decision makers at all levels rely on a consideration of costs and benefits to allocate their time, effort, and resources most efficiently to achieve the optimal set of outcomes. Decisions must be made about how capital budget dollars will be allocated, which drugs and procedures are eligible for reimbursement and payment, and numerous other resource choices at all levels of health care. In a world of scarce resources, health care organizations face difficult choices such as whether to invest in more intensive care capacity or an expanded emergency department. Formulary committees must decide which medications to include and which ones to exclude because resources are finite. This section focuses on four fundamental areas of concern to nurses: costs, quality of care, value, and technology.

Costs

Costs are resources required by the provider of services to produce health care products and services, as well as the amount a consumer pays to purchase the products and services. The costs to produce health care are the actual costs of inputs incurred for production, whereas the costs to purchase health care services are what the health care economy will bear (i.e., what the consumers and financiers are able and willing to pay) (Henderson, 2018). Thus, costs depend on supply and demand. Costs may be *monetary (pecuniary)* or *intangible (nonpecuniary)*. The pecuniary costs of care include salaries of health care providers, insurance premiums, the cost of supplies and equipment used during care, management overhead, pharmaceuticals, transportation, lost salary of the consumer, and construction and maintenance costs and research. Nonpecuniary costs are those associated with the personal loss, pain, suffering, and other consequences associated with the consumption of health care services.

The costs of health care are affected by many factors, including the supply of services, the demand for services, and the use of medical technology. An increase in the input costs of providing a service leads to an increase in health care expenditures, while the quantity and quality remain constant. Efforts are focused on reducing health care expenditures by reducing the input costs of care without sacrificing the quantity and quality of services (Henderson, 2018). The resources consumed to produce or purchase a product or service are no longer available for the production or purchase of an alternative product or service. The value of the alternative product or service forgone is known as the *opportunity cost* (McPake et al., 2020). The opportunity cost is the cost associated with the "alternative choice not taken" to afford the selected good or service. A hospital that can afford to purchase only one of two diagnostic or therapeutic technologies must, in choosing one, give up the known benefits of the other. The value of the forgone benefits (revenue generated, lives saved) is the opportunity cost. The concept of opportunity cost also can be applied to personal economic decision-making. In the case of RNs who decide to return to school full-time to pursue advanced education, the opportunity cost of this career decision includes any lost earnings resulting from reducing work hours to complete the educational program.

Quality of Care

Nurses historically have led and contributed to all aspects of quality improvement. The 2020 Future of Nursing Report builds on previous work to extend the nursing focus to improve safety, quality, and better outcomes, in the pursuit of health equity for individuals, families, communities, and populations (NASEM, 2021). The Report's recommendations are centered on nursing's role in numerous aspects, to be briefly discussed here. Beyond facilitating access to care, nurses improve the quality of care by coordinating person-centered care for preventive, acute, and chronic health needs within health settings and collaborating with social services to meet the social needs of individuals (NASEM, 2021). Nurses facilitate access to care across a wide variety of settings beyond hospitals, including federally qualified health centers (FQHCs), retail clinics, home health and home visiting, telehealth, school nursing, school-based health centers, as well as nurse-managed health centers. See Chapter 20: Health Care Quality and Safety for an expanded discussion of health care quality and safety concepts, principles, and practices relevant to present-day nursing and collaborative team-based health professions' practice and care delivery.

Nurses are especially prepared and positioned to improve the quality of care while assisting patients and families with navigating the health care system, providing close monitoring and follow-up across the care continuum, and focusing care on the whole person and providing care that is culturally respectful and appropriate (NASEM, 2021).

Specifically, nurses can help overcome barriers to quality care, structural inequities, and implicit bias, through care management, person-centered care, and cultural humility. Nurses engage in *care management, care coordination,* and *transitional care processes; work in teams* to *decrease fragmentation; bolster communication;* and *improve care quality and safety.* Nurses drive the **person-centered model** that incorporates personal choice and autonomy to meet the individual's needs in accordance with their abilities, needs, and preferences. Nurses are in a position to more systematically inject cultural humility into the profession through education, and to clinical settings through practice. *Cultural humility* enables nurses to partner more effectively with patients and families to improve team decision-making, communication and understanding, and improved quality outcomes. See Chapter 14: Diversity, Equity, and Inclusion—Impact on Health Care and Nursing Care Strategies for a more in-depth discussion of cultural humility.

Value

Value is the relationship between quality and cost. In the context of health care markets, *value* is defined as improved health outcomes in relation to the costs of producing services (Henderson, 2018). Stated more simply, value is the sum total of the benefits a provider promises that a consumer will receive in return for purchasing goods or services. In comparison with other industrialized nations, the U.S. health care system suffers from a large value gap. As previously noted, Table 7.1 provides a comparison of the health spending patterns of the major industrialized nations (Organization for Economic Cooperation and Development [OECD], 2021a; 2021b). Although comparisons of U.S. health expenditures with those of other industrialized nations are helpful, they should be interpreted with caution. Henderson (2018) points out that differences in population demographics, per-capita income, disease incidence, and institutional features make direct comparisons difficult.

Rising health care costs and limited health care resources have created a call for documenting the value of professional nursing services and the effect of nursing care on organizational and hospital outcomes. An understanding of the relationship between the quality and the cost of care is paramount because these data inform decisions about the appropriateness and effectiveness of nurses in achieving desired levels of patient care quality. Under the DRG prospective payment system used by the Medicare

TABLE 7.1 Comparison of Health Care Costs, Quality, and Outcomes	United States	OECD Average
Costs		
Percent of GDP (adjusted for cost of living)	16.9%	8.8%
Public spending[a]	$4993	$3038
Private spending[a]	$4092	$226
Out of pocket spending[a]	$1122	$716
Health Outcomes		
Life expectancy (years)	78.6	80.7
Suicide rate (deaths per 100,000)	13.9	11.5
Population Health		
Chronic disease burden (percent with 2 or more chronic medical conditions)	28.0%	17.5%
Obesity	40.0%	21.0%
Utilization		
Average physician visits (per capita, annually)	4.0	6.8
Average hospital length of stay (days)	5.5	6.4
Magnetic resonance imaging (MRI) (scans per 100,000)	111	65
Average hospital length of stay (days)	5.5	6.4
Inpatient hip replacements (per 1000 age 65 and older)	15.6	10.5
Quality and Care Outcomes		
Flu vaccines (percent of adults immunized, age 65 and older)	68%	44%
Breast cancer screening (percent of females screened, ages 50–69)	80%	60%
Breast cancer survival rate	90.2%	85.0%
Cervical cancer survival rate	62.6%	66.0%
Hospitalization rates from preventable causes (discharges per 100,000)		
Diabetes	204	135
Hypertension	159	105
Avoidable deaths (deaths per 100,000)		
2000	149	116
2016	112	70

[a]U.S. dollars, adjusted for cost of living.
Data from Health care costs, quality, and outcomes United States compared to Organisation for Economic Cooperation and Development (OECD, 2021; OECD, 2021a). 2019 Data.

program, hospitals are reimbursed a predetermined amount for services. Hospitals emphasize the daily costs of care, or the ratio of costs to charges for an episode of care, to align the expected reimbursement with profitability. Under this payment system, nursing services become vulnerable to cost-reduction efforts because nursing salaries and benefits make up a large portion of the per-day costs of hospital-based patient care. As discussed previously regarding payment systems, the focus for hospitals is to reduce the daily costs of care by reducing nurse staffing levels or substituting RNs with unlicensed personnel. Reducing nurse staffing levels emphasizes the cost of nursing without considering

how nurses contribute to the quality of patient care (Aiken, 2008). The impact of the intensity of direct nursing care and staffing levels, on the quality of patient care, has been well-documented since 1999 (Phillips et al., 2021). From the pioneering work of Linda Aiken (Aiken et al., 2002), to more recent studies and reviews (Needleman et al., 2020), substantial evidence has been accumulated to support the direct impact of nursing hours on patient, staff, and organizational outcomes (Aiken & Sloane, 2021).

Specifically, evidence demonstrates that patients suffer from higher mortality rates and overall failure-to-rescue rates in hospitals where nurses cared for more (rather than fewer) patients (Burke et al., 2022). *Failure-to-rescue* is the inability of a clinician to save a patient's life when a complication arises, and one of the presumed intermediaries between staffing levels and patient outcomes. Additionally, higher hours of care from all nursing care providers in conjunction with a higher proportion of RN hours of care are associated with better outcomes for hospitalized patients (Aiken et al., 2002). This research establishes that nurses create value. That is, the costs associated with nursing services bring increased returns to the consumer through nursing's contribution to patient care quality and safety. Failure-to-rescue comprises four key attributes: (1) errors of omission in care, (2) failures to recognize changes in patient condition, (3) failures to communicate condition changes, and (4) failures in clinical-decision making (Burke et al., 2022). Thus, nurses have a key role in preventing failure-to-rescue through early recognition, escalation of findings, and intervention of early changes signaling complications. The implication is that effective nursing resources, in terms of sufficient staffing, competencies, and effective management, all interact to shift failure-to-rescue.

Technology

In its broadest sense, *technology* is the application of scientific knowledge used to transform inputs into outputs with the goal of improving productivity or economic growth (Henderson, 2018). The expansion of health insurance since World War II has led to an interdependent relationship between health care technology and insurance and has had a dramatic effect on health care costs (NASEM, 2002). As the financing of services shifted from individuals to insurance companies, individuals became removed from, and insensitive to, the actual costs of health care technologies. Because of the retrospective payment system, in which all services rendered were reimbursed, health care providers (i.e., physicians and hospitals) had financial incentives to use all technologies available regardless of cost. Research and development markets also had the financial incentives of reimbursement to continue to produce new health care technologies at any cost (NASEM, 2002). Consequently, patient and provider demand for greater technology has heightened and become more widespread, as have soaring health care expenditures.

The abundant development and use of technologies have fueled the debate over the appropriateness of many disease-focused clinical interventions in improving health outcomes and overall health status. Because of how health technologies are financed, health care organizations have increased incentives to adopt new technologies, for many of which the long-term effectiveness or costs are not fully known. Once a new technology is integrated into clinical practice routines, it is very difficult for an organization to disengage from using that technology. Studies suggest that newer technologies tend to complement, rather than replace, older technologies and that hospitals with constrained financial resources are likely to retain ineffective clinical technologies, creating a reverse access problem in which disadvantaged populations have access to ineffective, less effective, or harmful treatments at a higher rate than the population at large (NASEM, 2002).

Technology assessment and *outcomes research* are intended to help decision-makers deal with the development, acquisition, and use of health care practices and technologies. The goal is to improve patient health, efficiency, and value. Technology assessment, as a form of policy research, evaluates the safety, effectiveness, and costs of technologies to provide the basis for clinical and social policies, including resource allocation. A *health technology assessment* (HTA) "provides a framework to determine whether prices of health interventions reflect the benefit to patients" (Mulligan et al., 2020). An HTA informs policy and decision-making regarding the allocation of limited resources using a multidisciplinary approach from the clinical, epidemiological, and health-economic perspectives (World Health Organization [WHO], 2020).

HTA has grown in popularity and use in response to cost containment pressures as a tool for evidence-based clinical and policy decision-making. HTA has evolved from a technique of synthesizing the best evidence for policymakers in national governments to disseminating information about the effectiveness of technologies to clinicians and managers to influence the costs, safety, and quality of patient care. Early assessments tended to focus on large, expensive, machine-based technologies, the scope of which has expanded to include "softer" technologies, such as counseling and other process-oriented health care services (Mulligan et al., 2020)

Technology assessments are time-consuming and costly. Traditional health care markets provide little incentive for investment in the process. During the 1990s technology assessment and the evidence-based practice movement gained importance as tools to inform policy, practice, and health care investment decisions. Nonetheless, these quality improvement methods are not without their limitations.

The AHRQ's Technology Assessment program has conducted technology assessments for the CMS since 2009 (AHRQ, n.d.). The assessments address current and emerging technologies to guide CMS decision-making in its national coverage decisions for the Medicare program. Private nongovernment insurance providers have access to this information as well. State-of-the-art methodologies are used to assess the clinical utility of medical interventions. Technology assessments are based on a systematic review of the literature, along with appropriate qualitative and quantitative methods of synthesizing data from multiple studies.

Nursing practice, education, and administration are directly affected by the application of new medical and health care practices and technologies. Nursing's participation in technology research has evolved significantly since 1990. In a systematic review of the literature, Ramacciati (2013) identified 70 technology assessment studies led by nurses. Nurses directly witness the individual and societal benefits and the burdens those various practices and technologies contribute to health care. Nurses offer a wealth of clinical knowledge and expertise that could advance technology assessment. Nurses can play an important part in interdisciplinary technology assessment teams, developing clinical practice guidelines, leading to organizational change initiatives focused on integrating evidence into clinical practice routines, and advocating social policy regarding health care technologies. In today's marketplace, payers are increasingly willing to pay only for those technologies that are cost-effective and medically appropriate. Within this context, the nursing profession has an opportunity to develop and demonstrate the effectiveness of nursing-specific interventions and service technologies.

Economic Evaluation in Health Systems

Economic efficiency in health care refers to the consideration of both health benefits and resource costs (Henderson, 2018). Evaluations are made in terms of costs and consequences. The two predominant methods of evaluating the economic costs of a service or program are cost-benefit analysis and cost-effectiveness analysis. Other analytical methods used to assess the economic effects of new health care interventions or technologies include cost-minimization analysis, cost-utility analysis, and a variety of combinations to suit a specific purpose (McPake et al., 2020).

Cost-Benefit Analysis. Cost-benefit analysis is an analytical technique that requires assessment and evaluation of the costs and benefits of a program to determine whether the benefits of a project outweigh its costs. In a cost-benefit analysis, all costs and benefits undergo valuation and are stated in monetary terms. This process places a dollar amount on both monetary and nonmonetary costs and benefits so a comparison can be made between competing projects or programs. In doing so, value or worth is assigned to nonmonetary aspects of the project's costs and benefits.

Cost-benefit analysis is a useful and powerful tool to justify the investment in nurse-managed services to managers responsible for resource allocation decisions. In this era of resource efficiency and service change, a critical skill for nurses across practice settings and role descriptions is the ability not only to speak the language of economics but also to demonstrate the unique value of nursing services in terms of cost, quality, and value. The widespread availability of personal computers and spreadsheet software makes cost-benefit analysis an accessible tool to a broad range of people. The calculations become effortless. Even so, quantification of the tangible and intangible costs is the difficulty of this method.

The comparative nature of the cost-benefit analysis is an attractive feature of this analytical technique, but in determining the "worthiness" of a project, it is also a pitfall and a drawback. The major limitation of the application of cost-benefit analysis in health care scenarios is that the valuation of intangible costs such as pain or grief or premature loss of life varies not only from case to case but also among analysts assigning the values. Economic evaluation methods can be applied across the continuum of strategic to operational, with the following two examples at each end of the continuum.

Cost-Effectiveness Analysis. Cost-effectiveness analysis is an analytical technique for comparing resource consumption between two or more alternatives that meet a particular objective (e.g., minimum quality of a product or production of a specific patient outcome) (Henderson, 2018). Cost-effectiveness analysis measures the costs involved with each alternative and determines the most cost-effective, or least costly, alternative (Henderson, 2018; McPake et al., 2020). In a cost-effectiveness analysis, only the monetary costs of inputs into each alternative are considered because the objective (or outcome) of the alternatives is assumed to be the same; the valuation of benefits is not considered. Thus, cost-effectiveness analysis avoids making valuations while providing an empirical evaluation of the costs of alternative health care interventions.

Other less widely used methods are *Cost-Utilization Analysis (CUA)* and *Cost-Minimization Analysis (CMA)*. CUA is a special case of CE analysis that addresses quality-of-life concerns using quality-adjusted life years (QALY). QALY assigns a value to identify the impact of a particular treatment and to compare treatment effectiveness. Providers and policymakers can use this type of analysis to guide decision-making when the clinical effectiveness of treatment options may be equivalent. Accordingly, when comparing several alternatives, the cost-minimization analysis approach may be most suitable.

THE SUPPLY AND DEMAND FOR NURSES: THE CYCLICAL NATURE OF THE NURSING WORKFORCE

In this section, we examine the market for nurses to illustrate the concepts of *supply and demand*. The concepts of *complements and substitutes* are also presented to examine the use of APRNs as an alternative to physicians as primary care providers (PCPs). *Supply* refers to the amount of a good or service available to consumers in the market and *demand* refers to a consumer's willingness to purchase a particular good or service (Henderson, 2018).

In economics, demand is different from "need" in the sense that we may predict that individuals require or need a particular service such as dental care, but without the willingness or ability to purchase these services, this need does not become a demand. Similarly, on the supply side, we may know that a certain number of RNs are licensed to practice, but if they do not make the decision to be employed in the workforce, they are not included in the supply. Economic principles drive decisions such as what services are offered in the health care system and how many and to what extent nurses participate in the workforce.

Economic theory predicts as demand increases, as will supply; the pricing mechanism, in the form of wages and other benefits, will create a balance (equilibrium) between firms in need of workers and individuals who are willing to work for the wage offered. When examining the market for labor, economists assume households have primary and secondary wage earners. Because a very high proportion of nurses are married, they are part of two-earner families and therefore may have more flexibility to respond to employment opportunities as real wages change or in relation to the employment situation of their spouses (Henderson, 2018).

The U.S. Nursing Workforce

The **NCSBN** and the **National Forum of State Nursing Workforce Centers (Forum)** conduct the only regular national-level survey focused on the entire U.S. nursing workforce, the *2020 National Nursing Workforce Survey* (NNWS) (Smiley et al., 2021). Their survey report provides data every two years on the supply of RNs and licensed practical nurses/licensed vocational nurses (LPNs/LVNs). These supply-side data provide information on emerging nursing workforce issues, especially important in 2020 during the coronavirus (COVID-19) pandemic (Smiley et al., 2021). As of December 2019, the total number of active RN and LPN/LVN licenses in the United States were 4,198,031 and 944,813, respectively. The number of RNs had increased by 6.3%, and the number of LPNs increased by 2.6%, since 2017. The NNWS of 2020 is based on a national randomized sample of 157,459 licensed RNs and 172,045 (LPNs/ LVNs, conducted between February and June 2020. It is important to put the data collection in context; on March 11, the WHO reported that COVID-19 had reached a pandemic level worldwide (WHO, 2020). In addition to the size of the workforce, key findings relate to the aging workforce;

gender, race, and ethnicity; education; licensure; employment and salary; and telehealth utilization.

Aging of the Workforce. The median age of RNs was 52 years, as compared to the median age of 51 in 2017. Nurses 65 years or older comprised 19.0% of the RN workforce, an increase from 14.6% in 2017, and 4.4% in 2013. Similarly, the average age of LPNs/LVNs was 53 years, an increase from 52 years in 2017. LPNs/LVNs over 65 comprise 18.2% of the workforce, an increase from 5.0% in 2017. Further impact from the aging workforce is expected as more than 20% of nurses surveyed plan to retire within the next 5 years.

Gender, Race, and Ethnicity. Males comprise 9.4% of RNs, and 8.1% of LPNs/LVNs, increasing from 9.1% and 7.7%, respectively, since 2017. In 2020, a third-gender option was offered and selected by 0.1% of nurses. Nearly 81% of RNs reported as White/Caucasian. Asians represented the second largest RN group at 7.2%, followed by Black/African American RNs at 6.7%. Hispanic/Latinx Ethnicity remained almost flat since 2017 at 5.6%.

Education. The percentage of baccalaureate-prepared RNs was 65.2%, an increase from 57.4% in 2017. The number of RNs with a doctor of nursing practice (DNP) degree increased from 0.4% to 1.4% in 2013. PhD-prepared RNs increased from 0.6% to 0.7% in 2017. Approximately 42% of RNs reported the baccalaureate as their entry-to-practice degree, an increase from 36.2% in 2013. RNs entering practice at the master's degree level decreased slightly from 3.9% to 3.6% in 2017. Interestingly, the percentage of LPNs/LVNs with associate and baccalaureate degrees was 12.7% and 3.1%, respectively.

Licensure. Over 750,000 RNs had duplicate licenses from more than a single jurisdiction, and over 2 million RNs are licensed in one of the 39 enhanced Nurse Licensure Compact (eNLC) states (NCSBN, 2022). The percentage of RNs with an APRN credential decreased from 10% to 6.6% in 2013. Almost 94% of RNs receive their license to practice in the United States, and 33% of nurses with a multistate license use it for physical cross-border practice. The percentage of LPNs/LVNs with a multistate license was 21.2%, with 4.4% of the total using the license for cross-border practice.

Employment and Salary. The percentage of RNs actively employed in nursing was 84.1%, with 64.9% working full-time (FT), a slight decrease in FT from 65.4% in 2017. The predominant primary practice setting was hospitals, with 54.8% of RNs, a slight decrease from 55.7% in 2017. Almost 10% of RNs practice in ambulatory settings, and approximately 4.5% in home health and nursing home/extended care settings. In terms of job title, 60.1% identified as a staff nurse, as compared to 58.0% in 2017. The percentage of APRN job titles decreased to 6.3% from 10.1% in 2017. Sixty-eight percent of RNs and 77.8% of LPN/LVNs reported spending the majority of their time providing direct patient care. Median pretax earnings for RNs increased to $70,000 from $60,000 in 2015, a 3.3% annual growth rate in earnings during the 5-year period. The median earnings for RNs have risen in all states since 2015. Almost two-thirds of LPN/LVNs are employed full-time in practice, which is like the 2017 results. Overall, the median pretax salary for this group increased to $44,000 from $38,000 in 2015, an annual rate of 3.1%.

Telehealth Utilization. Approximately half of all nurses reported using some type of telehealth technology in practice. It is important to again note the timing of the survey which was during the pandemic when many settings were transitioning to higher uses of telehealth. However, the percentage of nurses using telehealth has remained relatively unchanged since 2017.

Nurse Employment During the COVID-19 Pandemic

Using payroll and census data from before and during the first fifteen months of the pandemic, Buerhaus et al. (2022) examined the impact of the pandemic on the employment and earnings of RNs, nursing assistants (NA), and LPN/LVNs. While this study is unable to definitively attribute the impact to overall changes in supply or demand, it does identify trends to be further assessed. Overall, nurse employment remained low while wages increased during the first 15 months of the pandemic, which suggests a tightening labor market in which demand outpaced supply (Buerhaus et al., 2022).

Nurse employment decreased early in the pandemic as the demand for health care declined as health care organizations trimmed back or shuttered ambulatory and other non-critical services. As the pandemic progressed and the use of health care services resumed, nurse employment remained low while unemployment rates receded, and wages increased. As noted by Buerhaus et al. (2022), this suggests a tightening of the labor market for nurses in which demand exceeded supply. However, the employment rate did not rebound in nursing homes, with total employment remaining more than 10% below prepandemic levels. This may be in response to the proportion of nursing home residents' fatalities. As of March 2021, an estimated 10% of nursing home residents had died of COVID-19 (Long-term care Covid Tracker, 2021). Of note is that as employment rebounded overall as services resumed, RNs and NAs had higher initial unemployment and a lower rebound than Whites.

As Buerhaus et al. (2017) note, the important question for the longer term is whether the falling LPN employment rate and the plateaued RN rate will continue, and what will be the impact of the impending reduction in employed baby-boom RNs. The majority of the estimated 660,000 baby boom RNs still employed during the pandemic are expected to retire by 2030. The departure of such a large cohort of experienced RNs from the workforce will also represent a significant loss of nursing knowledge and expertise, which is likely to impact organizations for many years to come.

An extended analysis of employment data for the entirety of 2021 shows that the total supply of RNs decreased by more than 100,000 in that single year. This represents the greatest single-year decrease in the number of RNs over the past 40 years (Auerbach et al., 2022). Of specific concern is that the decrease resulted primarily from younger RNs. Compared to 2019, prior to the pandemic, the nursing workforce decreased by almost 2% overall, but an almost 4% reduction in hospital employment was partially offset by an approximate 2% increase in shifting to other practice settings (Auerbach et al., 2022).

Workforce Modeling and Forecasting Supply and Demand

Historically, forecasts for the supply and demand of nurses have been the responsibility of the National Center for Health Workforce Analysis (NCHWA), within the Bureau of Health Workforce of the Human Resources and Services Administration (HRSA). The Center constructed and shared models with stakeholders at the state, regional, and local levels to support decision-making related to the supply and demand of nurses. Beginning in 2013, the Center shifted toward greater collaboration with the **NCSBN** and the members of the **Forum**. The **NCSBN** is an independent nonprofit organization that supports and connects 59 boards of nursing. These include one board for each of the 50 states, the District of Columbia (DC), and four U.S. territories (American Samoa, Guam, Northern Mariana Islands, and the Virgin Islands). In addition, California, Louisiana, and West Virginia have separate boards for RNs and LPN/LVNs, and Nebraska has a separate board for APRNs. The **Forum** is a collaborative member organization that comprises the 34 state-level nursing workforce centers across the United States, supported through public and private funding sources. The Forum contributes to the national effort to "assure an adequate supply of qualified nurses to meet the health needs of the U.S. population" through long-range strategic planning (National Forum, n.d.).

As the NCHWA has partnered with NCSBN and The National Forum on sharing resources and the work related to surveys of the nursing workforce, its approach to constructing projection models for supply and demand has shifted. In 2015 the *Health Workforce Simulation Model* tool was introduced by NCHWA. The model is an integrated microsimulation tool that estimates the future supply and demand of health care workers in several professions, including nursing. The model provides state-level estimates with the ability for users to test the effects of policy decisions by customizing inputs through a web-based interface with the ability to export data sets to use at the micro level. In September 2021, the NCHWA launched the dynamic and interactive workforce projection site that is supported in the background by the microsimulation models (NCHWA, n.d.). Projections through 2030 are offered for behavioral health, long-term care, primary care, and women's health for various job titles, including nurse practitioners. However, projections, estimates, and the underlying assumptions do not reflect the impact of the pandemic, and data for RNs is not yet available on demand through the site. The latest national projections of supply and demand were published in 2017 using data from 2014. Although the source data is likely outdated now to draw any specific conclusions, the projections highlight the inequitable distribution of the nursing workforce across the United States (USDHHS, 2017).

The NCHWA most recently issued national- and state-level supply and demand projections for the nursing workforce, using the Health Workforce Simulation Model tool for through 2030 using 2014 as the base year (USDHHS, 2017). The projections highlight the inequitable distribution of the nursing workforce across the United States. Key findings from these projections identify substantial variation between states by 2030 (USDHHS, 2017). Seven states were projected to have deficits, including four states with deficits greater than 10,000 full-time equivalents (FTEs): (1) California (44,500), (2) Texas (15,900), (3) New Jersey (11,400), and (4) South Carolina (10,400) (USDHHS, 2017). States projected to experience the largest excess supply in terms of FTEs include: (1) Florida (53,700), (2) Ohio (49,100), (3) Virginia (22,700), and (4) New York (18,200) (USDHHS, 2017). Similar inequitable distribution patterns are projected for LPNs/LVNs (USDHHS, 2017). Thus, albeit somewhat outdated, projections demonstrate the existence of separate labor markets with an unknown degree of interaction.

The overall general model is shown in Fig. 7.5, with the supply model components on the left side and the demand components on the right (USDHHS, 2021). The major components of the *supply submodel* include: (a) microdata files containing the characteristics of the current workforce in the given profession, (b) annual estimates of the numbers and characteristics of those entering the workforce, and (c) equations that integrate workforce decisions such as retirement rates and the number of hours worked. On the *demand side*, the model simulates demand for services based on the individual characteristics of the U.S. population, including demographics, socioeconomics, health behavior, and health status. The major components of the demand submodel include: (a) databases that contain a representative sample of the population in each state by demographics, household income, medical insurance, and residency institution (e.g., community, residential care facility, or nursing home); (b) regression equations that relate health care use patterns by setting to an individual's characteristics; and (c) staffing ratios and patterns for emergency departments, hospitals, provider offices, outpatient departments, home health, nursing homes, and residential facilities (USDHHS, 2021). The Center allows individual users at the state and health system levels to use the model to upload data and explore alternative scenarios by modifying key parameters such as graduation rates, attrition rates, and retirement rates that pertain to the user's area of interest. Output from the model simulations can be downloaded and used as a foundation for planning tools for the recruitment and retention of the future nursing workforce.

Monopsony Power of Hospitals

In a well-functioning market, a shortage should be resolved by wage increases until a balance is restored (equilibrium) between organizations in need of workers and workers who are willing to participate in the labor force. One argument used to explain the chronic shortage of nurses is the notion that nurses are underpaid and it is the low wages, relative to those of other health professionals, and other job opportunities outside of nursing and health care, that keep individuals from participating in the workforce as RNs. From a purely economic perspective, linking the labor shortage to low wages is curious because it violates the basic assumptions of supply and demand.

In contrast, markets with many hospitals competing for nursing labor conform more closely to the predictions of supply and demand. As noted previously, the presence of multiple competitors (hospitals) in one market provides more favorable conditions for workers (nurses) in terms of the wages employers will offer to satisfy their demand for labor. Under competitive market conditions, when faced with a shortage of nurses, some hospitals will move faster than others and offer a higher wage for nurses. The wage increase brings about two important outcomes that, taken together, help alleviate the nursing shortage. In the short-term, increased wages are incentives for nurses who are currently unemployed to re-enter the workforce.

Although nurses are employed in several different practice settings, hospitals are the main employer of nurses. Approximately 55% of RNs are employed in acute care

Uninsured Rate by Poverty Status and Medicaid Expansion of State for Adults Aged 19 to 64: 2018 and 2020
(Population as of March of the following year, adults aged 19 to 64)

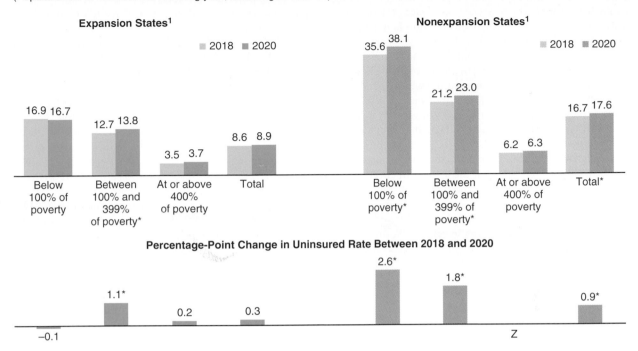

Fig. 7.5 Uninsured Rate by Poverty Status and Medicaid Expansion of State for Adults Aged 19 to 64.
(Used with permission Keisler-Starkey & Bunch, 2021.)

*Denotes a statistically significant change between 2018 and 2020 at the 90% confidence level.

Z rounds to zero.

[1]Medicaid expansion status as of January 1, 2020, for 2020 data, Medicaid expansion status as of January 1, 2018, for 2018 data. Expansion states on or before January 1, 2018, include AK, AR, AZ, CA, CO, CT, DC, DE, HI, IA, IL, IN, KY, LA, MA, MD, MI, MN, MT, ND, NH, NJ, NM, NV, NY, OH, OR, PA, RI, VT, WA, and WV. After January 1, 2018, and on or before January 1, 2020, ID, ME, UT, and VA expanded Medicaid. More information is available at www.medicaid.gov/state-overviews/index.html

Note: Information on confidentiality protection, sampling error, nonsampling error, and definitions, is available at https://www2.census.gov/programs-surveys/cps/techdocs/cpsmar21.pdf
Source: U.S. Census Bureau, Current Population Survey, 2019 and 2021 Annual Social and Economic Supplement (CPS ASEC).

hospital settings (Smiley et al., 2021). Therefore, much information about the market for nursing labor is understood within the context of hospitals. The monopsony model is based on the assumptions that the market has one dominant buyer (employer) or perhaps a few employers in a regional market who control the demand for workers and all persons who do the same work are paid the same wage. Because workers are paid the same wage, if the employer has to offer a higher wage to get additional workers, it must also raise the wages of the workers already employed. Eventually, higher portions of the operating budget would be expended on salaries and the hospital would not be able to make a sufficient surplus or profit. As discussed previously, organizations need to make a surplus to stay in business.

The hospital in the monopsony model considers the cost of hiring one more nurse in relation to the amount of revenue it will gain from the productivity of that nurse. In effect, the hospital sets nurses' wages, so it maximizes its ability to make a profit. In this situation, the wage level that satisfies the hospital's profit goal is lower than what nurses could be offered if there were more buyers in the market. Because nurses often have choices about participating in the labor force, they may decide the wage offered by a hospital is too low and decide to forgo working for a particular hospital. Thus, the hospital will continue to need nurses and the nurses' wages will be lower than those of other comparable workers. If nurses in sufficient numbers were willing to move to other communities with higher wages, or if they transferred their skills and experience to other types of work within the local labor market, competition could be restored which would raise wages (Henderson, 2018). An increased local demand for nurses outside the hospital would change the labor dynamic.

Traditionally, geographic mobility among nurses has been historically low. However, in a study of the willingness of nurses to travel for employment during the pandemic, Gottlieb and Zenilman (2020) found that as the market for travel nurses expanded, more nurses were willing to travel longer distances for work. This was viewed as an integrated national market expanded during the pandemic, resulting in a reallocation of RNs beyond their previous local market. It remains to be seen what the long-term effect on the monopsony in local nurse labor markets may be.

In examining economic issues related to the nursing labor market, it is important to also recognize and address the gender wage gap that occurs in nursing. Women's median salaries are lower than men's in nearly all occupations, nursing included. In the most recent report by the **Institute for Women's Policy Research** (IWPR, 2021), the median earnings by women were 96.9% as much as men's earnings. Similar discrepancies between men and women are seen as well in nonlicensed health care roles.

It is important to note nurses' decisions to participate in the workforce are complex and are not fully explained by economic theory. Managerial and public policies targeting cost containment, such as efforts to reduce in-patient length of stay (LOS), have had a greater effect on the working conditions of nurses and have contributed to the duration of the current shortage (Aiken, 2008). Strong evidence suggests attributes of the organizational environment, also referred to as the *nursing practice environment,* factor into individual nurses' decisions to stay employed at a particular hospital or participate in the workforce in the capacity of an RN. Organizational factors such as workload, managers' leadership style, autonomy over nursing practice, promotion opportunities, and work schedules also contribute to nurses' decisions to work (Nelson-Brantley et al., 2018). A recent integrative review of 43 studies suggests that nurse turnover has increased significantly during the pandemic. As the demand and workload have increased, stress, burnout, and psychological stress, present before the pandemic, were exacerbated (Falatah, 2021). The ongoing and future impact of the pandemic on nurse turnover will need to be incorporated into future nurse labor projections.

Nurses as Complements and Substitutes for Physicians

Complements are products or services that are usually consumed jointly so that an increase in the price of one decreases the demand for both (e.g., intravenous fluids and tubing) (Henderson, 2018). If nursing services are complements to physician services, an increase in the price of physician services will decrease the demand for both physician and nursing services.

Substitutes, on the other hand, are goods or services that satisfy the same want or need, so an increase in the price of one will increase the demand for the other (Henderson, 2018). One example of substitutes in health care occurs when two medications have the same therapeutic effect. Another example relates to an obstetrician and a nurse midwife. If nursing services are substitutes for physician obstetrical services, an increase in the cost of physician services will increase the demand for nurse-midwife services.

In the physician arena, an imbalance exists between generalists and specialists, resulting in a shortage of primary care physicians (Association of American Medical Colleges [AAMC], 2021). According to the AAMC, the United States could see an estimated shortage of between 21,400 and 55,200 primary care physicians by 2033, with RNs practicing in primary care centers as physician substitutes and possibly in hospitals. As the number of physicians in primary care practice falls short of the need, NPs and physician assistants (PAs) will partially fill the gap between supply and demand. The NPs will likely increase in overall number, and those employed in nonadvanced practice roles will have the opportunity to shift to primary care roles (CMS, n.d.-d). Similarly, health care delivery organizations, to reduce input costs, are incorporating the use of unlicensed personnel as substitutes for nurses for those activities that do not require licensure. For example, hospitals and other delivery organizations have changed the nursing staff skill mix to include RNs, LPNs/LVNs, and NA. Thus, nurses are both substituting for some types of providers and being substituted by other types of providers.

Physicians have traditionally held a monopolistic power as PCPs because regulations have prevented others from "practicing medicine." As alternative providers of health care services demonstrate their ability to provide comparable services, regulations are being changed to allow these substitutes to enter the market and compete with physicians. Such changes in regulation have come about because consumers have demanded more cost-effective providers, although the policy debate continues in the form of opposition from medical associations and physician groups (Kraus & Thompson, 2021).

With APRNs working as physician substitutes, competition between these two providers can occur based on cost-effectiveness. Numerous study findings suggest that care delivered by nurse practitioners, compared to the care delivered by physicians, probably generates similar or better health outcomes for a broad range of patient conditions

(Laurant et al., 2018). Butler et al. (2020) explored the impact of substituting nurses for physicians in various hospital roles on a patient, the process of care, and economic outcomes.

Another growing area in which NPs function as physician substitutes is in the retail clinic segment. Retail clinics differ from urgent care clinics because they are located within discount stores, grocery stores, or drug stores; are staffed by either NPs or PAs; offer a limited set of basic medical and preventive services. Retail clinics are an emerging trend in which APRNs act as substitutes for physicians to meet consumers' desire for more convenient and lower-cost medical care (Rand Corporation, 2016). Health care services typically offered at retail clinics include preventive care such as immunizations and blood pressure screening, as well as treatment for the upper respiratory tract, sinusitis, ear, or urinary tract infections. Clients mainly pay for retail visits out of pocket, although in recent years many insurance companies, including Medicare and Medicaid, will pay for these visits (Rand Corporation, 2016).

The numbers of retail clinics and urgent care centers have increased consistently each year since 2013. As of 2022, there were more than 3300 retail clinics in the United States, Canada, and Mexico, with the majority in the United States distributed across 44 states and the DC (Convenient Care Association [CCA], 2022). This is in addition to 9616 urgent care centers as of 2019, as patients seek convenience and affordability creating competition with traditional hospital and physician practice services (Finnegan, 2020).

Community-based nurse-led clinics led by APRNs are a growing trend in the United States, Sweden, the United Kingdom, New Zealand, Canada, and Australia (Dalia, 2018). Although a much smaller presence than in other settings, with 150 clinics in the United States in 2022, this model has shown promising results in terms of access, patient outcomes, and patient satisfaction (National Nurse-Led Care Consortium [NNLCC], n.d.; Randall et al., 2017). Cost-effectiveness is not well reported for this segment.

Generalist nurses may also be considered within the economic framework of substitution. Rutherford (2017) reports on the work of a group of Robert Wood Johnson Foundation (RWJF) Fellows who explored the use of RNs to provide behavioral health care. From an economic perspective, the cost of the current mental health crisis in the United States is estimated at $444 billion, including lost productivity. Early identification and treatment of mental illness would have a substantial effect on health care spending and overall economic effect. In this model, RNs are uniquely positioned to improve behavioral health through RN team leadership and care coordination across the care continuum (Rutherford, 2017).

Laurant et al. (2018) also identified numerous examples in which generalist nurses enhance service effectiveness and efficiency by reducing physician workload by assisting with history taking, screening, or ordering tests, prescription renewal, care planning with patients, and educational and psychological support. Many of these substitute activities could be accomplished through protocols.

THE ECONOMIC IMPACT OF COVID-19 ON THE HEALTH CARE INDUSTRY AND THE OVERALL ECONOMY

The COVID-19 pandemic that began in March 2020 has had a tremendous impact on most aspects of society across the world. This section will focus on the economic impact of the pandemic on the overall global and U.S. economies, insurance coverage, financial losses to providers, racial and ethnic disparities, the health care workforce, and public health infrastructure and capacity.

The Economy

The economy is the system through which goods and services are produced and consumed to fulfill the needs of its society members. Economies can be identified and described in global and individual nation terms, as well as more specific regarding regions, states, cities, and even personal households. At the national level, as discussed previously, the "size of the economy" is measured in terms of *gross domestic product* (GDP) (Henderson, 2018). In addition to its size or magnitude, the GDP can be characterized in terms of growth or decline as a rate, to determine how fast and by how much the economy changes. Measurement and reporting of the effects are typically retrospective, as economic impact occurs over time, but a current understanding by economists has developed (El Keshky et al., 2020).

On a global level, the production of goods and services declined, leading to a relatively shrinking economy. Declining sales due to the COVID-19 disruption impacts individuals and communities. When unemployed individuals are unable to contribute to the economy, multiple uncertainties arise, and overall disruption occurs. In the United States, several major legislative and government actions were taken to mitigate the economic effects of the pandemic on individuals and the nation. Since October 2020, $5.7 trillion has been authorized in Federal spending, tax cuts, loans, grants, and subsidies. An additional $7.1 trillion has been spent by the Federal Reserve to reinforce the money supply by purchasing additional long-term U.S. Treasury securities and mortgage-backed securities (Committee for a Responsible Federal Budget [CRFB], n.d.).

In 2021, federal spending was $6.82 trillion, equal to 30% of the GDP (U.S. Treasury Department, n.d.). Future debt was used to finance these current actions. Future economic impact will be measured in terms of the GDP and in terms of unemployment rates, spending, and interest rates.

Health insurance coverage was initially significantly undermined due to many individuals losing their employer-sponsored health insurance (Blumenthal et al., 2020). Many individuals may have found coverage with spouses, and others may have become eligible for Medicaid. Continued reliance on employer-sponsored plans for over half of the population is tenuous when employment is significantly affected as in the pandemic. The financial losses to health care providers have been well documented and reported. The AHA reported early in the pandemic hospitals faced tremendous strain, first from the closure or reduction in nonemergent services and then from the associated increased labor and nonsalary expense associated with caring for patients during the pandemic. Hospitals are expected to lose over $300 billion, after expenses. Longstanding racial and ethnic disparities and inequities were further exposed as the Black and Hispanic populations have been disproportionately affected by COVID-19 infection and deaths. In 2020, nearly 20% of U.S. counties are disproportionately Black, and these counties have accounted for more than half of COVID-19 cases and almost 60% of COVID-19 deaths nationally (Millett et al., 2020). The impact on the health care workforce has been discussed elsewhere in this chapter and is likely to be monumental and evolutionary in terms of how nursing emerges from this global health crisis. Finally, the need for a coherent public health capacity, at the national, state, and local levels, continues to be highlighted during the pandemic. Interstate collaboration and national direction will be required to prevent unnecessary suffering and deaths in this continuing pandemic and future pandemics.

SUMMARY

This chapter provides an overview of the many economic issues that are shaping the national discussion about health care service, its effect on our society, and, by extension, its effect on professional nursing practice. Professional nurses must have a basic understanding of economic forces and the ability to apply these principles if they are to effectively create a robust patient-centered, health-focused care delivery system. This chapter serves as a foundation on which to build knowledge and skills to participate in health system reform efforts. Keeping abreast of changes in the dynamic health care economy is one way in which new knowledge shapes the practice environment and professional decision-making. Journalistic accounts, professional publications, and Internet resources dedicated to the presentation and discussion of issues in health and nursing economics are widely available. Table 7.2 lists a variety of websites that address economic issues related to health care. Professional nurses have the knowledge and expertise to create a socially just health care system. Nursing participation in decision-making activities will occur by placing nursing services within an economic context.

TABLE 7.2   Online HealthCare System, Policy, and Economics Resources

Website	Description	Internet Address
AHRQ (Agency for Health Care Research and Quality)	Programs, tools, and data for health care professionals and policymakers to make informed health decisions	http://www.ahrq.gov/
ANA (American Nurses Association)	Current information related to nursing excellence, work environment, nurse workforce, and health policy	https://www.nursingworld.org/ana
CEVR (Center for the Evaluation of Health and Risk in Health)	Comprehensive database of health care economic analyses	https://cevr.tuftsmedicalcenter.org/databases/cea-registry
Commonwealth Fund (2021)	Independent research on health care issues and making grants to improve health care practice and policy	https://www.commonwealthfund.org/
Health Affairs Forefront	Health policy news, commentary, and analysis	https://www.healthaffairs.org/forefront

TABLE 7.2 Online HealthCare System, Policy, and Economics Resources—cont'd		
Website	**Description**	**Internet Address**
HRSA (Health Resources & Services Administration) Health Workforce	Health workforce research, data, tools, projections, grants, loan repayment, and scholarships	https://bhw.hrsa.gov/
Kaiser Family Foundation	A nonpartisan source of facts, analysis, and journalism for policymakers, the media, the health policy community, and the public	https://www.kff.org/
Paul Keckley Report	Independent health care industry current events blog	https://www.paulkeckley.com/the-keckley-report
Robert Wood Johnson Foundation	Information on research and demonstration projects, and statistics on population demographics and health insurance	https://www.rwjf.org/en/our-focus-areas/focus-areas/health-systems.html

SALIENT POINTS

- Economics in health care represents the relationships among the supply, demand, and costs of health care.
- The supply of health care refers to the amount of health care facilities, personnel, and financing available to consumers. Supply levels are affected by technological discoveries, costs for services, consumer demands, the level of competition in the marketplace, and the effect of government regulations.
- The demand for health care indicates what health care the consumer is willing to purchase. The demand level revolves around consumer needs and desires, the costs of health care, treatment selections ordered by health care providers, and general societal needs.
- The costs for health care reflect any financial expenditures contributed by providers or consumers to deliver and receive health care, as well as the intangible costs of seeking and receiving care. Factors influencing the cost of health care are numerous, ranging from consumer demands to advancements in medical technology to the status of the nation's economy.
- Economic concepts relevant to nursing practice include opportunity cost, complements and substitutes, and competition. Nurses must be able to incorporate these economic concepts into their management and clinical decision-making processes.
- Cost-containment pressures require that clinicians, managers, and researchers be able to incorporate economic methods such as cost-effectiveness analysis (CEA) and cost-benefit analysis (CBA) into practice routines. Such economically and clinically based research can serve as the basis for policy decision-making regarding regulatory reform, prioritization, rationing of health care technologies and services, and reimbursement for APNs.
- Nurses bring a unique perspective to the economic analysis of health care that can impact health care delivery systems, health policy, quality, and equity in terms of patient care access, processes, and outcomes.
- The rising costs of health care necessitate the provision of more cost-effective ways to provide comparable services. Nurses must continue to demonstrate their accessibility, quality of services, and cost-effectiveness to validate existing and expanding roles, broaden reimbursement policies for services that nurses are trained to provide and are capable of providing, and effectively compete with physicians and other providers of care.
- The fundamental framework of the Patient Protection and Affordable Care Act (ACA, 2010), commonly called the ACA, or Obamacare, remains in place. Many of its provisions and associated funding may still be altered through U.S. Supreme Court rulings, Executive Order by the President of the United States, further legislative action, and administrative and regulatory actions at the Federal and state levels. Its effect on access to health insurance, regardless of preexisting conditions or ability to pay, new models for payment, and accountability for outcomes persists. It is important to understand the original intent and framework of the ACA and its lasting imprint in the law and to keep apprised of its continually changing components.

CRITICAL REFLECTION EXERCISES

1. Discuss the economic concepts of supply, demand, and costs of health care as they relate to your nursing practice.
2. What are the implications for the nursing profession of the issues of:
   a. Access to health care.
   b. Cost containment.
   c. Quality of care.
3. Select one of the 10 guiding principles of economics from Box 7.1 and apply it to an analysis of health care delivery in your own organization.
4. Discuss the effect of the Patient Protection and Affordable Care Act on access to care, cost, and quality of care.
5. Estimating the nursing workforce in terms of supply and demand is a challenging and complex process.
   a. Discuss the effect on the demand for nursing by one of the following:
      • A major genetic breakthrough that leads to early identification of 50% of cancer cases
      • A widespread outbreak of Ebola in the United States
      • Advances in noninvasive medicine leading to a 75% reduction in cardiac surgery
   b. Discuss the effect on the supply of nursing by one of the following:
      • Implementation of a mandatory BSN for initial licensure
      • Mandatory overtime rules that restrict nurses from working more than 40 hours per week or more than 3 consecutive days
      • Implementation of minimum staffing ratios on medical-surgical units
      • Increase in the percentage of nurses who work in travel positions at significantly higher rates of pay
6. Applying the principles of supply and demand and data from the National Center for Health Workforce Analysis determine the effect of the salary differential between advanced practice registered nurses, including nurse practitioners and registered nurses on the future short- and long-term supply of both nursing workforce subgroups.

REFERENCES

Agency for Healthcare Research and Quality. (n.d.). *Technology assessment program.* https://www.ahrq.gov/research/findings/ta/index.html

Agency for Healthcare Research and Quality. (2019, January). *AHRQ national scorecard on hospital-acquired conditions.* https://www.ahrq.gov/sites/default/files/wysiwyg/professionals/quality-patient-safety/pfp/hacreport-2019.pdf

Aiken, L. H. (2008). Economics of nursing. *Policy, Politics, & Nursing Practice, 9*(2), 73–79. https://doi.org/10.1177/1527154408318253

Aiken, L. H., Clarke, S. P., & Sloane, D. M. (2002). Hospital staffing, organizational support, and quality of care: Cross-national findings. *International Journal for Quality in Health Care, 14*(1), 5–13. https://doi.org/10.1093/intqhc/14.1.5

Aiken, L. H., & Sloane, D. M. (2021). Nurses matter: More evidence. *BMJ Quality & Safety, 29*(1), 1–3. https://doi.org/10.1136/bmjqs-2019-009732

American Association of Colleges of Nursing. (2020). *Nursing fact sheet.* https://www.aacnnursing.org/News-Information/Fact-Sheets/Nursing-Fact-Sheet

American Hospital Association. (2020, June 30). *Losses deepen for hospitals and health systems.* [Press release]. https://www.aha.org/press-releases/2020-06-30-new-aha-report-losses-deepen-hospitals-health-systems

American Hospital Association. (2021). *Fast facts on U.S. hospitals.* https://www.aha.org/statistics/fast-facts-us-hospitals

Arrow, K. J. (1963). Uncertainty and the welfare economics of medical care. *The American Economic Review, 53*(5), 941–973.

Association of American Medical Colleges. (2021). *The complexities of physician supply and demand: Projections from 2019 to 2034.* https://www.aamc.org/media/54681/download?attachment

Auerbach, D. I., Buerhaus, P. I., Donelan, K., & Staiger, D. O. (2022, April 13). *A worrisome drop in the number of young nurses.* Health Affairs Forefront. https://www.healthaffairs.org/do/10.1377/forefront.20220412.311784

Babalola, O. (2017). Consumers and their demand for healthcare. *Journal of Health & Medical Economics, 3*(1), 6. https://health-medical-economics.imedpub.com/consumers-and-their-demand-for-healthcare.php?aid=21061

Beaulieu, N. D., Dafny, L. S., Landon, B. E., Dalton, J. B., Kuye, I., & McWilliams, J. M. (2020). Changes in quality of care after hospital mergers and acquisitions. *The New England Journal of Medicine, 382*(1), 51–59. https://doi.org/10.1056/NEJMsa1901383

Blumenthal, D., & Abrams, M. (2020). The Affordable Care Act at 10 years: Payment and delivery system reforms. *The New England Journal of Medicine, 382*(11), 1057–1063. https://doi.org/10.1056/NEJMhpr1916092

Blumenthal, D., Fowler, E., Abrams, M., & Collins, S. R. (2020). COVID-19: Implications for the health care system. *The New England Journal of Medicine*, *382*(15), 1483–1488. https://doi.org/10.1056/NEJMsb2021088

Bruch, J., Zeltzer, D., & Song, Z. (2021). Characteristics of private equity-owned hospitals in 2018. *Annals of Internal Medicine*, *174*(2), 277–279. https://doi.org/10.7326/M20-1361

Buerhaus, P. I., Auerbach, D. I., & Steiger, D. O. (2017, May 3). *How should we prepare for the wave of retiring baby boomer nurses?* Health Affairs Blog. https://www.healthaffairs.org/do/10.1377/forefront.20170503.059894/full/

Buerhaus, P. I., DesRoches, C., Applebaum, S., Hess, R., Norman, L. D., & Donelan, K. (2012). Are nurses ready for health care reform? A decade of survey research. *Nursing Economics*, *30*(6), 318–329.

Buerhaus, P. I., Steiger, D. O., Auerbach, D. I., Yates, M. C., & Donelan, K. (2022, January). Nurse employment during the first 15 months of the COVID-19 pandemic. *Health Affairs*, *41*(1), 79–85. https://doi.org/10.1377/hlthaff.2021.01289

Burke, J. R., Downey, C., & Almoudaris, A. (2022). Failure to rescue deteriorating patients: A systematic review of root causes and improvement strategies. *Journal of Patient Safety*, *18*(1), e140–e155. https://doi.org/10.1097/PTS.0000000000000720

Butler, M., Schultz, T. J., & Drennan, J. (2020). Substitution of nurses for physicians in the hospital setting for patient, process of care, and economic outcomes. *The Cochrane Database of Systematic Reviews*, *2020*(5), 1–16. https://doi.org/10.1002/14651858.CD013616

Center on Budget and Policy Priorities. (2020a). *Policy basics: Introduction to Medicaid*. https://www.cbpp.org/research/health/introduction-to-medicaid

Center on Budget and Policy Priorities. (2020b). *Policy basics: Top ten facts about Social security*. https://www.cbpp.org/research/social-security/top-ten-facts-about-social-security

Centers for Medicare and Medicaid. (n.d.-a). *Medicaid: About Section 1115 demonstrations-about*. Accessed January 30, 2023. https://www.medicaid.gov/medicaid/section-1115-demonstrations/about-section-1115-demonstrations/index.html.

Centers for Medicare and Medicaid Services. (n.d.-b). Hospital-acquired conditions. Accessed January 30, 2023. https://www.cms.gov/Medicare/Medicare-Fee-for-Service-Payment/HospitalAcqCond/Hospital-Acquired_Conditions.

Centers for Medicare and Medicaid Services. (n.d.-c). *The hospital value-based purchasing program (VBP)*. Accessed January 30, 2023. https://www.cms.gov/Medicare/Quality-Initiatives-Patient-Assessment-Instruments/Value-Based-Programs/HVBP/Hospital-Value-Based-Purchasing.

Centers for Medicare and Medicaid Services. (n.d.-d) *Shared savings program*. Accessed January 30, 2023. https://www.cms.gov/Medicare/Medicare-Fee-for-Service-Payment/sharedsavingsprogram/about.

Centers for Medicare and Medicaid Services. (2021a). *National health expenditure fact sheet-2020*. https://www.cms.gov/Research-Statistics-Data-and-Systems/Statistics-Trends-and-Reports/NationalHealthExpendData/NHE-Fact-Sheet

Centers for Medicare and Medicaid Services. (2021b). *Acute inpatient PPS: FY 2021 IPPS Final Rule Home Page. Table 16B Hospital Value-based Purchasing Program Adjustment factors* [Data set]. https://www.cms.gov/files/zip/fy-2021-ipps-fr-table-tables-16a-and-16b-hospital-value-based-purchasing-vbp-program-tables.zip

Centers for Medicare and Medicaid Services. (2021c). *CMS releases HVBP FY 2022 percentage Payment Summary Reports*. https://qualitynet.cms.gov/news/61955e7da91be5002238524a

Committee for a Responsible Federal Budget. (n.d.). *COVID money tracker*. https://www.covidmoneytracker.org/

Commonwealth Fund. (2021, May 20). *The economic and employment effects of Medicaid expansion under the American Rescue Plan*. https://www.commonwealthfund.org/publications/issue-briefs/2021/may/economic-employment-effects-medicaid-expansion-under-arp

Convenient Care Association. (2022). *About CCA*. http://ccaclinics.org/about-us/about-cca

Dalia, S. (2018). Nurse-led health clinics show positive outcomes. *American Journal of Nursing*, *118*(2), 12. https://doi.org/10.1097/01.NAJ.0000530229.30533.ce

Dayani, E. C. (1983). Professional and economic self-governance in nursing. *Nursing Economics*, *1*(1), 20–23.

Dierkes, A. M., Riman, K., Daus, M., Germack, H. D., & Lasater, K. (2021). The Association of hospital Magnet® status and pay-for-performance penalties. *Policy, Politics, & Nursing Practice*, *22*(4), 250–257. https://doi.org/10.1177/15271544211053854

Dummit, L. A., Kahvecioglu, D., Marrufo, G., Rajkumar, R., Marshall, J., Tan, E., Press, M. J., Flood, S., Muldoon, L. D., Gu, Q., Hassol, A., Bott, D. M., Bassano, A., & Conway, P. H. (2016). Association between hospital participation in a Medicare bundled payment initiative and payments and quality outcomes for lower extremity joint replacement episodes. *JAMA*, *316*(12), 1267–1278. https://doi.org/10.1001/jama.2016.12717

El Keshky, M., Basyouni, S. S., & Al Sabban, A. M. (2020). Getting through COVID-19: The pandemic's impact on the psychology of sustainability, quality of life, and the global economy—A systematic review. *Frontiers in Psychology*, *11*, 1–12. https://doi.org/10.3389/fpsyg.2020.585897

Ellis, R. P., Martins, B., & Zhu, W. (2017). Health care demand elasticities by type of service. *Journal of Health Economics*, *55*, 232–243. https://doi.org/10.1016/j.jhealeco.2017.07.007

Falatah, R. (2021). The Impact of the coronavirus disease (COVID-19) pandemic on nurses' turnover intention: An integrative review. *Nursing Reports*, *11*(4), 787–810. https://doi.org/10.3390/nursrep11040075

Feinberg, L. F., & Spillman, B. C. (2019). Shifts in family caregiving: And a growing care gap. *Generations: Journal of the American Society on Aging*, *43*(1), 73–77. https://www.jstor.org/stable/26632566

Finnegan, J. (2020, February 26). *Now more than 9,000 urgent care centers in the U.S., industry report says*. Fierce Healthcare. https://www.fiercehealthcare.com/practices/now-more-than-9-000-urgent-care-centers-u-s-industry-report-says

Fisher, E., Staiger, D., Bynum, J., & Gottlieb, D. (2006). Creating accountable care organizations: The extended hospital medical staff. *Health Affairs*, *26*, 44–57. https://doi.org/10.1377/hlthaff.26.1.w44

Folland, S., Goodman, A. C., & Stano, M. (2017). *The economics of health and health care* (8th ed.). Routledge.

Fronstin, P., Hagen, S., Hoppe, O., & Spiegel, J. (2021). *The more things change, the more they stay the same: An analysis of the generosity of employment-based health insurance, 2013–2019.* Employee Benefit Research Institute. https://www.ebri.org/docs/default-source/ebri-issue-brief/ebri_ib_545_av-28oct21.pdf?sfvrsn=86463b2f_12

Gottlieb, J. D., & Zenilman, A. (2020). *When workers travel: Nursing supply during COVID-19 surges.* National Bureau of Economic Research. https://www.nber.org/system/files/working_papers/w28240/w28240.pdf

Healthcare.gov. (n.d.). *Medicaid & CHIP: The Children's Health Insurance Program (CHIP).* Accessed January 30, 2023. https://www.healthcare.gov/medicaid-chip/childrens-health-insurance-program/.

Henderson, J. W. (2018). *Health economics and policy* (7th ed.). Cengage.

Herring, B., Gaskin, D., Zare, H., & Anderson, G. (2018). Comparing the value of nonprofit hospitals' tax exemption to their community benefits. *Inquiry, 55,* 1–11. https://www.ncbi.nlm.nih.gov/pmc/articles/PMC5813653/

Institute for Women's Policy Research. (2021). *The gender wage gap by occupation, race, and ethnicity 2020.* https://iwpr.org/iwpr-issues/esme/the-gender-wage-gap-by-occupation-race-and-ethnicity-2020/

Institute of Medicine. (2001). *Crossing the Quality chasm: A new health system for the 21st Century.* The National Academies Press. https://doi.org/10.17226/10027

Joynt Maddox, K. E., Orav, E. J., Zheng, J., & Epstein, A. (2018). Evaluation of Medicare's Bundled Payments Initiative for medical conditions. *The New England Journal of Medicine, 379*(3), 260–269. https://doi.org/10.1056/NEJMsa1801569

Kaiser Family Foundation. (2018). *Summary of the 2018 CHIP funding extension.* https://www.kff.org/medicaid/fact-sheet/summary-of-the-2018-chip-funding-extension/

Kaiser Family Foundation. (2019, February 13). *An overview of Medicare.* https://www.kff.org/medicare/issue-brief/an-overview-of-medicare/

Kaiser Family Foundation. (2021, November 10). *2021 Employer health benefits survey: Types of plans offered.* https://www.kff.org/report-section/ehbs-2021-section-4-types-of-plans-offered/

Kaufman, B. G., Spivack, B. S., Stearns, S. C., Song, P. H., & O'Brien, E. C. (2019). Impact of accountable care organizations on utilization, care, and outcomes: A systematic review. *Medical Care Research and Review, 76*(3), 255–290. https://doi.org/10.1177/1077558717745916

Keisler-Starkey, K., & Bunch, L. N. (2021, September 14). *Health insurance coverage in the United States: 2020.* U.S. Census Bureau. https://www.census.gov/library/publications/2021/demo/p60-274.html

Konar, H. (2018, February 2). *Health care is a public good.* https://readcommonground.com/topic/health-care-is-a-public-good/

Kraus, E. J., & Thompson, T. E. (2021). Debate continues around scope of practice expansion for APPs. *National Law Review, 12*(244), 1–4. https://www.natlawreview.com/article/debate-continues-around-scope-practice-expansion-apps

Lasater, K. B., Germack, H. D., Small, D. S., & McHugh, M. D. (2016). Hospitals known for nursing excellence perform better on value-based purchasing measures. *Policy, Politics, & Nursing Practice, 17*(4), 177–186. https://doi.org/10.1177/1527154417698144

Laurant, M., van der Biezen, M., Wijers, N., Watananirun, K., Kontopantelis, E., & van Vught, A. J. (2018). Nurses as substitutes for doctors in primary care. *The Cochrane Database of Systematic Reviews, 7*(7), 1–108. https://doi.org/10.1002/146511858.CD001271.pub3

Lown Institute. (2021). *Lown Institute Hospitals Index benefit metric.* https://lownhospitalsindex.org/2021-winning-hospitals-community-benefit/ - methodology

Mathauer, I., Saksena, P., & Kutzin, J. (2019). Pooling arrangements in health financing systems: A proposed classification. *International Journal for Equity in Health, 18,* 1–11. https://doi.org/10.1186/s12939-019-1088-x

McPake, B., Normand, C., Smith, S., & Nolan, A. (2020). *Health economics: An international perspective* (4th ed.). Routledge.

McWilliams, J. M., Hatfield, L. A., Landon, B. E., Hamed, P., & Chernew, M. E. (2018). Medicare spending after 3 years of the Medicare Shared Savings Program. *The New England Journal of Medicine, 279*(12), 1139–1149. https://doi.org/10.1056/NEJMsa1803388

Medicaid.gov. (2021). *Medicaid & CHIP enrollment data highlights.* https://www.medicaid.gov/medicaid/program-information/medicaid-and-chip-enrollment-data/report-highlights/index.html

Meyer, M. (2017). The ethics of universal health care in the United States. *Reflections on Healthcare Management, 1*(1), 1–6. https://doi.org/10.6083/m4sn082q

Millett, G. A., Jones, A. T., Benkeser, D., Baral, S., Mercer, L., Beyrer, C., Honermann, B., Lankiewicz, E., Mena, L., Crowley, J. S., Sherwood, J., & Sullivan, P. S. (2020). Assessing differential impacts of COVID-19 on black communities. *Annals of Epidemiology, 47,* 37–44. https://doi.org/10.1016/j.annepidem.2020.05.003

Muhlstein, D., Bleser, W. K., Saunders, R. S., Richards, R., Singletary, E., & McClellan, M. B. (2019, October 19). *Spread of ACOs and value-based payment models in 2019: Gauging the impact of pathways to success.* [Health Affairs Blog]. https://www.healthaffairs.org/do/10.1377/forefront.20191020.962600/full/

Mulligan, K., Lakdawalla, D., Goldman, D., Hlávka, J., Peneva, D., Ryan, M., Schaeffer Center Staff, Neumann, P. J., Wilensky, G., & Katz, R. J. (2020). *Health technology assessment for the U.S. healthcare system* [White paper]. https://healthpolicy.usc.edu/research/health-technology-assessment-for-the-u-s-healthcare-system/

National Academies of Sciences, Engineering, and Medicine. (2002). *The future of the public's health in the 21st century.* The National Academies Press. https://doi.org/10.17226/25982

National Academies of Sciences, Engineering, and Medicine. (2021). *The future of nursing 2020–2030: Charting a path to achieve health equity.* National Academies Press. https://doi.org/10.17226/25982

National Advisory Council on Nurse Education and Practice. (2019). *Promoting nursing leadership in the transition to value-based care*. Fifteenth Report to the Secretary of Health and Human Services and the U.S. Congress. https://www.hrsa.gov/sites/default/files/hrsa/advisory-committees/nursing/reports/2019-fifteenthreport.pdf

National Council of State Boards of Nursing. (2020, January 1). NCSBN's environmental scan: A portrait of nursing and healthcare in 2020 and beyond. *Journal of Nursing Regulation, 10*(4), S1–S35. https://doi.org/10.1016/S2155-8256(20)30022-3

National Council of State Boards. (2022). *eNLC fast facts*. https://www.ncsbn.org/public-files/NLC_Fast_Facts.pdf

National Forum of State Nursing Workforce Centers. (n.d.). *The leader for nursing workforce information*. https://nursingworkforcecenters.org/

National Nurse-led Care Consortium. (n.d.). *Nurse-led care*. https://nurseledcare.phmc.org/about/nurse-led-care.html

Needleman, J., Liu, J., Shang, J., Larson, E., & Stone, P. W. (2020). Association of registered nurse and nursing support staffing with inpatient hospital mortality. *BMJ Quality & Safety, 29*(1), 10–18. https://doi.org/10.1136/bmjqs-2018-009219

Nelson-Brantley, H. V., Park, S. H., & Bergquist-Beringer, S. (2018). Characteristics of the nursing practice environment associated with lower unit-level RN turnover. *The Journal of Nursing Administration, 48*(1), 31–37. https://doi.org/10.1097/NNA.0000000000000567

Norris, L. (2021). *Is there still a penalty for being uninsured?* https://www.healthinsurance.org/faqs/is-there-still-a-penalty-for-being-uninsured/

Organization for Economic Cooperation and Development. (2021a). *Health at a glance 2021: OECD indicators*. https://doi.org/10.1787/ae3016b9-en

Organization for Economic Cooperation and Development. (2021b). *Health statistics datasets*. [Data set]. https://www.oecd.org/health/health-data.htm

Patient Centered Outcomes Research Institute. (2020). *Annual report*. https://www.pcori.org/sites/default/files/PCORI-Annual-Report-2020.pdf

Patient Protection and Affordable Care Act. (2010). *111th US congress*. https://www.healthcare.gov/glossary/patient-protection-and-affordable-care-act/

Phillips, J., Malliaris, A. P., & Bakerjian, D. (2021). *Nursing & patient safety*. Patient Safety Network (PSNet). https://psnet.ahrq.gov/primer/nursing-and-patient-safety

Pollitz, K. (2022). *No surprises act implementation: What to expect in 2022*. https://www.kff.org/health-reform/issue-brief/no-surprises-act-implementation-what-to-expect-in-2022/

Ramacciati, N. (2013). Health technology assessment in nursing: A literature review. *International Nursing Review, 60*(1), 23–30. https://doi-org.proxy01.its.virginia.edu/10.1111/j.1466-7657.2012.01038.x

Ramakrishnudu, T., Prasen, T. S., & Chakravarthy, V. (2021). A framework for health status estimation based on daily life activities data using machine learning techniques. In S. N. Mohanty & G. Nalinipriya (Eds.), *Machine learning for healthcare applications* (pp. 19–32). Scrivener. https://doi.org/10.1002/9781119792611.CH2

RAND Corporation. (2016). *The evolving role of retail clinics*. https://www.rand.org/pubs/research_briefs/RB9491-2.html

Randall, S., Crawford, T., Currie, J., River, J., & Betihavas, V. (2017). Impact of community-based nurse-led clinics on patient outcomes, patient satisfaction, patient access and cost effectiveness: A systematic review. *International Journal of Nursing Studies, 73*, 24–33. https://doi.org/10.1016/j.ijnurstu.2017.05.008

Rau, J. (2021). *Medicare punishes 2,499 hospitals for high readmissions*. Kaiser Health News. https://khn.org/news/article/hospital-readmission-rates-medicare-penalties/

Rutherford, M. (2017). Enhanced RN role in behavioral health care. *Nursing Economics, 35*(2), 88–95.

Salmond, S. W., & Echevarria, M. (2017). Healthcare transformation and changing roles for nursing. *Orthopedic Nursing, 36*(1), 12–25. https://doi.org/10.1097/NOR.0000000000000308

Sankaran, R., Sukul, D., Nuliyalu U., Gulseren, B., Engler, T. A., Arntson, E., Zlotnick, H., Dimick, J. B., & Ryan, A. M. (2019). Changes in hospital safety following penalties in the U.S. Hospital Acquired Condition Reduction Program: Retrospective cohort study. *BMJ, 366*. https://doi.org/10.1136/bmj.l4109

Shorr, R. I., Staggs, V. S., Waters, T. M., Daniels, M. J., Liu, M., Dunton, N., & Mion, L. C. (2019). Impact of the hospital-acquired conditions Initiative on falls and physical restraints: A longitudinal study. *Journal of Hospital Medicine, 14*, E31–E36. https://doi.org/10.12788/jhm.3295

Smiley, R. A., Ruttinger, C., Oliviera, C. M., Hudson, L. R., Allgeyer, R., Reneau, K. A., Silvestre, J. H., & Alexander, M. (2021, April 1). The 2020 National Nursing Workforce Survey. *Journal of Nursing Regulation, 12*(1), S1–S96. https://doi.org/10.1016/S2155-8256(21)00027-2

Sovie, M. D. (1985). Managing nursing resources in a constrained economic environment. *Nursing Economics, 3*(2), 85–94.

Spatz, I. (2018, February 22). *Health affairs forefront: IPAB RIP*. https://www.healthaffairs.org/do/10.1377/forefront.20180221.484846/full/

Spaulding, A., Hamadi, H., Moody, L., Lentz, L., Liu, X. A., & Wu, Y. J. (2020). *Do Magnet®-designated hospitals perform better on Medicare's Value-Based Purchasing Program?* https://doi.org/10.1097/NNA.0000000000000906

Starr, P. (1982). *The social transformation of American medicine*. Basic Books.

Sullivan, G., & Feore, J. (2019). *Physician-led accountable care organizations outperform hospital-led counterparts*. [Press release]. https://avalere.com/press-releases/physician-led-accountable-care-organizations-outperform-hospital-led-counterparts

The White House. (2021, July 9). *Fact sheet: Executive order on promoting competition in the American Economy*. https://www.whitehouse.gov/briefing-room/statements-releases/2021/07/09/fact-sheet-executive-order-on-promoting-competition-in-the-american-economy/

U.S. Department of Health and Human Services. (2018). *Report to Congress: Evaluation of the independence at home demonstration*. https://innovation.cms.gov/files/reports/iah-rtc.pdf

U.S. Department of Health and Human Services, Health Resources and Services Administration, & National Center for Health Workforce Analysis. (2017). *National and regional supply and demand projections of the nursing workforce: 2014–2030*. https://bhw.hrsa.gov/sites/default/files/bureau-health-workforce/data-research/nchwa-hrsa-nursing-report.pdf

U.S. Department of Health and Human Services, Health Resources and Services Administration, & National Center for Health Workforce Analysis. (2021). *In Technical documentation for HRSA's health workforce simulation model, Version 3.18.2021*. https://bhw.hrsa.gov/sites/default/files/bureau-health-workforce/data-research/technical-documentation-health-workforce-simulation-model_092921.pdf

U.S. Treasury Department, (n.d.). *Fiscal date: Spending*. https://datalab.usaspending.gov/americas-finance-guide/spending/

Veterans Affairs. (n.d.) *The clinical nurse leader role (CNL)*. Office of Nursing Services (ONS). https://www.va.gov/NURSING/practice/cnl.asp

Veterans Health Administration. (2021). *2021 VA Agency financial report*. https://www.va.gov/performance/

Weiss, A. J., Elixhauser, A., & Steiner, C. (2010). *Statistical brief #155: Readmissions to U.S. hospitals by diagnosis. Healthcare Cost and Utilization Project (HCUP)*. Agency for Healthcare Research and Quality. https://www.ncbi.nlm.nih.gov/books/NBK154385/

Welton, J. (2006). Paying for nursing care in hospitals. *American Journal of Nursing, 106*(11), 67–69. https://doi.org/10.1097/00000446-200611000-00022

Welton, J. M., Fischer, M. H., DeGrace, S., & Zone-Smith, L. (2006). Hospital nursing costs, billing, and reimbursement. *Nursing Economics, 24*(5), 239–262.

World Health Organization. (2020, March 11). *WHO director-general's opening remarks at the media briefing on COVID-19*. https://www.who.int/director-general/speeches/detail/who-director-general-s-opening-remarks-at-the-media-briefing-on-covid-19—11-march-2020

8

Nurse as Interprofessional Collaborator

Karen J. Saewert, PhD, RN, CPHQ, ANEF and
Gerri Lamb, PhD, RN, FAAN

ⓔ http://evolve.elsevier.com/Friberg/bridge/

"Imagine a future in which patients can routinely expect collaborative,
coordinated care from an interprofessional team."

Source: Team-Based Competencies: Building a Shared Foundation for Education
and Clinical Practice (Interprofessional Education Collaborative, 2011, p. 14)

OBJECTIVES

After completion of this chapter, the reader will be able to:

- Reflect on the role and importance of interprofessional collaboration and teamwork in nursing practice.
- Define core concepts related to interprofessional collaboration and teamwork in health care delivery.
- Recognize key organizations and influential works advancing interprofessional education, practice, and teamwork in the nursing and health professions workforce.

- Discuss key characteristics and core competencies essential for nurses and nursing as a discipline in interprofessional collaboration and teamwork.
- Recognize theories, models, and key concepts that contribute to the effectiveness of interprofessional collaboration and teamwork.

INTRODUCTION

The call to change and transform the health care system has been sounding for decades. All health care professionals, regardless of their level of education, title, discipline, or type of service, are called to be *change agents* (Noureddine et al., 2022a). Nursing and other health professions are positioned to advance and facilitate health care delivery and practice, health care education, and formal and informal health care systems. Dramatic changes are essential in both systems to address the quality, safety, equity, and value of care delivery required to respond effectively and efficiently to the ubiquitous needs of our patients, their families, communities, and populations.

The complexity of health care makes the active involvement and collaboration and synergistic knowledge, skills,

and values from a diverse professional and disciplinary workforce necessary. Patient care—and our performance—can be improved by pooling insights and experiences to problem-solving, enhanced care delivery, and quality improvement (Disch, 2017a). Nursing education also needs to be transformed in many ways to prepare nursing graduates to work collaboratively and effectively with other health professions in a complex and evolving health care system across a variety of settings (Institute of Medicine [IOM], 2011). An envisioned future calls for cross-profession partnerships and support—where *interprofessional collaboration and coordination* are the norm (National Academies of Sciences, Engineering, and Medicine [NASEM], 2021).

Nursing plays a critical role in this interprofessional dialogue and brings its unique perspective (Box 8.1) to the core competencies for *all* health care professionals: *patient-centered care, teamwork and collaboration, evidence-based practice, quality improvement,* and *informatics* (Institute of Medicine [IOM], 2011). When a patient is at risk for a problem, it is often the bedside nurse who alerts the interprofessional team and begins the problem-solving process on their behalf (Hughes, 2018). (See Chapters 5, 20, and 13, respectively, for more detailed information and discussion related to evidence-based practice, health care quality and safety, and information management.)

Building a foundation of understanding about key concepts (Table 8.1) and processes related to how interprofessional collaboration aligns with nursing practice requires an openness to examining one's understanding of self and gaining self-knowledge in relation to others. So, what does

being interprofessional mean? Why does it matter? What motivates nurses to commit to advancing the interprofessional agenda in nursing? How do you see yourself within the broader landscape of health care? What does it mean to be a nursing professional now and into the future?

Clarifying answers to these and other questions may support current efforts to break down the silos of health professions education, establish a shared identity, and intentionally teach and practice methods for improving care through interprofessional collaboration (Noureddine et al., 2022b). These efforts are at a starting point. Change is possible. What role will you choose?

This chapter provides you with opportunities to consider how you might expand your vision of what this means.

INTERPROFESSIONAL IDENTITY FORMATION

Cultivating an identity as a nurse and nurse leader that includes interprofessionalism (Box 8.2) requires *intentionally* learning, developing skills, and nurturing beliefs and attitudes that will allow you as a nurse to invest yourself as a collaborative partner in optimizing valuable outcomes for patients, families, communities, and populations (Saewert, 2018). The *Interprofessional Socialization Framework* developed by Khalili et al. (2013) conceptualized a dynamic, progressive, and iterative three-stage process for the development and adoption of a dual professional and interprofessional identity—a dual identity—to ultimately advance interprofessional practice cultures.
- Stage 1: Breaking Down Barriers
- Stage 2: Interprofessional Role Learning—Interprofessional Collaboration
- Stage 3: Dual Identity Formation

TABLE 8.1 Key Concepts

Concept	Definition
Interprofessional Education	"When students from two or more professions learn about, from and with each other to enable effective collaboration and improve health outcomes" (World Health Organization [WHO], 2010, p. 7).
Interprofessional Collaborative Practice	"When multiple health workers from different backgrounds work together with patients, families, carers, and communities to deliver the highest quality of care" (World Health Organization [WHO], 2010, p. 7).
Interprofessional Teamwork	"The level of cooperation, coordination and collaboration characterizing the relationships between professions in delivering patient-centered care" (Interprofessional Education Collaborative [IPEC], 2016, p. 8)
Interprofessional Team-Based Care	"Care delivered by intentionally created, usually relatively small work groups in health care who are recognized by others as well as by themselves as having a collective identity and shared responsibility for a patient or group of patients" (Interprofessional Education Collaborative [IPEC], 2016, p. 8).

BOX 8.2 Cultivating an Interprofessional Identity

Cultivating an identity as a nurse and nurse leader that includes interprofessionalism requires intentional learning, developing skills, and nurturing beliefs and attitudes that will allow you as a nurse to invest yourself as a collaborative partner in optimizing valuable outcomes for patients, families, communities, and populations (Saewert, 2018, p. 118).

The dismantling of existing misconceptions across professions facilitates moving toward adopting a dual (vs. uniprofessional) identity takes place in Stage 1. Preparation for building an interprofessional identity occurs in Stage 2 through interprofessional role learning and collaboration. Stage 3 occurs when a sense of belonging to one's own profession and the interprofessional community is achieved (dual identity formation).

Being interprofessional—how we are, how we act, what we do—is an *active* state and not the last resort when things go wrong or problems need to be solved (Hammick et al., 2009). To achieve that *active* state, interprofessional role learning and collaboration must take place. Let's transition our attention in the next section from self-knowledge to role learning and competency as an effective team member.

INTERPROFESSIONAL COLLABORATION AND TEAMWORK

Interprofessional learning experiences prepare future health care professionals for enhanced team-based care of patients, which will lead to improved population health outcomes (Zorek et al., 2021). However, not all teams are created equal. Brashers et al. (2020) stipulated:

> Some teams produce a synergy that others lack. It is the relationships that exist among these individuals that are the secret ingredient. It becomes imperative that the interprofessional members of teams learn how to quickly establish relationships, work together, and manage conflicts when they arise. (p. 129)

So, what are the professional competencies that constitute the overarching interprofessional collaboration domain? The Interprofessional Education Collaborative's (IPEC) core competencies have become the gold standard (Zorek et al., 2021).

Interprofessional Competencies

The interprofessional competencies and subcompetencies provide a comprehensive blueprint for preparing all health professionals with a common core of knowledge, skills, and values for effective collaboration and teamwork in all settings. Each of the competencies is grounded in principles, like patient and family-centeredness, that are closely aligned with the goals and context for collaboration in health care today. They incorporate attention to the processes inherent in team building as well as their outcomes since both are essential to effective teamwork performance. They were written to guide learners at all levels and to be applied in all professions and across all settings. Importantly, they were purposely written using words and concepts that would be understood and meaningful to those in the health care practice.

The IPEC's core competencies include knowledge, skills, and values across four major areas: (1) values and ethics required for interprofessional practice, (2) roles and responsibilities of each team member, (3) interprofessional communication, and (4) teams and teamwork. IPEC's definition for each of these areas is provided in Box 8.3.

Values and Ethics. Long-held health care values, beliefs, attitudes, and new ethical questions can be put to the test by rapid shifts and sharp pivots in our systems of care. The COVID-19 pandemic serves as a sobering reminder of the challenges and obstacles to the safe, timely, efficient, effective, and equitable provision of safe and quality care delivery.

The value and ethics of core competency is foundational to collaboration. They call for all team members to recognize and respect each other's diverse backgrounds and contributions. We know from past research that stereotyping among the health professions may be a barrier to effective teamwork and the implementation and achievement of all four IPEC competencies (Conroy, 2019) (see Box 8.3). We also know that some of these stereotypes and biases may originate from misinformation or portrayals of different professions in the media. Others may come from a lack of information about how other health professionals are educated. Looking at possible stereotypes you may have about nursing and other professions is a good place to start thinking about your values surrounding teamwork. Take a moment to reflect on what you believe about other health professions, including the potential source(s) of those beliefs.

For changes in health care to take place at the national and organizational levels it involves the willingness of individuals to reflect on their biases and prejudices (Noureddine & Hagge, 2022a, 2022b). *Interprofessional socialization* (see Chapter 3) and *dual-identify formation* addressed earlier in this chapter drew attention to the importance of *breaking down barriers* of existing misconceptions within and across professions. Failure to identify and eliminate these barriers:

BOX 8.3   Interprofessional Collaboration

Competency 1: Values/Ethics for Interprofessional Practice
Work with individuals of other professions to maintain a climate of mutual respect and shared values.

Competency 2: Roles/Responsibilities
Use the knowledge of one's own role and those of other professions to appropriately assess and address the health care needs of patients and to promote and advance the health of populations.

Competency 3: Interprofessional Communication
Communicate with patients, families, communities, and professionals in health and other fields in a responsive and responsible manner that supports a team approach to the promotion and maintenance of health and the prevention and treatment of disease.

Competency 4: Teams and Teamwork
Apply relationship-building values and the principles of team dynamics to perform effectively in different team roles to plan, deliver, and evaluate patient/population-centered care and population health programs and policies that are safe, timely, efficient, effective, and equitable.

Source: Interprofessional Education Collaborative. (2016). *Core competencies for interprofessional collaborative practice: 2016 update.* Author. https://ipec.memberclicks.net/assets/2016-Update.pdf

(1) promotes turf battles, (2) maintains professional silos, and (3) hinders the ability to collaborate, communicate, and function as a team (Noureddine & Hagge, 2022a).

Campoe (2020) asserts that "nurses are bound professionally to collaborate" (para. 3). Our influence as nurses was built on years of developing respect, trust, ethical communication, and collaboration that created a foundation of global respect for nurses. Strengthening this foundation through growing competence in interprofessional values and ethics positions nurses to leverage interprofessional collaboration strategically, shape future successes, and bring mutually supportive recognition to nursing and other health professions—all while continuing to learn about, from, and with one another. All boats rise. The need is urgent.

Roles and Responsibilities. Given the complexity of the health care environment and the threats to patient safety and quality care, collaboration with other members of the team is vital (Disch, 2017b). Vega and Bernard (2016, March 8)

made nine recommendations for establishing roles and responsibilities for interprofessional team-based care:

1. Communicate one's role and responsibilities clearly to patients, families, and other professionals.
2. Recognize one's limitations in skills, knowledge, and abilities.
3. Engage diverse health care professionals who complement one's professional expertise, as well as associated resources, to develop strategies to meet specific patient care needs.
4. Explain the roles and responsibilities of other care providers and how the team works together to provide care.
5. Use the full scope of knowledge, skills, and abilities of available health professionals and health care workers to provide care that is safe, timely, efficient, effective, and equitable.
6. Communicate with team members to clarify each member's responsibility in executing components of the treatment plan or public health intervention.
7. Forge interdependent relationships with other professions to improve care and advance learning.
8. Engage in continuous professional and interprofessional development to enhance team performance.
9. Use unique and complementary abilities of all members of the team to optimize patient care.

Teams and Teamwork. What makes or breaks the work of an interprofessional team? The growing complexity of tasks frequently surpasses the cognitive capabilities of individuals and, thus, necessitates a team approach (Cooke et al., 2000). Nurses must be able to demonstrate leadership by initiating and maintaining effective working relationships using mutually respectful communication and collaboration within interprofessional teams (AACN, 2011). However, interprofessional collaboration is more than cooperation and coordination (Eisler & Potter, 2014). The World Health Organization (2010) clarifies the difference:

Many health workers believe themselves to be practicing collaboratively, simply because they work together with other health workers. In reality, they may simply be working within a group where each individual has agreed to use their own skills to achieve a common goal. Collaboration, however, is not only about agreement and communication, but about creation and synergy. Collaboration occurs when two or more individuals from different backgrounds with complementary skills interact to create a shared understanding that none had previously possessed or could have come to on their own. (p. 36)

How willing are you to commit to being an *active* and engaged team member?

Interprofessional Communication. We each have a powerful opportunity to revolutionize patient safety by recreating how health care is delivered as a team, as a system, and as a champion (Sheridan, 2017). Critical to effective communication are the following elements (IPEC, 2011):

- Routine, reliable, and secure forms of communication should be established. The precise tools for communication may vary from practice to practice, but they should be planned thoughtfully. All team members should have a voice in establishing a communication system to ensure feasibility and increase buy-in.
- Clinical practice is always busy. Communication systems should emphasize technology to facilitate interaction and improve team efficiency. Timely communication of important health data can avoid injuries and prevent severe consequences.
- Communication should include patients and caregivers, and these conversations should avoid jargon to provide clear information. There is a long history of hierarchy on the health care team. Interprofessional communication should emphasize good listening skills and mutual respect for all team members. All team members should have the opportunity to contribute.
- Team members should feel comfortable providing constructive feedback to one another.
- There should be a consistent emphasis on the importance of team in patient-centered and community-focused care.

Unfortunately, it is not difficult to find media that share heartbreaking stories related to health care errors—simple yet catastrophic system failures due to communication breakdowns and uncoordinated teamwork. Listening to them is hard. Living them defies description. It is in the *telling*, that we are gifted. The gift is the inability to *unhear* the words, *unfeel* the emotions, and *unsee* the impact. Let it spur our commitment to lead *for* change.

The preceding sections of this chapter engaged in discussions related to self-knowledge and self-understanding in anticipation of interprofessional collaboration and teamwork. Practice theories that can help you understand and improve teamwork and guide you in the process of interprofessional role learning and interprofessional collaboration competency development are presented in the next section.

THEORETICAL MODELS FOR COLLABORATION

While your intuition and predisposition to be collaborative can be helpful guides to becoming a good team member or leader, finding and using team theories provides you with important conceptual anchors for understanding and improving your team practice. Team theories describe and explain common experiences in teams, such as the stages that teams go through in becoming effective or how team members can create safe environments for working together. How well your team functions is pivotal to your well-being as well as to achieving patient outcomes. Becoming aware of team theories provides a useful starting place for developing effective teams and gaining insights into what may be happening when your team is not working as well as you expected or hoped. Team theories also can help you with ways to communicate your contribution to team outcomes (Will & Lamb, 2021).

Team theories include many different concepts that are core to effective team functioning, like communication, collaboration, roles, conflict, and trust. They can help you define important aspects of these concepts to look for in your teams, regardless of where you practice or the role you play as a nurse on the team. Some theories focus on challenging aspects of teamwork, like power or conflict, and propose how and why these challenges may evolve. Importantly, team theories, through connecting concepts and relationships among them, provide meaningful strategies for navigating through problem areas in teamwork. For instance, one of the most used theories in team science, Tuckman's (1965) theory of small group development, describes common stages of team development. According to this theory, teams go through predictable steps from "forming" to "norming" to "storming" to "performing" to "adjourning." Notice that storming or conflict is an expected stage of teamwork and is necessary to get to effective performance. Think about how you might feel as a member of a storming team if you didn't have Tuckman's theory in your conceptual toolkit to understand "this conflict is ok. It's a sign of progress if we can manage it effectively together."

Table 8.2 provides a sample of the range of team theories available to guide you in your nursing and interprofessional practice. There are theories, as shown in the table, that can help you understand different aspects of teamwork, including the stages of team development and strategies for effective communication and conflict management. A way to get familiar with the theories you may want to know and use is to select one or two that focus on questions about teams and collaboration that you find interesting or, perhaps, challenging or stressful.

The theories in Table 8.2 come from several different fields of study, including sociology, psychology, engineering, and even crisis management. Each field uses a *different lens* to illuminate important aspects of teamwork. For instance, sociologists who study teams commonly focus on the team as a small group. They ask questions about what makes groups effective or ineffective and how leaders can

TABLE 8.2   Teamwork and Collaboration Theories

Questions of Interest	Theory/Framework/ Model	Brief Description	Learn More

• What are the stages that teams commonly go through?
• How can I recognize the stages?
• How can I help my team move through the stage and get to performing well together?
	Tuckman's small group development theory (also referred to as the Tuckman model)	This theory started as a model to explain the predictable stages of small groups.
		It has become one of the most popular models for interpreting team dynamics.
			Resource:
			  Tuckman, B. W. (1965). Developmental sequence in small groups. *Psychological Bulletin, 63*(6), 384. https://doi.org/10.1037/h0022100
			Search Terms:
			  Tuckman theory, stages of group development, team theories, examples of team stages

• Why are relationships important to effective teams?
• What are strategies for improving team coordination and communication?
	Relational coordination	Understanding of some of the core elements of team relationships emerged from Jody Hoffer Gittell's study of airline flight teams.
		This theory has been used to guide research and practice in health care and many other settings.
		It incorporates important team concepts like shared goals and mutual respect.
			Resource:
			  Gittell, J. H. (2016). *Transforming relationships for high performance: The power of relational coordination.* Stanford Business Books. https://doi.org/10.1515/9780804797047
			Search Terms:
			  Relational coordination theory, Jody Hoffer Gittell, high-performance teamwork

• How can I boost my confidence as a team member?
• Why does feeling safe make a difference in team outcomes?
• What can leaders in my setting do to encourage trust and risk-taking on our teams?
	Psychological safety	This theory connects trust in team members with the willingness to speak up and take risks.
		It calls out the importance of feeling safe among team members and the factors that can influence it.
			Resource:
			  Edmondson, A. C. (2019). *The fearless organization: Creating psychological safety in the workplace for learning, innovation and growth.* John Wiley & Sons.
			Search Terms:
			  Psychological safety, trust, risk-taking

• How do I prepare myself to be a good team leader?
• What do courage and vulnerability have to do with leadership?
• What if I'm scared?
	Transformational leadership	There are many different leadership theories and models.
		The group of theories about transformational leadership focus on leader characteristics and behaviors that inspire and motivate others.
			Resource:
			  Brown, B. (2018). *Dare to lead: Brave work, tough conversations, whole hearts.* Random House.
			Search Terms:
			  Courage, change, values, innovation, becoming

Questions of Interest	Theory/Framework/ Model	Brief Description	Learn More

• What are important areas for me to think about to improve my team's performance?
• What are my choices for interventions to help my team when we are having difficulty working together?
	The nine "Cs"	This framework identifies nine pivotal areas to consider when developing a new team or working to improve existing teams.
		Based on decades of research, it brings together core elements of teamwork using a practical way to think about them.
			Resource:
			  Salas, E., Shuffer, M. L., Thayer, A. L., Bedwell, W. L., & Lazzara, E. H. (2015). Understanding and improving teamwork in organizations: A scientifically based practical guide. *Human Resources Management, 54*(4), 599–622. https://doi.org/10.1002/hrm.21628
			Search Terms:
			  Teams, groups, 9 Cs, cooperation, collaboration, coaching

TABLE 8.2 Teamwork and Collaboration Theories—cont'd

support the development of effective groups. Team theories emerging from sociology can help you understand and develop strategies to get your teams off to a good start. Theories from psychology tend to look at team dynamics and key aspects of collaboration, like communication or managing conflict. These theories can also provide important insights into how the organizational culture and leadership in your practice setting can support or create barriers to effective teamwork. Changing your lens—and the theories you use—can offer new insights about your team performance and ways to help your team members improve their impact and satisfaction working together.

RELEVANCE TO NURSING PRACTICE

You can expect to be a member of and possibly lead many intraprofessional and interprofessional teams in your nursing career. As discussed earlier in this chapter, we know from considerable research on team performance how team members that work together can have a major impact on quality outcomes for patients and families and the well-being of team members. During the COVID-19 pandemic, nurses, doctors, and other team members have frequently commented on the importance of their teams for both personal and professional support. How you prepare for and collaborate as a team member can and should be a key element of your professional development and identity.

Collaborative competencies, including communication and coordination, are central to the conduct of nursing care in every health care setting. Nursing assessments and interventions must be communicated to have an impact. As the major connectors between team members within and across settings, teams rely on nurses to communicate and coordinate key elements of the patient's care effectively and efficiently. Your interactions with team members educate them about what nurses contribute to patient care and enhance your ability to improve the quality of your care to patients.

Strategies to Enhance Team Effectiveness

Here are some strategies to enhance team effectiveness:
- Recognize that interprofessional identity is an important part of your nursing identity and practice. Most nursing functions occur in the context of relationships and teamwork.
- Make the time and effort to practice and improve your teamwork skills. Competencies for teamwork discussed earlier in this chapter are an integral part of nursing education and continuing professional education for practicing nurses and health professionals.
- Look for content and exercises to build your comfort in articulating your role as a nurse and your knowledge of the roles and contributions of other team members.
- Integrate strategies to enhance effective team performance in your daily practices.
- Think about how you can prepare to step up as a team leader when the situation calls for it. Many situations call for nursing expertise, such as coordinating a patient-centered care plan or assuring that a patient's and family's voices are consulted in deciding a course of action.
- Use your role as team leader to model effective teamwork and involve all team members including patients and families in planning and decision-making.

SUMMARY

Nurses have a significant leadership role to play in care delivery. Effectively navigating from within the interprofessional context of health care to provide safe, timely, efficient, effective, and equitable provision of safe and quality care delivery to individuals, families, communities, and populations requires a commitment to advance the interprofessional agenda in nursing. Possessing knowledge of self and knowledge of self in relation to others extends one's interprofessional role learning, collaboration competency achievement, and capacity to engage as an effective team member. These efforts are further aided by leveraging theoretical models for collaboration to optimize knowledge, skills, and strategies for making meaningful contributions to team effectiveness.

SALIENT POINTS

- Now, as ever, is the time to be interprofessional.
- Dramatic changes are needed in education and practice systems to address the quality, safety, equity, and value of care delivery.
- Knowledge of self is foundational to being an effective nurse and team member.
- The ability to see oneself within the broader landscape of health care contributes to an understanding of self in relation to others.
- Practice theories can guide you in the process of interprofessional role learning, competency development, and confidence-building.
- A foundation of understanding about interprofessional collaboration aligns with health care quality and safety minded nursing practice and health care delivery.
- Commitment to advancing the interprofessional agenda in nursing is critical to advancing the role of nurses as collaborative leaders in the interprofessional health care system.
- Dual identity formation occurs when a sense of belonging to one's profession and the interprofessional community is achieved.

CRITICAL THINKING EXERCISES

1. Think about a time when you had an outstanding experience as a member of a clinical team. What do you think was important to your being able to contribute to the work of this team?
2. What aspects of collaboration and teamwork are most stressful for you? What would help you feel more confident about managing them?
3. You are asked to lead an interprofessional team meeting to review and refine the care plan for a complex patient who is not doing well. What knowledge, skills, and values do you bring to this discussion as a nurse and as a team leader?
4. Quality improvement and safety initiatives are optimized by their interprofessional team-based nature. Identify something about the health care you would like to change. Describe your early thinking related to forming an interprofessional team best suited to lead the change.
5. Reflect on interdisciplinary attitudes, stereotypes, and/or biases you have that may serve as barriers to the development and adoption of a dual professional identity. Consider approaches to reducing the identified barriers in a manner that would allow you to possess a discipline-specific professional identity and the identity of belonging to an interprofessional team.

REFERENCES

American Association of Colleges of Nursing (AACN). (2011). *Essentials of master's education in nursing.* https://www.aacnnursing.org/portals/42/publications/mastersessentials11.pdf

Brashers, V., Haizlip, J., & Owen, J. A. (2020). The ASPIRE model: Grounding the IPEC core competencies for interprofessional collaborative practice within a foundational framework. *Journal of Interprofessional Care, 34*(1), 128–132. https://doi.org/10.1080/13561820.2019.1624513

Brown, B. (2018). *Dare to lead: Brave work, tough conversations, whole hearts.* Random House.

Campoe, K. (2020). Interprofessional collaboration during COVID-19. *MedSurg Nursing, 29*(5), 297–298. https://www.thefreelibrary.com/Interprofessional+Collaboration+During+COVID-19.-a0638989875

Conroy, C. (2019). Stereotyping as a major barrier to achievement of interprofessional education competencies: A narrative literature review. *The Internet Journal of Allied Health*

Sciences and Practice, 17(3), Article 8. https://nsuworks.nova.edu/ijahsp/vol17/iss3/8

Cooke, N. J., Salas, E., Cannon-Bowers, J. A., & Stout, R. J. (2010). Measuring team knowledge. *Human Factors, 42*(1), 151–173. https://doi.org/10.1518/001872000779656561

Disch, J. (2017a, July 31). Interprofessional education: Combining skills and knowledge from different disciplines enhances patient care. [Newsletter]. *American Nurse Today, 12*(7), 26–30.

Disch, J. (2017b). Teamwork and collaboration. In G. Sherwood & J. Barnsteiner (Eds.), *Quality and safety in nursing: A competency approach to improving outcomes* (2nd ed., pp. 85–107). John Wiley & Sons.

Edmondson, A. C. (2019). *The fearless organization: Creating psychological safety in the workplace for learning, innovation and growth.* John Wiley & Sons.

Eisler, R., & Potter, T. M. (2014). *Interprofessional education and practice: A call for partnership. In transforming interprofessional partnerships: A new framework for nursing and partnership-based health care* (pp. 27–46). Sigma Theta Tau International.

Gittell, J. H. (2016). *Transforming relationships for high performance: The power of relational coordination.* Stanford Business Books. https://doi.org/10.1515/9780804797047

Hammick, M., Freeth, D., Copperman, J., & Goodsman, D. (2009). *Being interprofessional: Models and meaning. In being interprofessional* (pp. 7–24). Polity.

Hughes, R. G. (2018). Overview of patient safety and quality of care. In P. Kelly, B. A. Vottero, & C. A. Christie-McAuliffe (Eds.), *Introduction to quality and safety education for nurses: Core competencies for nursing leadership and management* (2nd ed., pp. 3–38). Springer.

Institute of Medicine (IOM). (2011). *Transforming education. The future of nursing: Leading change, advancing health.* National Academies Press. https://doi.org/10.17226/12956

Interprofessional Education Collaborative (IPEC). (2011). *Team-based competencies: Building a shared foundation for education and clinical practice.* https://ipec.memberclicks.net/assets/Team-Based.pdf

Interprofessional Education Collaborative. (2016). *Core competencies for interprofessional collaborative practice: 2016 update.* https://ipec.memberclicks.net/assets/2016-Update.pdf

Khalili, H., Orchard, C., Laschinger, H. K. S., & Farah, R. (2013). An interprofessional socialization framework for developing an interprofessional identity among health professions students. *Journal of Interprofessional Care 27*(6), 448–453. https://doi.org/10.3109/13561820.2013.804042

National Academies of Sciences, Engineering, and Medicine (NASEM). (2021). *The future of nursing 2020–2030: Charting a path to achieve health equity.* National Academies Press. https://doi.org/10.17226/25982

Noureddine, N., & Hagge, D. K. (2022a). A call to action for advancing IPE. In N. Noureddine, W. Ofstad, & D. K. Hagge (Eds.), *Interprofessional education toolkit* (pp. 151–162). Plural Publishing.

Noureddine, N., & Hagge, D. K. (2022b). Interprofessional bias and dual professional identity in IPE. In N. Nouredine, W. Ofstad, & D. K. Hagge (Eds.), *Interprofessional education toolkit* (pp. 49–62). Plural Publishing.

Noureddine, N., Ofstad, W., & Hagge, D. K. (2022a). Leading the change. In N. Nouredine, W. Ofstad, & D. K. Hagge (Eds.), *Interprofessional education toolkit* (pp. 27–47). Plural Publishing.

Noureddine, N., Ofstad, W., & Hagge, D. K. (2022b). Why IPE? Why now? In N. Nouredine, W. Ofstad, & D. K. Hagge (Eds.), *Interprofessional education toolkit* (pp. 1–5). Plural Publishing.

Saewert, K. J. (2018). Leading interprofessionally. In J. M. Adams, J. Mensik, P. R. Ponte, & J. Sommerville (Eds.), *Lead like a nurse: Leadership in every healthcare setting* (pp. 101–121). American Nurses Association.

Salas, E., Shuffer, M. L., Thayer, A. L., Bedwell, W. L., & Lazzara, E. H. (2015). Understanding and improving teamwork in organizations: A scientifically based practical guide. *Human Resources Management, 54*(4), 599–622. https://doi.org/10.1002/hrm.21628

Sheridan, S. (2017). *Sue Sheridan video on patient safety* [Video]. AHRQ. https://www.ahrq.gov/teamstepps/instructor/videos/ts_Sue_Sheridan/Sue_Sheridan-400-300.html

Tuckman, B. W. (1965). Developmental sequence in small groups. *Psychological Bulletin, 63*(6), 384. https://doi.org/10.1037/h0022100

Vega, C. P., & Bernard, V. (2016). Interprofessional collaboration to improve health care: An introduction. http://www.medscape.org/viewarticle/857823

World Health Organization (WHO). (2010). *Framework for action on interprofessional education & collaborative practice.* https://apps.who.int/iris/handle/10665/70185

Will, K. K., & Lamb, G. (2021). A theory-based approach for identifying nurse and team member contributions in the electronic health record. *Journal of Nursing Scholarship, 53*(6), 1–9. https://doi.org/10.1111/jnu.12702

Zorek, J. A., Lacy, J., Gaspard, C., Najjar, G., Eickhoff, J., & Ragucci, K. R. (2021). Leveraging the Interprofessional Education Collaborative Competency Framework to transform health professions education. *American Journal of Pharmaceutical Education, 85*(7), 493–496. https://doi.org/10.5688/ajpe8602

9

Think Like a Nurse

Brenda C. Morris, EdD, MS, RN, CNE

ⓔ http://evolve.elsevier.com/Friberg/bridge/

OBJECTIVES

At the completion of this chapter, the reader will be able to:

- Contrast the concepts of critical thinking, clinical judgment, clinical reasoning, and nursing judgment.
- Describe strategies to develop critical thinking, clinical judgment, and clinical reasoning.
- Apply the universal intellectual standards of thought to nursing practice.
- Describe the steps of Tanner's (2006) clinical judgment model.
- Discuss nursing activities associated with developing clinical judgment.

- Describe the steps of the nursing process and the relationships among those steps.
- Discuss nursing activities associated with each step of the nursing process.
- Discuss the relationships among critical thinking, clinical judgment, clinical reasoning, and the nursing process.
- Apply critical thinking, clinical judgment, and clinical reasoning skills in nursing practice situations.

INTRODUCTION

As you read this chapter, you may wonder what makes thinking like a nurse different than the ordinary types of thinking we do daily. The cognitive processes used in ordinary thinking, such as processing information, using reasoning skills, and making decisions, are the same as those nurses use to think like a nurse. However, thinking like a nurse requires disciplined, focused, reflective, structured, systematic thinking to assess and evaluate client care information and make effective clinical judgments.

Nurses use critical thinking and clinical reasoning skills to make clinical judgments about client care situations or nursing judgments about nursing practice. Critical thinking and clinical reasoning are examples of disciplined, focused, reflective, structured, and systematic thinking approaches that facilitate decision-making, judgment, and problem-solving. These thinking approaches allow nurses to examine situations from different perspectives, identify alternative solutions to problems, and apply knowledge to

new situations. Nurses need thinking skills that prepare them to manage client care situations for conditions that are known as well as unknown future conditions. Think about the beginning of the pandemic and how nurses used their critical thinking, clinical reasoning, and clinical judgment skills to face the unknown when learning how to care for clients diagnosed with COVID-19.

Using a systematic approach to decision-making facilitates effective decision-making.

Nurses make frequent decisions requiring clinical judgment in the provision of care to clients. Over 46% of tasks performed by first-year nurses required the use of clinical judgment (Hensel & Billings, 2020). Bucknall (2000) observed the number and type of decisions critical care nurses made in the first 2 hours of their shift and found that these nurses made 238 decisions per hour, or one decision every 30 seconds. Nurses who lack sound clinical judgment skills are more likely to make client care errors (Hensel & Billings, 2020). Hence, it is critical for nurses to have sound clinical judgment.

Why is it important for nurses to use disciplined, focused, reflective, structured, and systematic thinking? The health care system and nursing practice are changing at a rapid pace due to advances in medical treatment; the emergence of new infectious diseases (COVID-19, Zika) and health conditions; pressures to contain health care costs; clients living longer with more chronic illnesses, thus increasing the complexity of care; and the continued shift to move health care from in-client, acute care settings to out-client community-based settings. These changes require nurses to apply content-specific knowledge and use their thinking skills to rapidly process information from multiple sources to make complex clinical judgments in planning, managing, delivering, and evaluating the health care of their clients. According to the American Nurses Association's (2015b) *Scope and Standards of Practice for Nurses*, nurses are accountable for their decisions, even when they may be following a physician's order. This requires that nurses demonstrate proficiency in critical thinking, clinical reasoning, clinical judgment, and nursing judgment to make effective decisions for client care and nursing practice.

This chapter covers both classic and current sources to examine the processes nurses use "to think like a nurse," including critical thinking, clinical reasoning, clinical judgment, nursing judgment, and the nursing process.

WHAT IS CRITICAL THINKING?

The concept of critical thinking first emerged when Watson and Glaser (1964) described it as the ability to define a problem, recognize stated and unstated assumptions, formulate and select hypotheses, draw conclusions, and judge the validity of inferences. Scriven and Paul (1987) included the role of intellectually disciplined thinking, as well as specific cognitive processes, such as conceptualizing, applying, analyzing, synthesizing, and evaluating information, in their definition of critical thinking. Ennis (1989) added the dimension of self-reflection, when he described critical thinking as "reasonable reflective thinking focused on deciding what to believe or do" (p. 4).

Delphi research project produced the following consensus definition of critical thinking as:

> *Purposeful, self-regulatory, judgment which results in interpretation, analysis, evaluation, and inference, as well as explanation of evidential, conceptual, methodological, criteriological, or contextual considerations upon which that judgment is based.*
> **American Philosophical Association (1990)**

Examples of the cognitive and metacognitive skills and subskills associated with critical thinking are presented in Box 9.1.

BOX 9.1 Critical Thinking Cognitive Skills and Subskills

Interpretation
Categorization
Decoding sentences
Clarifying meaning

Inference
Querying evidence
Conjecturing alternatives
Drawing conclusions

Analysis
Examining ideas
Identifying arguments
Analyzing arguments

Explanation
Stating results
Justifying procedures
Presenting arguments

Evaluation
Assessing claims
Assessing arguments

Self-Regulation
Self-examination
Self-correction

Facione and Facione (1996) recognized that critical thinking has two elements, including a disposition to think critically, as well as specific cognitive and metacognitive processes. Some characteristics consistent with the disposition to think critically include the following:

- *Inquisitiveness* is the demonstration of intellectual curiosity and a true desire for learning. Nurses who routinely ask, "I wonder why…" in the absence of a specific problem display inquisitiveness.
- *Systematicity* is the tendency toward organized, orderly, focused, and diligent inquiry. Nurses who use a systematic approach to gathering data demonstrate systematicity.
- *Analyticity* is the application of reasoning and the use of evidence to resolve problems. Nurses who use an analytic approach connect clinical observations with the theoretical knowledge to anticipate clinical events and intervene to prevent complications.
- *Truth seeking* is the desire to seek the best knowledge in each context. Nurses who engage in truth seeking demonstrate courage in asking questions, strive to remain objective, and continually reevaluate new information.
- *Open-mindedness* is being tolerant of divergent views and being sensitive to one's own biases. Nurses who practice open-mindedness support the provision of culturally competent care to diverse populations.
- *Self-confidence* is trusting in one's own reasoning processes and judgments. Nurses who demonstrate self-confidence effectively present their clinical reasoning and judgments to improve client care.
- *Maturity* is the ability to approach problems, inquiry, and decision-making with the understanding that some problems are ill defined and some situations have more than one plausible option. It is important for nurses to

demonstrate maturity to facilitate ethical decision-making in nursing.

Scheffer and Rubenfeld (2000) replicated the Delphi study with a panel of 55 nurse educators to obtain a consensus definition of critical thinking for nursing as:

An essential component of professional accountability and quality nursing care. Critical thinkers in nursing exhibit these habits of the mind: confidence, contextual perspective, creativity, flexibility, inquisitiveness, intellectual integrity, intuition, open-mindedness, perseverance, and reflection. Critical thinkers in nursing, practice the cognitive skills of analyzing, applying standards, discriminating, information seeking, logical reasoning, predicting, and transforming knowledge. (p. 7)

Elder and Paul (2010) defined critical thinking as self-directed, self-disciplined, and self-corrective thinking, implying that individuals apply intellectual standards to their thinking and engage in a reflective thinking process. Critical thinkers formulate clear and precise questions, gather information and assess its relevance, develop conclusions, think open-mindedly and explore alternative solutions to problems, and communicate effectively with others. Critical thinkers routinely apply the universal intellectual standards of clarity, accuracy, precision, relevance, depth, breadth, logic, and fairness to assess the quality of reasoning about a problem, issue, or situation.

Alfaro-LeFevre (2013) defines critical thinking in nursing as "purposeful, informed, outcome-focused thinking" (p. 8).

Critical thinking applies logic, intuition, creativity, and reflective thinking to identify problems, issues, and risks and make judgments based on evidence. Critical thinking is guided by standards and laws and incorporates elements of the nursing process, problem-solving, the scientific method, clinical reasoning, and clinical judgment.

Niewoehner (2016) states that "critical thinking monitors and questions the health of our thinking" (p. 71). Critical thinking challenges one to validate observations, identify biases, evaluate assumptions, consider alternative points of view, and clarify and refine thoughts. These are essential skills for nursing practice.

There is consensus among most authors that critical thinking processes are generalizable and transferable across disciplines (Elder & Paul, 2010; Facione & Facione, 1996; Watson & Glaser, 1964). However, the difference lies in the discipline-specific context in which the critical thinking processes are applied. For example, professional nurses apply critical thinking to client care situations to make sound clinical judgments, whereas engineers apply critical thinking to business or industrial situations to make sound decisions. To effectively apply critical thinking to a discipline, the individual must have discipline-specific knowledge, in addition to understanding how to use critical thinking processes.

Although a universally accepted definition of critical thinking has not emerged, agreement exists that it is a complex process. The variety of definitions helps provide insight into the myriad dimensions of critical thinking. The definitions presented earlier are summarized for comparison in Table 9.1.

TABLE 9.1   Select Definitions of Critical Thinking

Author	Definition
Watson and Glaser (1964)	The combination of abilities needed to define a problem, recognize stated and unstated assumptions, formulate and select hypotheses, draw conclusions, and judge the validity of inferences.
Scriven and Paul (1987)	An intellectually disciplined process of conceptualizing, applying, analyzing, synthesizing, and evaluating information.
Ennis (1989)	"Reasonable reflective thinking focused on deciding what to believe or do" (p. 4).
American Philosophical Association (1990) Delphi research project	Purposeful, self-regulatory, judgment that results in interpretation, analysis, evaluation, and inference, as well as explanation of evidential, conceptual, methodological, criteriological, or contextual considerations upon which that judgment is based.
Scheffer and Rubenfeld (2000)	"An essential component of professional accountability and quality nursing care. Critical thinkers in nursing exhibit these habits of the mind: confidence, contextual perspective, creativity, flexibility, inquisitiveness, intellectual integrity, intuition, open-mindedness, perseverance, and reflection. Critical thinkers in nursing practice the cognitive skills of analyzing, applying standards, discriminating, information seeking, logical reasoning, predicting, and transforming knowledge" (p. 7).
Elder and Paul (2010)	Self-directed, self-disciplined, and self-corrective thinking, implying that individuals apply intellectual standards to their thinking and engage in a reflective thinking process.
Alfaro-LeFevre (2013)	"Purposeful, informed, outcome-focused thinking" (p. 8).

INTELLECTUAL TRAITS OF CRITICAL THINKERS

Eight interdependent traits of mind are essential to becoming a critical thinker. These are presented in Box 9.2 (Elder & Paul, 2012):

- *Intellectual integrity:* Application of rigorous and consistent standards of evidence and the admission of errors when they occur
- *Intellectual humility:* Awareness of the limits of one's knowledge and sensitivity to the possibility of self-deception
- *Confidence in reason:* Confidence in one's ability to think fairly
- *Intellectual perseverance:* Willingness to seek intellectual insights continually over a period of time and in the face of difficulties
- *Fair-mindedness:* Consciousness of the need to treat all viewpoints alike, without reference to one's own feelings or vested interests

---

BOX 9.2 Intellectual Traits of Critical Thinkers

Intellectual Integrity
- Application of standards of evidence and the admission of errors when they occur

Intellectual Humility
- An awareness of the limits of one's knowledge

Confidence in Reason
- Confident in one's ability to think fairly

Intellectual Perseverance
- Seek intellectual insights continually over a period of time

Fair-Mindedness
- Ability to treat all viewpoints alike, without reference to one's own feelings

Intellectual Courage
- Willingness to listen and examine all ideas

Intellectual Empathy
- Ability to reason from the viewpoint of others

Intellectual Autonomy
- Have control of one's beliefs, values, and inferences

Source: Elder, L., & Paul, R. (2012). Critical thinking: Competency standards essential to the cultivation of intellectual skills, part 4. *Journal of Developmental Education, 35*(3), 30–31.

- *Intellectual courage:* Willingness to listen and examine all ideas, including those that trigger a negative reaction
- *Intellectual empathy:* Imagining oneself in the place of others to better understand them; allows reasoning from the viewpoint of others
- *Intellectual autonomy:* Having rational control of one's beliefs, values, and inferences

STRATEGIES TO BUILD CRITICAL THINKING SKILLS

Critical thinking is enhanced in environments that are caring, nonthreatening, flexible, and respectful of diverse points of view. Nurses who are familiar with the nursing process, the scientific method, evidence-based practice, and research methods already know much about critical thinking because they are based on some of the same principles as critical thinking.

Strategies to enhance critical thinking include fostering the development of critical thinking dispositions, the intellectual traits of critical thinkers, and taking time to reflect upon one's thinking and nursing practice. Becoming a critical thinker is a lifelong process; everyone can improve by working at it.

CLINICAL REASONING

Definitions of clinical reasoning are presented in Table 9.2. Alfaro-LeFevre (2013) defines clinical reasoning as "ways of thinking about client care situations" (p. 8). Clinical reasoning applies the thought processes associated with critical thinking, such as problem-solving, diagnostic, ethical and moral reasoning, decision-making, and evidence-based practice to make judgments about client care situations.

Tanner (2006) defines clinical reasoning as the "processes by which nurses and other clinicians make their judgments and includes both the deliberate process of generating alternatives, weighing them against the evidence, and choosing the most appropriate" (pp. 204–205).

Benner et al. (2010) define clinical reasoning as "ability to reason about a clinical situation as it unfolds, as well as the client and family concerns and the context" (p. 46). Contextualization is important in developing clinical reasoning because it allows the nurse to consider the multiple variables that affect the client's situation, such as the client's history, responses to the environment, interventions, and treatments; interrelationships between physiological systems, social interactions with others, and the presence/absence of a support system (Benner et al., 2010). Contextualization helps the nurse apply clinical reasoning to a specific client situation and make appropriate client-specific clinical judgments.

TABLE 9.2 Definitions of Clinical Reasoning	
Author	**Definition**
Alfaro-LeFevre (2013)	"Ways of thinking about client care situations" (p. 8).
Tanner (2006)	"Processes by which nurses and other clinicians make their judgments and includes both the deliberate process of generating alternatives, weighing them against the evidence, and choosing the most appropriate" (pp. 204–205).
Benner et al. (2010)	"The ability to reason about a clinical situation as it unfolds, as well as the client and family concerns and the context" (p. 46).
Simmons (2010)	"Complex process that uses cognition, metacognition, and discipline-specific knowledge to gather and analyze client information, evaluate its significance, and weigh alternative actions" (p. 1151).

Simmons (2010) defines clinical reasoning as a "complex process that uses cognition, metacognition, and discipline-specific knowledge to gather and analyze client information, evaluate its significance, and weigh alternative actions" (p. 1151). The attributes of clinical reasoning include analysis, deliberation, inference, metacognition, logic, cognition, information processing, and intuition. Nurses use clinical reasoning cognitive processes when applying the nursing process to client care situations. Many variables affect clinical reasoning, such as cognitive ability, life experience, professional expertise, and maturity.

The cognitive and metacognitive thought processes used to develop critical thinking, as well as contextualization, help the nurse develop clinical reasoning. For example, when assessing the client, the nurse uses metacognition to reflect upon data collection to ensure that all essential information has been gathered and that appropriate analysis and interpretation have occurred. The nurse uses contextualization to assess for cues to better understand the client's specific situation and to guide the clinical reasoning process. Another helpful strategy to develop clinical reasoning is learning how to anticipate potential complications or outcomes and how to respond to prevent the onset of the complications or untoward outcomes.

In summary, clinical reasoning is a complex cognitive process that involves metacognition, contextualization, and discipline-specific knowledge to make decisions about client care. Clinical reasoning is similar to critical thinking in that many of the same cognitive and metacognitive processes are used. However, critical thinking is broader than clinical reasoning and may be applied in both clinical and nonclinical situations.

CLINICAL JUDGMENT

"Sound nursing clinical judgment is at the core of competent and safe client care" (Dickison et al., 2019, p. 72).

Critical thinking and clinical reasoning are the processes used to make a clinical judgment, which is "the conclusion you come to, the decision you make, or the opinion you form" (Alfaro-LeFevre, 2013, p. 70). Tanner (2006, p. 204) defines clinical judgment as "an interpretation or conclusion about a patient's needs, concerns or health problems, and/or the decision to take action (or not), use or modify standard approaches, or improvise new ones as deemed appropriate by the patient's response."

To make good clinical judgments, the nurse must "understand not only the pathophysiological and diagnostic aspects of a patient's disease but also the illness experience for the patient and family, and their physical, social, and emotional strengths and coping resources" (Tanner, 2006, p. 205). Several factors influence a nurse's ability to make clinical judgments, including prior experience and knowledge, assessment of the situation, knowing the patient's typical pattern of responses, and understanding the political and social contexts in which the situation occurs. Nurses use one or more different types of reasoning to make clinical judgments. The analytical approach to reasoning involves breaking down a situation into its elements and comparing the elements to the desired clinical outcomes or textbook outcomes for a similar situation. Other reasoning approaches include the use of intuition or narrative thinking.

Tanner (2006) developed a four-step model that describes the major phases of clinical judgment (noticing, interpreting, responding, and reflecting) for use in rapidly changing clinical situations. The first step in the model is noticing; during this phase, the nurse assesses the clinical situation based on knowledge of the patient, including the patient's usual response patterns and prior experience with similar types of situations. The nurse uses reasoning skills to interpret the meaning of these data and respond to the situation by determining the appropriate course of action during the interpreting and responding phases. The nurse

TABLE 9.3   Definitions of Clinical Judgment

Author	Definition
Alfaro-LeFevre (2013)	Critical thinking and clinical reasoning are the processes used to make a clinical judgment, which is "the conclusion you come to, the decision you make, or the opinion you form" (p. 70).
Tanner (2006)	"An interpretation or conclusion about a patient's needs, concerns or health problems, and/or the decision to take action (or not), use or modify standard approaches, or improvise new ones as deemed appropriate by the patient's response" (p. 204).

reflects upon the situation during the final phase (reflection). The initial reflection-in-action occurs during the noticing, interpreting, and responding phases when the nurse evaluates the assessment of the patient, the patient's response to nursing interventions, and outcomes (Lasater, 2007). After responding to the clinical situation, the nurse performs reflection-on-action, in which the nurse retrospectively evaluates the overall situation and connects nursing actions with outcomes. It is during the reflection-on-action phase that new clinical learning occurs. Table 9.3 presents definitions of clinical judgment.

The National Council of State Boards of Nursing introduced its *Nursing Clinical Judgment Measurement Model* to measure the development of clinical judgment and decision-making on the National Council Licensure Examination for Registered Nurses. Clinical judgment is viewed as a higher-order thinking process that nurses are required to demonstrate to provide safe client care. To form clinical judgment, nurses recognize and analyze cues; form, refine, and prioritize hypotheses; generate solutions; take action; and evaluate outcomes in the context of environmental and individual factors (Dickison et al., 2019). Nurses who "recognize, analyze, hypothesize, respond, and evaluate" are prepared to deliver excellent care by making effective clinical judgments in varied contextual client care situations (Dickison et al., 2019, p. 73).

NURSING JUDGMENT

The development of nursing judgment is essential to nursing practice. Provision 4 of the American Nurses Association (ANA) (2015a, p. 15) *Code of Ethics for Nurses with Interpretative Statements* assigns the nurse "authority, accountability, and responsibility for nursing practice." Inherent in the responsibility to deliver optimal client care, the nurse is "accountable for decisions made and actions taken in the course of nursing practice" (ANA, 2015a, pp. 15–16). Nurses use nursing judgment to make client care decisions (ANA, 2015a). "Nursing judgment is the culmination of education, experience, and insight that allows nurses to execute the best action possible on behalf of clients" (de Tantillo & De Santis, 2019, p. 266).

Nurses use critical thinking, clinical judgment, clinical reasoning, and the nursing process to inform nursing judgments about client care. For example, when the nurse prepares to administer a prescribed medication to a client, they begin with the first step of the nursing process, which is assessment. The nurse uses their critical thinking, clinical judgment, and clinical reasoning skills to assess the client to make a nursing judgment about whether it is safe to administer the medication as prescribed. If, in the nurse's judgment, it is not safe to administer the medication, the nurse will withhold the medication and notify the prescriber. Another example to illustrate this point occurs when the nurse is preparing to delegate a nursing task to another health care worker. The nurse uses their nursing judgment to determine if the individual to whom the task will be delegated has the knowledge, skills, and experience to safely carry out the delegated task.

THE NURSING PROCESS

The nursing process is a systematic, problem-solving approach that provides the framework for nursing practice in the United States and Canada. The nursing process has five steps, including:

- *Assessment:* Gathering and validating client health data, strengths, risks, and concerns
- *Diagnosis:* Analyzing and processing client data to identify appropriate nursing diagnoses[1]
- *Planning:* Developing interventions to solve identified problems and build on client strengths
- *Implementation:* Delivering nursing interventions and documenting the planned care
- *Evaluation:* Determining the effectiveness of the care delivered

---

[1]Outcomes identification may be included as part of the diagnosis phase, or it may be recognized as a separate step in the nursing process.

The ANA, in its publication *Nursing: Scope and Standards of Practice* (ANA, 2015b), uses the nursing process as the framework for professional nursing practice. Outcome identification, which follows the nursing diagnosis phase and precedes the planning phase, is identified as a separate step in the ANA model. "Critical thinking underlies each step of the nursing process, problem-solving, and decision-making" (ANA, 2015b, p. 8).

The nursing process is sometimes depicted as a systematic, linear model proceeding from assessment through diagnosis, planning, implementation, and evaluation. It is more appropriately conceptualized as a continuous and interactive model, thereby providing a flexible and dynamic approach to client care. This model can accommodate changes in the client's health status or failure to achieve expected outcomes through a feedback mechanism. The interactive nature of the model with its feedback mechanism permits the nurse to reenter the nursing process at the appropriate stage to collect additional data, restructure nursing diagnoses, design a new plan, or change implementation strategies. This model is consistent with the concepts of critical thinking and clinical reasoning as ways of processing thinking about client care issues. Further examination of the elements of the nursing process reveals the multiple activities embedded in each step.

Assessment

In the assessment phase, the nurse systematically collects and analyzes data to determine the client's health status (ANA, 2022, https://www.nursingworld.org/practice-policy/workforce/what-is-nursing/the-nursing-process/). Data are collected to assess the cultural, emotional, functional, physiological, psychological, and spiritual dimensions of the client. Data collection centers on the use of multiple sources and types of data, a variety of data collection techniques, and the use of reliable and valid measurement instruments. All these elements are critical to a comprehensive assessment of the client.

Sources of Data. The primary source of data is the client, whether the client is defined as the individual, the family, or the community. Secondary sources of data include written records, other health care providers, and significant others (e.g., family members, friends). To strengthen the overall assessment and validate client data, it is important to use primary and secondary data sources.

Data Collection Techniques. Assessment techniques include measurement, observation, and interview. Measurement is used to determine the dimensions of a given indicator (e.g., blood pressure) or to ascertain characteristics such as quantity, size, or frequency. Measurement may require the use of

specialized equipment (e.g., stethoscope, thermometer) or specialized assessment tools (e.g., pain scale, depression scale) to assess functional, behavioral, social, or cognitive domains. Data collection by observation requires the use of the senses, including visual observation and tactile (palpation) and auditory techniques (auscultation). Observation provides a variety and depth of data that may be difficult to obtain by other methods. A structured or unstructured interview may be used to obtain information such as a health history and demographic data. A structured interview is commonly used in emergency situations when the nurse needs to gather specific information. An unstructured interview is commonly used in situations in which the nurse wishes to elicit information from the client's perspective or gain insight in to the client's understanding of a problem. The unstructured interview allows the nurse to use active listening skills while building rapport with the client through the use of an open-ended interview format. These interprofessional collaboration techniques are discussed in more detail in Chapter 8.

Types of Data. To complete a comprehensive assessment, objective and subjective data are obtained. Objective data are factual data, usually obtained through observation or measurement. An example of objective data occurs when the nurse uses an otoscope to assess the client's tympanic membrane and observes that it is reddened and inflamed. Subjective data are based on the client's perception of the health problem. An example of subjective data occurs when the client states he has pain in his right ear. It is important to collect both objective and subjective data to complete a comprehensive assessment. Care should be taken to record data factually and avoid personal or biased interpretations.

Data Collection Instruments. The use of selected data collection measures and instruments can assist the nurse in compiling a comprehensive database and organizing data into meaningful patterns. Assessment usually begins by taking a nursing history and conducting a physical examination. The nursing history is comprehensive and includes an assessment of the social determinants of health, which are "nonmedical factors that influence health outcomes," such as "the conditions in which people are born, grow, work, live, and age" (World Health Organization, n.d.). Additionally, the nursing database should include the following categories of information:

- Demographic data
- Current and past medical problems
- Family medical history
- Surgical and (if appropriate) obstetrical history
- Childhood illnesses

- Allergies
- Current medications
- Psychological status
- Social history
- Environmental background
- Physical assessment

The amount of detail may vary; for example, a history obtained in an emergency department may be different from one taken in an extended care facility. The focus of the assessment and history also may vary based on the type of client served. For example, on an oncology unit emphasis may be placed on assessment of pain, social support networks, and coping skills, whereas in a prenatal clinic the focus would be on assessment of fetal growth, knowledge of nutrition, and the need for community resources such as childbirth education classes. The nurse conducts a focused assessment to address the area of concern and a holistic assessment to assess the cultural, emotional, functional, physiological, psychological, and spiritual dimensions of the client.

To ensure appropriate identification of client health problems, it is important to perform a comprehensive assessment. The nurse may also use the assessment phase as a time to establish the nurse-client and nurse-family relationships and begin the discharge planning process. Completion of a comprehensive assessment lays the foundation for making effective clinical judgments and implementing appropriate nursing care to meet the client's identified health needs. To accurately assess a client, the nurse must apply the critical thinking skills of observing, distinguishing relevant from irrelevant data, validating the accuracy and completeness of the data, and organizing the data to provide the basis for subsequent analysis and diagnosis.

Analysis/Nursing Diagnoses

Analysis involves processing the data by organizing, categorizing, and synthesizing the information. The nurse uses critical thinking skills to make inferences in the data from which conclusions can be drawn. Analysis gives meaning to the data as client strengths, problems, and risks are identified. Client data may be compared against known norms, such as the stages of growth and development or disease-specific behaviors or expectations. Gaps or incongruities in the data are identified, and patterns of behavior are ascertained. Analysis occurs while the nurse is actively listening and questioning the client and, later, when the nurse processes the information to formulate a plan of care. Analysis is an ongoing process that is initiated when new information is obtained or changes in the client's health status occur. The end result of data analysis is the formation of a *nursing diagnosis.*

A nursing diagnosis is "the nurse's clinical judgment about the client's response to actual or potential health conditions or needs" (ANA, 2022, https://www.nursingworld.org/practice-policy/workforce/what-is-nursing/the-nursing-process/). In this case, the client may be an individual, family, or community. The nursing diagnosis provides the basis for the nurse's care plan and the selection of nursing interventions. During the diagnosis step, the nurse uses critical thinking and clinical reasoning skills to draw conclusions from identified patterns in the data and make nursing clinical judgments. The nurse uses inductive and deductive reasoning to determine an appropriate nursing diagnosis. A nurse uses *inductive reasoning* when making the observation that clients who underwent bowel resection surgery experience intense postoperative pain. From this observation, the nurse concludes that all clients who undergo bowel resection surgery will probably experience pain postoperatively and therefore will have the nursing diagnosis of acute pain. *Deductive reasoning* is used to draw specific conclusions from generalized data or facts. If the nurse accepts the premise that pain in the left arm and jaw is a cardinal sign of a myocardial infarction, then when a client presents to the emergency department complaining of left arm and jaw pain, the nurse uses deductive reasoning to suspect that the client is having a myocardial infarction until it can be proved otherwise. Diagnosis entails back-and-forth movement between these two modes of reasoning.

A nursing diagnostic statement differs from a medical diagnosis in both content and context. The medical diagnosis describes a pathological condition or symptom that requires treatment aimed at curing the disease or alleviating the symptom. The nursing diagnosis, on the other hand, describes the client's response to actual or potential health conditions or needs.

It is important for the nurse to accurately identify the client's nursing diagnoses and to validate these nursing diagnoses with the client. If the nursing diagnoses are not validated with the client before nursing interventions are implemented, the nursing care plan may be ineffective and may not meet the client's health care needs. The client's nursing diagnosis guides the planning, implementation, and evaluation phases of nursing care.

Planning

During the planning phase of the nursing process, the nurse collaborates with the client to determine the priority nursing diagnosis or diagnoses, establish the client's short- or long-term outcomes, and identify nursing interventions to assist the client toward achieving the outcomes. It is important to involve the client, family, and significant others in the planning process, when appropriate, to gain their support for implementing the plan of care.

Prioritizing nursing diagnoses consists of ranking them according to importance. In general, the highest-priority nursing diagnoses address basic survival needs, life-threatening client problems, and safety. Additional considerations in setting priorities are the need for early resolution of health problems that have the potential to impair functioning or normal growth and development; the client's individual needs, values, and overall health status; and constraints of time and resources. Ideally, the client and nurse mutually determine the priority nursing diagnoses; however, this is not always possible.

Once priorities are established, desired outcomes are identified. Behavioral *outcomes* are client-centered and meet the SMART criteria (specific, measurable, achievable, realistic, and include a time frame). Outcomes are written to reflect attainment of an optimal level of health, alleviation or minimization of a health problem, or modifications of lifestyle. It is recommended to begin the outcome statement with the phrase "The client will… ." This helps the nurse write the outcome from the client's perspective rather than the nurse's perspective. It is helpful to use the following format when writing an outcome statement: "The client will *(insert action verb and behavioral criterion)* by *(insert time frame)*." This format adheres to the SMART criteria. An example of a well-written outcome is as follows: "The client will ambulate 50 feet with the assistance of a walker by the first postoperative day." In this example, the phrase "ambulate 50 feet with the assistance of a walker" includes the action verb and behavioral criterion; the phrase "by the first postoperative day" describes the time frame. In clinical situations a specific date and time (e.g., 9 a.m. on month/day/year) may be used. See Table 9.4 for another example of a well-written client outcome.

Each outcome must be accompanied by one or more *nursing interventions* aimed at helping the client achieve the outcome. Nursing interventions require the use of critical thinking, clinical reasoning, and clinical judgment because the nurse is legally responsible for intervening appropriately (ANA, 2015b). Nursing interventions may be performed by the nurse or delegated to assistive personnel as appropriate. It is important to select nursing interventions that are specific to the nursing diagnosis, acceptable

to the client, feasible to implement, realistic, and supported with scientific rationale or evidence.

Nursing diagnoses, client outcomes, and nursing interventions are incorporated into a nursing care plan. *The nursing care plan* is used as a communication tool between nurses and other health professionals and serves as a guide for nursing care. Clinical agencies may use standardized care plans or care maps created by clinical experts, which contain common nursing diagnoses, client outcomes, and nursing interventions for clients experiencing common medical and surgical illnesses. Nurses customize the standardized care plans or care maps to meet the specific needs of their client.

Implementation

During the implementation phase, the nurse executes the previously identified plan of care by using intellectual, interpersonal, and technical skills to provide care that is client-focused and outcome-oriented and meets the needs of the client. Common nursing interventions initiated during the implementation phase include performing assessments to monitor client health status, providing or assisting the client with personal care, assisting the client to perform activities of daily living, administering medications or other prescribed treatments, teaching the client, or consulting with other health care professionals. During implementation, the nurse uses critical thinking and clinical reasoning skills to apply knowledge to client care situations, reflect upon implementation of the plan of care by assessing for changes in the client's condition, evaluating the effectiveness of the nursing interventions, and making changes to the plan of care based on this assessment.

The final step in the implementation phase is careful documentation. The system of documentation may be agency specific, but the content should reflect the client's concerns and the nursing process. It is important to include the following information in the record:

- A description of the nursing intervention that was performed
- The client's response to the intervention
- Any new data that may have emerged
- Progress (or lack of it) toward the achievement of client care outcomes

Documentation should also include a description of any planned interventions that did not occur and the reasons why they were not implemented. It is very important to ensure that all information is documented correctly; therefore, it is recommended that nurses review their documentation for errors before finalization. Additional discussion on the legal aspects of nursing documentation can be found in Chapter 11 (Legal Aspects of Nursing Process).

TABLE 9.4 **Example of a Measurable Behavioral Outcome That Meets the SMART Criteria**	
Outcome	**Characteristic**
The client will walk	Performance
One-half the length of the hall	Criterion
Unassisted	Condition
On the second postoperative day	Condition

Evaluation

Evaluation is an ongoing activity that occurs at each stage of the nursing process. The overall purpose of the evaluation phase of the nursing process is to determine whether the client met the identified outcomes. The nurse evaluates the attainment of outcomes by comparing the predicted outcome with the client's actual progress toward meeting the outcome.

Evaluation occurs within each step of the nursing process. During the assessment phase, evaluation focuses on the appropriateness and completeness of data collection. During the analysis and diagnosis phase, evaluation centers on whether the data are appropriately clustered; whether the nursing diagnoses reflect the data and the client's health concerns; and whether the nursing diagnoses are clear, concise, and relevant. During the planning process, evaluation activities are directed toward determining the appropriateness of the outcomes, nursing diagnosis priorities, and selected nursing interventions. During the implementation stage, evaluation focuses on the relevance and effectiveness of specific nursing interventions. The nurse and client continue to evaluate these components until the client's health concerns are resolved, the outcomes are achieved, or the episode of care ends.

Another way to focus evaluation activities is to judge the appropriateness, effectiveness, and efficiency of the plan of care and its implementation. The ideal plan of care is relevant to the client's health concerns and focuses on mutually desirable outcomes, is effective in achieving desired outcomes within the specified time frame, and is efficient in maximizing the use of client, provider, and agency resources.

Guidelines for Evaluation. As previously mentioned, evaluation includes comparing actual outcomes against predicted outcomes and evaluating the nursing care plan. If the outcomes are not met, the nurse and client must determine the reason. The following questions may be asked:

- Were the assessment data appropriate and complete?
- Were the data interpreted correctly?
- Were the nursing diagnoses appropriate?
- Were the outcomes realistic, attainable, and measurable?
- Was the nursing care plan directed toward resolution of nursing diagnoses?
- Was the implementation of the plan individualized in accordance with the client's strengths and limitations?
- Were both the nurse and the client working toward the same outcome?

Based on the answers to these questions, the nurse will modify the plan of care.

The nursing process principles discussed in this chapter as they relate to nursing care for individuals and families can be applied to communities, populations, systems, and organizations to address health status, care environments, or delivery of services.

CRITICAL THINKING, CLINICAL REASONING, CLINICAL JUDGMENT, AND THE NURSING PROCESS: PUTTING IT ALL TOGETHER IN NURSING PRACTICE

What is the significance of critical thinking, clinical reasoning, and clinical judgment to professional nursing practice?

Nurses have become more autonomous in their practice and responsible for the outcomes of client care during the past few decades. The use of technology in providing health care and the acuity of hospitalized clients have increased significantly, requiring more complex nursing care management. The ongoing shift from acute care to community-based care requires nurses to become experts in coordinating complicated transitions of care with clients and families. Because of these fast-paced changes in the health care environment and the increased complexity of nursing practice, it is imperative for nurses to have strong critical thinking, clinical reasoning, and clinical judgment skills to provide safe, effective nursing care.

The American Association of Colleges of Nursing (AACN) establishes nursing program standards and defines competencies for entry-level and advanced professional nursing education and recognizes the significance of producing nurse graduates who demonstrate strong clinical judgment skills (AACN, 2021). One of the core concepts for all professional nurses is clinical judgment. Nurses use critical thinking and clinical reasoning skills to form clinical judgment. The integration, translation, and application of nursing knowledge form the foundation for clinical judgment (AACN, 2021). Manetti (2019), as cited in AACN (2021), describes nurses who demonstrate clinical judgment as "the process by which nurses make decisions based on nursing knowledge (evidence, theories, ways/patterns of knowing), other disciplinary knowledge, critical thinking, and clinical reasoning" (p. 108). This process is used to understand and interpret information in the delivery of care. Clinical decision-making based on clinical judgment is directly related to care outcomes (AACN, 2021).

Professional standards, such as the ANA's (2015a, 2015b) *Code of Ethics for Nurses With Interpretive Statements Scope and Standards of Practice for Nurses,* and state nurse practice acts, further define required competencies for professional nursing practice. These professional standards use the nursing process as the framework for nursing practice. These standards recognize the importance of critical thinking and clinical reasoning as cognitive and metacognitive processes required to successfully implement the nursing process and make sound clinical judgments.

The nursing process serves as a framework for applying critical thinking, clinical reasoning, and clinical judgment to nursing practice. The nurse uses the cognitive and metacognitive processes inherent in critical thinking and clinical reasoning throughout the nursing process to sort and categorize data, identify patterns in the data, draw inferences, develop hypotheses that are stated in the form of outcomes, test these hypotheses as care is delivered, and make criterion-based judgments of effectiveness. Therefore, critical thinking and clinical reasoning can distinguish between fact and fiction, providing a rational basis for clinical judgments and the delivery of nursing care. Although the components of the nursing process are described as separate and distinct steps, they become an integrated way of thinking as nurses gain more clinical experience. A thorough understanding of the nursing process reveals that critical thinking, clinical reasoning, and clinical judgment are integral parts of its most effective use.

APPLICATION OF TANNER'S FOUR-STEP CLINICAL JUDGMENT MODEL AND CRITICAL THINKING TO A CLINICAL SITUATION

Clinical judgment is an interpretation or conclusion about a patient's needs, concerns or health problems, and/or decisions to take action (or not), use or modify standard approaches, or improvise new ones as deemed appropriate by the patient's response.

Tanner (2006, p. 204)

Situation

An elderly male client was admitted to the medical unit with diagnoses of congestive heart failure, chronic obstructive pulmonary disease, and diabetes. The client's wife notifies the nurse that there is "something wrong with her husband" when he stops talking to her in the middle of a conversation and does not respond to her attempts to awaken him.

Noticing. The nurse assesses the client and obtains the following data. The client is:
- Diaphoretic
- Skin is pale
- Nonresponsive to verbal stimuli
- Blood glucose = 25 mg/dL
- Blood glucose values have ranged from 120 to 240 mg/dL for the past 48 hours
- Baseline mental status is alert and oriented to person, place, and time

Interpreting. The client has diabetes and is displaying symptoms consistent with a severe hypoglycemic reaction (decreased blood glucose value, diaphoretic, nonresponsive).

Responding. The nurse reviews the standing orders for this client and implements the orders for managing a severe hypoglycemic reaction in a nonresponsive client. The nurse administers dextrose intravenously per the standing order.

The client becomes responsive to verbal stimuli and follows simple commands within 2 minutes of the intravenous administration of dextrose. The client's blood glucose is 100 mg/dL after treatment.

Reflecting

Reflecting in action. The nurse uses reflecting in action to evaluate assessment findings, determine the client's response to the nursing interventions implemented, and evaluate client outcomes.

Reflecting on action. The nurse uses reflection on action to retrospectively evaluate the overall clinical situation. The nurse uses the critical thinking skill, deductive reasoning, and clinical judgment skill of contextualization to reflect upon why this client may have experienced a severe hypoglycemic reaction, when the client's most recent blood glucose levels have been in the normal to hyperglycemic range. Upon further evaluation, the nurse learns that the client received his usual dose of insulin lispro 15 minutes before the delivery of his lunch tray. However, he did not eat his lunch because he felt nauseous. The severe hypoglycemic reaction occurred 45 minutes after the insulin administration.

SUMMARY

It is crucial for the nurse to be able to think critically and apply clinical reasoning skills to provide a safe environment and deliver optimal client care. As nurses enhance their critical thinking and clinical reasoning skills, they will make sound clinical judgments based on evidence.

Today's health care environment requires nurses to solve complex problems, explore unique client situations, and evaluate the effectiveness of a wide range of interventions. Critical thinking and clinical reasoning are integral parts of effective nursing action. They are complex cognitive and metacognitive processes that nurses use to make clinical judgments. The conscious application of critical thinking principles and clinical reasoning can result in effective decision-making and ultimately enhance the quality of care.

SALIENT POINTS

- The American Nurses Association (2015b) *Scope and Standards of Practice for Nurses* calls upon nurses to use critical thinking in each step of the nursing process and to use critical thinking when making judgment (nursing judgments) about client care.
- Critical thinking incorporates thinking skills and a disposition to think critically.
- Critical thinking skills are transferable and may be applied across disciplines.
- Nursing process is a systematic problem-solving approach used by nurses to manage client care situations.
- Nurses use critical thinking and clinical reasoning skills to make clinical judgments about client care.

- Appraisal, problem-solving, creativity, and decision-making are interrelated concepts in critical thinking.
- Nurses with expert clinical judgment display characteristics of high-level critical thinking.
- To think critically, nurses must be able to see connections; use logic; differentiate fact, inference, and assumptions; evaluate arguments; consider many sides of an issue; be creative; and believe in their ability to think and reason.
- Becoming a critical thinker is a lifelong process that involves acquiring a set of skills and developing a disposition toward critical thinking.

CRITICAL REFLECTION EXERCISES

1. Contrast the terms critical thinking, clinical reasoning, clinical judgment, and nursing judgment.
2. Think about a client care situation that you have recently encountered.
   a. Apply Tanner's (2006) four-step clinical judgment model to this situation.
   b. What did you learn from this situation?
3. An elderly client is admitted to the hospital. In conducting their initial assessment, the nurse notices that the client is somewhat confused. The admitting notes indicate that they take digoxin and furosemide (Lasix). The nurse suspects that the client may be experiencing side effects from their medications.
   a. Use critical thinking and clinical reasoning skills to apply the nursing process to this situation.
   b. What are the common side effects of digoxin and furosemide?
   c. What additional assessment data will you gather?

4. Evaluate the nursing assessment instrument used in your current area of practice in terms of its adequacy for your clinical setting, usefulness in other clinical settings, and comprehensiveness. What additional data would be useful and how might you collect this information?
5. Describe the best and worst decision-making you have seen by a nurse in a client care situation.
   a. Compare these two situations in terms of the thought process used, the underlying assumptions of the nurses, the accuracy of available information, the interpretation of information, and the soundness of the decision reached.
6. Describe strategies you can use to enhance critical thinking.
7. Discuss the interrelationships among critical thinking, clinical reasoning, clinical judgment, nursing judgment, and the nursing process.

(e) EVOLVE WEBSITE/RESOURCES LIST

American Nurses Association. This website provides the *Code of ethics for nurses with interpretive statements* for online viewing at no charge.

Foundation for Critical Thinking. This website provides classic definitions and references discussing the concept of critical thinking.

National Council of State Boards of Nursing. View the *Nursing Clinical Judgment Measurement Model*, which serves as a foundation for the Next Generation NCLEX.

REFERENCES

Alfaro-LeFevre, R. (2013). *Critical thinking, clinical reasoning, and clinical judgment: A practical approach* (5th ed.). Elsevier.

American Association of Colleges of Nursing (AACN). (2021). *The essentials: Core competencies for professional nursing education.* https://aacnnursing.org/Portals/42/AcademicNursing/pdf/Essentials-2021.pdf

American Nurses Association. (2015a). *Code of ethics for nurses with interpretive statements.*

American Nurses Association. (2015b). *Nursing: Scope and standards of practice.*

American Nurses Association. (2022). *The nursing process.* https://www.nursingworld.org/practice-policy/workforce/what-is-nursing/the-nursing-process/

American Philosophical Association. (1990). *Critical thinking: A statement of expert consensus for purposes of educational assessment and instruction. The Delphi Report: Research findings and recommendations prepared for the Committee of Pre-college Philosophy.*

Benner, P. A., Sutphen, M., Leonard, V., & Day, L. (2010). *Educating nurses: A call for radical transformation.* Jossey-Bass.

Bucknall, T. K. (2000). Critical care nurses' decision-making activities in the natural clinical setting. *Journal of Clinical Nursing, 9*(1), 25–35.

de Tantillo, L., & De Santis, J. (2019). Nursing judgment. *Advances in Nursing Science, 42*(3), 266–276. https://doi.org/10.1097/ANS.0000000000000245

Dickison, P., Haerling, K. A., & Lasater, K. (2019). Integrating the National Council of State Boards of Nursing Clinical Judgment Model into nursing educational frameworks. *The Journal of Nursing Education, 58*(2), 72–78. https://doi.org/10.3928/01484834-20190122-03

Elder, L., & Paul, R. (2010). Critical thinking: Competency standards essential for the cultivation of intellectual skills, part 1. *Journal of Developmental Education, 34*(2), 38–39.

Elder, L., & Paul, R. (2012). Critical thinking: Competency standards essential to the cultivation of intellectual skills, part 4. *Journal of Developmental Education, 35*(3), 30–31.

Ennis, R. H. (1989). Critical thinking and subject specificity: Clarification and needed research. *Educational Researcher, 18*(3), 4–10. https://doi.org/10.3102/0013189X018003004

Facione, N. C., & Facione, P. A. (1996). Externalizing the critical thinking in knowledge development and clinical judgment. *Nursing Outlook, 44*(3), 129–136. https://doi.org/10.1016/s0029-6554(06)80005-9

Hensel, D., & Billings, D. M. (2020). Strategies to teach the National Council of State Boards of Nursing Clinical Judgment Model. *Nurse Educator, 45*(3), 128–132. https://doi.org/10.1097/NNE.0000000000000773

Lasater, K. (2007). Clinical judgment development: Using simulation to create an assessment rubric. *Journal of Nursing Education, 46*(11), 496–503. https://doi.org/10.3928/01484834-20071101-04

Manetti, W. (2019). Sound clinical judgment in nursing: A concept analysis. *Nursing Forum, 54*(1), 102–110. https://doi.org/10.1111/nuf.12303

Niewoehner, R. (2016). Portaging Richard Paul's model to professional practice: Ideas that integrate. *Inquiry: Critical Thinking Across the Disciplines, 31*(1), 69–85. https://doi.org/10.5840/inquiryct20163116

Scheffer, B. K., & Rubenfeld, M. G. (2000). A consensus statement on critical thinking in nursing. *Journal of Nursing Education, 39*(8), 352–359. https://doi.org/10.3928/0148-4834-20001101-06

Scriven, M., & Paul, R. (1987). National Council for Excellence in Critical Thinking: Critical thinking defined. Paper presented at the Eighth Annual International Conference on Critical Thinking and Education Reform. http://www.criticalthinking.org/pages/defining-critical-thinking/766

Simmons, B. (2010). Clinical reasoning: Concept analysis. *Journal of Advanced Nursing, 66*(5), 1151–1158. https://doi.org/10.1111/j.1365-2648.2010.05262.x

Tanner, C. A. (2006). Thinking like a nurse: A research-based model of clinical judgment in nursing. *Journal of Nursing Education, 45*(6), 204–211. https://doi.org/10.3928/01484834-20060601-04

Watson, G., & Glaser, E. M. (1964). *Critical thinking appraisal.* Harcourt Brace Jovanovich.

World Health Organization. (n.d.). *Social determinants of health.* http://www.who.int/health-topics/social-determinants-of-health#tab=tab_1

10

The Continuum of Learning and Teaching in Nursing

Heidi C. Sanborn, DNP, RN, CNE

 http://evolve.elsevier.com/Friberg/bridge/

OBJECTIVES

At the completion of this chapter, the reader will be able to:
- Examine the concepts that influence the quality of learning.
- Summarize the gaps that create inequity in education and health care.
- Identify theories that support teaching strategies across settings.
- Distinguish the main considerations of educational design.
- Contrast the elements of various teaching modalities.

INTRODUCTION

The concepts of teaching and learning are ubiquitous within the practice of nursing. There is virtually no scenario in which a nurse would not embody these roles. For that reason, the topics explored in this chapter are relevant to any learner audience, regardless of the stage and trajectory of their nursing pathway. Consider the importance of education in each of these scenarios:
- A high school student interested in a career in health care talks with their mother's friend who is a nurse to learn more about the nursing role.
- A nursing student in a postclinical conference is asked to present their care plan for a patient with recurrent chronic foot ulcers.
- A medical/surgical nurse precepting a nursing student is demonstrating how to provide tracheostomy care to an adult patient.
- A nurse is approached by a colleague asking what they can do about an increasing sense of stress and burnout due to chronically short staffing on the unit.
- A nursing instructor is developing the learning plan for three simulation days that will supplement a pediatric clinical rotation.

In each of these cases, the nurse must be aware of the factors that can influence learning while demonstrating effective teaching. These factors include the attributes that influence how people learn; the challenges of addressing justice, equity, diversity, and inclusion (JEDI) in education; the theories that can guide the design of teaching and learning experiences; and the influence of educational design and teaching modalities on the development of new knowledge and behaviors.

These scenarios provide examples of how nurses reside at the center of the three Cs of nursing education (community, client, and colleagues) with clear links to the four goals of the Quadruple Aim (Fig. 10.1). Each of the four elements of the Quadruple Aim emerges in the dynamic interactions among each of the three Cs:
1. Educating individuals and communities to better manage their health, nurses can reduce the cost of care delivery and improve their experience within the health care system.
2. Providing education on preventive care and wellness strategies can improve population health and enhance the experience for individuals interacting with the health care system.
3. Educating other health care colleagues to improve care delivery will reduce costs and improve the health of the communities we serve (Berwick et al., 2008).

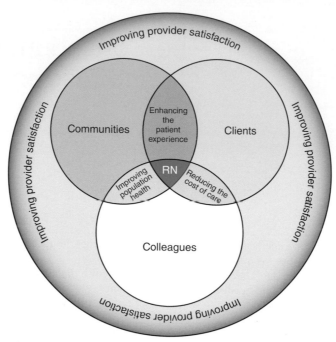

Fig. 10.1 Three Cs of Nursing Education That Influence the Quadruple Aim. *Note.* The nurse's role as an educator places them at the center of the three Cs. Their work in these realms directly influences the achievement of all four elements of the Quadruple Aim which are shown in this Venn diagram.

4. Preventing clinician burnout through more efficient workflows, effective care outcomes, and improved relationships with those being served (Bodenheimer & Sinsky, 2014).

THE CONTINUUM OF LEARNING

Learning is a process that should begin long before a student enters a nursing program and continue throughout the entire professional nursing lifecycle (National Academies of Sciences, Engineering, and Medicine [NASEM], 2016). Many nurses can articulate a desire to learn that began well before they received admission to a nursing program. For some, it started through a meaningful encounter with a nurse that sparked a desire to enter the profession. Regardless of how it begins, the nursing career follows a steep trajectory of learning to master the art and science of nursing. But graduation and licensure as a new nurse are just the beginning of a path of lifelong learning. The complexity of health care means even the most seasoned nurses will always have more to learn, and the

responsibility to become master learners is inherent to any position a nurse may hold (Halstead, 2018; NASEM, 2021).

An additional aspect of learning is an obligation for nurses to better understand the factors that foster effective learning. One of the fundamental roles of the nurse is to be a teacher, a topic explored in more detail later in this chapter. But delivering education must begin by understanding the concepts that promote optimal learning, regardless of who a nurse is teaching. Nurses should understand these concepts so that they can have a positive influence on learning outcomes. To effectively educate the nursing workforce to address health inequities and to teach patients and communities to promote healthy outcomes, one must first consider the attributes of learners that can have an impact on how and why they learn.

Commitment to Lifelong Learning

The nursing profession has, for many decades, explored the impact of education on patient care outcomes. Many autonomous nursing organizations across practice and education have come together to support and promote strategies that facilitate the educational advancement of the nursing profession (American Association of Colleges of Nursing [AACN], 2019; AACN et al., 2012). There is a significant body of research that demonstrates the association between improved outcomes and reduced costs with increased education (Aiken et al., 2017). There is also an advancement in quality and safety knowledge that comes with higher degree levels in nursing, which can improve care delivery among nurses (Djukic et al., 2019). The continued growth of nursing knowledge optimizes the health and well-being of nurses as well as the individuals and communities they care for (NASEM, 2021).

Concepts That Influence Learning

Learning occurs throughout the lifecycle of a nursing career, underscoring a need to facilitate learning across settings and contexts. There are a variety of attributes and conditions that, when cultivated, can create the ideal conditions necessary for deep learning and lead to sustained changes in knowledge, behaviors, and attitudes. Learner characteristics—motivation, literacy, learning styles, and generational attributes—can all influence the ability to learn. Before any nurse can embrace the responsibility of teaching, they must first understand how these characteristics affect learning.

Deep Versus Surface Learning

The goal of building and reinforcing knowledge is to develop deep learning. Surface learning implies nothing more than rote memorization of content, whereas deep learning enables the critical application of concepts across a variety of contexts (Asikainen & Gijbels, 2017; Nielsen, 2016). This is important whether in the context of a teacher-student exchange in a nursing course or a patient-client education session in a clinical encounter. Developing deep learning requires active engagement in the material through critical thinking and the integration of concepts to enable the transfer of knowledge to new situations (Biwer et al., 2020; Nielsen, 2016).

Motivation

Understanding the link between motivation and learning is crucial to becoming an effective teacher. This is true for nurses embarking on continuing education as well as the patients, colleagues, and community members they will teach throughout their careers. Learners can be motivated extrinsically, like when they want to avoid failing an exam, or intrinsically, such as when discharge home necessitates following a specific care regimen (Takase et al., 2020). Adults will choose to learn based on their intrinsic desires and will learn best when fueled by that motivation rather than responding to orders or threats of failure (Candela, 2020).

To tap into motivation, the educator must articulate the value of what is being taught within the context of the learner's world and then guide the learner through the process of building new knowledge (Wentzle, 2021). Motivational interviewing (MI) is a widely used technique to identify an individual's intrinsic motivation to learn. In the context of helping patients learn, MI can uncover what will prompt a patient to change their behaviors and facilitate engagement in learning. Regardless of the context (nurse to patient, nurse to nurse, or faculty to student), uncovering and tapping into motivation is critical to facilitating learning.

Literacy

There are many facets to literacy within the context of learning. Health literacy is defined as the ability to understand health information needed to make decisions about health behaviors for themselves and others (Institute of Medicine, 2014). Nearly one in five adults in the United States is functionally illiterate (Rampey et al., 2016) and as much as 80% of information learned during a primary care visit is immediately forgotten (MedStar Health Research Institute [MedStar], 2018). Even those individuals with higher levels of literacy can find complex health information difficult to understand (Brach et al., 2012). This has consequences for nurses who are responsible for teaching the skills needed to maintain health, prevent readmissions, and manage complex illnesses at home. Five decades of Healthy People reports (1990 through 2030) explore and address the barriers to population health and well-being. These reports call out health literacy as a foundational principle. Because complex health information can be difficult to understand, clear, accessible communication can improve outcomes, especially for those with impaired health literacy skills (Office of Disease Prevention and Health Promotion, n.d.).

Many techniques have been developed to overcome literacy-related barriers to learning. The National Academy of Medicine has provided a set of recommendations to improve health literacy, including:
- simplifying communications (written and verbal) to ensure universal comprehension.
- involving the target audience in the development and evaluation of health communication tools.
- providing user-friendly electronic sources that are universally easy to access and use.
- verifying comprehension through techniques, including teach-back and show-me (Brach et al., 2012).

Teach-back is used to confirm that intended learning has occurred (Brach & Borsky, 2020; MedStar, 2018). It involves having the learner teach back information, in their own words, so that gaps in knowledge or misinformation can be corrected before the encounter is over. This technique is useful when educating patients, nursing students, and practicing nurses. Teaching back a new skill or concept can confirm the level of health literacy needed to improve outcomes.

Learning Styles

Learning styles refer to the ways that individual learners perceive, interact with, and recall new knowledge (Kitchie, 2019). There are numerous models to characterize learning styles. One of the most recognizable is the VARK model, which describes learner preferences for receiving and sharing information through (**V**)isual, (**A**)uditory, (**R**)eading/writing, and (**K**)inesthetic modalities (Fleming & Mills, 1992). If a learner retains more material when listening to a podcast than when assigned reading from a textbook, this indicates a preference for auditory learning. While the literature does not support the notion that teaching methods should be adjusted to match a learner's identified learning style (Newton & Miah, 2017), it is important to understand how preferences for learning styles should influence education. Preferences for various styles do not mean that learning cannot occur across styles. Rather, the focus should be on varied materials and instructional techniques to engage a wide variety of learners and learning styles (Kitchie, 2019). This has become increasingly important with the growing shift to digital learning, both in online and hybrid learning modalities. Instead of focusing on a learner's preferred style, educators should offer multiple types of instructional materials which can promote engagement with the information (Rice & Ortiz, 2021).

Generational Attributes

There is a large body of literature, dating back more than a century, that has defined generational differences in learners which can be used to guide teaching strategies. It is thought that economic, social, and cultural characteristics experienced during youth will influence the way people learn (Shorey et al., 2021). One generation that receives a significant amount of attention is Millennials. This generation now comprises most learners in the college classroom and they are seen as tech-savvy multitaskers who prefer frequent and instant feedback (Cantrell & Farer, 2019). However, just as with any other attempt to categorize a large cohort of diverse individuals into a single stereotype, generational labels have the potential for bias that misses the individualization and nuance of modern learners (Jauregui et al., 2020). A better strategy is to embrace generational humility that allows for the recognition of how eras in time can influence worldviews and behaviors while also understanding that every learner will have unique preferences that can impact how they should best be taught (Jauregui et al., 2020).

Closing the Learning Gap

Education requires more than understanding the attributes that contribute to learning. Awareness of the factors that cause inequity, both in health and learning, is critical. Factors outside the learning environment can have a significant impact on one's ability to learn. This is true for patients, who may not have the resources necessary to act upon new knowledge. Think of the patient being discharged with a new and complex regimen for managing cardiac health after suffering a myocardial infarction. Proper care requires multiple medications, which cost money, and requires a car to drive to the pharmacy. Lack of resources is also an issue for the student nurse who, after COVID, is expected to attend classes online, requiring a laptop and webcam, broadband internet, and a quiet, dedicated space to virtually attend class. Awareness of these inequities is an obligation for all nurses who must ensure that the knowledge they are sharing can be effectively received by the learner. Education will otherwise fail to lead to changes in behavior, which should be the primary outcome of any learning experience.

Justice, Equity, Diversity, and Inclusion

The interrelated concepts of JEDI have become central to nursing education as important considerations for closing learning gaps. Increasing diversity within nursing, both in practice and education, will help build a future workforce that better reflects the lived experiences of the patients we serve. A resemblance to, and appreciation of, the communities nurses serve will arguably improve understanding of the social and environmental influences on health and will continue to position nurses as advocates for well-being (NASEM, 2021). JEDI plays an important role in ensuring that learners have fair access to education and that learning environments are designed to enable success for all. This begins with a drive toward holistic admission criteria that enables nontraditional students more equitable access to nursing programs. Equity in the admission and education of nurses from diverse communities and backgrounds will lead to a more representative nursing workforce that is better prepared to address JEDI in education, practice, leadership, and policy (AACN, 2017).

THE ART OF TEACHING IN NURSING

Teaching others, whether clients or colleagues, is something that all nurses will do countless times throughout their careers. Sometimes teaching is informal, occurring without a nurse being aware. This can happen when a nurse works alongside a less experienced colleague who is helping on the unit for the day, or when a student nurse observes other nurses responding to a critical event during their clinical rotation. Formal teaching is more overt, often requiring intentional preparation before the teaching takes place. Regardless of whether teaching is delivered formally or informally, it is helpful to understand the theoretical underpinnings that guide how teaching occurs and what is needed for it to be effective. Also important is knowledge of the principles that guide the design, delivery, and evaluation of teaching. A final consideration is the unique application of specific modalities of learning such as classroom or online, clinical or simulation, and, most recently, in the metaverse.

Teaching Theories and Models

Theories are frameworks that help describe specific phenomena of interest. Grand or macro theories are broad and abstract, whereas middle-range theories are more narrowly focused on a specific set of interrelated concepts. Models, also referred to as frameworks or schema, are less formal and structured than theory but are useful for organizing abstract ideas into a format that more easily predicts relationships between concepts (Polit & Beck, 2021). Within the frame of teaching and learning, theories and models can help guide or predict how people best learn in various contexts (Braungart et al., 2019). The following section provides a brief exploration of the many theories that exist, organized within the settings where nurses function in a teaching role. When using this lens, some theories have broad applicability across settings, while others will have singular relevance to a specific audience. (Broader discussion of theories, models, frameworks, and schema can be found in Chapter 5.)

Teaching Students in the Academic Setting

Cognitive and behavioral learning are two main types of learning theories. Cognitive learning theory focuses on the learner and how they build new knowledge (Bandura, 2001). The process is driven by the learner and their internal motivations for learning (Richards, 2019), and should be inclusive of the learner's stage between novice and expert based on Benner's model (Benner, 1982). Theorists such as Piaget (1954), Lewin (1951), Gagné (1974), and Bloom (1956) examined cognition and the ways that learners process information. Behaviorist theory, derived from the classic work of Thorndike (1913), Pavlov (1927), Skinner (1953), and Wolpe and Lazarus (1966), as well as some of Bruner's (1966) earliest writings, focuses on observable behaviors that result from teaching.

By the mid-20th century, a new method of teaching and learning, known as constructivism, appeared in the literature (Bruner, 1966). This method of teaching and learning proposes that learners construct new ideas based on previous knowledge and experiences. Today, many cognitive and behavioral psychologists support this view, which asserts that learners engage or become active in the learning process instead of passively receiving information. In this view, learners actively seek information, problem-solve, collaborate with others, and apply information to authentic problems that reflect real-world complexity (Reiser, 2001). Most cognitive and learning experts believe that active learning is superior to passive learning.

Teaching Students in the Clinical Setting

Learning within a social environment, like those that occur in simulation labs and clinical learning environments, often calls on psychological theories to understand how social interactions influence learning and change behaviors (Hilgard & Bower, 1975). Teaching in the clinical environment is influenced by the dynamic relationships between nurses, students, and patients. Bandura's more recent theoretical work focuses on the social context and how human interactions influence learning (Bandura, 2001). This includes the concept of role modeling, where teachers and peer learners exert influence over learning (Fitzgerald & Keyes, 2019). Vygotsky's (1978) social constructivism theory suggests that learning occurs through the meanings that result from social interactions.

Another important aspect of learning in the clinical environment is psychomotor skills (Anderson & Krathwohl, 2001). Much of the teaching that occurs, both for nurses and their patients, involves the motor skills needed to perform a physical action (Gubrud-Howe, 2020). This could be a nursing student learning to start an IV, a nurse learning to operate a defibrillator, a patient learning to perform self-catheterization, or a family member learning to assist with tracheostomy care. Motor learning, which promotes the capability for a specific set of movements, is guided by many theories (Adams, 1971; Newell, 1991; Schmidt, 1975). Fitts and Posner (1967) explain motor learning as occurring through stages of sequential learning. These stages move from the initial cognitive stage of *knowledge acquisition*, into the *associative stage* of slower but consistent performance, and finally into the *autonomous stage*, where a physical skill is performed consistently with speed and accuracy.

Teaching Online

Theories are an important guide for driving learner engagement when the teacher and learner are distant, as is the case for online learning. Adult Learning Theory, or andragogy, is a common frame for learning in the online classroom since, until the pandemic, remote learning was mostly within the realm of postsecondary education of adult learners. The main assumptions of andragogy are that adult learners are self-directed and intrinsically motivated to learn. They view learning through the lens of their own experiences and approach learning as a way to solve real-life problems or tasks (Kennedy, 2017; Knowles, 1980). Understanding this can help the online educator frame the delivery of online learning.

With the exponential growth in online nursing education in the past decade, Garrison et al. (2000) provided a framework based on their Community of Inquiry model to develop collaborative learning environments when teachers and learners are physically distant and even communicating asynchronously. Designing effective online courses requires an understanding of the learner's stage along the continuum of novice to expert (Benner, 1982) and their cognitive load (Sweller & Chandler, 1991) to intentionally scaffold learning. Many frameworks serve to guide the development of an online course, a discipline known as Instruction Design (ID). Gagné's conceptual model that defines the nine events of instruction (Gagné et al., 1998) serves as a foundation for instructional design (Seel et al., 2017), paving the way for ADDIE (Branson, 1977), Structural Learning Theory (Scandura, 2003), Four-Component Instruction-Design ([4C/ID], Van Merriënboer et al., 2002), and the Backward Design framework (Wiggins & McTighe, 2006). The common theme in each of these models is that successful learning in the online environment requires an intentional and structured design that focuses on learner needs and experiences.

Designing Education

The design, delivery, and evaluation of learning is a process involving several stages. Each stage requires consideration as it must relate to all other stages to achieve the intended effect of the education. This is true whether designing discharge teaching for a newly diagnosed diabetic patient in an acute care unit, or a lesson on diabetes care and management in a nursing program. The main considerations for course design include what you want to teach (*content*), how you plan to teach it (*process*), and what you expect to achieve by teaching it (*outcome*). These elements can be ordered in either forward, central, or backward design (Richards, 2013). While each of these design orders has value, backward design is favored when it is necessary to meet specific outcomes (Wiggins & McTighe, 2006). Such is the case in health care, where patient care and medication regimens must meet specific evidence-based procedures and protocols.

Developing Objectives and Outcomes

Outcomes and objectives form the roadmap that shows both the destination (*outcome*) and route (*objectives*) that comprise the teaching/learning experience. Outcomes are

the characteristics that a learner should demonstrate at the end of a learning period, be it a discharge teaching session, an 8-week unit orientation, or a semester-long nursing course. Objectives, sometimes referred to as competencies or goals, are the specific behaviors that lead toward the outcome (Sullivan, 2020). Objectives should be both measurable and observable statements about what a learner should be doing with the new knowledge delivered to them (Mager, 1962). Bloom's (1956) taxonomy, a categorization of action verbs, is a widely adopted strategy for categorizing behavior domains (cognitive, psychomotor, and affective) into scaffolded levels of increasing complexity requiring higher orders of thinking (Anderson & Krathwohl, 2001). See Bloom's Taxonomy Resources at the end of this chapter to access publicly available lists of Bloom's verbs. Fig. 10.2 shows the learning domains along a continuum of complexity with examples of increasingly complex thinking needed to care for patients using a clinical example of heart failure.

Learning Activities and Assessments

Once the framework of objectives and outcomes has been created, the focus of course design turns to the activities that can be used to both deliver knowledge and evaluate learning. Passive learning, such as reading a textbook chapter and watching videos, leads to the acquisition of information, whereas active learning, such as discussions, simulations, and problem-based learning, involves student engagement with the material (Phillips, 2020). Learning can be accomplished through individual or group activities with learners working together at the same time (*synchronously*) or with each learner participating individually on their own time (*asynchronously*). Finally, these learning activities form the basis for the evaluation of learning. *Formative* evaluation is used to confirm knowledge acquisition during learning and *summative* evaluation confirms that an outcome or objective has been met (Worral, 2019). Consider these concepts together as part of a learning activity designed to teach disaster preparedness to nurses (Fig. 10.3). Learning occurs both individually and with peers, using both passive and active strategies, to deliver foundational knowledge about the role of a nurse during a disaster (*formative*) that will then be used to create a disaster plan at the end of the learning activity (*summative*). In this example, the foundational assessment confirming understanding of nursing roles ensures students can successfully apply that knowledge in the summative presentation.

Alignment and Evaluation of Learning

The alignment of any educational activity speaks to the intentional selection of outcomes, and the associated activities and assessment of learning, to directly influence

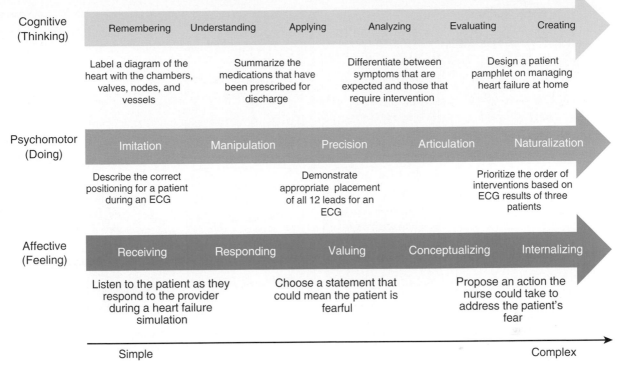

Fig. 10.2 Bloom's Revised Taxonomy. *Note*. The verbs used in Bloom's revised taxonomy are sorted within three domains of learning and ordered from simple to complex. They can be used to construct objectives to ensure increasingly higher-ordered thinking, like the examples shown here.

the skills and abilities of learners beyond the classroom. In this context, alignment means that learning is situated in the real world, leading to improvements in performance outside the classroom and long after learning has occurred (Biggs & Tang, 2011). In a simple example, proper alignment of an outcome for the learner to *demonstrate the proper technique for subcutaneous injection of insulin* would include a final or summative assessment requiring that the learner perform an injection rather than pass a quiz on the pharmacokinetics of short-, medium-, and long-acting insulins. The broader implications of alignment would be to confirm (evaluate) that the learner can perform the injection correctly at home without assistance after being discharged from the hospital.

Evaluation of this alignment confirms that the desired knowledge and skills have been delivered and led to sustained behavior change. A commonly used model for evaluating education is Kirkpatrick's Evaluation Model. Kirkpatrick's (2007) model describes the strategy of measuring *reaction, learning, behavior,* and *results*. *Reaction* is a measurement of the honest impression of learners immediately following the

event. This is commonly done in a postlearning survey. The next two levels are *evaluating learning* and *behaviors.* Learning, such as through a knowledge-based exam, and behaviors, such as measuring performance in the short term after the class has finished, are both important to ensure that the learner gained the knowledge needed to achieve the desired outcomes. The final stage, *evaluating results*, requires a long-term look at the return on investment of the course. These often look at measures beyond the learner, such as organizational and care delivery metrics. Consider the example of a newly developed breastfeeding class developed by a lactation consultant and delivered by all nurses on a postpartum unit. The four levels of evaluation might look like this:

1. Level 1 (*Reaction*): All mothers will complete a learner satisfaction survey immediately at the end of the class.
2. Level 2 (*Learning*): Mothers will be assessed for knowledge of breastfeeding practices during the in-patient consult with the lactation consultant before discharge.
3. Level 3 (*Behavior*): The nurse will observe breastfeeding during the 1-month postdischarge home visit.

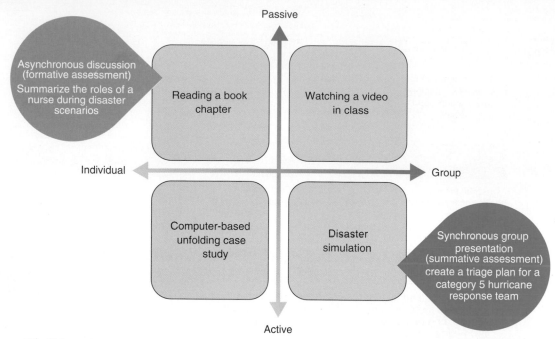

Fig. 10.3 Learner Activities and Assessments. *Note.* Course design requires the selection of learning activities that fit the delivery (active or passive, individual or group) and lead to an assessment of learning during (formative) and at the end (summative) of the activity.

4. Level 4 (*Results*): Metrics will be tracked for all patients 1 year after discharge to determine if breastfeeding rates and duration have changed since the initiation of the new course.

Teaching Modalities

The final consideration for teaching is the modality used for learning. There are enduring concepts that remain unchanged regardless of where education is delivered. Many of these have been discussed earlier in this chapter, including understanding the strategies to promote learning and close learning gaps; identifying characteristics that influence learning; applying the theoretical foundations of teaching and learning; and designing effective educational delivery. Despite this synergy, there are some unique attributes to the various learning modalities that are important to consider.

Classroom (Ground and Online)

Whether teaching face to face, online, or using a combination of both (called hybrid learning), some universal, best-practice strategies drive deep learning. These include:

- delivering information through lectures and supplemental materials, in written, visual, and audio format;

- building knowledge through activities that engage learners, such as seminars and discussions in either synchronous or asynchronous formats;
- applying new knowledge through problem-based learning, either individually or as a team; and
- evaluating knowledge acquisition in the short and long-term (Worral, 2019).

Delivery of education to promote critical thinking requires engagement and interaction between the nurse educator and the learner. There is no escaping the need for learning material (handouts, readings, videos, lectures, podcasts, etc.) as a vehicle to deliver new knowledge. Both ground and online modalities can take advantage of these materials. However, learning activities that promote interaction with these materials are what elevate education from rote memorization to active learning (Phillips, 2020). The goal should be the creation of new knowledge based on peer and faculty interactions that are designed to actively engage in learning, as shown in Fig. 10.4.

Simulation and Clinical Settings

Nursing education necessarily requires opportunities to perform skills in a hands-on, realistic way. These can occur through in-class role-plays and demonstrations, hands-on

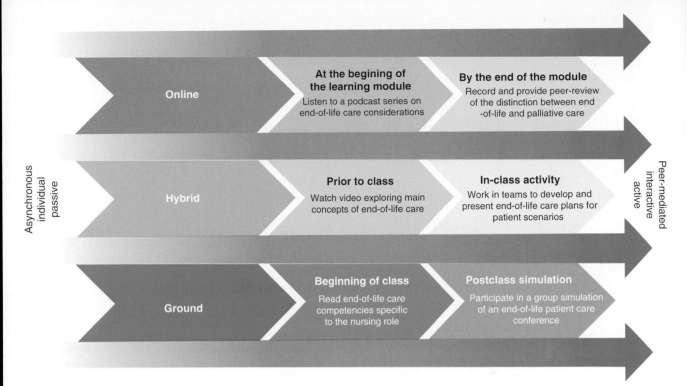

Fig. 10.4 **Learning Activities Across Modalities.** *Note.* The delivery of, and interaction with, knowledge follows a continuum of learning from passive to active. Deep learning, regardless of modality, occurs most readily through meaningful activities that promote engagement with the material, the nurse educator, and peer learners.

lab practice, and scenarios with simulated participants. Role-plays and demonstrations enable the performance of a targeted element of a complex skill, such as demonstrating the proper technique for drawing up injectable medications. They facilitate the safe practice of isolated skills that can then be applied as a step in a broader patient care scenario. Lab practice and simulated patient scenarios enable the practice of more complex skills such as mock codes and full head-to-toe examinations. Simulation offers skill-based learning that promotes critical thinking in a highly controlled setting that is free of risk and fosters the transferability of skills to the real world (Forneris, 2020; Roberts et al., 2019).

Over the past several decades, simulated learning has evolved from a technological game to a validated mainstay for teaching critical thinking and decision-making as a step toward functioning in a live clinical environment (Fitzgerald & Keyes, 2019). Clinical sites have been increasingly difficult to secure over the past decade. But during the pandemic, when clinical learning environments were closed to all students, simulation became the only means of preparing the future health care workforce. The data does show a year-over-year decline in NCLEX-RN pass rates in the years immediately following the pandemic's start (National Council of State Boards of Nursing, n.d.), combined with decreasing confidence in practice readiness for new graduate nurses while clinical sites were closed to students (Powers et al., 2021). While this may indicate that fully simulated nursing education is not optimal, there is broad agreement that simulation is a critical adjunct for students to safely learn a wide range of clinical skills (Aebersold, 2018). High-quality simulation as a supplement to clinical education is now widely accepted, with many state boards of nursing taking a position on the optimal blend of clinical and simulation time for nursing students (Hungerford et al., 2019).

Clinical and practicum experiences offer real-world environments for students to practice and perfect skills and are a requirement for all nursing programs that lead to licensure. The ideal clinical educator is an expert in their field, with an established track record of clinical judgment and skills (Gubrud-Howe, 2020). Preferably, students will have had the opportunity to learn the background knowledge and practice and validate skills in a simulated environment before participating in clinical experiences to mitigate the risk of real-world practice with vulnerable populations (Aebersold, 2018). In addition, nurses functioning in the clinical educator role should have not only clinical expertise but also a solid understanding of teaching and learning principles such as those outlined in this chapter (Bastable & Alt, 2019; Gubrud-Howe, 2020). This is true of nurse educators as well as practicing nurses who are functioning in a preceptor or mentor capacity with learners.

Teaching in the Metaverse

There has been a long history of exploration into alternate realities to gamify learning or replicate in-person education. In the 1990s, platforms like Second Life were used in health professions' education, allowing students to interact in a virtual world with their faculty and peers for problem-based learning and simulation (Sanborn et al., 2019). Since then, there has been an explosion of interest in this concept, paving the way for experimentation with virtual reality (VR), augmented reality (AR), mixed reality (MR), extended reality (XR), and now the metaverse—a space where many of these technologies work together seamlessly to bring real-world experiences to learners wherever they are situated (Yoon, 2021).

While these terms can be used in disparate or interchangeable ways, the overall intent is to enable realistically collaborative learning that overcomes the barriers of time and distance. Learners can interact with these technologies, either alone or with multiple users, through a computer, mobile device, or special platforms such as immersive headsets or holographic glasses (Scavarelli et al., 2020). Virtual education is quickly moving from simple avatars and roughly rendered second worlds into fully immersive and highly realistic virtual environments capable of delivering simulated patient care experiences. It is only a matter of time before every nurse is exposed to one of these technologies at some point in their learning trajectory.

SUMMARY

The exploration of both learning and teaching as foundational elements of the nursing role is an undoubtedly broad topic. This chapter provided a high-level exploration of the concepts and best-practice strategies available to all nurses to better understand what promotes learning, and how best to teach in the nursing role. The primary message in this chapter is that all nurses play a role in learning and teaching across the lifecycle of their careers. They are positioned to influence future generations of nurses, their nursing and interprofessional colleagues, and the patients and communities they serve. Education is so fundamental to nursing that it should not be considered a specialty role for only a few nurses to master. All nurses need to drive teaching and learning as an inextricable part of their role. There is a universal obligation to learn how to effectively design and deliver education across settings, learners, and modalities.

SALIENT POINTS

- The role of the nurse as an educator across the three spheres of influence (three Cs) can have a direct and positive impact on meeting the goals of the Quadruple Aim.
- The nursing scope of practice requires an understanding of teaching and learning principles across settings and audiences.
- A nurse is responsible for understanding and addressing the different learner characteristics that can influence the quality of learning outcomes.
- Deep learning is desirable because it leads to the critical application of concepts across a variety of contexts.
- Adults are motivated to learn based on their intrinsic desires and learn best when fueled by that motivation rather than in response to being told what to do.
- Teach-back, used to confirm that intended learning has occurred, involves having the learner teach back information, in their own words, so that gaps in knowledge or misinformation can be corrected in real time.
- Rather than focusing on a learner's preferred style, educators should offer multiple types of instructional materials to promote engagement with the information.
- Generational humility allows for the recognition of how eras in time can influence worldviews and behaviors while also understanding that every learner will have unique preferences that can impact how they should best be taught.
- The nurse of the future must consider new ways to positively influence JEDI for the learners they will support.
- There is a significant body of theories and models that can be used to guide the nurse educator in their role across settings and audiences.
- Educational design should be accomplished through a methodical design of objectives, outcomes, activities, and assessments, that are aligned and can be evaluated for effectiveness.

- The underlying elements of education (knowledge delivery, application, and assessment) are present across modalities of teaching (online, face-to-face, hybrid).
- Regardless of the format used to deliver education, education should be designed to promote interaction with learning materials to create and expand knowledge.
- Virtual reality (VR), augmented reality (AR), mixed reality (MR), and extended reality (XR) are part of the metaverse, a space where these technologies work together to bring real-world experiences to learners wherever they are situated.
- Simulation is an important and effective modality for teaching clinical skills.

CRITICAL REFLECTION EXERCISES

1. Think about a class you have taken in your current program of study. Reflect on how each of the four concepts that influence the quality of learning—motivation, literacy, learning styles, and generational attributes—can impact learners in this class.
2. Consider that you are tasked with providing discharge teaching to a patient with newly diagnosed heart failure. What inequities and lack of resources could influence their ability to receive and act upon your instructions? How could you address these in your discharge instructions?
3. Reflect on a recent patient care scenario you have experienced or learned about. Provide your rationale for choosing a nursing theory that could help guide your actions as you teach the patient.
4. Write a learning outcome that would be appropriate for a class designed to teach patients how to use an insulin sliding scale (refer to the website resources for help choosing your Bloom's verb). Choose one example of learning material and an assessment that would align with this outcome.
5. Identify a disease process that you have either cared for or learned about that you could teach to a new nursing student. Choose a teaching modality you feel would be best suited to deliver this education. Discuss your rationale for this choice over other modalities.

BLOOM'S TAXONOMY RESOURCES

There is no singularly definitive list of Bloom's verbs. When using Bloom's verbs to develop objectives and outcomes, it is helpful to choose one list and reference the source. Following are a few of many lists that universities have made freely available for use by their faculty.

Arizona State University Office of Evaluation and Educational Effectiveness: https://uoeee.asu.edu/blooms-taxonomy

Azusa Pacific University Revised Bloom's Taxonomy Action Verbs: https://www.apu.edu/live_data/files/333/blooms_taxonomy_action_verbs.pdf

The Ohio State University Sample Bloom's Verbs: https://teaching.resources.osu.edu/examples/sample-blooms-verbs

University of Arkansas Teaching and Innovation Pedagogical Support Bloom's Taxonomy Verb Chart: https://tips.uark.edu/blooms-taxonomy-verb-chart/

University of Pittsburgh Bloom's Taxonomy Verbs: http://www.rstce.pitt.edu/RSTCE_Resources/RSTCE_Res_Doc/BloomsTaxonomyVerbs.pdf

Utica University Bloom's Taxonomy of Measurable Verbs: https://www.utica.edu/academic/Assessment/new/Blooms%20Taxonomy%20-%20Best.pdf

Vanderbilt University Bloom's Taxonomy: https://cft.vanderbilt.edu/guides-sub-pages/blooms-taxonomy/

REFERENCES

Adams, J. A. (1971). A closed-loop theory of motor learning. *Journal of Motor Behavior, 3,* 111–115.

Aebersold, M. (2018). Simulation-based learning: No longer a novelty in undergraduate education. *OJIN: The Online Journal of Issues in Nursing, 23*(2). https://doi.org/10.3912/OJIN.Vol23No02PPT39

Aiken, L. H., Sloane, D., Griffiths, P., Rafferty, A. M., Bruyneel, L., McHugh, M., Maier, C. B., Moreno-Casbas, T., Ball, J. E., Ausserhofer, D., & Sermeus, W. (2017). Nursing skill mix in European hospitals: Cross-sectional study of the association with mortality, patient ratings, and quality of care. *BMJ Quality & Safety, 26,* 559–568. https://doi.org/10.1136/bmjqs-2016-005567

American Association of Colleges of Nursing. (2017). *Diversity, equity, and inclusion in academic nursing [Position statement].* https://www.aacnnursing.org/Portals/42/News/Position-Statements/Diversity-Inclusion.pdf

American Association of Colleges of Nursing. (2019). *The impact of education on nursing practice [Fact sheet].* https://www.aacnnursing.org/Portals/42/News/Factsheets/Education-Impact-Fact-Sheet.pdf

American Association of Colleges of Nursing, American Association of Community Colleges, Association of Community College Trustees, National League for Nursing, & National Organization for Associate Degree Nursing. (2012). *Joint statement on academic progression for nursing students and graduates.* https://www.aacnnursing.org/NewsInformation/Position-Statements-White-Papers/Academic-Progression

Anderson, L. W., & Krathwohl, D. R. (2001). *Taxonomy for learning, teaching, and assessing: A revision of Bloom's Taxonomy of educational objectives.* Longman.

Asikainen, H., & Gijbels, D. (2017). Do students develop towards more deep approaches to learning during studies? A systematic review on the development of students' deep and surface approaches to learning in higher education. *Educational Psychology Review, 29*(2), 205–234. https://doi.org/10.1007/s10648-017-9406-6

Bandura, A. (2001). Social cognitive theory: An agentic perspective. *Annual Review of Psychology, 52,* 1–26. https://doi.org/10.1146/annurev.psych.52.1.1

Bastable, S. B., & Alt, M. F. (2019). Overview of education in health care. In S. B. Bastable (Ed.), *Nurse as educator: Principles of teaching and learning for nursing practice* (4th ed., pp. 3–30). Jones & Bartlett

Benner, P. (1982). From novice to expert. *American Journal of Nursing, 82*(3), 402–407.

Berwick, D. M., Nolan, T. W., & Whittington, J. (2008). The Triple Aim: Care, health, and cost. *Health Affairs (Millwood), 27*(3), 759–769. https://doi.org/10.1377/hlthaff.27.3.759

Biggs, J., & Tang, C. (2011). *Teaching for quality learning at university: What the student does* (4th ed.). Society for Research in Higher Education & Open University Press.

Biwer, F., Egbrink, M. G. A. oude, Aalten, P., & de Bruin, A. B. (2020). Fostering effective learning strategies in higher education: A mixed-methods study. *Journal of Applied Research in Memory and Cognition, 9*(2), 186–203. https://doi.org/10.1016/j.jarmac.2020.03.004

Bloom, B. S. (1956). *Taxonomy of educational objectives: The classification of educational goals* (1st ed.). Longman: Green.

Bodenheimer, T., & Sinsky, C. (2014). From Triple to Quadruple Aim: Care of the patient requires care of the provider. *Annals of Family Medicine, 12*(6), 573–576. https://doi.org/10.1370/afm.1713

Brach, C., & Borsky, A. (2020). How the U.S. Agency for Healthcare Research and Quality promotes health literate health care. *Studies in Health Technology and Informatics, 269,* 313–323. https://doi.org/10.3233/SHTI200046

Brach, C., Keller, D., Hernandez, L. M., Baur, C., Parker, R., Dreyer, B., Schyve, P., Lemerise, A. J., & Schillinger D. (2012). *Ten attributes of health literate health care organizations.* National Academy of Medicine. https://doi.org/10.31478/201206a

Branson, R. K. (1977). *Interservice procedures for instructional systems development: Task V Final Report.* ERIC Clearinghouse.

Braungart, M. M., Braungart, R. G., & Gramet, P. R. (2019). Applying learning theories to healthcare practice. In S. B. Bastable (Ed.), *Nurse as educator: Principles of teaching and learning for nursing practice* (4th ed., pp. 63–110). Jones & Bartlett.

Bruner, J. (1966). *Toward a theory of instruction.* Harvard University.

Candela, L. (2020). Theoretical foundations of teaching and learning. In D. M. Billings & J. A. Halstead (Eds.), *Teaching in nursing: A guide for faculty* (6th ed., pp. 247–269). Elsevier.

Cantrell, M. A., & Farer, D. (2019). Millennial nursing students' experiences in a traditional classroom setting. *The Journal of Nursing Education, 58*(1), 27–32. https://doi.org/10.3928/01484834-20190103-05

Djukic, M., Stimpfel, A.W., & Kovner, C. (2019, March). Bachelor's degree nurse graduates report better quality and safety educational preparedness than associate degree graduates. *Joint Commission Journal on Quality and Patient Safety, 45*(3), 180–186. https://doi.org/10.1016/j.jcjq.2018.08.008

Fitts, P. M., & Posner, M. I. (1967). *Human performance.* Brooks/Cole.

Fitzgerald, K., & Keyes, K. (2019). Instructional methods and settings. In S. B. Bastable (Ed.), *Nurse as educator: Principles of teaching and learning for nursing practice* (4th ed., pp. 469–515). Jones & Bartlett.

Fleming, N. D., & Mills, C. (1992). Not another inventory, rather a catalyst for reflection. *To Improve the Academy, 11*(1), 137–155. https://doi.org/10.1002/j.2334-4822.1992.tb00213.x

Forneris, S. G. (2020). Teaching and learning using simulations. In D. M. Billings & J. A. Halstead (Eds.), *Teaching in nursing: A guide for faculty* (6th ed., pp. 353–373). Elsevier.

Gagné, R. M. (1974). *Essentials of learning for instruction.* Dryden.

Gagné, R. M., Briggs, L. J., & Wager, W. W. (1998). *Principles of instructional design* (3rd ed.). Holt, Rinehart, and Winston.

Garrison, D. R., Anderson, T., & Archer, W. (2000). Critical inquiry in a text-based environment: Computer conferencing in higher education. *The Internet and Higher Education, 2*(2–3), 87–105.

Gubrud-Howe, P. (2020). Teaching in the clinical setting. In D. M. Billings & J. A. Halstead (Eds.), *Teaching in nursing: A guide for faculty* (6th ed., pp. 328–352). Elsevier.

Halstead, J. A. (Ed.). (2018). *NLN core competencies for nurse educators: A decade of influence.* National League for Nursing. https://nln.lww.com/

Hilgard, E. R. & Bower, G. H. (1975). *Theories of learning* (4th ed.). Prentice-Hall.

Hungerford, C., Blanchard, D., Bragg, S., Coates, A., & Kim, T. (2019). An international scoping exercise examining practice experience hours completed by nursing students. *The Journal of Nursing Education, 58*(1), 33–41. https://doi.org/10.3928/01484834-20190103-06

Institute of Medicine. (2014). *Implications of health literacy for public health: Workshop summary.* The National Academies Press. https://doi.org/10.17226/18756

Jauregui, J., Watsjold, B., Welsh, L., Ilgen, J. S., & Robins, L. (2020). Generational "othering": The myth of the Millennial learner. *Medical Education, 54*(1), 60–65. https://doi.org/10.1111/medu.13795

Kennedy, S. (2017). *Designing and teaching online courses in nursing.* Springer. https://doi.org/10.1891/9780826134097

Kirkpatrick, D. (2007). *The four levels of evaluation: Measurement and evaluation* (1st ed.). American Society for Training & Development.

Kitchie, S. (2019). Determinants of learning. In S. B. Bastable (Ed.), *Nurse as educator: Principles of teaching and learning for nursing practice* (4th ed., pp. 113–163). Jones & Bartlett.

Knowles, M. S. (1980). *The modern practice of adult education: From pedagogy to andragogy.* Association Press/Follett.

Lewin, K. (1951). *Field theory in social science.* Harper & Row.

Mager, R. (1962). *Preparing instructional objectives.* Fearon Publishers.

MedStar Health Research Institute. (2018, April). *Guide to improving patient safety in primary care settings by engaging patients and families.* Agency for Healthcare Research and Quality. https://www.ahrq.gov/patient-safety/reports/engage.html

National Academies of Sciences, Engineering, and Medicine. (2016). *A framework for educating health professionals to address the social determinants of health.* The National Academies Press. https://doi.org/10.17226/21923

National Academies of Sciences, Engineering, and Medicine. (2021). *The future of nursing 2020–2030: Charting a path to achieve health equity.* The National Academies Press. https://doi.org/10.17226/25982

National Council of State Boards of Nursing. (n.d.). *NCLEX pass rates.* https://www.ncsbn.org/

Newell, K. M. (1991). Motor skill acquisition. *Annual Review of Psychology, 42*(1), 213–237. https://doi.org/10.1146/annurev.ps.42.020191.001241

Newton, P. M., & Miah, M. (2017). Evidence-based higher education: Is the learning styles "myth" important? *Frontiers in Psychology, 8,* 1–9. https://doi.org/10.3389/fpsyg.2017.00444

Nielsen, A. (2016). Concept-based learning in clinical experiences: Bringing theory to clinical education for deep learning. *The Journal of Nursing Education, 55*(7), 365–371. https://doi.org/10.3928/01484834-20160615-02

Office of Disease Prevention and Health Promotion. (n.d.). *Health communication. Healthy People 2030.* U.S. Department of Health and Human Services. https://health.gov/healthypeople/objectives-and-data/browse-objectives/health-communication

Pavlov, I. (1927). *Conditioned reflexes* (G. V. Anrep, Trans.). Oxford University Press.

Phillips, J. M. (2020). Strategies to promote student engagement and active learning. In D. M. Billings & J. A. Halstead (Eds.), *Teaching in nursing: A guide for faculty* (6th ed., pp. 286–303). Elsevier.

Piaget, J. (1954). *The language and thought of the child* (3rd ed.). Routledge & Kegan Paul.

Polit, D. F., & Beck, C. T. (2021). *Nursing research generating and assessing evidence for nursing practice* (11th ed.). Lippincott, Williams & Wilkins.

Powers, K., Montegrico, J., Pate, K., & Pagel, J. (2021). Nurse faculty perceptions of readiness for practice among new nurses graduating during the pandemic. *Journal of Professional Nursing, 37*(6), 1132–1139. https://doi.org/10.1016/j.profnurs.2021.09.003

Rampey, B. D., Finnegan, R., Goodman, M., Mohadjer, L., Krenzke, T., Hogan, J., & Provasnik, S. (2016). *Skills of U.S. unemployed, young, and older adults in sharper focus: Results from the Program for the International Assessment of Adult Competencies (PIAAC) 2012/2014: First look (NCES 2016-039).*

U.S. Department of Education, National Center for Education Statistics. https://nces.ed.gov/pubs2016/2016039.pdf

Reiser, R. A. (2001). A history of instructional design and technology: Part II: A history of instructional design. *Educational Technology Research and Development, 49*(2), 57–67. https://doi.org/10.1007/BF02504928

Rice, M. F., & Ortiz, K. R. (2021). Evaluating digital instructional materials for K-12 online and blended learning. *Tech Trends, 65*(6), 977–992. https://doi.org/10.1007/s11528-021-00671-z

Richards, J. C. (2013). Curriculum approaches in language teaching: Forward, central, and backward design. *RELC Journal, 44*(1), 5–33. https://doi.org/10.1177/0033688212473293

Richards, E. (2019). Compliance, motivation, and health behaviors of the learner. In S. B. Bastable (Ed.), *Nurse as educator: Principles of teaching and learning for nursing practice* (4th ed., pp. 217–253). Jones & Bartlett.

Roberts, E., Kaak, V., & Rolley, J. (2019). Simulation to replace clinical hours in nursing: A meta-narrative review. *Clinical Simulation in Nursing, 37*(2), 5–13. https://doi.org/10.1016/j.ecns.2019.07.003

Sanborn, H., Cole, J., Kennedy, T., & Saewert, K. J. (2019). Practicing interprofessional communication competencies with health profession learners in a palliative care virtual simulation: A curricular short report. *Journal of Interprofessional Education & Practice, 15,* 48–54. https://doi.org/10.1016/j.xjep.2019.01.010

Scandura, J. M. (2003). *Structural Learning Theory: Current status and new perspectives.* ERIC Clearinghouse.

Scavarelli, A., Arya, A., & Teather, R. J. (2020). Virtual reality and augmented reality in social learning spaces: A literature review. *Virtual Reality: The Journal of the Virtual Reality Society, 25*(1), 257–277. https://doi.org/10.1007/s10055-020-00444-8

Schmidt, R. A. (1975). A schema theory of discrete motor skill learning. *Psychological Review, 82*(4), 225–260. https://doi.org/10.1037/h0076770

Seel, N. M., Lehmann, T., Blumschein, P., & Podolskiy, O. A. (2017). *Instructional design for learning: theoretical foundations.* BRILL. https://doi.org/10.1007/978-94-6300-941-6

Shorey, S., Chan, V., Rajendran, P., & Ang, E. (2021). Learning styles, preferences and needs of generation Z healthcare students: Scoping review. *Nurse Education in Practice, 57,* 1–11. https://doi.org/10.1016/j.nepr.2021.103247

Skinner, B. (1953). *Science and human behavior.* Macmillan.

Sullivan, D. T. (2020). An introduction to curriculum development. In D. M. Billings & J. A. Halstead (Eds.), *Teaching in nursing: A guide for faculty* (6th ed., pp. 103–134). Elsevier.

Sweller, J., & Chandler, P. (1991). Evidence for cognitive load theory. *Cognition and Instruction, 8*(4), 351–362. https://doi.org/10.1207/s1532690xci0804_5

Takase, M., Niitani, M., & Imai, T. (2020). What educators could do to facilitate students' use of a deep approach to learning: A multisite cross-sectional design. *Nurse Education Today, 89,* 1–7. https://doi.org/10.1016/j.nedt.2020.104422

Thorndike, E. (1913). *The psychology of learning.* Teachers College Press.

van Merriënboer, J. J. G., Clark, R. E., & de Croock, M. B. M. (2002). Blueprints for complex learning: The 4C/ID-Model. *Educational Technology Research and Development*, *50*(2), 39–64. https://doi.org/10.1007/BF02504993

Vygotsky, L. S. (1978). *Mind in society: The development of higher psychological processes*. Harvard University Press.

Wentzle, K. R. (2021). *Motivating students to learn* (5th ed.). Routledge. https://doi.org/10.4324/9780429027963

Wiggins, G. P. & McTighe, J. (2006). *Understanding by design* (Expanded 2nd ed.). Pearson Education, Inc.

Wolpe, J., & Lazarus, A. (1966). *Behavior theory techniques: A guide to the treatment of neurosis*. Pergamon Press.

Worral, P. S. (2019). Evaluation in healthcare education. In S. B. Bastable (Ed.), *Nurse as educator: Principles of teaching and learning for nursing practice* (4th ed., pp. 601–636). Jones & Bartlett.

Yoon, H. (2021). Opportunities and challenges of smartglass-assisted interactive telementoring. *Applied System Innovation*, *4*(3), 1–18. https://doi.org/10.3390/asi4030056

11

Legal Aspects of Nursing Practice

Elizabeth E. Friberg, DNP, RN

 http://evolve.elsevier.com/Friberg/bridge/

OBJECTIVES

At the completion of this chapter, the reader will be able to:

- Describe the basic law principles foundational to nursing practice.
- Discuss basic laws that interface with a nurse's employment relationships.
- Differentiate torts of relevance to nursing practice.
- Discuss strategies the nurse can use to reduce legal exposure.

INTRODUCTION

Nurses practice within a framework of legal principles on a daily basis. Legal concepts, expectations, and consequences surround all health care professionals in the United States. To reduce exposure to adverse legal consequences, an informed and safe nurse must be aware of the effect these legal aspects have on nursing practice. Learning the basics of civics education provides a foundation for understanding how societies establish order and settle problems as well as the governmental policy structure of a country. In the United States, this structure is distributed between the federal government and the state and local governing bodies. Formal definitions of legal terms are provided in Box 11.1. A summary of the relationships between the terms as they might relate to nurses and nursing practice is provided later.

Law is the sum of human-made binding or enforceable rules of conduct or action designed to help people maintain order in their society and settle their problems in a nondestructive manner. *Statutory law* is established through the legislative process and expands each time Congress (federal) or state legislatures pass new legislation. *Common law*, also known as *case law*, as opposed to statutory law, is established by previous court decisions and expands each time a judge makes a legal ruling in a case.

The function of law is to create and interpret relationships. *Public law* applies to the public at large and defines and interprets relationships between individuals and the government (public powers, rights, capacities, and duties). The major categories of public law are constitutional law, administrative law, and criminal law. *Private law* defines and interprets the relationship between individuals (private rights, duties, and liabilities). Private law includes contract law and tort law.

These areas of law have an effect on the practice of nursing. *Constitutional law*, embedded in the written text of state and federal constitutions, defines the clients' and nurses' constitutional rights and remedies. *Administrative law*, created by the administrative agencies of federal, state, and local governments, includes the licensing and regulation of nursing practice as well as areas such as collective bargaining. *Criminal law* encompasses the body of rules and statutes that define conduct prohibited by the government, because it threatens and harms public safety and welfare, and establishes imposed punishments for the commission of such acts. Nurses may be involved as a witness; however, criminal law can also involve the nurse as a defendant who is accused of a criminal offense. *Contract law* involves contracts, either written or oral, that identify the common types of employer–employee relationships and determines the risks and protections inherent in each type

BOX 11.1   Legal Terms

Term	Definition
Law	A binding custom or practice of a community; a rule of conduct or action prescribed or formally recognized as binding or enforced by a controlling authority. https://www.merriam-webster.com/dictionary/law
Statutory law	The law that exists in legislatively enacted statutes, especially as distinguished from common law. https://www.merriam-webster.com/legal/statutory%20law
Common law	The body of law developed in England primarily from judicial decisions based on custom or precedent, unwritten in statute or code, and the basis of the English legal system and of the system in all of the United States except Louisiana (Napoleonic or civil code). Merriam-Webster *Case law:* Law established by judicial decisions in cases before the courts. https://www.merriam-webster.com/dictionary/case%20law
Public law	A legislative enactment affecting the public at-large; concerned with the relations of individuals with the government and the organization and conduct of the government itself. https://www.merriam-webster.com/dictionary/public%20law *Constitutional law:* A body of statutory and case law that is based on, concerns, or interprets a constitution. https://www.merriam-webster.com/legal/constitution%20law *Administrative law:* Law dealing with the establishment, duties, and powers of and available remedies against authorized agencies in the executive branch of the government. https://www.merriam-webster.com/dictionary/administrative%20law *Criminal law:* The law of crimes and their punishments. https://www.merriam-webster.com/dictionary/criminal%20law *Case law and civil law feature different burdens of proof.*
Private law	A branch of law concerned with private persons, property, and relationship. https://www.merriam-webster.com/dictionary/private%20law *Contract law:* Concerned with a binding (legally enforceable, agreement between two or more persons or parties). https://www.merriam-webster.com/dictionary/contract#legalDictionary *Tort law:* Concerned with a wrongful act other than a breach of contract for which "relief" may be obtained in the form of damages or an injunction. https://www.merriam-webster.com/dictionary/torts *Civil law:* The body of private law developed from Roman law (Justinian code) and used in Louisiana and in many countries outside the English-speaking world. https://www.merrian-webster.com/dictionary/case%20law *Case law and civil law feature different burdens of proof.*

of relationship. ***Tort law*** is the body of rights, obligations, and remedies that is applied by the courts in civil proceedings to provide relief for persons who have suffered harm from the wrongful acts of others, and it is concerned with the reparation of wrongs or injuries inflicted by one person on another. It defines the legal liability for the practice of nursing and identifies the elements essential for each tort. Criminal law and civil law feature different burdens of proof when one is attempting to persuade the judge or a jury with sufficient evidence. This chapter describes the interaction between law and nursing in three major areas: (1) administrative law, (2) employment law (contract), and (3) civil (or tort) law. This approach provides a basic framework for informed and safe nursing practice.

ADMINISTRATIVE LAW IN NURSING

All states have a "police power" to enact legislation to protect the health, safety, and welfare of their citizens. The power of the state to license nurses and other health care professionals originates in the 10th Amendment (reserved powers) of the U.S. Constitution (Library of Congress, 2021) that allows the states to enact legislation that is not preempted or prohibited by federal law. Each state constitution has a health-and-welfare clause that empowers it to pass such legislation.

Each jurisdiction has a law and related regulations (rules) called the **Nurse Practice Act (NPA)**, which is enforced by each jurisdiction's **Board of Nursing (BON)**. The NPA describes the qualifications for licensure, nursing titles, scope of practice, and actions that can happen if the nurse does not follow the nursing law (National Council of State Boards of Nursing [NCSBN], 2021a).

National professional organizations' guidelines serve as useful references for state jurisdictions and nurses in proposing and implementing state laws. The American Nurses Association (ANA), the American Association of Colleges of Nursing (AACN), the National Organization of Nurse Practitioner Faculties (NONPF), and other professional groups develop definitions and standards of nursing education, practice, and ethics often incorporated into state NPAs.

BONs are jurisdictional government agencies in the 50 states, the District of Columbia, and the four U.S. territories. They are created by the state NPAs. The BONs are responsible for protecting the public's health and welfare through oversight activities. The BONs (1) oversee and ensure the safe practice of nursing through regulations (rules) outlining safe nursing care, (2) issue licenses to practice nursing and monitor license compliance with jurisdictional laws (implementation), and (3) take action on the licenses of nurses who have exhibited unsafe nursing practices (enforcement; NCSBN, 2021a).

Since 1978, all 59 BONs in the United States are members of the **National Council of State Boards of Nursing (NCSBN)**. In 2019, the NCSBN stated (https://www.ncsbn.org/about.htm) that its mission was to empower and support nursing regulators in their mandate to protect the public. The **NCSBN 2020–2030 Strategic Plan** stated four initiatives: (1) promote *agile* regulatory systems for relevance and responsiveness to change, (2) champion regulatory solutions to address *borderless* health care delivery, (3) expand the *active engagement and leadership* potential of all members, and (4) pioneer *competency assessments* to support the future of health care and the advancement of regulatory excellence (https://ncsbn.org/strategic-plan.htm). NCSBN convened the **International Regulator Collaborative (INRC)**, an eight-nation member collaboration to explore standardization and borderless health care delivery. NCSBN also participates in the **Tri-Regulator Collaboration**, which includes the Federation of State Medical Boards (FSMB); the National Association of Boards of Pharmacy (NABP); and the Tri-Council on Nursing, which comprises the AACN, ANA, American Organization of Nurse Executives (AONE), and the National League for Nursing (NLN). The NCSBN also maintains the **National Nursing Database (NURSYS)**, an electronic information system (https://www.nursys.com) that reports active nursing licenses and supports nursing workforce analyses; it is shared by 57 of the 58 U.S. nursing regulatory bodies. The **e-Notify** component of NURSYS allows State Boards of Nursing to update information, employers to verify licensure,

and nurses to manage their nursing licenses. In collaboration with the **National Forum of State Nursing Workforce Centers**, NCSBN conducts the only national-level survey every 2 years focused on the entire nursing workforce, which generates data on the supply of registered nurses (RNs) and licensed practical nurses/licensed vocational nurses (LPNs/LVNs), data that are critical to planning for enough adequately prepared nurses to ensure a safe, diverse, and effective health care delivery system. In addition, the NCSBN supports the **National Council Licensure Examination (NCLEX) Administration**, **NCSBN Learning Extension**, **National Practitioner Data Bank** (a reporting/query discipline agent), and the *Journal of Nursing Regulation*.

For most nurses, licensing is their only direct contact with the BON; however, many find themselves tangentially involved with the board through some level of conflict about the definition of nursing in that state. Even fewer nurses have direct contact with the board's disciplinary unit. A nurse should be aware of the state NPA regulations in ***all*** the jurisdictions in which they practice.

Licensure

Licensure is an exercise of the state's "police power" to grant or revoke a permission (license) to act or practice, which the state legislature uses to protect the health, safety, and welfare of its citizens. Through state licensure statutes, the state controls (1) entry into the profession, (2) the discipline of licensees who fail to comply with minimal standards, and (3) the nursing activities of unlicensed practitioners ("nurse imposters"). Boards are composed largely of the professionals whom they regulate. Nurses themselves, typically with some consumer representation and input, implement the standards of nursing practice because their specialized knowledge best qualifies them to evaluate and oversee nursing practice. This approach ensures that "nursing practice is controlled by the nursing profession with consumer oversight and input."

The most visible function of NPAs is the control over entry of new members into the nursing profession. Entry requirements typically include completion of an approved nursing education program, satisfactory performance on a standardized licensure examination, competency in spoken English, and strong moral character. Laws regulating nursing practice vary from state to state, with each state placing its individual requirements on the profession. All state NPAs, however, are designed to ensure the health and safety of the patients receiving care from nurses. Many issues have been raised related to NPAs and state licensure activities; the following questions are some of those issues. Licensing is supposed to protect the public from incompetence and abuse. Does a blanket license, covering practice over a broad range of specialties, accomplish that purpose?

Do recredentialing tests scrutinize actual competence? Other licensure questions facing the nursing profession include the following: Is licensure too restrictive in its limits on entry into the profession? Do the tests and criteria used actually identify the individuals who are safe and competent nurses, or do they shut out good nurses who are different from a homogenized stereotype? Do licensure requirements protect the public, or do they protect nursing professionals by eliminating competition? Should national licensure for nurses be established so that nurses can easily practice across state boundaries?

Although a national nursing license is not currently available, an interstate mutual recognition model of nurse licensure, also known as the **Nurse Licensure Compact** (NLC), was approved by the NCSBN in 1998. To participate in the NLC, each state legislature must enact the NLC model legislation. The first state to pass the NLC into law was Maryland, in 1999. The NLC allows a nurse who holds a license in the state of legal residency (the state used as residence on the federal tax return) to practice in other states that have enacted the NLC. The NLC is the result of technological advances, including the Internet and the increasing ease of transportation and communication in health care. The goal of the NLC is to ensure public protection and enhance access to safe and competent nursing care for patients who are across state lines from their nurse. The state-based licensure system creates regulation, oversight, and enforcement accountability for the practice of nursing on the basis of the location of the patient. These patients may be receiving services through telenursing, by a traveling nurse, or by a nurse who regularly drives across a state line to get to work. By adopting a uniform NLC model legislation, license portability supports critical access to care. This became a critical issue during the COVID-19 pandemic and allowed for movement of the nursing workforce to address severe shortage events. This portability of health care workforce resources to address surges and shortages is now considered a national security issue. Nurses must have state-based licenses in all of the nonNLC (outside the Compact) states where the nurse may practice. Because the nurse who is practicing with an NLC license is subject to each state's laws, the NLC nurse must be familiar with and comply with the NPA for each state in which he or she works. In 2018, the NCSBN began an initiative to reconstruct licensure mobility in response to a U.S. Department of Health and Human Services (2018) report published in collaboration with the Departments of Treasury and Labor, the Federal Trade Commission, and the White House. The report, *Reforming America's Healthcare System Through Choice and Competition*, addressed scope of practice, worker mobility, and telehealth. The NCSBN established an **Enhanced NLC** (eNLC) that strives to unlock access to nursing care across the nation. As states adopt the enhanced regulatory model, multistate license holders will come under the enhanced framework. As of June 2021, 39 states have passed the eNLC model legislation (https://www.ncsbn.org/nurse-licensure-compact.htm).

In addition, discussions related to a **unique nursing identifier** (**UNI**) to enhance mobility and patient access to care have received increased attention because of the COVID-19 pandemic. The NCSBN responded to that need to identify nurses across educational programs, care settings, and individual state licensures by maintaining an NCSBN unique identifier that is matched exclusively to a nurse and not to a state or organization. This UNI is assigned to each nursing student when they register to take the NCLEX exam. Nurses who took the NCLEX before 1994 have been retroactively assigned a UNI. The NCSBN maintains these identifiers in the NURSYS database, and nurses can look up their UNI by logging into the NURSYS e-Notify database and selecting "As a nurse" to create an account on the site (https://www.nursys.com/EN/ENDefault.aspx). UNIs may be used within electronic health records for documentation, research, education, and training purposes, to bring visibility to nursing's contribution to health delivery and health outcomes.

Because state laws governing advanced practice registered nurses (APRNs) vary more significantly than those governing entry into nursing, setting standards for multistate certification took longer to develop. In September 2008, the NCSBN endorsed a new *Consensus Model for APRN Regulation: Licensure, Accreditation, Certification, and Education*. In 2015, the NCSBN approved an APRN Compact, allowing APRNs to hold a multistate license with a privilege to practice in other compact states. However, until 10 states pass the APRN Compact model legislation, APRNs must continue to obtain APRN certification (a procedure that is in addition to, and separate from, RN licensure) in each state where they are practicing. As of June 2021, only a few states have passed the APRN Compact model legislation (https://www.ncsbn.org/aprn-consensus.htm).

The **National Provider Identification** (**NPI**), implemented in 2004 by the Department of Health and Human Services, is a unique 10-digit number required for providers or organizations that transmit financial transactions electronically to federal and private health programs (direct billing to payers). The NPI is granted through an online process using the National Plan and Provider Enumeration System (NPPES), and a discussion of it is beyond the scope of this chapter because it does not relate to licensure to practice. The NPPES can be accessed at https://nppes.cms.hhs.gov/#/. APRNs who direct bill for services seek an NPI to facilitate payment.

More recent topics are *micro-credentials,* which are earned by demonstrating competency in a specific practice area, and *badges,* which are a simple visual representation of that credential to display as part of your personal digital file or put on your curriculum vitae or resume to showcase your talents and accomplishments. The accrual of micro-credentials and badges speaks to the lifelong learning required of nurses in practice. This is an area to watch as it evolves because it speaks to the assurance of ongoing competency in the profession.

Control Over Practice

The *power to control entry into the profession* and the *power to take disciplinary action on the license of practitioners* were developed to assure the public of safe, qualified practitioners. An indirect result of those powers is that the state nursing boards have some ability to exert control over the nursing market. Licensure grants a privileged place in the occupational hierarchy, but it is a position challenged both by the public and by other professionals who fear the surrender of power. Nurses also control the quality and standards of nursing care in the state through the disciplinary process of nurses in the NPAs. Thus, as in many other professions, NPAs leave public consumers of nursing care dependent, to a large degree, on members of the profession to control access to nursing services and to maintain the quality of nursing care. The result is that nurses have the duty to advocate for patients, at the point-of-care and before the licensing board, and for high-quality care from competent licensed practitioners. The ability of nurses to meet this great responsibility is sometimes challenged by members of the public who fear competing professional incentives. Some have also argued this is too much power to give any profession because professionals may be reluctant to discipline their own colleagues.

This power is also challenged by other professionals, from physicians to wound care specialists and lay midwives, who are afraid nursing's scope of practice will compete with their own professional and financial incentives. NPAs permit nurses to function under a broad definition of nursing while restricting the practice of nonnursing personnel who might otherwise deliver many services provided by nurses.

Enforcement of the prohibition against the unauthorized practice of nursing is exemplified by the practice of lay midwifery. Some states define *midwifery* as an advanced practice area within nursing and prohibit the practice of midwifery by nonnurses. Some nursing boards have administrative fining powers for unlicensed practitioners, which they can impose on lay midwives. These powers are invoked regardless of client satisfaction and often in spite of public protest. Nursing boards argue that a threat to the public safety and welfare is inherent whenever unlicensed practice

occurs, regardless of the specific situation. Similar policies and procedures have prevented nursing from taking over functions that have been absorbed into medical specialties. The jurisdiction of the nursing board may overlap with other professions that perform some of the same functions as nursing. Several issues have arisen related to the restrictive nature of licensing laws and raise some of the following questions. Is licensing too restrictive, or is licensing too permissive by granting blanket licenses? Does licensure today permit nurses to practice beyond their actual competence? No individual nurse can competently perform all the services nurses are licensed to deliver. Although most nurses practice in only a limited field (e.g., surgery, obstetrics, oncology), a nursing license permits a nurse to practice in all areas of nursing. In addition, after initial licensure, many states require little or no demonstration of continuing competency to practice. Although some states have moved in the direction of mandatory continuing education for licensure, others question the validity of continuing professional education to maintain clinical competence. Some jurisdictions are considering models that use simulation or other measures to ensure the ongoing safety and protection of the public. These are issues to watch.

Delegation in Nursing Practice

Most state NPAs authorize RN to delegate, or assign, certain nursing care tasks to a nonnurse, although the nursing process itself cannot be delegated. Some nurses, knowing they are accountable for the care they delegate to their nursing assistants and other nursing extenders, are fearful of delegation. However, nurses who delegate reasonably and responsibly do not need to fear the task of delegating. In early 2015, the NCSBN convened two panels of experts to develop national guidelines to facilitate and standardize the nursing delegation process across the various levels of nursing licensure, which they did, building on the previous work done by the NCSBN and the ANA regarding delegation in 2006. Delegation is a multifaceted process that begins at the administrative level with the employer and nurse leader and involves the licensed nurse and the delegate; all parties have specific responsibilities. The *Delegation Model* and *National Guidelines for Nursing Delegation*, as well as the associated literature review to support the guidelines, can be found on the NCSBN website (https://ncsbn.org/1625.htm). Because each state has its own NPA, it is the responsibility of all licensed nurses to know what is permitted in their own NPA and the rules, regulations, and policies (NCSBN, 2021b).

Disciplinary and Administrative Procedures

A BON usually has both regulatory and adjudicatory power. The *regulatory power* authorizes the board to develop rules and regulations for nursing licensure, nursing education, and nursing practice. The ***adjudicatory power*** authorizes the board to investigate, hear, and decide the outcomes of complaints that involve violations of the NPA and of the rules and regulations promulgated by the board. As mandated by the NPA, the board must ensure that a licensed nurse continues to practice within the standard of care, behaves professionally and ethically, and obeys all relevant state laws. The NPA contains or incorporates a number of grounds to achieve this. ***Disciplinary actions*** are noted on the license of the nurse, and that license may be suspended or revoked by the nursing board.

It is important to understand that the responsibility of state boards is to protect the current and future safety of the public. Their delegated powers are to protect the public from unfit nurses, not to punish bad nurses. Boards can only limit or deny a nursing license. They cannot incarcerate a nurse, and they cannot require a nurse to compensate a patient for damages—financial or otherwise. Most board actions cannot be used in a lawsuit against a nurse. If an injured patient does seek monetary damages, he or she must file a civil lawsuit against the nurse. If an individual thinks a nurse has acted criminally, that person must contact the office of the state attorney.

A **professional license** is property protected by the U.S. Constitution. This means it cannot be limited or taken away without due process. Each state has an **Administrative Procedure Act** that guides the procedures within state agencies to guarantee this due-process right. Each state agency has its own regulations that describe how the agency implements the law. These regulations can vary greatly from state to state and even among professional boards within a state. A BON in one state may hear all arguments concerning nursing issues. The board in a neighboring state may delegate this action to an administrative law judge or a hearing officer. Within a state, a BON may hear its own cases, whereas another professional board in the same state may have its cases heard by an outside hearing officer.

Due process requires the right to be heard, and it requires notice. A licensed nurse has a duty to be aware of the state's NPA. The NPA is considered notice to nurses in that state about the grounds for which they may lose their license to practice. Further notice comes when a nurse receives a charging document. This paper advises the nurse that the board has probable cause to believe the nurse is violating the NPA. It has to be specific enough to give the nurse notice about what a feasible defense could be and about the time and place of the hearing.

Due process further requires that a nurse be afforded the right to appeal any decision made by the board that seems improper. This appeal is usually made to the state civil courts. An appeal is typically limited to procedural issues, such as whether the board had a right to hear the case or whether the board gave the nurse proper due-process rights.

Although all NPAs have commonalities, each state has its own unique legislation. Nurses who move from one state to another or practices in multiple states through the NLC should obtain a copy of each state's NPA. The differences in state NPAs can be significant. For example, one state may impose no legal duty on a nurse to report the incompetence of a physician. In the next state, the nurse may find that failure to report such a physician can result in the loss of the nurse's license. Nurses need to be familiar with the requirements of the local NPA for licensure, the boundaries and definitions of practice, the areas for discipline on practice, and the procedures in place to protect the nurse in case the board challenges the license.

The Americans With Disabilities Act

In 1990, the federal government enacted the **Americans With Disabilities Act (ADA)**, which was revised in 2010 and again in 2016, adding Titles II and III, respectively. The ADA prohibits discrimination based on disability in employment. It also prohibits disability-related discrimination by state and local governments, by private companies, and by commercial facilities. This is a federal law and, like the constitutional right to due process, it applies to all state boards. Current information and the entire text of the ADA and its requirements can be found online at the website of the U.S. Department of Justice, Civil Rights Division (https://www.ada.gov/2010_regs.htm).

Substance abuse disorder is recognized by the NCSBN as a chronic and progressive disease that encompasses a pattern of behavior ranging from misuse to dependence or addiction (NCSBN, 2021c). This disease creates significant legal and ethical responsibilities for colleagues. Nurses have the same prevalence of this disorder as the general public but are at higher risk for developing it because of their relatively easy access to controlled substances in the workplace and the high-stress nature of nursing roles. Nurse managers and nurse colleagues need to be aware of the warning signs of potential substance abuse, act to identify and report the problem, and take the necessary action to obtain appropriate referral and treatment for the nurse in a transparent and supportive manner. The sooner this is done, the sooner patients are protected and the better the chance is that the nurse can return to work safely. Substance abuse is treatable, and long-term recovery is possible. The NCSBN maintains a suite of online resources to support nurses' knowledge about the problem; guidance on identification, reporting, investigation, intervention, and treatment; alternatives to disciplinary programs;

recovery; and return to practice. These resources can be found on the NCSBN website (https://ncsbn.org/substance-use-disorder.htm).

The ADA also requires professional boards to make any special arrangements necessary to facilitate nurses' access to practice. Examples are special communication services for people with sensory impairments and reasonable accommodations at the entrance to the site for licensure examinations or disciplinary hearings.

NURSING AND EMPLOYMENT LAW

Most nurses work as employees rather than as employers or independent contractors. Nurse employees deal daily with the tension of being professionally independent and responsible for their actions in practice while simultaneously being constrained by the standards and requirements of their employer. Nurses may also work under independent contracts for per diem work or under travel nursing arrangements. Nurses need to be aware of the arrangements under which they are employed. At some point, every nurse will be faced with making a decision about accepting a work assignment. Similarly, nurses are likely to be faced with decisions about delegation of nursing functions to unlicensed assistive personnel. These practice challenges raise several considerations for licensed nurses. How can nurses' voices be heard and valued in creating work environments that promote the delivery of high-quality care? What avenues of redress do nurses have if they experience employee and/or management problems, such as hospital downsizing or cross-training of nonprofessionals to carry out nursing functions under their supervision? How can nurses tell, for bargaining purposes, whether they are employees or part of management?

Contract Law

Nurses who are employed work under some form of contract. A **contract** is a promissory agreement between two or more parties that creates (or modifies or destroys) a legal relationship (Bix, 2012). A contract can be in writing, or it can be in spoken language with specific terms, in which case it is called an **express contract.** A contract also can be solely on the basis of the conduct of the parties. These contracts are referred to as **implied contracts.**

An enforceable contract must first be for the performance of legal goods or services. A nurse cannot contract to practice medicine. Second, the parties must have legal capability to agree to the contract. For example, they must all have the mental ability to understand their actions and must be old enough to make a legal agreement. Third, all parties at the time of the contract must agree to do something, and they must agree on what that something is.

Finally, there must be *consideration* (i.e., some kind of trade in which each party gets something from the contract). In a typical nurse employment situation the employer receives nursing services, and the employee receives financial reimbursement.

All states have a statute of frauds that limits the enforcement of some contracts that are not written. These vary and are usually not significant to a nurse employee situation. However, a nurse who wants to prove the specific terms of a contract will obviously have difficulty with an oral contract. Of more significance is the state *parole evidence rule*, which provides that if oral agreements are made that differ from the written contract, the courts will not allow them to add to or change the written contract. Overcoming a written contract can be difficult for nurses, although it can be done—for example, by showing fraud or duress by the employer. When a nurse agrees to an employment position, he or she should be familiar with the employment contract, obtain it in writing, and not rely on oral agreements that are not part of the written contract. What about the role of the contract when the nurse is being terminated from employment or wants to leave employment? A contract can be legally terminated when it has been completely performed, its terms have been met, both parties agree to a change, it becomes impossible (e.g., through the death of a party or the destruction of the subject matter), or both parties agree to annul the contract. A contract can also be terminated by a *breach*, which means one of the parties fails to meet the terms of the agreement. When that happens, the other party can sue in civil court for any damages. For instance, an employee could sue for lost wages, and an employer could sue for lost profits. The **Fair Labor Standards Act of 1938 (FLSA)** sets standards for overtime pay, minimum wage, family and medical leave, child labor, and workers' compensation. The U.S. Department of Labor provides a detailed description and up-to-date information on the provisions of the FLSA online (https://www.dol.gov/agencies/whd/compliance-assistance/toolkits/flsa). A nurse employee in a private setting could also file a grievance with the National Labor Relations Board (NLRB). Of utmost importance for nurses to understand is that most employment contracts are not individual contracts but are *at will*. The following section clarifies this concept.

Employment at Will

Employment at will means the employee has the right to quit employment at any time for any reason, or "at will." The employer has the parallel right to terminate the employee at any time for any reason, also "at will." The law of employment at will considers the employee and employer to have equal power, an assumption that nurse employees know does not reflect employee–employer realities. For this reason, it is a harsh legal doctrine. An example is an employee who is terminated for reasons that are against the public good, such as for joining a union or serving on a jury. Courts have found ways to restrict this doctrine, but they are limited to public policy, implied contract, and good faith. Employees terminated against an implied contract are those who can show that this contract included hospital procedural manuals and personnel handbooks, an employer's conduct or policy, or (rarely) oral promises. An informed nurse employee must be familiar with such manuals and handbooks, document any oral promises, and get them in writing as soon as possible. What else can nurses do to enhance their protection as employees?

Labor Law

Collective bargaining by nurses is an evolving activity. In 1974 Congress extended coverage of the **National Labor Relations Act (NLRA)** to apply to workers in certain health care organizations. According to the American Federation of Labor and Congress of Industrial Organizations (AFL-CIO), in 2014, 17% of RNs were union members. This means they had formed a collective bargaining unit and could bargain with the employer as a group, in good faith, to make an agreement regarding similar interests in wages, hours, and working conditions. Collective bargaining agreements contain grievance procedures guaranteed to all employees. Furthermore, they usually contain a clause protecting the nurse employee from discharge except for "good cause." Nurses who work in a unionized facility cannot bargain individually with the employer. Because the NLRA is federal law, its protections apply in all states.

Only nurses who are employees can participate in collective bargaining with the union. The NLRA defines "employee," "supervisor," and "professional employee" and their ability to participate in collective bargaining. Nurses should understand how the NLRA applies to their specific employment position. As a result, every nurse should ask whether supervision of other employees might be interpreted as "management," thereby depriving the nurse of the right to collective bargaining and its protections.

Compliance Programs

Nurses are often employees of health care organizations, which have to comply with multiple state and federal laws and programs. A compliance office is responsible for developing and implementing related policies and procedures. The purpose of the **compliance program** is to promote conformity with legal requirements in the institution by identifying potential concerns and correcting and preventing the recurrence of any identified problems. Compliance programs should include a confidential disclosure program,

such as a toll-free telephone line, that allows employees to report suspected violations of federal or state health care program requirements or of the company's policies and procedures to the compliance officer. Nurses should be able to make these reports anonymously and be protected from retaliation or any other adverse action for making a report in good faith. Nurses should become familiar with their employer's written standards of conduct and compliance program. Nurse employees typically receive annual training that covers health care compliance policies, procedures, and related legal requirements.

Government Employees

The NLRA applies only to privately employed nurses. Federal employees, such as nurses who work for the Veterans Administration, are covered under the **Civil Service Reform Act of 1978**. The employment rights of state employees are governed by each state's public employee statutes.

TORT LAW IN NURSING

Another area of the legal system of particular importance to nurses is that of tort law. **Torts** are private or civil wrongs, in contrast to crimes, which are wrongs committed against the state (Goldberg et al., 2012; Schwartz et al., 2010). The plaintiff, or person filing the lawsuit, files a tort action to recover damages for personal injury or property damage occurring from negligent conduct or unintentional misconduct (Schwartz et al., 2010). **Unintentional torts** are those in which persons incur harm or injury as a consequence of an unintended, wrongful act by another person. **Negligence** and the related legal concept of **malpractice** are examples of unintentional torts (Goldberg et al., 2012; Schwartz et al., 2010). Several types of torts are often encountered in legal actions against nurses. These include negligence, assault, battery, false imprisonment, lack of informed consent, and breach of confidentiality. A brief discussion of each of these types of torts follows.

Negligence and Malpractice

Negligence occurs when a person fails to act in a reasonable manner under a given set of circumstances (Schwartz et al., 2010). For example, if a person drinks excessively at a party, drives down the highway, and injures another motorist, the injured motorist could file a tort suit for negligence. Driving a car under the influence of alcohol or drugs is not considered reasonable conduct. Consequently, in addition to possible criminal action by the state where the accident happened, a negligence lawsuit probably also would result.

Unreasonable conduct by a nurse or other professional is a specific type of negligence, one referred to as **malpractice**.

The nurse has the legal duty to provide the patient with a reasonable standard of care. This is usually described as "what the reasonably prudent nurse would do under the same or similar circumstances." In malpractice cases, the issue is whether the conduct of the nurse is below the standard established by law for the protection of others or whether the care given by the nurse involves an unreasonable risk for causing damage to another (Goldberg et al., 2012; Schwartz et al., 2010). The courts usually, on the basis of long-established legal precedent, place the responsibility of establishing that the nurse acted wrongly on the injured patient. The nurse is initially assumed to be innocent of the malpractice charge. Consequently, the plaintiff patient has the responsibility of proving that the nurse's conduct was unreasonable. In some cases, the nurse is able to resolve the patient's charges out of court, through an alternative dispute resolution (ADR) strategy (Philipsen, 2008). To successfully negotiate a settlement or defend in court, the nurse responds to a patient complainant or plaintiff who must provide evidence related to four elements:

1. *Duty*. A duty is a legal obligation toward the patient (Schwartz et al., 2010). A nurse's signature in the patient's medical record may be enough to prove that the nurse had a duty to the patient. For purposes of establishing the element of duty in a malpractice case against a nurse, the question is, "Did the nurse have a legal obligation toward this patient?"

2. *Breach of duty*. This element of negligence and malpractice considers whether the nurse's conduct violated the duty to the patient (Schwartz et al., 2010). To determine whether a breach of duty occurred, the plaintiff must show that the nurse's conduct did not comply with reasonable standards of care rendered by an average, like-specialty provider under similar circumstances (Schwartz et al., 2010). A number of methods are used to determine whether the nurse's care was reasonable. Expert witness testimony, nursing textbooks, professional journals, standards developed by professional organizations, institutional procedures and protocols, and equipment guidelines developed by manufacturers can all be used to decide whether the nurse's care complied with reasonable care (Glannon, 2010; Guido, 2013; Schwartz et al., 2010). Use of careful documentation techniques, such as those specified in the documentation guidelines of their institutions, or generic sources, such as regulatory agencies or professional organizations, provides documented evidence that the nurse's conduct complied with reasonable standards of care.

3. *Causation*. This element addresses two issues: whether the nurse's action or inaction caused the patient's injury and whether the patient's injury was foreseeable (Glannon, 2010; Guido, 2013; Schwartz et al., 2010). To determine whether the nurse's action or inaction caused the injury to the patient, lawyers frequently use the "but for" test (Schwartz et al., 2010), which asks, "But for the acts or inaction of the nurse, would the injury to the patient still have occurred?" The second part of the causation element looks at whether the nurse could have reasonably anticipated that his or her conduct might lead to patient harm (Guido, 2013).

4. *Damages*. For a patient to recover damages from a nurse in a malpractice suit, he or she must have suffered some type of damage (i.e., injury, harm). For example, if the nurse gave the patient the wrong medication, but the patient did not experience any adverse effects, the damage element would be missing and the malpractice suit would be unsuccessful.

Assault and Battery

The common law has long recognized the right to be free from offensive touching or even the threat of offensive touching. An *assault* is a deliberate act in which one person threatens to harm another person without his or her consent and has the ability to carry out the threat (Schwartz et al., 2010). A *battery* is a nonconsensual touching, even if the touching may be of benefit to the patient (Schwartz et al., 2010). For example, a lawsuit for assault could result when a nurse threatens to medicate a competent person against his or her will. Battery would occur when the nurse actually administers the medication to the unwilling patient.

In some circumstances, such as restraint situations, the law allows providers to touch patients without their consent. However, special circumstances and procedural safeguards must be adhered to so as to excuse the battery. Courts first look at whether the battery was needed to protect the patient, health care team members, or the property of others (e.g., a patient threatens to set a fire in an emergency department). Next, courts examine whether restraining the patient was the least intrusive method to control the patient. For example, could the patient have been placed in a quiet room rather than being placed in a restraint? Finally, courts typically inquire whether the health care team regularly reassessed the need to continue using the restraint. If the health care team can demonstrate that it has complied with these requirements and with institutional procedure, nonconsensual touching will be excused. Consequently, nurses need to be sure they provide detailed documentation to indicate that (1) the patient was a threat to self, others, or the property of others; (2) the restraint was the least intrusive means of controlling the patient; (3) regular reassessment of the need to continue the restraint occurred; and (4) the restraint was discontinued as soon as possible. Many hospitals and clinical facilities have specific procedures and protocols dealing with the application of restraints. Every nurse needs to be familiar with applicable agency policies.

Informed Consent

Informed consent lawsuits focus on whether the patient was given enough information before a treatment to make an informed, intelligent decision, including the decision to refuse treatment. The legal mandate for informed consent in the United States is unambiguous and overwhelming. It is based on the 14th Amendment, the constitutional right to privacy and self-determination and the liberty interest, on the First Amendment's constitutional Free Exercise Clause, and on state and federal legislation, as well as on common law. Informed consent requires that the patient receive adequate information concerning the nature of the proposed treatment and its purposes, the material risks and benefits of the proposed treatment and of doing nothing (based on best evidence, and including discomfort), and the choice to refuse or accept (Farmer & Lundy, 2017). In other words, did the patient get enough information so that he or she was the ultimate decision maker regarding whether to pursue or abandon the proposed treatment?

Consent may be expressed or implied. *Express consent* is given in spoken or written direct words. *Implied consent* is inferred from the patient's conduct. Even if the patient does not sign a consent form expressly consenting to a proposed treatment or procedure, courts sometimes find that the patient gave implied consent to the treatment or procedure by coming to the health care facility and submitting to the treatment or procedure. For example, coming to an emergency department implies the patient is seeking emergency treatment, or holding out an arm to receive a vaccination implies consent to the vaccination. In most circumstances, express written consent is the standard.

The patient may accept or refuse any treatment, even lifesaving procedures. Nearly all states today treat the failure to provide the necessary information so a patient can make an informed decision regarding the risks and benefits of care as negligence under the informed consent doctrine. In other states, the plaintiff files a battery action, alleging that the failure to give adequate treatment information constituted nonconsensual touching. The right to informed consent and informed refusal was affirmed at the federal level by the Patient Self-Determination Act of 1991.

Recognized exceptions to the doctrine of informed consent exist. If a patient was admitted to an emergency department with a severe, hemorrhaging abdominal injury that required the immediate removal of his spleen, this would be considered an *emergency exception* to the mandate to provide the usual explanation of the splenectomy and obtain informed decisions about care from the patient. Some courts have allowed a provider to avoid full disclosure to a patient if disclosure of information might lead to further harm to the patient. This exception is known as *therapeutic privilege*. For example, if the provider thought a psychiatric patient's knowledge of terminal cancer would lead the patient to commit suicide, the provider might exert therapeutic privilege and not reveal the cancer to the patient.

Consent must be obtained from the patient or the patient's legal representative. In any exception, the practitioner must seek the best possible substitute for informed consent by the patient. In emergencies, implied consent permits the caregiver to save a life but does not waive the patient's right to informed consent as expeditiously as practical. Patients who are unconscious, incompetent, or minors are unable to provide their own informed consent. The caregiver must locate the person with (1) the patient's power of attorney for health care, (2) the next of kin designated by state law, or (3) the court-appointed guardian who has the power to make decisions for the patient, in that order. Parents are generally responsible for making the health care decisions for their minor children, unless the parents are not acting in the child's best interest. The caregiver must inform the patient, the patient's guardian, or the patient's surrogate for health care decisions of the patient's care options and must obtain consent for treatment. A true exception is court-ordered care, for example, drug treatment or psychiatric care ordered during sentencing by a criminal court. When in doubt, the nurse should consult with the facility's attorney.

Responsibility for the consent procedure typically rests in the hands of the practitioner who will be performing the treatment, which frequently is a physician, with the nurse serving as a witness. When the nurse signs the witness portion of the consent form, he or she is attesting that the signature on the consent form is the patient's signature. If the nurse witnesses the physician giving the pertinent information regarding the treatment or procedure, the nurse may want to write "consent procedure witnessed" below his or her signature. If a lawsuit later develops concerning whether the provider gave the patient information concerning the procedure or treatment, the "consent procedure witnessed" statement can furnish powerful evidence that the patient did receive adequate information. Today's APRNs often perform procedures and treatments that require consent, such as suturing, obstetrical care, and administration of medications. In these circumstances, the APRN is the practitioner who must ensure the patient has enough information to make an informed decision regarding a proposed treatment.

False Imprisonment

False imprisonment occurs when a person is unlawfully confined within a fixed area. The confined person must be aware of the confinement or be harmed as a result of the confinement. To prevail in a false imprisonment action, the patient must prove that he or she was physically restrained or restrained by threat or intimidation and that he or she did not consent to the restraint (Schwartz et al., 2010). False imprisonment suits may involve situations in which a patient was kept in a mental health facility against his or her will and without a judicial order, or a restraint device was applied to a patient against his or her will.

The laws on false imprisonment vary from state to state. Most states allow some degree of patient confinement if the patient poses a serious threat of harm to self, others, or the property of others. In deciding whether a valid confinement occurred, judges and juries often look at the reasonableness of the decision to confine the patient, how long the patient was confined, whether the need for the confinement was regularly reassessed, and whether the least restrictive methods for detention of the patient were used.

Breach of Confidentiality

Confidentiality is the duty of health care providers to protect the secrecy of a patient's information, no matter how it is obtained (Murray et al., 2011). Until recently, patients had few legal remedies when the privacy of their medical records was breached. Today, state and federal laws provide patients with legal remedies to compensate them for confidentiality breaches.

One such law is the **Health Insurance Portability and Accountability Act (HIPAA;** PL 104-191; 42 U.S.C. §§1320d et seq.), which was enacted by Congress in 1996, along with the regulations issued under HIPAA governing the privacy of personal health information (the Privacy Rule, at 45 C.F.R. §§160 and 164) and the security of such information (the Security Rule, at 45 C.F.R. §164.302 et seq.), which set a minimum standard governing uses and disclosure of this information. This legislation also protects individuals from losing their health insurance when leaving or changing jobs (portability), and it increases the government's authority over health care fraud and abuse (accountability). HIPAA established that although the health care practitioner who created a health record owns that record, the information that it contains belongs to the patient. The HIPAA Privacy Rule prohibits the release of *identifiable personal health information* (*PHI*) in any form without the patient's permission. Penalties for failure to comply with the Privacy Rule involve a substantial fine and/or prison term for those who use individual health information for commercial or personal gain or to inflict harm. The Security Rule provides two standards to ensure the authenticity of electronic patient records: the Integrity Standard and the Person or Entity Authentication Standard (45 C.F.R. §§164.31). As the electronic medical record becomes commonplace and new patient privacy issues surface, nurses should expect that additional regulations will be promulgated under HIPAA.

The **ANA Position Statement on Privacy and Confidentiality** addresses issues related to computerized medical databases, telehealth, social media, genetic information, and other Internet-based technologies (American Nurses Association, 2015). The position statement establishes the role of the nurse in protecting privacy and confidentiality and provides recommendations to avoid a breach. The relationship to internal scope and standards of practice, code of ethics, and other ANA essential documents, as well as relevant federal regulations, is provided.

A strict level of confidentiality typically exists for patients receiving drug or alcohol abuse treatment. Providers are usually prohibited from even disclosing information on whether a certain person is a patient. In addition, the state where a nurse is practicing may have laws that identify who has authority to control access to the medical records of patients who are incapacitated, incompetent, minors, or deceased. Information concerning special situations is available through the office of the state's attorney general and through the employer's legal counsel.

The use of social media by nurses raises additional issues related to privacy and confidentiality. Although nurses are welcome to use social media in their personal lives or use electronic media to share workplace experiences, in particular those that are challenging or emotionally charged, nurses must not mention patient names or use any other information that might identify patients or the institution. The NCSBN (2021d) provided guidance on the use of social media by nurses in the workplace and the potential consequences of inappropriate use. Vigilance in self-regulating the use of blogs, online chat rooms, and other online communication forums must balance professional responsibility with freedom of expression … be wise. Issues related to privacy and confidentiality are also addressed in Chapter 12: Ethical Dimensions of Nursing and Health Care.

Disaster/Emergency Nursing

Nurses who respond to disaster are typically volunteer nurses, working either through a recognized nonprofit organization, such as the American Red Cross, or through a government agency. As long as the volunteer nurse acts in good faith and within his or her scope of practice, he or she is protected from tort actions. Special provisions in most NPAs permit practice across state borders for emergencies. *Good Samaritan Acts,* which were designed to encourage individuals to volunteer to help in emergencies, also protect volunteer nurses. In addition, special tort laws protect nurses who may be working as disaster volunteers under the coordination of a state or federal government agency, in the same way employees of that agency are protected

(Howie et al., 2012). As discussed earlier in this chapter, during the COVID-19 pandemic, the NCSBN provided access to state-level emergency actions that allowed nurses to return to practice or have license mobility to respond to the need for workforce supplementation for surge events.

CRIMINALIZATION OF UNINTENTIONAL ERROR

In rare cases, officials of the local criminal courts have charged health care providers criminally for patient deaths that resulted from unintentional error. This is an extreme example of a common response to error: to punish the individual who made the error. Errors are seldom due to one individual failure, and that reaction is unlikely to make the system safer. In addition, one element of a crime is that it must include the *intent to do wrong*. Carelessness is not a crime, unless the individual was so reckless as to show intentional disregard for others, as in the case of drunk driving or waving a loaded handgun. All nurses make mistakes, but mistakes do not create criminal intent, regardless of patient outcome. Criminalization of health care providers in the past decade has been initiated by complaints related to medication errors, patient abandonment, and disaster care.

When bad outcomes in health care are criminalized, they are likely to receive public attention. These cases discourage the recruitment of nurses and other caregivers, the reporting of errors, and participation in lifesaving organ donation, and they discourage caregivers from volunteering in disasters. In response, authoritative bodies have begun to emphasize the need to stop blaming the individual for bad outcomes in health care systems. The Institute of Medicine, in their 2000 report *To Err Is Human: Building a Safer Health System*, stated

> *The focus must shift from blaming individuals for past errors to a focus on preventing future errors by designing safety into the system … when an error occurs, blaming an individual does little to make the system safer and prevent someone else from committing the same error. Health care is a decade or more behind other high-risk industries in its attention to ensuring basic safety.*
>
> *(Institute of Medicine, 2000, p. 5)*

Nurses and other health care professionals must work together to enforce a policy against the criminalization of error. Belonging to an authoritative professional organization, such as the ANA, is one act every nurse can take to effectively advocate for nursing and for patients. In 2022, professional nursing organizations at national and state levels responded to the conviction of a registered nurse for criminal negligent homicide and impaired adult abuse. The organizations noted the harmful consequences for patient safety of discouraging the voluntary reporting of errors when effective and just mechanisms to examine errors, establish system-level improvements, and take corrective action already exist within the health care delivery system ANA conviction response (https://www.nursingworld.org/news/news-releases/2022-news-releases/statement-in-response-to-the-conviction-of-nurse-radonda-vaught/). This issue is further discussed in Chapter 20: Health Care Quality and Safety.

SUMMARY

A basic understanding of the effect of legal principles on nursing practice is essential to safe and effective performance as a nurse. An understanding of the role of the state BON in the control and regulation of nursing practice is also important. A thorough knowledge of employment rights and responsibilities when nurses enter into employment contracts can make them better negotiators. Knowledge of tort law is crucial to understand the duties and liabilities in our system and to serve as both a professional and patient care advocate.

SALIENT POINTS

- The power of the state to license nurses is derived from the U.S. Constitution.
- Licensing of health professionals is intended to protect the health, safety, and welfare of the public.
- Nurse practice acts (NPAs) define the practice of nursing, identify the scope of nursing practice, set the requirements for licensure, and provide guidelines for licensure disciplinary action.
- A nurse who is charged with a violation of a state's NPA has a right to due process in the investigation and hearing of the charge.

- The Americans with Disabilities Act (ADA) grants special confidentiality to nurses who are in treatment for protected disabilities.
- Nurses work under a contract, which is an express or implied agreement with an employer that creates a legal relationship.
- A collective bargaining agreement establishes a contractual relationship between the union and the employer.
- Torts are private civil wrongs against individuals, in contrast to crimes, which are wrongs against the state.

- Negligence occurs when a person fails to act in a reasonable manner.
- Malpractice occurs when the conduct of a nurse or other professional practices is below the established standard.
- Assault is a threat to touch or harm another person.
- Battery is nonconsensual touching, even if the touching is beneficial to the patient.
- The principle of informed consent requires that the patient be given enough information before treatment to make an informed, intelligent decision about whether to pursue or abandon treatment.
- False imprisonment occurs when a person is unlawfully confined within a fixed area.
- Information about a patient belongs to the patient; the health care provider is duty bound to keep information about a patient confidential and generally cannot share it unless the patient gives permission.
- Disaster nurses who act in good faith and within their scope of practice are protected from tort claims.
- The criminalization of nursing errors is rare and a violation of public policy.
- One way that nurses can advocate for changes in health care policy or law is to join an authoritative professional organization such as the American Nurses Association (ANA).

CRITICAL REFLECTION EXERCISES

1. Review your state's nurse practice acts (NPA) and delineate the definition and scope of nursing practice. Evaluate its relevance to today's health care environment.
2. Discuss the administrative and disciplinary functions of state boards of nursing (BONs).
3. How does the right of due process protect the nurse? How does it protect the public?
4. What must a plaintiff prove to recover damages in the following situation?
   An IV was left in place for 5 days, although the hospital policy specified 2 days. As a result, the patient sustained a thrombosis and inflammation at the site.
5. Discuss the concepts of employment law as they relate to your employment situation.
6. Apply knowledge of tort law to formulate risk reduction strategies that could protect a nurse against legal action.

e WEBSITE RESOURCES

- *American Nurses Association:* https://www.nursing-world.org/. The professional organization for registered nurses is a resource for standards for practice and safety, policy, and advocacy.
- *Merriam-Webster's On-Line Law Dictionary:* https://www.merriam-webster.com/legal. Legal terms in plain English.
- *National Council of State Boards of Nursing:* https://www.ncsbn.org/index.htm. The nonprofit organization where state boards come together, share goals and concerns, and develop policy statements and model laws, as well as the national nursing licensure examination (NCLEX).
- *National Institutes of Health, Institute of Medicine. To err is human: Building a safer health system:* https://nap.nationalacademies.org/catalog/9728/to-err-is-human-building-a-safer-health-system. This report by the Institute of Medicine estimates that as many as 98,000 people in the United States die each year as a result of medical errors. The report examines primarily hospital-based errors. Common errors and suggested solutions are addressed.
- *National Labor Relations Board (NLRB):* https://www.nlrb.gov. Facts about the NLRB, labor law, weekly summaries, press releases, rules and regulations, and decisions are all available on this free government website. Information is available in Spanish and English.
- *U.S. Department of Health and Human Services. Laws & Regulations:* https://healthit.gov/topic/laws-regulation-and-policy/health-it-legislation. The HHS website includes links to statutes related to nursing and health care such as HIPAA and HITECH.
- *U.S. Department of Justice. Americans with Disabilities Act:* https://www.ada.gov. The ADA website gives valuable information on the history of the ADA, provisions of the Act, enforcement considerations, settlement information, technical assistance, new or proposed regulations, and ADA mediation information.
- *VersusLaw:* http://www.versuslaw.com. VersusLaw is a legal search engine. Cases from all states and the federal government are available. There is a modest fee to use the site.

REFERENCES

American Nurses Association. (2015, June). *American Nurses Association position statement on privacy and confidentiality.* ANA Position Statement on Privacy & Confidentiality.

Bix, B. H. (2012). *Contract law: Rules, theory & context.* Cambridge University Press.

Farmer, L., & Lundy, A. (2017). Informed consent: Ethical and legal considerations for advanced practice nurses. *Journal for Nurse Practitioners, 13*(2), 124–130. https://doi.org/10.1016/j.nurpro.2016.08.011

Glannon, J. W. (2010). *The law of torts* (4th ed.). Wolters Kluwer.

Goldberg, J. C. P., Sebok, A. J., & Zipursky, B. C. (2012). *Tort law: Responsibilities and redress* (3rd ed.). Wolters Kluwer.

Guido, G. W. (2013). *Legal and ethical issues in nursing* (6th ed.). Prentice Hall.

Howie, W. O., Howie, B. A., & McMullen, P. C. (2012). To assist or not assist: Good Samaritan considerations for nurse practitioners. *Journal for Nurse Practitioners, 81*(9), 688–692. https://doi.org/10.1016/jnurpra.2012.07.002

Institute of Medicine. (2000). *To err is human: Building a safer health.* National Academies Press. https://doi.org/10.17226/9728

Library of Congress: Congressional Research Service. (2021). The Constitution of the United States of America: Analysis and interpretation: Tenth Amendment. In G. Lawson & R. Schapiro (Eds.), *U.S. Constitution Tenth Amendment.* https://constitution.congress.gov/constitution/amendment-10/

Murray, T. I., Calhoun, M., & Philipsen, N. (2011). Privacy, confidentiality, HIPAA, and HITECH: Implications for the health care practitioner. *Journal for Nurse Practitioners, 7*(9), 747–752. https://doi.org/10.1016/j.nurpra.2011.07.005

National Council of State Boards of Nursing. (2021a). *About U.S. Boards of Nursing.* Retrieved June 16, 2021, from NCSBN: About.

National Council of State Boards of Nursing. (2021b). *Delegation.* https://www.ncsbn.org/1625.htm

National Council of State Boards of Nursing. (2021c). *Substance use disorder.* https://www.ncsbn.org/sud

National Council of State Boards of Nursing. (2021d). *Professional boundaries: Social media.* Retrieved June 14, 2021, from NCSBN Professional Boundaries.

Philipsen, N. (2008). Resolving conflict: A primer for nurse practitioners on alternatives to litigation. *Journal for Nurse Practitioners, 4*(10), 766–772. https://doi.org/10.1016/j.nurpra.2008.09.005

Schwartz, V. E., Kelly, K., & Partlett, D. F. (2010). *Prosser, Wade, and Schwartz's torts: Cases and materials* (12th ed.). Foundation Press.

U.S. Department of Health and Human Services. (2018). https://www.hhs.gov/sites/default/files/Reforming-Americas-Healthcare-System-Through-Choice-and-Competition.pdf

12

Ethical Dimensions of Nursing and Health Care

*Beth Epstein, PhD, RN, HEC-C, FAAN and
Frances Rieth Maynard, PhD, MBE, APN*

 http://evolve.elsevier.com/Friberg/bridge/

OBJECTIVES

At the completion of this chapter, the reader will be able to:

- Identify resources and strategies to address ethical problems in practice.
- Define key terms in ethics language.
- Describe the nursing role in ethically challenging situations, including the use of an ethical framework.

- Define moral distress and moral residue and how they commonly arise in nursing.
- Identify the nursing contribution to ethics on four professional levels: patient, unit, organization, and national/global.

INTRODUCTION

We are sometimes asked why nurses must learn about ethics. In the questioner's words, "Aren't nurses 'by definition' ethical? What should we expect to learn?" Gallup surveys repeatedly find that the American public believes nurses to be the most honest and ethical of all professions (Gallup, 2020). Are those who are truly ethical attracted to the nursing profession and thus imbue the discipline with innate morality? Why should nurses and nursing students spend their time appraising ethics theories or reasoning if we are "already there?" A nurse may mean well and be a caring and highly skilled clinician but, without ethics knowledge, is unprepared for the complex and ethically challenging clinical situations that occur every day in health care. The ethical issues nurses face are at the patient level, unit level, and organizational level and involve not only patients but families, interprofessional colleagues, and administrators. Health care professionals must learn about ethics—not to help them be ethical people but to help them understand and contribute to ethically

challenging clinical and organizational situations that arise and to recognize the ethical aspects of their profession with every patient encounter. Good intentions are insufficient for ethical problem-solving. Nurses may be reluctant to participate in discussions regarding ethical decisions because of their own presumed knowledge deficits. This is changing, thankfully, as recognition that the nursing role is critical in identifying ethically justifiable solutions to clinical problems and ethical issues at the organizational level. In today's health care system, learning ethics is as important as learning pathophysiology and pharmacology.

Given that the writings about health care ethics are vast both in number and scope, what is important—indeed, essential—for the nurse practicing at the bedside to know and understand? Nurses must have a foundational understanding of the language of ethics, applied frameworks for ethical reasoning, and resources to facilitate effective ethical problem-solving. This chapter is intended to build the student's knowledge base about ethics in general and nursing ethics more specifically. We discuss the nurse's role in ethically challenging clinical and organizational situations and provide resources for further learning.

TO BEGIN: WHAT IS ETHICS?

Ethics is a form of philosophy derived from the Greek word *ethos,* which is roughly interpreted as "character." In a broad sense, ethics is an attempt to establish a foundation for determining good and bad conduct. When referring to an individual's behavior, it has become common practice to use the term *morals* instead of *ethics. Normative* ethics describes the accepted ways of conducting ourselves and asks the question, "What should I do?" For example, suppose a nurse made a medication error that resulted in no harm to a patient. Should they tell the patient about the mistake? If the nurse were to draw on normative ethics in this situation, they would arrive at the answer, to tell the truth. Telling the truth is accepted ethical practice. Normative ethics attempts to provide standards for determining what is morally right or wrong. Conversely, *descriptive* ethics describes the actual practices that occur. The questions, "How are problems solved?" and "How do people behave?" are addressed with these types of ethics (Vaughn, 2019). In a study of nurse and physician experiences with infant death in the neonatal intensive care unit [NICU] (Epstein, 2008), an expected (normative ethic) finding was that decisions to withdraw aggressive treatment from terminally ill infants would be based largely on the best interests of the infant. In reality, however, end-of-life decision-making is much more nuanced and involves not only the best interests of the infant, but the best interests of the family, the team's relationship with the parents, and the team's skill in end-of-life discussions. This is descriptive ethics— the ethical reasoning that occurs in reality. Therefore, normative ethics might describe how we *ought* to behave and descriptive ethics describes how we *do* behave. How does a health care team determine what *should* be done? This is the practice of *applied* ethics—the use of ethical frameworks to identify ethically justifiable solutions to thorny clinical issues. A judicious appreciation of applied ethics depends on conceptual precision (Paul & Elder, 2013). Is it ethics or is it religion? Is it ethics or is it law? Consider the case of Bradley and Mary. Bradley and Mary are adult siblings whose mother is critically ill and has little hope of recovery. They are in a heated discussion about whether to withdraw aggressive treatment (mechanical ventilation) and Bradley states, "Mary, withdrawal is a sin! How can you suggest such a thing? This goes against my religious beliefs and it's unethical." Nuanced deliberation may well come to a halt with Bradley's claims that treatment withdrawal is unethical on religious grounds. Reflecting on the religious pronouncements of sin related to feeding tube withdrawal in the case of Terry Schiavo (Roig-Franzia, 2005), where decisions were framed by discussions of "quality of life" versus "sanctity of life," it is unsurprising that public commentary developed religious overtones. Sin is a religious construct. Religious traditions may delineate the construct differently, but each expects their own view to be regarded as an ethical construct. This perspective fails to appreciate that sin and many other concepts (e.g., miracle, salvation) are theological concepts with varied interpretations and do not constitute an ethical perspective (Paul & Elder, 2013). Importantly, the practice of applied ethics would not take the pronouncement of religious beliefs as a trump card that inhibits further discussion. Instead, applied ethics might allow for redirection of the discussion to ethically grounded concepts (e.g., mother's preferences, risks, harms, benefits, quality of life) and away from a topic as sensitive and unresolvable as religion.

Ethics and the law may be similarly confused. What would be the reason for ethical deliberation if any dilemma could be reduced to whether it was against the law? Confusion may exist because ethics and the law share many features. Both use a similar language. Both try to regulate individual actions, and both present behavioral standards from which individuals and society may learn. Law and ethics do have distinct differences. The law defines the floor of acceptable behaviors, and punishments for infractions are often public. Goals of ethics, on the other hand, are aspirational—the ceiling of acceptable behavior, the "what ought we do." In historical observations of health care, law and ethics seldom reach a decision at the same time. Situations in which law has followed ethics' pronouncements include tort law evolution and practice guidelines. Conversely, the law weighed in on issues dealing with informed consent, standards of care, and health care provider duties (Gostin, 2002) before the literature on ethics related to these concepts was established. Ethics has an active presence in case law (court rulings that may be cited as precedent). The New Jersey Supreme Court established a patient's right to refuse treatment (McFadden, 1995) and influenced the requirement of access to mechanisms for resolution of ethics disputes at accredited health care institutions; the U.S. Supreme Court impelled the emphasis of advance directives and health care proxies (Lewin, 1990) and determined that there is no constitutional right to die, thus opening the door for state regulation of physician-assisted suicide. A discussion of basic law principles foundational to nursing practice can be found in Chapter 11 (Legal Aspects of Nursing Practice).

Given that applied ethics is the practice of using ethical frameworks to solve dilemmas and that it is a separate process from consideration of religious beliefs or legal aspects, the next question is, "What is an ethical dilemma?" Beauchamp and Childress (2019) define ethical or moral dilemmas as those "circumstances in which moral obligations demand or appear to demand that a person adopt each of two (or more) alternative but incompatible actions, such that the person cannot perform all the required actions" (p. 11). In a particular situation, a person could take action A or action B, but not both, and neither A nor B alone is entirely satisfactory. The first step in applied ethics is to identify the actions that are justifiable. This is where the law and religion may need to be considered. For example, suppose an 18-year-old patient comes to the clinic concerned that she may be pregnant. A pregnancy test confirms that she is indeed pregnant. An ethical analysis of the situation may conclude that an abortion is an ethically justifiable solution. However, if the patient herself is against abortion on religious grounds, the abortion option drops from the list of ethically justifiable solutions. Additionally, if abortion were illegal, it would not be an ethically justifiable solution either. Once ethically justifiable solutions are identified, the next step is attempting to discover which action (A or B) is the better of the two. To help guide reasoning in terms of identifying appropriate actions and determining which is best, engaging ethical theory and ethical frameworks can be useful.

ETHICAL THEORY

Normative ethics address classifications of ethical theories, including those that are act-based (e.g., deontology), outcomes-based (e.g., utilitarianism), or agent-based (e.g., virtue ethics). These theories of morality provide a foundation for understanding what we ought to do in a certain circumstance and a rationale for why the actions identified are morally right or morally wrong. Although there are many ethical theories, three are commonly used in the health care field. Each has significant strengths and, unfortunately, each has significant drawbacks as well. None of the theories will produce all of the morally right (or wrong) actions in every situation. The first theory, *virtue ethics,* centers on the character of the person acting. Historically, Western nursing and medicine were highly virtue-centric. A "good" doctor or a "good" nurse would know the right action to take. In the early 1900s, "good" (in nursing) involved many characteristics, such as being obedient, attentive to detail, caring, sturdy, Christian, and White (Robb, 2008). We now understand that most of these "goods" are not moral goods and that a good doctor or nurse cannot possibly know the right thing to do based on his or her virtues alone. However, might it help the doctor or nurse identify right and wrong actions if they are

capable of empathy? Of kindness? Of trustworthiness? Many would argue that possessing certain virtues can be helpful in that they are alerted to moral problems in the workplace—that is, they can recognize moral issues because they can feel that something is not quite right. In addition, a highly compassionate nurse may be able to find morally right and wrong actions that an uncaring or hard-hearted nurse may never see. Virtue-based ethics can be helpful, but in terms of being a reliable ethical theory that will provide the guidance that today's clinicians need to resolve complex ethical challenges, it is insufficient. Theresa Drought (2002) described that being a nurse is to experience the privilege of bearing witness and that witnessing suffering, death, hope, and recovery cannot help but change how one sees the world and his or her place in it. As nurses, we have undoubtedly been changed by what we have experienced and we exhibit the behaviors of our profession as a result.

The second ethical theory centers on the duties of the person acting. What is one obligated to do? This theory is called *deontology* and arises largely from Immanuel Kant (1724–1804). This theory begins with the acknowledgment that every person has inherent dignity and worth and that acting ethically means acting in such a way that respects others' (and one's own) dignity and worth. Kant's categorical imperative (the foundational principle upon which all obligations rest) is to act such that you always treat others and yourself as an end and never only as a means (Degrazia et al., 2011). For example, Mike is interested in meeting a famous musician. He learns that the musician is going to a big party at a neighbor's house down the street from where he lives. This neighbor is not Mike's friend and, although they have lived on the same street for 15 years, the disparate election stickers on their cars have not facilitated substantial conversation between them. Mike could introduce himself to the neighbor and be very friendly in the hopes that the neighbor would offer an invitation to the party. According to the deontological perspective, this would be wrong because Mike would be using his neighbor only as a means of getting what he really wants, which is to meet the famous musician.

The strengths of this theory are that they make intuitive sense to make use of identified duties (do not lie, do not kill, keep your promises) that most who are morally minded value. It also emphasizes our need to reason through problems to identify the proper duty and apply it. Rather than relying on personal character (kindness, empathy), this theory calls on us to draw on common rules of conduct. The drawbacks are many, however. When more than one duty is apparent in a given situation, there is no method of prioritizing them to discern which duty to follow. For instance, suppose you had promised your professor that you would help her collect data this afternoon. However, when you called home to check on your infant son, the babysitter informed you that he had a fever and had vomited twice. Your duties here are in conflict—keeping a promise versus attending to one's sick child. How do you know which duty to follow to be morally right? Deontology cannot help you here. In addition, deontology does not take into consideration the outcomes of acting on duties. Suppose the year is 1943 and you are a German citizen living in Nazi Germany. A family of Jews is hiding in your attic. One day the Nazis come to your door and ask if you are hiding anyone. As a deontologist, you might determine that your duty is to tell the truth. The outcome would be disastrous, however. So, again, deontology provides little guidance in terms of identifying duties to which we should adhere to resolve moral problems. However, this theory cannot always identify the "right" action to take.

The third ethical theory, *utilitarianism,* places emphasis on the outcomes of a situation. Mill (1806–1873) and Bentham (1748–1832) suggested that right action is determined by identifying actions that yield the greatest good for the greatest number (Beauchamp & Childress, 2019). If that goal is met, the action is morally right. Many utilitarians accept rules as guidelines and do not discount them entirely. However, unlike a deontologist, a utilitarian could justify lying to the Nazis because the outcome, saving the lives of the Jews in the attic, is far better than allowing them to be discovered.

Utilitarian applications abound in health care. Examples include the Patient Protection and Affordable Care Act and vaccination programs. Both seek to achieve the greatest good (health care insurance for most Americans and a reduced risk for the spread of disease, especially to those who are particularly vulnerable) for the greatest number of people. Another example would be planning for the COVID-19 pandemic or natural disaster. These plans include complex *triaging* algorithms addressing decision points such as the likelihood of survival, the likelihood of severe disease or death, and prioritization due to the essential nature of work. In the COVID-19 pandemic as with previous epidemics, those living with fewer socioeconomic resources, including access to health care, are at higher risk of getting COVID-19 and of dying from it (DeBruin et al., 2012; Hawkins et al., 2020; Johns Hopkins Coronavirus Resource Center, 2022). Further discussion relating to social determinants of health is addressed in Chapter 14 (Diversity, Equity, and Inclusion: Impact on Health Care and Nursing Care Strategies) and Chapter 15 (Health and Health Promotion).

Utilitarian thinking allows attention to be paid to the greater good. On an individual level, utilitarian thinking can be helpful in considering the potential outcomes of several treatment plans. Which outcomes are desired? Which are possible? Which of the treatment plans might help the patient achieve his or her desired outcome? Weaknesses of this theory include the potential to downplay the needs of the minority or even harm the minority to achieve the greatest good for the greatest number. An extreme oft-used example would be the following: Nurse Peters is caring for four patients: (1) Mr. Frederickson, a homeless man with no support system and a belligerent personality who is admitted with serious injuries after a pedestrian accident; (2) Ms. Delaney, a married housewife and mother of two young children who is on the kidney transplant list; (3) Mr. Pfeffercorn, a 78-year-old healthy man who is in need of a corneal transplant; and (4) Mrs. Divers, a 58-year-old woman with liver failure who is on the liver transplant list. A utilitarian could (conceivably) determine that not treating Mr. Frederickson (allowing him to die) would be an appropriate action to take because, in doing so, three lives (Delaney, Pfeffercorn, and Divers) could be saved or improved by harvesting his organs. This action does not sit well, however. It might be justifiable using utilitarian thinking, but we know that something is not quite right about this action.

In summary, there are many ways to think about ethical problems. We could consider the problem in terms of the person who will act and whether that person possesses virtues that would assist in making the right decision. Alternatively, we could consider the actions themselves. Given a certain situation, what are our obligations and duties? What rules shall we live our lives by and how should we apply those rules? Finally, we could consider the outcomes of whatever action we take. Which action will yield the greatest good?

A BRIEF HISTORY OF NURSING ETHICS

Caring for sick, suffering, recovering, and dying patients and their families is inescapably a moral practice. Nurses have been considering the question, "What ought I do now for my patient," for generations. *How* they have considered this question, given the context of their practice, has changed dramatically over the years. However, important lessons are learned from every stage in nursing ethics' history. In the early years of professional nursing, the nurse's personal behavior and values were the foundation of nursing ethics. A nurse of high moral character was one who would provide ethically grounded care. This was a time when nurses were subservient to doctors, when there were few technological aspects to nursing, and when nursing was extraordinarily "hands on." Thus, virtues such as obedience, sincerity, and graciousness (Fowler, 1997) were important. This was also a time when nurses were primarily White women from upper-class families, so virtues like Christian, good posture, and poise (Fowler, 1997) were not so surprising. Nursing schools were charged with providing a "moral training ground" designed to promote the development of nurses with strong moral character (Fowler, 1997, p. 24). Although it is easy to brush many of the stated virtues off as irrelevant for today, the nursing profession actually carries forward many lessons learned from this era (see Chapter 1: A Brief History of the Professionalization of Nursing in the United States). Although nursing schools are no longer considered "moral training grounds," much honing of moral character occurs during training. Attending to the ideas of respect for the dignity of persons and for privacy, rules about appearance during clinicals (i.e., no crop tops), and mindfulness about not expressing job dissatisfaction to patients are all grounded in the early virtues of nursing. Conversely, some of the virtues extolled so reverently in the past have remained there. Gone, thankfully, is the misbelief that the White, upper-class, Christian woman is the ideal nurse. We have learned that diversity brings creativity and broadened perspectives so critical to effective nursing practice. Nursing ethics developed from these early days as nursing became increasingly viewed as a profession, and as nursing in the context of society and health care shifted. The first code of ethics was written in the 1920s and centered on nursing duties—to self, to patient, and to doctors.

It was not until 1950 that the American Nurses Association (ANA) adopted a Code of Ethics and, by then, significant shifts in the nurse's role had occurred. This and later versions reflected a sense of empowerment and accountability, as military nurses served in the world wars and, especially, in Vietnam, and as health care technologies became increasingly complex. The independence, professionalism, and accountability achieved during these difficult times were here to stay. The current Code of Ethics speaks to the nurse's obligations to patient, self, colleagues, and professional practice and is a valuable guide for nurses in all roles—researchers, bedside nurses, nurse practitioners, policymakers, and teachers. The *ANA Code of Ethics for Nurses* (2015) is available to ANA members and nonmembers at the following link: https://www.nursingworld.org/practice-policy/nursing-excellence/ethics/.

The International Council of Nurses (ICN), a federation of national nurses' associations serving nurses in more than 128 countries, also published a code of ethics in 1953, with its most recent revision appearing in 2021 (ICN, 2021). The *ICN Code of Ethics for Nursing* can be accessed at: https://www.icn.ch/system/files/2021-10/ICN_Code-of-Ethics_EN_Web_0.pdf.

NURSING ETHICS IN PRACTICE: FOUR LEVELS

The *ANA Code of Ethics* provides a foundation for understanding nursing ethics today. There are essentially four levels of nursing ethics: the patient, professional, organizational, and national/global levels. Each level brings a different perspective of nursing ethics to light and involves a different way of ethical thinking as well. Here, we review each of the four levels, highlighting the important features and the ethical contribution from nursing.

Historically, nurses have not viewed themselves as key players in these types of situations because they are not the medical decision-makers, and often nurses and other staff shy away from involvement because they feel they lack the knowledge about ethics that is necessary to analyze the situation and arrive at appropriate solutions. It is critical, however, that today's nurse recognizes himself or herself as an important contributor in ethically challenging clinical situations. As so beautifully put by nurse and ethicist, Theresa Drought (2002):

> *In all of our work we bear witness to the experience of others. We witness the inexorable wear of disease, the environment and time on the human body. We witness the love that binds humankind: the mother stroking the cheek of her newborn child; the son stroking the cheek of his dying mother; the friend holding a hand during a bout of pain. We witness the wonton senselessness of vice and violence: the victim of a drunken driver; the woman beaten by her husband; the teenage victim of a gang shooting. The moral challenge for us as nurses is to explicate meaning and identify the duties that follow from what we are privileged to witness. (p. 238)*

The nurse is in the unique position of being able to see clinical situations from many angles at once. The nurse learns from the patient and family about their past experiences, their deepest fears, their beliefs, and how they interpret the current situation. At the same time, the nurse understands the pathophysiological basis of the disease, treatment options, likely outcomes, and expected clinical trajectory. All of this is important information and can be very helpful in assessing and analyzing an ethical dilemma. To participate in finding solutions, the nurse must know himself or herself to be an ethical practitioner (Taylor, 2011) and must be able to convey relevant and important information in a constructive way.

Carol Taylor (2011) has delineated the features of an ethical practitioner; these include clinical competence, trustworthiness, demonstration of commitment to advancing the patient's best interests, accountability, ability for collaboration and conflict mediation, and capacity to recognize the ethical aspects of practice, including patient care, technology, resource use, and care delivery. Engaging these features on a daily basis ensures that nurses seek circumstances in which they can contribute to resolution of ethical problems and be accountable for their actions. A key factor is conveying relevant information to other team members. This is critical and does not, surprisingly, require a tremendous amount of ethics knowledge. It does, however, require that nurses be able to identify relevant features of a case. Cases can be at the patient level, the unit level, the organizational level, or the national/global level.

Patient-Level Ethics

Most commonly, we think of ethics as being at the bedside—encountering a difficult patient situation as it unfolds. To illustrate the potential for nursing input, we provide the following case.

Father (Fr.) Frank Fowler is a 70-year-old Roman Catholic priest. His power of attorney for health care was his long-time colleague and friend, Fr. Jeremy Lewis. Fr. Fowler is a patient in the intensive care unit (ICU) after surgery for a gastrointestinal (GI) obstruction. He has a history of diverticulitis, coronary artery disease, and hypertension. He has experienced several complications after surgery, including respiratory failure and pseudomonas sepsis. He was intubated and on a ventilator while critically ill. He now has a tracheostomy and remains ventilator-dependent. His sepsis is improving dramatically, and he is alert and oriented. He cannot speak but can write and has a good relationship with you, his nurse.

Fr. Fowler is described by his colleagues, including the nuns from the convent associated with his church, as ornery and difficult, even in the best of circumstances. However, he has devoted friends and, to many congregants, he is a beloved leader.

At one point, early on in his admission, Fr. Fowler refused to cooperate with treatment recommendations. These refusals were believed to be part of an arduous postoperative adjustment. At the time, in fact, Fr. Fowler agreed that the postoperative course had been difficult and that he was unafraid to die—both of these led him to refuse aggressive treatments. However, after talking with his friend, Fr. Lewis, he felt better and stronger and expressed a wish to carry on and to "see things through." For the past several weeks, Fr. Fowler has been ill-tempered and uncooperative, but he has been accepting treatments. This week, he is again unwilling to continue treatment. His condition has improved, though, and there is hope for a good outcome. The critical care and surgical teams acknowledge his right to refuse treatment, but they are a bit perplexed given his current clinical picture.

He has stated to the nurse and to the critical care physician that he wants the ventilator stopped. The physician told him that if the ventilator was stopped, he would die, and Fr. Fowler expressed that he understood this outcome by nodding his head appropriately.

He had seemed to several nurses to be depressed during this hospitalization. When he had become septic and critically ill, the focus was on sustaining his life, and antidepressants were never started. Now, Fr. Fowler is refusing to talk to a psychiatrist or to take antidepressants. He did say, however, that he wanted to continue treatment until Fr. Lewis could visit. He also wanted to speak with his longtime friend and colleague, Sister Mary Jane. He enjoyed their company and wanted to hear their perspectives.

The critical care physician and surgeon are concerned about his clinical picture and his desire to withdraw from the ventilator. This would take a huge emotional toll on the staff and on them to withdraw life-sustaining treatment for a completely lucid person who seemed to be doing so well. They are considering contacting the ethics consult service. (Case adapted from Ford & Dudzinski [2008].)

What can Fr. Fowler's nurse contribute in this situation? Most importantly, the nurse can provide information and interpretation. The *Four Topics* approach to ethical decision-making (Jonsen et al., 2022) can be effective for both. The *Four Topics* approach involves ordering the information that is known about a case in to four discrete sections: medical indications, patient preferences, quality of life, and external factors (Table 12.1). By separating the relevant facts of the case into these four categories, the nurse is able to identify key issues that require further investigation or that will play a role in the ethical analysis of the case. In Fr. Fowler's case, the quadrant might go as follows.

Medical Indications. This section includes relevant medical data. Fr. Fowler is currently in the ICU after surgery for a GI obstruction. He has a history of diverticulitis, coronary artery disease, and hypertension and has experienced complications after surgery, including respiratory failure and pseudomonas sepsis. He now has a tracheostomy and is ventilator dependent. His condition is improving. He is alert and can communicate through writing. His health care providers are concerned that he is suffering from depression.

Patient Preferences. This section is intended to provide a clearer picture of how the patient is thinking about his or her treatments, what his or her stated preferences are, and whether there are any directives that could be helpful.

TABLE 12.1 Four Topics Approach

Medical Indications
The Principles of Beneficence and Nonmaleficence

1. What is the patient's medical problem? Is the problem acute? Chronic? Critical? Reversible? Emergent? Terminal?
2. What are the goals of treatment?
3. In what circumstances are medical treatments not indicated?
4. What are the probabilities of success of various treatment options?
5. In sum, how can this patient be benefited by medical and nursing care, and how can harm be avoided?

Patient Preferences
The Principle of Respect for Autonomy

1. Has the patient been informed of benefits and risks, understood this information, and given consent?
2. Is the patient mentally capable and legally competent, and is there evidence of incapacity?
3. If mentally capable, what preferences about treatment are the patient stating?
4. If incapacitated, has the patient expressed prior preferences?
5. Who is the appropriate surrogate to make decisions for the incapacitated patient?
6. Is the patient unwilling or unable to cooperate with medical treatment? If so, why?

Quality of Life
The Principles of Beneficence, Nonmaleficence, and Respect for Autonomy

1. What are the prospects, with or without treatment, for a return to normal life, and what physical, mental, and social deficits might the patient experience even if treatment succeeds?
2. On what grounds can anyone judge that some quality of life would be undesirable for a patient who cannot make or express such a judgment?
3. Are there biases that might prejudice the provider's evaluation of the patient's quality of life?
4. What ethical issues arise concerning improving or enhancing a patient's quality of life?
5. Do quality-of-life assessments raise any questions regarding changes in treatment plans, such as forgoing life-sustaining treatment?
6. What are plans and rationale to forgo life-sustaining treatment?
7. What is the legal and ethical status of suicide?

Contextual Features
The Principles of Justice and Fairness

1. Are there professional, interprofessional, or business interests that might create conflicts of interest in the clinical treatment of patients?
2. Are there parties other than clinicians and patients, such as family members, who have an interest in clinical decisions?
3. What are the limits imposed on patient confidentiality by the legitimate interests of third parties?
4. Are there financial factors that create conflicts of interest in clinical decisions?
5. Are there problems of allocation of scarce health resources that might affect clinical decisions?
6. Are there religious issues that might affect clinical decisions?
7. What are the legal issues that might affect clinical decisions?
8. Are there considerations of clinical research and education that might affect clinical decisions?
9. Are there issues of public health and safety that affect clinical decisions?
10. Are there conflicts of interest within institutions or organizations (e.g., hospitals) that may affect clinical decisions and patient welfare?

Adapted by Julia Taylor, MD from "Four Quadrants" Jonsen, A. R., Siegler, M., & Winslade, W. J. (2022). *Clinical ethics: A practical approach to ethical decisions in clinical medicine* (9th ed.). McGraw-Hill; and Schumann, J. H., & Alfandre, D. (2008). Clinical ethical decision making: The four topics approach. *Seminars in Medical Practice, 11,* 36–42.

Fr. Fowler has stated that he wants the ventilator to be stopped. In the past he has refused treatments, but he changed his mind after speaking with his friends. Now, Fr. Fowler seems sure of himself, although again, he would like to speak with his friends before making his final decision. He understands that treatments can be removed or withheld.

Quality of Life. This section provides some idea of the quality of the patient's life before the illness, during the illness, and after the illness. Health care providers often discuss quality of life issues, but they must be careful to acknowledge that they cannot judge another person's quality of life. Only the patient can make this judgment. For example, a young patient who suffers severe spinal injuries in a motor vehicle accident and who is now quadriplegic may, in fact, perceive herself to have a very good quality of life. It might not be the life she had imagined or hoped for, but she (and many others in her situation) may find her life to be entirely worth living. We, as health care providers, have no say in how one perceives quality of life. In Fr. Fowler's case, we are unsure of his *past* quality of life, but the evidence is there that he led a parish, has parishioners who cherish him, and has deeply valued friendships. His *current* quality of life might be perceived by him to be poor. What is making his quality of life poor, especially when his condition has improved substantially? What would need to change to help him see his life differently? Might clinical depression be influencing his decision? Finally, what is his *future* quality of life likely to be? The health care team believes that he is likely to have a "good outcome," but what does that mean? What are they expecting his future life to be like, and, more importantly, will that qualify as a "good outcome" for Fr. Fowler?

Contextual Factors. This section includes other factors that are or could be relevant to the case, such as insurance coverage, home safety/conditions, companionship, availability of caregivers, financial issues, and so on. For Fr. Fowler, we know little about his financial issues. We can assume he is covered by Medicare but do not know his insurance status beyond this. His insurance status will dictate any long-term care decisions that are made. He is unmarried but has dear friends. Their ability to provide care for Fr. Fowler is unknown.

Having completed the four sections, we can see gaps in our current knowledge about Fr. Fowler and can interpret some of the important factors. A significant gap is our lack of understanding of Fr. Fowler's past, current, and future quality of life. Here, the nurse can play an important role. The nurse can ask Fr. Fowler about what his life was like before his illness, what he enjoyed, what he looked forward to, and what gave him purpose. The nurse could ask about what, in his current state, is so dissatisfying. What kinds of things are burdensome? Why does he want the ventilator stopped when his condition is improving? What is keeping him from talking with a psychiatrist? The nurse could investigate the meaning of a "good outcome." Further clarification of this is certainly necessary. A good outcome could mean anything from a ventilator-dependent patient being discharged to a skilled nursing facility to an independently functioning patient being discharged home. The

goals of care must be clarified and then articulated to Fr. Fowler. Would the expected outcomes be satisfactory and allow him to enjoy his life? Other gaps in the case include whether he has an advance directive, what his insurance status is, and whether he is concerned about his financial status. The nurse certainly can be helpful in finding this information. So, Fr. Fowler's nurse plays an important role in filling out the picture as it is presented. Once this is done, the work of analysis begins.

Case Analysis. There are myriad ways in which an ethically challenging case can be analyzed. Most familiar to health care providers is using the *principlism theory* articulated by Beauchamp and Childress in the 1970s. This approach has since become the foremost used framework for analysis in health care settings. Four principles are applied to cases: *respect for autonomy, beneficence, nonmaleficence,* and *justice.* Within each principle are content areas that provide further guidance in applying the principle to the case. Briefly, let us discuss Fr. Fowler's case using the principlist approach and incorporating information gleaned from the *Four Topics* approach.

Respect for Autonomy. This principle addresses the idea that a person's wishes ought to be respected (assuming they do not overly burden others or violate the law [there are limits]). This is true for people who are capable of making autonomous decisions. Such people must have *liberty* (be free from influencing factors), *agency* (be able to make decisions), and *understanding* (have enough information to make decisions) (Beauchamp & Childress, 2019). Factors that influence another's decision may render that person unable to make independent decisions. Others who demand a person act a certain way (i.e., the grandmother of an infant who insists that the mother bottle feed the infant rather than breastfeed) or severe depression can be influencing factors. Not included in this category, generally, are religious beliefs, even very restrictive religious beliefs. For example, a patient who practices as a Jehovah's Witness may request that no blood products be used, even if this means that they may die. This is not to say that this patient's request should not be explored a bit more deeply to ensure that it is truly their belief and not the demands of others influencing their opinion, but, if this is truly what the patient believes, their wishes ought to be followed. In Fr. Fowler's case, there is no reason to question his ability to make decisions. He is alert and conversant. If his mental outlook is appropriately investigated during the assessment phase, it may or may not be deemed to be an influencing factor, which speaks to his liberty in terms of decision-making. Fr. Fowler appears to have an understanding of the benefits and burdens of continuing treatment, especially if the vague concept of a good outcome has been explored. If Fr. Fowler has liberty, agency, and understanding, he may choose to have aggressive treatments withdrawn.

Also, within the principle of respect for autonomy are guidelines for surrogate decision makers and the informed consent process. Suppose that Fr. Fowler was unable to make decisions about his medical treatment. He would require someone to decide for him; this is a person he can designate while he has decision-making capacity, as he did when he chose Fr. Lewis. For those who have not designated someone to make decisions for them, individual states have determined who the surrogate decision makers should be and in what order they would become surrogates. In the Commonwealth of Virginia, for example, surrogate decision-makers are prioritized as follows: designated guardian, patient's spouse, adult child, patient's parent, adult sibling, and other relative in descending order of blood relationship (Virginia Statutes Health Care Decisions Act). This means that if a patient has been living with someone for 20 years but is not married, that person may not legally be able to make decisions for the patient. The nurse can play an important role in this by ensuring that patients have designated the person they wish to make decisions for them, should they become unable to do so while in the hospital. In Fr. Fowler's case, it would be important to include Fr. Lewis in discussions about treatment withdrawal (if that was acceptable to Fr. Fowler).

Beneficence. This principle calls on us as health care providers to do good for our patients—to prevent and remove harm. First, it is incumbent upon health care providers to identify the potential harms and benefits of the different options available. In Fr. Fowler's case, withdrawing treatment would lead to his death, certainly a harm and an irreversible one, but there are worse harms than death for many patients. Death is not necessarily the worst possible outcome. One harm of not withdrawing aggressive treatment may be that Fr. Fowler goes on to have a lifelong disability that he would rather not endure. The "rather not endure" aspect of this harm is important because it too is a harm in and of itself. Purposely refusing to follow a capable person's wishes is called *paternalism*. Sometimes, paternalism is acceptable. Examples include situations in which safety is a primary concern (e.g., insisting that a patient who is in traction after orthopedic surgery use the bedpan rather than following their wish to get up to use the commode) or when a patient asks that the health care provider do something that is not legal (e.g., the patient asks the provider to administer opioids for the purpose of ending their life). Many times, however, overriding a patient's wish is unacceptable. Fr. Fowler may be one such case, but this is not entirely clear. We do not know why Fr. Fowler is asking for discontinuation of aggressive treatment and we do not know what he considers to be harms and benefits of continued treatment versus discontinuation.

Nonmaleficence. This principle also involves harms, similar to beneficence. The difference is that the focus is on not inflicting harm rather than preventing or removing harm. It is not difficult to think of situations in health care in which pain or suffering is actually inflicted on patients, such as getting a patient up to walk soon after a surgical procedure. There is little doubt that this is painful. However, *not* doing so leads to much greater harms. These actions matter little in the context of the principle of nonmaleficence. Inflicting *unnecessary* harm is central to this principle. So, in Fr. Fowler's case, would we be inflicting harm if we discontinued treatment? How about if we continued treatment? Again, Fr. Fowler's view of "harms" would be helpful here.

Justice. This final principle speaks to the idea of distribution of goods, particularly scarce goods. It generally applies to communities, societies, or even organizations rather than individual patients and hence has little relevance in Fr. Fowler's case. The usefulness of this principle comes into play when considering unit, organization, or national/global levels of ethics.

Using the principlist approach, it is clear that Fr. Fowler is a capable decision-maker and thus health care providers ought to abide by his wishes. However, it is much less clear why he wants these treatment modalities to be stopped. What does he consider the harms of the current treatments? Before proceeding with withdrawal per his wishes, a fuller understanding of Fr. Fowler's perceived harms and benefits seems necessary. The nurse could take the lead in investigating this. What if Fr. Fowler writes, "This tracheostomy makes my ability to talk to my friends and congregants impossible; I can't write everything I want to say. If I can't communicate with my congregants, how am I going to do the work I set out for myself to do?" How enlightening! The issue is not that he wants to die or that the treatments are too burdensome but that he cannot see how he can continue to do the work he loves to do. Is there a different tracheostomy tube he could use that would enable him to speak? Is there hope that he may, with time and therapy, be able to have the tracheostomy tube removed? This new information sets the case on a different path, leading the team and the patient down a different road than the one on which they all had been. The nurse's work of breaking out the important aspects of the case into the four topics helped identify key features of the case and gaps in knowledge. The case analysis targeted those key features and gaps and framed them in such a way as the team could understand what information was needed and for what purpose. The team needed Fr. Fowler's perspective on harms and benefits to fully understand the case.

Beyond the Principles: Rules for Health Care Providers. In addition to the four principles, several rules apply to health care situations, including *privacy* and *confidentiality, veracity,* and *fidelity.* Privacy involves not only treating a patient's information as private but protecting the patient's privacy as well. Most nurses are now familiar with the requirements of the Health Insurance and Portability and Accountability Act (HIPAA) (USDHHS, 1996), and its stipulations certainly should be followed. More troublesome are the situations that seem quite minor but are violations of *privacy* or *confidentiality*—the elevator or hallway discussions about patients, telephone conversations that can be overheard, the presence of patients at the nurses' station where patient information is exchanged. The nurse must be mindful of what is being said in public areas and is obligated to take action when violations of privacy or confidentiality occur.

The principle of *veracity* is defined as the obligation to tell the truth and to not lie or deceive others (Fry & Veatch, 2006). Truthfulness has long been regarded as fundamental to the existence of trust among individuals and has special significance in health care relationships (Fry & Grace, 2007). Over and over again, studies have shown that patients and families want to receive honest information and that this is what health care teams ought to strive for (Institute of Medicine [IOM], 2001).

Fidelity is another rule that speaks to the obligations of persons to others or to organizations. Nurses have multiple simultaneous obligations, and often it is difficult to determine which obligations are strongest. The ANA 2015 *Code of Ethics* would say that one's obligation to the patient is most important. However, there are many situations in which maintaining a commitment to the patient jeopardizes future relationships with colleagues, and this risk is not insubstantial. Gordon and Hamric (2006) found that nurses' experiences of being in situations where they could choose to call an ethics consult often involved an assessment of risk in terms of relationships with medical colleagues. Some took the risk and others declined to call a consult because the perceived risk was too high. Thus, identifying one's obligations and considering them is not such an easy task. It is not so simple as just putting the patient first.

Unit-Level and Organizational-Level Ethics

Much of what nursing ethics is extends beyond the patient. Daniel Chambliss' sociological study of ethical issues faced by nurses in the hospital setting revealed that the most problematic issues are derived not from individual patients but from the system itself (Chambliss, 1996). Chambliss noted that the repeated situations of poor communication, planning, and follow-through are what challenge the nurse's ability to do the work that needs to be done.

The ethical environment certainly influences perceptions and behavior. Penticuff and Walden (2000) found that nurses were more likely to get involved in resolving ethically challenging cases if they perceived their unit to be supportive of such work. Other studies have shown that nurses who perceive their units to have a better ethical climate (more collegial, administrative support, good avenues of communication) tend to have lower levels of moral distress (Epstein et al., 2019; Hamric & Blackhall, 2007; Hamric et al., 2012; Whitehead et al., 2015). This is a growing area of research interest and one where nursing's contribution could be substantial and influential because nurses are called on to contribute to the building and maintenance of strongly ethical health care environments (ANA Code of Ethics, 2015, provision 6).

Moral Distress. Moral distress was first defined in the 1980s but only recently has it begun to be studied and better understood. First described in nurses, moral distress is now known to affect every type of health care provider, including physicians, respiratory therapists, psychologists, chaplains, social workers, and more (Austin et al., 2005; Bruce et al., 2015; Dodek et al., 2016; Fantus et al., 2017; Laabs, 2012; Pauly et al., 2009; Penny et al., 2016; Schwenzer & Wang 2006; Sporrong et al., 2005; Whitehead et al., 2015). Moral distress is a phenomenon occurring when:

> *Clinicians are constrained from taking what they believe to be ethically appropriate actions or are forced to take actions they believe are ethically inappropriate. As a result, they feel complicit in acting unethically and are unable to fulfill important professional obligations.* (Epstein et al., 2020, p. 149)

Many providers who experience moral distress note that what is so damaging is that they believe they are forced to do something that is morally wrong. There are two stages to moral distress: initial moral distress and moral residue (Jameton, 1993). Initial moral distress occurs in the moment, while the problematic situation is taking place. The level of moral distress may rise (crescendo) over time as the situation becomes more entrenched and difficult to resolve (Fig. 12.1). Then, once the situation has passed, the level of moral distress drops dramatically, but it never returns to zero (or to the level it was before the problematic situation). This residual moral distress is called *moral residue.* We know this exists because when we ask health care

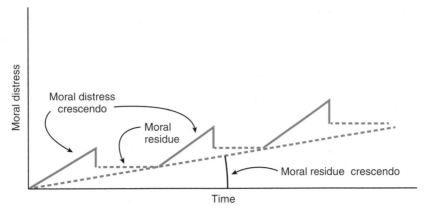

Fig. 12.1 Crescendo Effect (*solid lines* indicate moral distress; *dotted lines* indicate moral residue). (Permission received from Epstein, E. G., & Hamric, A. B. [2009]. Moral distress, moral residue, and the crescendo effect. *Journal of Clinical Ethics, 20*[4], 330–342. https://www.journals.uchicago.edu/doi/pdf/10.1086/JCE200920406?download=true. Used with permission *Journal of Clinical Ethics*.)

providers who had been in morally distressing situations 5, 10, or 30 years ago what they recall about the situation, they can recount in vivid detail the complexities of the case, where they were, and how they felt (frustrated, angry, hurt, trapped). Repeated exposure to morally distressing situations may lead to burnout or to providers becoming less engaged in the ethical aspects of their work. Some, but not all, studies of nurses have shown that moral distress levels increase with increasing years in a position (Elpern et al., 2005; Epstein & Hamric, 2009; Hamric & Blackhall, 2007). Several studies have now shown that higher levels of moral distress are associated with burnout or are an independent predictor of burnout (Fumis et al., 2017; Johnson-Coyle et al., 2016; Neumann et al., 2018). The crescendo effect is a model that requires more testing but is supported by significant qualitative and quantitative evidence, especially for nurses (Epstein & Hamric, 2009).

Few studies have published strategies to address moral distress. However, one of the most powerful strategies we have found is that naming the problem when it arises can be empowering and can decrease the amount of anxiety. It is not uncommon to hear providers say that they believed themselves to be weak or to be unable to handle the stresses of the job before they understood the concept of moral distress. Knowing one is not alone is a relief to many providers. In addition to recognizing moral distress in oneself and others, beginning dialogue within the unit about moral distress is important. Building supportive networks, learning more about moral distress, and working together to identify the sources of moral distress and design strategies to reduce moral distress—all of these are good steps

toward being prepared to work in units in which morally distressing situations tend to occur. Health care organizations are beginning to address moral distress in various ways. One method being used at several institutions is moral distress consultation (Hamric & Epstein, 2017). Typically, under the umbrella of an institutional Ethics Consult Service, moral distress consultation promotes open discussion of the issues causing moral distress in the moment and helps teams identify ways to directly address them, thus decreasing the source of the moral distress. For resources related to moral distress and moral distress consultation, please see the website for the Moral Distress Consultation Collaborative (https://med.virginia.edu/biomedical-ethics/moral-distress-collaborative/).

Ethics Consult Services and Committees. One prospect for facilitation of ethical reflection and understanding for practicing nurses is consultation with the organization's ethics committee (EC). Daily decisions that nurses make often have ethical components and mirror the values of both the persons making those decisions and the profession of nursing. Articulation of those values may require careful consideration and may be assisted by those who are expert in the language and nuance of ethical deliberation.

The Joint Commission requires hospitals to have structures in place to resolve situational conflict with ethical components (Joint Commission International [JCI], 2020); ECs at most hospitals have become the means for doing so. Mandates for ECs include education (of members and other employees), consultation and mediation of conflict, policy generation and review, and research/quality improvement to ensure policies are working as envisioned. An EC is often comprised of various disciplines and the community but is not required to do so. However, the multiplicity of perspectives, experiences, and professional disciplines facilitate collaboration in creditable ethical decision making and policy development. Nursing is an integral part of these committees, and those who are members should be experienced in clinical practice, expert in communication, and practiced in the art of negotiation. Price (1995) observes that nurses as members of ECs provide a specific perspective that includes a "holistic view" of patients and families, an appreciation of power differentials experienced by families and staff, and a pragmatic understanding of proposed solution implementation for conflicts about ethical issues.

Ideally, members of ECs are consulting and writing policy on issues including guidelines for end-of-life, informed consent, treatment refusal, professionalism, and resource allocation. Through EC member presentation on ward rounds or grand rounds, awareness may permeate the entire organization; this education allows for sensitization to issues of ethics. EC resources ought to be available to all members of the health care team and to patients and families; organizational mechanisms should allow anyone to ask for case consultation.

Gordon and Hamric (2006) studied nurses' perceptions of "risk, power dynamics, and regret" with requests for ethics consultation. These researchers found that even with those nurses who were aware of EC resources, a majority of them did not know how to request ethics consultation. Nurses in this study expressed reluctance to ask for ethics consultation primarily because of their fears of disrupting collegial relationships with attending physicians and other members of the health care team. The small group of nurses who stated they did feel comfortable making a request for an ethics consultation were the ones who reported supportive colleagues and managers and trusting relationships with their attending physicians. This notion of ethical climate's relation to constructive working conditions and relationships evokes Walker's (1993) conception of keeping "moral space" open within health care environments. The purpose of this kind of space is to facilitate an "integrated and inclusive process of moral negotiation" (Walker, 1993, p. 40). Achieving this kind of inclusiveness is difficult with interdisciplinary expectations and conflict. Shannon (1997) explored possible origins for the nature of interdisciplinary ethics conflict, noting that nurturing sensitivity to disciplinary perspectives may help attenuate discord. An organizational commitment to respect for the knowledge and accountability of colleagues, well-designed systems to detect and act on problems and errors, curiosity and honesty with regard to ethical discourse, and effective leadership promotes a culture of safety for patients and providers.

National and Global Levels

Numerous resources in health care ethics are available to nurses on national and international levels. The ANA, for example, is the professional organization representing the interests of all registered nurses in the United States. Membership in this organization provides access to extensive (including print) copies of texts relevant to discussions of ethics in nursing. Even without membership, it is possible to read the ANA Code of Ethics for Nurses and the various position papers on ethics and human rights (e.g., medical aid in dying, forgoing nutrition, and access to therapeutic marijuana) on the ANA website (https://www.nursing-world.org/practice-policy/nursing-excellence/official-position-statements/). A search of the position statements of the ANA illustrates the distinction in application between law and ethics. Capital punishment, although legal in more than a few states, is firmly opposed by the ANA. In fact, the 2016 position statement extends the role of the nurse from one of nonparticipation to one of open opposition. The current statement on medical aid in dying, in contrast, toes the tenuous line between ethics and the law by drawing a clear distinction between medical aid in dying and euthanasia and promoting a compassionate, informed approach to the nurses' role in end-of-life conversations and patients' requests for aid in dying. The ANA cites core values as espoused in the Code of Ethics for Nurses that undergird these position statements. The ANA website also provides extensive dialogue and further resources for ethical issues experienced by nurses.

The ICN, founded in 1899 by nurses in Germany, the United Kingdom, and the United States, is a federation of more than 128 national nurses' associations providing international guidelines for nursing practice and policy worldwide. This organization works with the World Health Organization and represents nursing at the annual World Health Assembly. The ICN Code of Ethics for Nurses (2021), freely available on their website (https://www.icn.ch/system/files/2021-10/ICN_Code-of-Ethics_EN_Web_0.pdf), emphasizes working collegially with coworkers to advance the health of individual patients, communities, and the natural environment. Policy statements (approved by all member associations) include those on ethical nurse recruitment, health care waste, and elimination of female genital mutilation.

In 2021, the National Academies of Sciences, Engineering, and Medicine published the Future of Nursing 2020–2030: Charting a Path to Achieve Health Equity (National Academies of Sciences, Engineering, and Medicine [NASEM], 2021), a comprehensive summary of key issues facing nursing and health care for the next decade. Among the recommendations for action are at least two that have ethical implications. Recommendation 3 addresses the need for nursing education programs, employers, nursing leaders, and others to ensure systemic structures that promote well-being among nurses. Given today's high-stress, high-pressure, high-stakes health care settings, maintaining a culture of safety, respect, and ethical practice for every health care provider (not only nurses) is essential for safe patient care. The Future of Nursing Report also addresses social determinants of health and health equity, critical issues that have been underemphasized, even ignored, for far too long.

Nursing education is changing, too, adopting the new American Association of Colleges of Nursing Essentials (American Association of Colleges of Nursing [AACN], 2021), which focuses on attainment of competency at the prelicensure and advanced practice levels. Within these Essentials, ethics finds itself in good company with foundational concepts for nursing such as clinical judgment, communication, compassionate care, diversity/equity/inclusion, evidence-based practice, health policy, and social determinants of health—all of which are threads that run throughout the ten competency domains.

SUMMARY

Nurses in today's health care system need a foundational understanding of ethics to practice. The health care system is complex, patient situations are complex, and the nurse's role in both is critical and often not intuitive. Understanding moral philosophy, professional ethics, nursing professional values, and nursing ethics provides a foundation for ethical nursing practice and decision making. As we recover physically, emotionally, and socially from the COVID-19 pandemic, we have begun to recognize the impact of nearly 2 years of exhaustion on health care providers. We have learned important lessons about health care organizations as moral communities, where all stakeholders—doctors, nurses, pharmacists, lab technicians, housekeeping, transportation, and organizational leaders—understand themselves to be obligated to the well-being and success of every other stakeholder in order to provide good, safe patient care (Epstein et al., 2020). The deepest underpinnings of health care systems are rooted in ethics. When confronted with a challenging situation, it is not necessary for the nurse to be able to analyze the situation and identify ethically appropriate actions. However, it is necessary for the nurse, as a member of a moral community, to provide information (perhaps using the Four Topics approach) to participate in the resolution of the case to the extent possible, to be accountable for that participation, and to know when to call the ethics consult service. It is also important that the nurse be aware that although the ethical challenge may be centered on the patient, there are often unit and organizational components at play. These should certainly be considered carefully and seriously, and the nurse can play an influential role in that, too. Finally, the ANA Code of Ethics for Nurses calls on us to be active on the national and global levels as well—to speak up, to work for social justice, to advance nursing practice, and to be engaged.

SALIENT POINTS

- Nurses play an important role in identifying and framing ethical problems at the bedside, on the unit, within the organization, within the nation, and on a global scale.
- Frameworks are available to help make sense of clinical, psychosocial, economic, and other contextual details so that they can be thoroughly considered in the process of finding good solutions to ethical problems.
- All health care providers can experience moral distress. Recognizing moral distress in self and others and acting on it may promote a healthy work environment.

CRITICAL REFLECTION EXERCISES

1. Think through the following scenario: Mr. Jones was a 64-year-old dying patient. Nurse Stiles cared for Mr. Jones on many occasions and learned that Mr. Jones had been a musician "back in the day" and that he had once had a close-knit family, including two siblings. About 10 years ago, there had been an argument and this divided Mr. Jones from his siblings. Since then, he has had very little contact with them. Mr. Jones and Nurse Stiles talk frequently about the old days and about the way he wants his life to end. He has not told either sibling that he is dying and says he "wants to keep it that way." Nurse Stiles has two siblings also, with whom she gets along well. Although Nurse Stiles understands Mr. Jones' wishes, she feels that if his siblings knew of their brother's situation, they could come and see him and make amends before Mr. Jones dies.
   - What actions would be appropriate if you considered only Nurse Stiles' virtues?

- What actions would be appropriate if you considered only Nurse Stiles' duties and obligations?
- What actions would be appropriate if you considered only the potential outcomes of the situation?

2. Consider what resources are available to you if you were to encounter an ethically challenging case at your institution. Discuss with your student peers what the available resources are and how you access them as a professional nurse.

ⓔ EVOLVE WEBSITE/RESOURCES LIST

American Medical Association: Principles of Medical Ethics: https://www.ama-assn.org/delivering-care/ama-principles-medical-ethics

American Nurses Association: http://www.nursingworld.org/MainMenuCategories/EthicsStandards
This site contains information on general ethics and moral distress.

American Society for Bioethics and Humanities: http://www.asbh.org

End-of-Life Nursing Education Consortium: https://www.aacnnursing.org/ELNEC

End-of-Life/Palliative Education Resource Center: http://www.caringcommunity.org/helpful-resources/models-research/end-of-lifepalliative-care-education-resource-center-medical-college-of-wisconsin-milwaukee/

International Council of Nurses: http://www.icn.ch

International Medical Interpreters Association Code of Ethics: http://www.imiaweb.org/code/default.asp

Kennedy Institute of Ethics: http://kennedyinstitute.georgetown.edu/

National Association of Social Workers Code of Ethics: https://www.socialworkers.org/About/Ethics/Code-of-Ethics/Code-of-Ethics-English

National Hospice and Palliative Care Organization: https://www.nhpco.org

National Human Genome Research Institute: http://www.genome.gov/issues/

National Institute of Health, State of Science Conference Statement on Improving End of Life Care: https://pubmed.ncbi.nlm.nih.gov/16219618/

Nuffield Council on Bioethics: http://www.nuffieldbioethics.org/

Respecting Choices®: https://respectingchoices.org/

Society of Critical Care Medicine: http://www.sccm.org

The Hastings Center: http://www.thehastingscenter.org/

U.S. National Library of Medicine Bioethics Information Resources: http://www.nlm.nih.gov/bsd/bioethics.html

Journal Resources

American Journal of Bioethics
Cambridge Quarterly Journal of Ethics
Hastings Center Report
HEC Forum
Journal of Clinical Ethics
Journal of Medical Ethics
Journal of Medicine and Philosophy
Kennedy Institute of Ethics Journal
Nursing Ethics

REFERENCES

American Association of Colleges of Nursing. (2021). *The essentials: Core competencies for professional nursing education.* https://www.aacnnursing.org/Portals/42/AcademicNursing/pdf/Essentials-2021.pdf

American Nurses Association. (2015). *Code of ethics for nurses.* https://www.nursingworld.org/practice-policy/nursing-excellence/ethics/

Austin, W. M., Rankel, M., & Kagan, L. (2005). To stay or to go, to speak or to stay silent, to act or not to act: Moral distress as experienced by psychologists. *Ethics and Behavior, 15*(3), 197–212. https://doi.org/10.1207/s15327019eb1503_1

Beauchamp, T., & Childress, J. (2019). *Principles of biomedical ethics* (8th ed.). Oxford University Press.

Bruce, C. R., Miller, S. M., & Zimmerman, J. L. (2015). A qualitative study exploring moral distress in the ICU team: The importance of unit functionality and intrateam dynamics. *Critical Care Medicine, 43*(4), 823–831. https://doi.org/10.1097/CCM.0000000000000822

Chambliss, D. F. (1996). *Beyond caring: Hospitals, nurses, and the social organization of ethics.* University of Chicago Press.

DeBruin, D., Liaschenko, J., & Marshall, M. F. (2012). Social justice in pandemic preparedness. *American Journal Public Health, 102*(4), 586–591. https://doi.org/10.2105/AJPH.2011.300483

Degrazia, D., Mappes, T. A., & Brand-Ballard, J. (2011). *Biomedical ethics* (7th ed.). McGraw-Hill.

Dodek, P. M., Wong, H., Norena, M., Ayas, N., Reynolds, S. C., Keenan, S. P., Hamric, A., Rodney, P., Stewart, M., & Alden, L. (2016). Moral distress in intensive care unit professionals is associated with profession, age, and years of experience. *Journal of Critical Care, 31*(1), 178–182. https://doi.org/10.1016/j.jcrc.2015.10.011

Drought, T. (2002). The privilege of bearing witness. *Nursing Ethics, 9*(3), 238–239. https://doi.org/10.1191/0969733002ne505xx

Elpern, E. H., Covert, B., & Kleinpell, R. (2005). Moral distress of staff nurses in a medical intensive care unit. *American Journal of Critical Care: An Official Publication, American Association of Critical-Care Nurses, 14*(6), 523–530.

Epstein, E. G. (2008). End-of-life experiences of nurses and physicians in the newborn intensive care unit. *Journal of*

Perinatology: Official Journal of the California Perinatal Association, 28(11), 771–778. https://doi.org/10.1038/jp.2008.96

Epstein, E. G., & Hamric, A. B. (2009). Moral distress, moral residue, and the crescendo effect. *The Journal of Clinical Ethics, 20*(4), 330–342. https://www.journals.uchicago.edu/doi/pdf/10.1086/JCE200920406?download=true

Epstein, E. G., Haizlip, J., Liaschenko, J., Zhao, D., Bennett, R., & Marshall, M. F. (2020). Moral distress, mattering, and secondary traumatic stress in provider burnout: A call for moral community. *AACN Advanced Critical Care, 31*(2), 146–157. https://doi.org/10.4037/aacnacc2020285

Epstein, E. G., Whitehead, P. B., Prompahakul, C., Thacker, L. R., & Hamric, A. B. (2019). Enhancing understanding of moral distress: The measure of moral distress for healthcare professionals. *AJOB Empirical Bioethics, 10*(2), 113–124. https://doi.org/10.1080/23294515.2019.1586008

Fantus, S., Greenberg, R. A., Muskat, B., & Katz, D. (2017). Exploring moral distress for hospital social workers. *The British Journal of Social Work, 47*(8), 2273–2290. https://doi.org/10.1093/bjsw/bcw113

Ford, P. J., & Dudzinski, D. M. (2008). *Complex ethics consultations: Cases that haunt us.* Cambridge University Press.

Fowler, M. (1997). Nursing's ethics. In A. J. Davis, M. A. Aroskar, J. Liaschenko, & T. S. Drought (Eds.), *Ethical dilemmas and nursing practice* (4th ed., pp. 17–34). Appleton & Lange.

Fry, S. T., & Grace, P. J. (2007). Ethical dimensions of nursing and health care. In J. L. Creasia, & B. J. Parker (Eds.), *Conceptual foundations: The bridge to professional nursing practice* (4th ed., pp. 273–299). Mosby.

Fry, S. T., & Veatch, R. M. (2006). *Case studies in nursing ethics* (3rd ed.). Jones & Bartlett.

Fumis, R. R. L., Junqueira Amarante, G. A., de Fátima Nascimento, A., & Vieira, J. M., Jr. (2017). Moral distress and its contribution to the development of burnout syndrome among critical care providers. *Annals of Intensive Care, 7*(71), 1–8. https://doi.org/10.1186/s13613-017-0293-2

Gallup. (2020). https://news.gallup.com/poll/274673/nurses-continue-rate-highest-honesty-ethics.aspx

Gordon, E. J., & Hamric, A. B. (2006). The courage to stand up: The cultural politics of nurses' access to ethics consultation. *The Journal of Clinical Ethics, 17*(3), 231–254.

Gostin, L. O. (2002). *Tarasoff v. Regents of California: Duty to warn.* https://web.archive.org/web/20141220125650/http://adoctorm.com/docs/tarasoff.htm

Hamric, A. B., & Blackhall, L. J. (2007). Nurse-physician perspectives on the care of dying patients in intensive care units: Collaboration, moral distress, and ethical climate. *Critical Care Medicine, 35*(2), 422–429. https://doi.org/10.1097/01.CCM.0000254722.50608.2D

Hamric, A. B., Borchers, C. T., & Epstein, E. G. (2012). Development and testing of an instrument to measure moral distress in healthcare professionals. *AJOB Primary Research, 3*(2), 1–9. https://doi.org/10.1080/21507716.2011.652337

Hamric, A. B., & Epstein, E. G. (2017). A health system wide moral distress consultation service: Development and evaluation. *HEC Forum, 29*(2), 127–143. https://doi.org/10.1007/s10730-016-9315-y

Hawkins, R. B., Charles, E. J., & Mehaffey, J. H. (2020). Socioeconomic status and COVID-19 related cases and fatalities. *Public Health, 189,* 129–134. https://doi.org/10.1016/j.puhe.2020.09.016

Institute of Medicine. (2001). *Crossing the quality chasm: A new health system for the 21st century.* National Academies Press.

International Council of Nurses. (2021). *ICN Code of ethics for nurses.* https://www.icn.ch/system/files/2021-10/ICN_Code-of-Ethics_EN_Web_0.pdf

Jameton, A. (1993). Dilemmas of moral distress: Moral responsibility and nursing practice. *AWHONN'S Clinical Issues in Perinatal and Women's Health Nursing, 4*(4), 542–551.

Johns Hopkins Coronavirus Resource Center. (2022). https://coronavirus.jhu.edu/data/disparity-explorer

Johnson-Coyle, L., Opgenorth, D., Bellows, M., Dhaliwal, J., Richardson-Carr, S., & Bagshaw S. M. (2016). Moral distress and burnout among cardiovascular surgery intensive care unit healthcare professionals: A prospective crosssectional survey. *Canadian Journal of Critical Care Nursing, 27*(4), 27–36.

Joint Commission International. (2020). *Joint Commission International accreditation standards for hospitals: Including standards for Academic Medical Center Hospitals* (7th ed.). Joint Commission Resources.

Jonsen, A. R., Siegler, M., & Winslade, W. J. (2022). *Clinical ethics: A practical approach to ethical decisions in clinical medicine* (9th ed.). McGraw-Hill.

Laabs, C. A. (2012). Confidence and knowledge regarding ethics among advanced practice nurses. *Nursing Education Perspectives, 33*(1), 10–14. https://doi.org/10.5480/1536-5026-33.1.10

Lewin, T. (1990). Nancy Cruzan dies, outlived by a debate over the right to die. *The New York Times.* http://www.nytimes.com/1990/12/27/us/nancy-cruzan-dies-outlived-by-a-debate-over-the-right-to-die.html

McFadden, R. D. (1995, June 12). Karen Ann Quinlan, 31, dies. *New York Times.* http://www.nytimes.com/1985/06/12/nyregion/karen-ann-quinlan-31-dies-focus-of-76-right-to-die-case.html

National Academies of Sciences, Engineering, and Medicine. (2021). *Future of nursing 2020–2030: Charting a path to achieve health equity.* National Academies Press.

Neumann, J. L., Davis, L. & Jernigan, C. (2018). Methods to address moral distress experienced by stem cell transplantation nurses and build resiliency. *Biology Blood Marrow Transplant, 24*(3), S117–S118. https://doi.org/10.1016/j.bbmt.2017.12.690

Paul, R., & Elder, L. (2013). *Ethical reasoning.* Foundation for Critical Thinking.

Pauly, B., Varcoe, C., Storch, J., & Newton, L. (2009). Registered nurses' perceptions of moral distress and ethical climate. *Nursing Ethics, 16*(5), 561–573. https://doi.org/10.1177/0969733009106649

Penny, N. H., Bires, S. J., Bonn, E. A., Dockery, A. N., & Pettit, N. L. (2016). Moral Distress Scale for Occupational Therapists: Part 1. Instrument development and content validity. *American Journal of Occupational Therapy, 70*(4), 7004300020. https://doi.org/10.5014/ajot.2015.018358

Penticuff, J. H., & Walden, M. (2000). Influence of practice environment and nurse characteristics on perinatal nurses' responses to ethical dilemmas. *Nursing Research, 49*(2), 64–72. https://doi.org/10.1097/00006199-200003000-00002

Price, D. (1995). An ethical perspective: ethics committees and nurses. *Journal of Nursing Law, 2*, 57–64.

Robb, I. (2008). *Nursing ethics for hospital and private use (1900)*. Kessinger.

Roig-Franzia, M. (2005, March 22). Schiavo case goes to federal judge. *The Washington Post*. http://www.washingtonpost.com/wp-dyn/articles/A53153-2005Mar21.html

Schumann, J. H., & Alfandre, D. (2008). Clinical ethical decision making: The four topics approach. *Seminars in Medical Practice, 11*, 36–42.

Schwenzer, K. J., & Wang, L. (2006). Assessing moral distress in respiratory care practitioners. *Critical Care Medicine, 34*(12), 2967–2973. https://doi.org/10.1097/01.CCM.0000248879.19054.73

Shannon, S. E. (1997). The roots of interdisciplinary conflict around ethical issues. *Critical Care Nursing Clinics of North America, 9*(1), 13–28.

Sporrong, S. K., Höglund, A. T., Hansson, M. G., Westerholm, P., & Arnetz, B. (2005). We are white coats whirling around: Moral distress in Swedish pharmacies. *Pharmacy World & Science, 27*(3), 223–239. https://doi.org/10.1007/s11096-004-3703-0

Taylor, C. (2011). *Fundamentals of nursing: The art and science of nursing care* (7th ed.). Lippincott Williams & Wilkins.

U.S. Department of Health and Human Services. (1996). *Health information privacy*. http://www.hhs.gov/ocr/privacy/

Vaughn, L. (2019). *Bioethics: Principles, issues, and cases* (4th ed.). Oxford University Press.

Virginia Statutes Health Care Decisions Act §54.1-2981-§54.1 2993. http://www.nrc-pad.org/images/stories/PDFs/virginia_adstatute.pdf

Walker, M. U. (1993). Keeping moral space open: New images of ethics consulting. *Hastings Center Report, 23*, 33–40. https://doi.org/10.2307/3562818

Whitehead, P. B., Herbertson, R. K., Hamric, A. B., Epstein, E. G., & Fisher, J. M. (2015). Moral distress among healthcare professionals: Report of an institution-wide study. *Journal of Nursing Scholarship: An Official Publication of Sigma Theta Tau International Honor Society of Nursing, 47*(2), 117–125. https://doi.org/10.1111/jnu.12115

13

Information Management

Daniel Todd Wilson, MLS

 http://evolve.elsevier.com/Friberg/bridge/

OBJECTIVES

At the completion of this chapter, the reader will be able to:
- Describe the qualities of an "information literate" person.
- Recognize the need for standardized languages for information retrieval in electronic systems.
- Understand the differences between keyword searching and searching using a controlled vocabulary in a citation database.

- Recognize the importance of citation management.
- Describe and give examples of the advantages of evidence-based practice to patient care.
- Explain the process of developing an answerable clinical question for improved information retrieval.
- Understand the expanding use of personal health records and describe some concerns that consumers may have with them.

INTRODUCTION

Information from all disciplines is expanding rapidly. In health care, the flood of electronic data may be compromising providers' abilities to find and use the best information. For clinicians, the "danger of missing key information while drowning in data is real" (Flood et al., 2010, p. 101). Internet search engines, like Google, return millions of hits per search term. Databases such as MEDLINE, the bibliographic database from the National Library of Medicine, contain millions of references from health sciences journals, and health care records systems are generating giant data sets that are being used to develop targeted treatments based on an individual's genetic makeup. For nurses, the skills and resources needed to filter and process this abundant information have become essential to improving patient care.

Recognizing that health care providers need to be equipped with basic computer skills, information literacy, and an understanding of informatics and information management, the Technology Informatics Guiding Education Reform (TIGER) initiative was formed in 2006. This summit brought together over 70 stakeholders who, after extensive evaluation of the state of informatics research,

education, and practice, developed the TIGER Nursing Informatics Competencies Model. This model contains three parts: Basic Computer Competencies, Information Literacy, and Information Management (The TIGER Initiative, 2008). The TIGER Initiative, along with the National League for Nursing 2008 position statement, and the best practices from the American Association of Colleges of Nursing (AACN) (2008), strongly urges the nursing profession to develop informatics competencies to deliver safer and more efficient care through the use of information technology. This chapter will describe the skills and concepts nurses need to know to manage information in the technology-based health care world.

INFORMATION MANAGEMENT

Health informatics includes the study of systems and information technology in health care, but "its focus is information management, not computers" (Sewell & Thede, 2013, p. 4). Information management is a process consisting of collecting data, processing data, and communicating that data as information or knowledge (The TIGER Initiative, 2008). Nurses have always managed patient data and are central to the communication of the information needed for ongoing patient care. Nurses must organize and develop medication records, orders, and care plans, whether that information is found in a written chart or an electronic medical record (EMR). The evolving information landscape, however, requires students and nurses to develop a renewed interest in best practices and processes and a desire to use online resources to answer the many questions that arise in nursing education, practice, and research.

INFORMATION LITERACY

Information literacy incorporates informatics and information management processes. To improve these nursing skills, it is helpful to establish connections with a librarian, especially a health sciences librarian, because they are important sources of instruction for nurses and faculty learning about the ever more complex world of information retrieval and management.

Basic Information Literacy Skills

When searching for scholarly journal literature, nurses will find that the best source for organized information on a topic is a citation database because, unlike an Internet search, content in a database has been evaluated for authority and accuracy. A citation in a bibliographic database is a record that contains details about a publication, such as the title, the authors' names, the journal name and volume, and often an abstract of the article. The citation record may link to the full text of an article if it is freely available or if the institution owns a subscription to the online version of the journal. It is essential that nurses be able to retrieve an article from a citation database. Once an article is found, nurses should be able to evaluate the reliability, validity, accuracy, authority, timeliness, and point of view or bias of the article (ACRL, 2013). Not all literature is of high quality, even if published in a journal, and the ability to evaluate an article is an important component of information literacy. Obtaining the skills to appropriately find and use scholarly information will enhance the nurse's ability to conduct research and implement quality improvements.

Information Retrieval

To be useful, information must be logically categorized and easily retrievable. Libraries have traditionally collected and cataloged nursing and medical information in books and databases, but now information can be stored in multiple places and retrieval has become an exercise in critical thinking. Where to go to find the correct source to answer a question is a complex task. A student's need to access information for an academic assignment in a baccalaureate nursing program will differ from that of a registered nurse (RN) in a hospital unit required to find and evaluate the evidence available for recommending a change in practice. Whether the information is accessed from the EMR on a bedside computer or the student's laptop, tablet computer, or mobile phone, the nurse must assess the reliability of the resource retrieved and effectively search through its content for the appropriate data, document, or website.

Nursing Languages. Nurses have collected information since Florence Nightingale began conducting her research in 1882, yet Sewell and Thede (2013) comment on the "invisibility of nursing" wherein, historically, nursing's contributions to patient care have not been adequately described or documented and nursing's value has not been easily measured. There are many groups working to standardize nursing terminologies to make the value of nursing care explicit and comparable in electronic systems. Nurses understand that the terms *decubitus ulcer* and *bed sore* are the same, but various information systems might not classify them in the same way. A common language allows for quality improvement based on data that are retrievable and equivalent to that of other hospitals and health care providers.

Primary Databases. A database is usually defined as a large collection of data organized for rapid electronic computer-based search and retrieval (Merriam-Webster, n.d.). The Cumulative Index to Nursing and Allied Health Record (CINAHL) is a database that provides the most comprehensive coverage of nursing literature (EBSCO, 2022). It indexes the contents of more than 3600 journals and also includes records of nursing dissertations, book chapters, and some conference proceedings. CINAHL is available only through a specific vendor, and it requires a paid subscription through a school or other institution. CINAHL can be searched using keywords and subject headings (controlled vocabulary). MEDLINE is the world's largest database for finding biomedical literature. MEDLINE can be searched by using either PubMed or Ovid MEDLINE. PubMed, the freely available version of MEDLINE (http://www.pubmed.gov), contains 33 million citations from MEDLINE, life science journals, and online books. Ovid MEDLINE (http://www.ovid.com) is a for-cost commercial database that searches MEDLINE. Both PubMed and Ovid MEDLINE can be searched using keywords or controlled vocabulary.

CINAHL and MEDLINE are the major databases needed for searching the medical and nursing literature; in addition, there are numerous other databases such as PsycINFO (http://www.apa.org/psycinfo/), Web of Science (http://webofknowledge.com/), and Education Resources Information Center (ERIC) (http://eric.ed.gov/) that can be helpful for nurses, especially now that there is an increasing focus on interdisciplinary research in health care.

Controlled Vocabularies in Journal Article Databases.

A database that organizes and arranges terms in subject headings is considered a controlled vocabulary database. PubMed, Ovid MEDLINE, and CINAHL each use controlled vocabularies. The Advanced Search option in CINAHL aids students and nurses by connecting natural language terms used by a searcher to an index of preferred subject terms. This is called *mapping*. If a student inputs the term *bed sores* into the search box in CINAHL, the term is mapped to the preferred Subject Heading *pressure ulcer*. The same mapping would take place if other synonyms were used in the initial search such as *decubitus ulcers* or even if alternative spellings and singular rather than plural terms were used, as when inputting the term *bedsore* instead of *bed sores*. The controlled vocabulary in PubMed and Ovid MEDLINE is called MeSH, which stands for Medical Subject Headings. PubMed automatically maps terms to MeSH, whereas Ovid MEDLINE requires the user to select MeSH based on a list of suggested MeSH terms. Scope Notes that define the subject term are also included in CINAHL, PubMed, and Ovid MEDLINE. These databases are set up with a hierarchical structure that allows searchers to narrow or expand their search. Expanding a search is known as exploding a term. Exploding the subject term *pressure ulcer* in CINAHL would result in a search that also contains citations related to specific types of pressure ulcers such as heel ulcers and deep tissue injuries. A broader term to use would be *skin ulcer*. To explode the term *skin ulcer* would result in citations about all types of skin ulcers, not just pressure ulcers. In MeSH and CINAHL, subheadings are available to limit a search even more precisely. When searching for articles about pressure ulcers, nurses may choose to limit their retrieval by using one or more of 40 narrower subheadings, ranging from "complications" to "prevention and control." There is also an ability to limit retrieval in CINAHL and MEDLINE to only those articles in which the topic is the major subject of an article by choosing "Major Concept" in CINAHL, "Focus" in Ovid MEDLINE, or "Major Topic" in PubMed.

Combining and Limiting Searches.

In most databases, searches can be combined using Boolean operators. The two most used Boolean operators are AND and OR. Fig. 13.1 shows how a search for *skin ulcer* AND *diabetes mellitus, type 2* will decrease the number of citations retrieved because the articles have to include both terms, but searching for *skin ulcer* OR *diabetes mellitus, type 2* will increase the number of results because the search will include all the articles that are about either one of these terms or both. Using the OR Boolean operator can result in a large number of irrelevant citations and hours of frustration for searchers. However, most databases include helpful ways to filter results using various limits to the articles retrieved. In MEDLINE and CINAHL, searches can be limited to article type and publication years, among other filters. For example, searchers may specify that their results only include publication types such as systematic reviews or randomized controlled trials (RCTs), or they may want to limit to research articles in CINAHL. For students, another valuable limit in CINAHL is a filter for only those journals that are peer-reviewed. This helps the searcher know that the articles retrieved are from scholarly sources and therefore more authoritative.

Using keywords for searching in a database or search engine is often the simplest way to find journal citations. Keep in mind that using keywords may miss other related terms that are captured using controlled vocabulary. An advantage to using keywords is that the most recent articles will be retrieved because it takes some time for an article to be indexed by an indexer. For the most thorough search, use a combination of keywords and controlled vocabulary. If the search requires a comprehensive literature search or a search for evidence-based information, it is helpful to consult with a librarian for help developing appropriate search strategies. It is important to save any search terms that were used and the results so as not to have to recreate the search from memory at a later time. Most databases have a "save search" option so search results can be saved temporarily or permanently, or results can be emailed or saved in a file.

Gray Literature

Gray literature encompasses all literature not found in journals. It includes dissertations; reports; documents from local, state, and federal agencies; conference proceedings; and white papers. Because gray literature does not go through the publishing process, which takes time, it may contain more current information. However, because it does not go through the publishing process, its authority and accuracy need to be assessed before using it as evidence to support changes. The value in using gray literature is the ability to compare data across international, national, regional, and local parameters; access to large survey data and results; expert opinion, guidelines, standards, or protocols; access to public domain technical and research reports; or issue briefs that supplement your scholarship. A simple process for finding gray literature is to use the Advanced Search option in Google. Enter search terms and then enter .edu, .gov, or .org in the site or domain field.

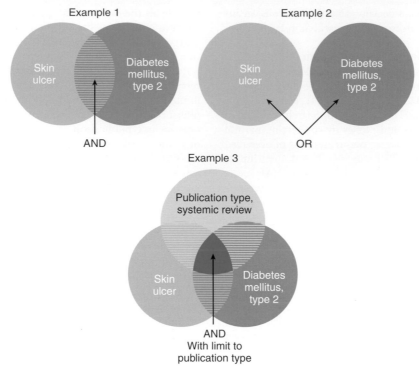

Fig. 13.1 Boolean Operators.

Mobile Computing Resources

Tablets and smartphones play an important role in nursing education and bedside care. Nurses use these devices to talk directly with other clinicians, use text messaging, or use e-mail (Broussard & Broussard, 2013). Some institutions allow access to the EMR and the Internet through wireless devices, and they may be used in education to provide podcasts, instructional videos, evidence-based guidelines, and reference materials. A common use of these devices is for retrieving drug information at the point of care. A popular free drug information resource for nurses is Epocrates Rx (http://www.epocrates.com/). Along with quick access to information, this resource allows users to include local formularies in search results. Other drug information resources include mobile Micromedex and Lexicomp. These and hundreds of other medical "apps" are available either for free or often for a low cost for Apple iOS (iPad, iPhone, iPod Touch) and Android-powered devices. Despite the many advantages of mobile devices in the workplace and education, there are concerns when implementing these new technologies such as "cost, frequent releases of new products, accessibility, interference, disease transmission, and confidentiality" (Phillippi & Wyatt, 2011, p. 451). With the

rapid development of medical apps, it can be difficult to assess their quality. Wu et al. (2011) found that though clinicians perceived an increase in efficiency from the use of smartphones, nurses in their study noted a perceived decrease in the quality of interprofessional relationships because of overreliance on electronic communication. Nurses may be very comfortable with the use of these devices for social connections in their personal lives, but because of these concerns, institutions must develop the appropriate infrastructure for the implementation of mobile devices in practice and clear policies for their use. In 2011, the ANA published *Principles for Social Networking and the Nurse: Guidance for the Registered Nurse*, which can be used as a general guide for nurses and nursing students to maintaining professional standards in new media environments (see https://www.nursingworld.org/~4af4f2/globalassets/docs/ana/ethics/social-networking.pdf).

Citation Management

Once a searcher has found relevant citations for a paper or project from a database search, whether the search was done from a desktop computer or smartphone, keeping these expanding collections stored in files on a computer is no longer adequate (Glassman & Sorensen, 2012).

Information-literate nurses must now understand the use of citation management software. Sometimes referred to as bibliographic or reference management software, these programs allow users to store, organize, output, and share their bibliographic citations online and on a local device (Childress, 2011). Most allow users to gather references automatically from article databases and format papers and citations instantly in a variety of styles, such as the American Psychological Association (APA) style. Users can generate bibliographies and save references in a personal database that they may then share with others. Glassman and Sorensen (2012) noted that, traditionally, citation management software was developed for desktop and laptop computers, but now there is a new focus on the use of these tools on mobile devices for easier "sharing, collaborating and social bookmarking" (p. 223). Some common citation management tools are EndNote, Mendeley, RefWorks, and Zotero. EndNote and RefWorks are commercial products, whereas Zotero (http://www.zotero.org) and Mendeley (http://www.mendeley.com/) are freely available online. Once again, it is important to collaborate with a librarian for help with answering questions about the basic features of these products, such as how to import citations from different databases, how to use word processors to input citations during the writing process, and how to generate a bibliography in a preferred output style.

EVIDENCE-BASED PRACTICE

Evidence-based practice (EBP) has been called the "key to delivering the highest quality of health care and ensuring the best patient outcomes" (Melnyk & Fineout-Overholt, 2011, p. 3). Learning the steps for retrieving, analyzing, and using best evidence tests the information literacy skills of any clinician, but Melnyk and Fineout-Overholt (2011) note that if clinicians can find and use information about best practices and if patients are confident that their providers use the best evidence in their care, outcomes are better for all. Research has clearly established that there are numerous advantages to basing nursing practice on evidence. EBP results in improvements in the quality of patient care, better patient outcomes, decreased health care costs, and enhanced work satisfaction for nurses (Brockopp et al., 2013; Melnyk et al., 2009, 2010; Poe et al., 2010). In addition, EBP is a standard for Magnet Recognition, the measure awarded by the American Nurses Credentialing Center as a means of recognizing hospitals that offer excellent nursing care (Drenkard, 2013). The standards contain a renewed focus on outcomes and stress more relevant data collection. The National Academy of Medicine also encourages nurses to lead and manage collaborative efforts with physicians and other members of

the health care team, conduct research, and redesign and improve practice environments and health systems (Institute of Medicine [IOM], 2011). However, even with these institutional calls to incorporate EBP into all nursing care, barriers to implementing these practices are still present. Challenges to implementing EBP include a lack of time, resources, and organizational support (Shaffer et al., 2013). The EBP process has been comprehensively described by many authors (Melnyk & Fineout-Overholt, 2011; Poe et al., 2010; Rosswurm & Larrabee, 1999; Sackett, 2000; Titler et al., 2001) and models have been developed to help clinicians understand the components and implementation of EBP. The Johns Hopkins Nursing Evidence-Based Practice Process involves three major components called PET: Practice Question, Evidence, and Translation (Poe et al., 2010), whereas Melnyk et al. (2010) list the following seven steps of EBP:

Step 0: Cultivate a spirit of inquiry.
Step 1: Ask clinical questions in PICOT format.
Step 2: Search for the best evidence.
Step 3: Critically appraise the evidence.
Step 4: Integrate the evidence with clinical expertise and patient preferences and values.
Step 5: Evaluate the outcomes of the practice decisions or changes based on evidence.
Step 6: Disseminate EBP results.

The steps of EBP often begin with the formulation of an answerable clinical question, yet, as Levin and Feldman (2013) found, clarifying that question still can be a challenge for clinicians. Learning to articulate a clearly defined question is a skill that should be practiced because it will aid in the selection of the best resource to consult for an answer. When choosing a resource to search, it is important to know if the information needed is a background question or a foreground question (Noble, 2001). Background questions are those that look for general knowledge or summary information about a disease, a problem, or a population. An example of a background question would be, "What is the pathophysiology of pressure ulcers?" These types of questions may be best answered by a textbook, an online textbook such as UpToDate (http://www.uptodate.com/), or a review article. Foreground questions ask for specific knowledge to inform clinical decisions and these types of questions tend to be more complex than background questions (Fineout-Overholt & Johnston, 2005). Quite often, foreground questions investigate comparisons. A foreground question might be, "Are there special beds or mattresses that are more effective than standard hospital beds for preventing pressure ulcers in nursing home populations?" Foreground questions are best answered by searching scholarly journal databases such as MEDLINE and CINAHL, or specific evidence-based collections such as the Cochrane Database of Systematic Reviews (http://www.cochrane.org/) and Joanna Briggs Institute (http://www.joannabriggs.org). See Chapter 4: Fostering a Spirit of Inquiry—The Role of Nurses in Evidence-Based Practice for more information about evidence-based practice.

Framing the Clinical Question

Framing and focusing a question in a structured way helps the nurse search for and retrieve relevant answers. The Cochrane Collaboration recommends that the clinical question should specify the types of population (participants), types of interventions (and comparisons), and the types of outcomes that are of interest. The acronym PICO (Participants, Interventions, Comparisons, and Outcomes) helps serve as a reminder of these (Higgins & Green, 2011). Other formulations use the PICOT template (Population, Intervention, Comparison or Control, Outcomes, and Time). The T in this format stands for "time frame." This component is included when it is important to know the time it takes for the intervention to achieve the outcome or when a population has been followed for a particular length of time (Huang et al., 2006; Melnyk & Fineout-Overholt, 2011). An example of using the PICO format with the question of whether there are special types of mattresses that help prevent pressure ulcer formation in nursing home residents would be organized like this:

Population—Nursing home residents
Intervention—Special mattresses
Comparison—Standard mattresses
Outcome—Prevention of pressure ulcers

A librarian is important to include in any group searching for evidence to initiate or change clinical practice because formulating a well-developed question and conducting a comprehensive search using controlled vocabulary can be challenging.

Levels of Evidence

After a literature search for evidence has been completed, the next step is to review the citations by scanning the abstract or retrieving and reading the full text of articles to determine which articles best answer the clinical question. The searcher must then assess the level of evidence each article represents. Organizations such as the Cochrane Collaboration and the Joanna Briggs Institute develop systematic reviews and metaanalyses considered to be the "gold standard" of health care evidence. A systematic review finds all the existing primary research on a topic that meets certain criteria, and this is assessed using stringent guidelines to establish whether there is conclusive evidence about a specific treatment or test. Cochrane only selects RCTs to combine for their systematic reviews or metaanalyses because RCTs are considered to have the most rigorous study design. Randomly assigning subjects in an experiment is like flipping a coin as to who receives an intervention or not. This minimizes the bias inherent in other types of studies. Metaanalysis is the statistical combination of results from two or more separate studies (Higgins & Green, 2011), and this can represent an even higher level of evidence because the combined number of participants increases the certainty of the results. Qualitative studies represent a lower level of evidence because this type of research is not generalizable as is quantitative research such as RCTs. Many organizations and authors have developed various frameworks for establishing their own levels of evidence. Levels range from 1 through 8 in Melnyk and Fincout-Overholt's scale (Melnyk et al., 2010), 1 to 3 in DynaMed (https://dynamed.ebscohost.com/content/levels-of-evidence), or 1 to 5 at the Oxford Center for Evidence-Based Medicine (CEBM, 2013) (http://www.cebm.net/?o = 1025). Usually, the lowest level of evidence on a scale is considered to be case studies or narrative opinions of experts, although some put animal studies at the bottom (Fig. 13.2).

After completing a comprehensive database search, research evidence for a decision may be lacking, so it is important in the decision-making process to examine and evaluate other types of available evidence, such as those guidelines found in a gray literature search. Other sources of evidence may come from clinical guidelines and recommendations from national and local professional organizations. It is important to remember that not all clinical guidelines can be considered evidence-based. It is necessary to read the guideline to determine how the guideline was classified and which ranking scale was used for its recommendations.

Critical Appraisal

Establishing the evidence level of an article is important, but this is only part of critically appraising the quality of a study. Critical appraisal requires specific skills. Time is needed to establish if a study provides valid and reliable evidence that can be applied to the clinician's and the patient's specific circumstances. To assist busy clinicians, new consolidated resources are available that can be quickly accessed at the point of care. These resources, including DynaMed, Essential Evidence Plus (http://www.essentialevidenceplus.com/), Mosby's Nursing (https://systematicreviewsjournal.biomedcentral.com/), the Joanna Briggs Institute (http://www.joannabriggs.org), and Evidence Summaries (https://systematicreviewsjournal.biomedcentral.com/), contain prefiltered evidence based information in which all content has been evaluated and given a strength of evidence or strength of recommendation rating.

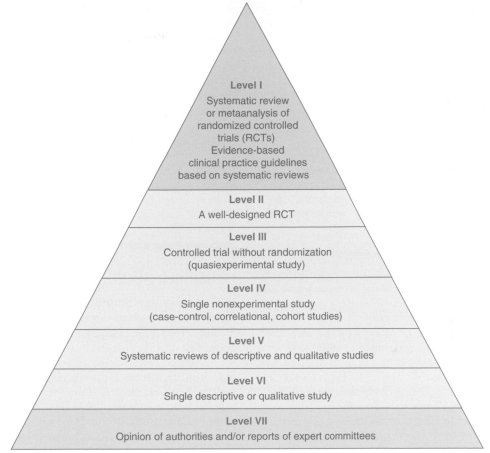

Fig. 13.2 Levels of Evidence Pyramid. (From LoBiondo Woods, G., & Haber, J. [2010]. *Nursing research* [7th ed.]. Mosby.)

One way for nurses to learn more about critical appraisal of research studies is to institute a journal club. Journal clubs usually meet face to face to discuss a particular article of interest with a group. Berger et al. (2011) note that journal clubs both educate nurses and improve clinical practice by helping them learn how to translate research into improved patient care. Nurses learn to analyze the quality of studies and become more familiar with the process of critical appraisal in a supportive setting. Nurses may be too busy to meet face-to-face, however, so the authors suggest forming a virtual journal club using a video conferencing platform such as Teams or Zoom, or a blog format that allows text-based interactions among participants. In addition, publishers may have online journal clubs as one of their evidence-based tools available to users. Such online journal clubs often guide the user through an appraisal of different types of literature for their quality.

Implementing Evidence-Based Practice

Once the evidence has been gathered and appraised, clinical judgment is required before implementation is considered. Describing the process of implementing evidence into clinical practice has been comprehensively outlined by Melynk and Fineout-Overholt, Sackett, Poe, and others (Melnyk & Fineout-Overholt, 2011; Poe et al., 2010; Sackett, 2000). Expert support and guidance from administration and experienced research mentors will always be necessary to promote the collaborative effort and find the time in a busy unit schedule needed to complete an EBP project. Shaffer et al. (2013, pp. 359–360) developed a set of recommendations for the bedside nurse to consider when implementing an evidence-based project:

- Realize that the EBP process will take longer than anticipated.

- Identify and involve staff nurses who are invested in the project. The group should include five to eight nurses, depending on the scope of the project.
- Involve clinical and research experts to help identify the scope of the project, assist with the process, and establish a realistic timeline to understand the concept and to plan accordingly.
- Identify an EBP model to follow that all can easily understand and use.
- Set goals and a timeline. Be prepared to modify the timeline as needed.
- Communicate the plan not only to each member of the team but also to the nurse manager and all appropriate staff members responsible for project implementation.
- Remember the following three key words: *time*, *patience*, and *perseverance*.

Keeping Current With New Evidence

Results of new studies are published every day; so many databases such as CINAHL, PubMed, and the search engine Google Scholar allow users to save their searches so they can be updated as new information appears. In these databases, searches may be saved as alerts and users then receive an e-mail or a rich site summary (RSS) feed with any new citations that match the search strategy. Nurses also may sign up for journal table-of-contents services either through a database or directly through the publisher's website. Many journals are published for specialty areas such as critical care or perianesthesia nursing, so receiving information about the current contents of a specific journal can help nurses keep up on the latest topics in their field. Online services such as QxMD (https://qxmd.com/) and Medscape (http://www.medscape.com/) deliver free journal articles and news to users based on a personalized registration profile. The commercial product BrowZine (http://www.browzine.com) is available at many academic health systems. BrowZine provides the user the ability to create a personalized bookshelf of favorite journals and alerts them when a new issue is available.

Dissemination

It is important to the nursing profession that information from new research and programs be widely disseminated. There are various venues for presenting content to an audience. Poster sessions are presentations of information by individuals or representatives of teams at a congress or conference with an academic or professional focus. Poster guidelines are determined by the specific event and will dictate the size, orientation, or other features identified by the event sponsors such as deadlines for submission. Along with poster presentations, nurses are often called upon to give individual or panel presentations about their research

at a meeting or asked to write an article for publication in a scholarly journal. To encourage authors to submit information about their scholarly activities, conference providers will often send out a "call for abstracts" for posters or presentations. *An abstract* is defined as a brief written statement of the main points or facts in a longer report, speech, etc. (Merriam-Webster, n.d.). Weinert (2010) notes that the importance of the abstract is often overlooked and a well-crafted abstract is essential for having nursing research and writing noticed and accepted. Faculty and clinical mentors must be readily available for new nurse authors learning the article submission process. One method of providing this type of support is described by Hoke and Papa (2014), who developed a three-part workshop that included a process of peer review to provide authors with guidance and encouragement for the development of successful abstracts.

CONSUMER HEALTH INFORMATION

Personal Health Records

Personal health records can be part of the Medicare and Medicaid Electronic Health Record (EHR) Incentive Programs that provide financial incentives for the meaningful use of certified EHR technology to improve patient care. To receive an EHR incentive payment, providers must show that they are "meaningfully using" their EHRs by meeting thresholds for a number of objectives. The meaningful use objectives are grouped into five patient-driven domains that relate to health outcomes policy priorities (HealthIT.gov, 2019):

- Improve Quality, Safety, Efficiency
- Engage Patients and Families
- Improve Care Coordination
- Improve Public and Population Health
- Ensure Privacy and Security for Personal Health Information

The "Blue Button" is a technology that allows consumers to download their personal health information online and U.S. military veterans have had access to their online records since 2010. The Veterans Administration (VA) was the first to display the Blue Button symbol on its patient portal, but now many other health care providers and plans are using this technology. Leadership of the initiative to promote this technology is by the Office of the National Coordinator for Health Information Technology. Technology is being developed that will allow consumers to better share their Blue Buttoned information with others they trust and plug them into new apps and tools. "With more than half of Americans using smartphones today and an abundance of popular health apps and tools such as digital pedometers, glucose monitors, and sleep sensors, consumers are becoming an undeniable part of the equation for better health and health care through health information technology" (Ricciardi, 2013, para. 8).

Health Literacy

It is hoped that the information accessible through a PHR will help health care consumers in making informed health decisions, although concerns need to be addressed around the issue of the literacy level of its users. The Patient Protection and Affordable Care Act of 2010, Title V, defines *health literacy* as the degree to which an individual has the capacity to obtain, communicate, process, and understand basic health information and services to make appropriate health decisions. Concerns regarding health literacy were described in 2004 by the Institute of Medicine (IOM), which convened the Committee on Health Literacy to write *Health Literacy: A Prescription to End Confusion*. The report notes that while individuals are expected to maintain their own health and the health of their families and communities, consumers rely heavily on the health information that is available to them. This information is at the core of the partnerships that patients and their families forge with today's complex modern health systems. Yet many Americans cannot understand the information given to them by health care personnel (Institute of Medicine [IOM], 2004). The National Assessment of Adult Literacy (NAAL) has found that more than a third of U.S. adults would have trouble with common health tasks, such as following directions on a prescription drug label or adhering to a childhood immunization schedule using a standard chart (U.S. Department of Education, 2006). Berkman et al. (2011) found that low health literacy was consistently associated with decreased ability to understand health messages, less ability to understand labels and take medication appropriately, lower receipt of screening mammograms and flu vaccinations, more hospitalizations, greater use of emergency care, and, among elderly people, worse overall health status and higher mortality rates. Health literacy is also discussed in Chapter 15: Health and Health Promotion and Chapter 17: Global Rural Nursing Practice.

Nurses can recognize the diverse information needs of their patients and use tested strategies to assist them. Koh et al. (2012, pp. 2–3) found that certain procedures help patients deal with complicated and confusing forms and instructions:

- Simplifying and making written materials easier to understand using things such as simple pictograms when educating about medications.
- Improving providers' communication skills by having providers receive feedback on their education methods with low literacy patients.
- Improving patients' self-management skills by developing self-care, picture-based educational materials, and

using scheduled telephone follow-ups to reinforce adherence to necessary medication regimens and instructions.

Patient education information is provided by hundreds of different vendors. Some commercial vendors such as Krames StayWell (http://kramesstaywell.com) can be integrated into the EMSR. Many commercial products provide information at a targeted reading level—usually fifth to eighth grade—and often provide their patient information in multiple languages.

Consumer Health Information Resources on the Internet

In 2013 Fox and Duggan found that 72% of U.S. patients searched for online health information. Most used search engines such as Google or Bing to begin their search. Though patients persistently use the Internet for information, they still turn for help to health care providers for serious health concerns or questions (Fox & Duggan, 2013). This raises an opportunity for nurses not only to provide tailored education to patients seeking information at the point of care but also to educate patients on how to access quality information when searching on their own. The National Library of Medicine's consumer health database, MedlinePlus (http://medlineplus.gov/), is considered to be one of the most reliable sources of advertisement-free health information on the Internet. MedlinePlus contains information on more than 900 health topics in English and Spanish, plus videos, tutorials, and other multimedia content. It has easy-to-read information and links to information in multiple languages. This is a resource that should be recommended to patients and consumers as a place to start a search for health care information. There are also thousands of other competing health information sources found on the Internet, such as the popular and authoritative Mayo Clinic (http://mayoclinic.org/). Many are commercial sites such as WebMD, which permit advertisements on their pages, and many are provided by organizations such as the American Academy of Family Physicians (http://www.familydoctor.org/) or the American Cancer Society (http://www.cancer.org/). The information seeker needs, at a minimum, to be aware of the authority of the authors of such sites and the currency of the information, and users need to be able to verify the information they find at a site by finding similar information from other sources. Many consumers like to use the Internet to find others who share a particular medical condition. Websites such as PatientsLikeMe (http://www.patientslikeme.com/) allow patients to connect with others online to discuss concerns about symptoms and medical treatments. These sites promote open sharing, but there is always a need to understand the level of privacy afforded by the site before disclosing personal health information.

SUMMARY

Health care resources and processes are rapidly evolving. Nurses must learn the most effective ways to manage the information generated by new electronic systems to provide quality care. Although sometimes challenging in practice, students and bedside nurses need well-developed information retrieval skills to ensure they are finding the best available evidence. Nurses should also take an active part in synthesizing and critically appraising information to implement best practices in their settings. Health care consumers are now seeking health information at expanding rates and nurses can offer essential guidance in helping these consumers find quality resources that are appropriate to their level of health literacy.

SALIENT POINTS

- Nurses must position themselves to manage the expanding amount of information being generated in academic and health care settings.
- Information literacy requires the development of skills to find, analyze, and use electronic information.
- Information can be retrieved from multiple formats, including the Internet, bibliographic databases, EMR, and personal health records.
- Mobile resources will continue to play a large part in data entry and point-of-care retrieval.
- Nursing stakeholders must continue to improve the cross-mapping of nursing terminologies in larger electronic records systems to ensure the interoperability and inclusion of critical nursing data.
- Learning effective strategies for finding reliable information will become increasingly important as the majority of health care institutions broaden their focus on the provision of evidence-based care.
- Collaboration with a librarian, especially a medical librarian, is important when developing a comprehensive literature search for medical or nursing information.
- Evidence-based practice requires time for skill development and support from administrators for bedside nurses to be successful in its implementation.
- Personal health records are improving consumers' access to personal medical information, although privacy concerns should continue to be addressed.
- Research has shown that limited health literacy leads to poorer health care outcomes, so nurses have an obligation to make sure the information they provide is understandable and sensitive to the patient's unique needs.

CRITICAL REFLECTION EXERCISES

1. Find the website of an academic medical library such as the Hardin Library of the Health Sciences (http://www.lib.uiowa.edu/hardin/) or the Duke Medical Center Library (https://mclibrary.duke.edu/) and determine whether they provide subject guides for nursing or evidence-based practice.
2. Conduct a search for a topic (e.g., pressure ulcer) that can be mapped to a Subject Heading in CINAHL. Compare the results to a keyword search for the same topic in a search engine such as Google.
3. Develop a clinical question in the PICOT format and consider how you would begin to search for the answer to this question in a database such as MEDLINE or CINAHL.
4. Search http://medlineplus.gov/ for the topic "asthma." Find and review an interactive tutorial on this topic and determine how you might use this resource for patient care.
5. Using Google Advanced Search, find the gray literature item *New Ways to Identify and Treat Sepsis* from the Texas Medical Center. *Hint:* Type *sepsis* in a search field and then limit your search by typing .edu in the site or domain field.

ⓔ EVOLVE WEBSITE/RESOURCES LIST

- *American Academy of Family Physicians:* http://familydoctor.org
- *American Cancer Society*: http://www.cancer.org/
- *BrowZine*: http://www.browzine.com
- *Cochrane Database of Systematic Reviews*: http://www.cochrane.org/
- *DynaMed*: https://dynamed.cbscohost.com/content/LOE
- *Epocrates Rx*: http://www.epocrates.com/
- *ERIC*: http://eric.ed.gov/

- *Essential Evidence Plus*: http://www.essentialevidenceplus.com/
- *Evidence Summaries*: https://systematicreviewsjournal.biomedcentral.com/
- *Google Scholar*: http://scholar.google.com/
- *Joanna Briggs Institute*: http://joannabriggs.org
- *Krames StayWell*: http://kramesstaywell.com
- *MedlinePlus*: http://medlineplus.gov
- *Medscape*: http://www.medscape.com
- *Mendeley*: http://www.mendeley.com/
- *Mosby's Nursing Consult*: https://www.clinicalkey.com/nursing/#!/
- *Ovid MEDLINE*: http://www.ovid.com
- *Oxford Center for Evidence-Based Medicine*: http://www.cebm.net/?o = 1025
- *PatientsLikeMe*: http://www.patientslikeme.com/
- *PsycINFO*: http://www.apa.org/psycinfo/
- *PubMed*: http://www.pubmed.gov
- *QxMD*: https://qxmd.com/
- *UpToDate*: http://www.uptodate.com/
- *Web of Science*: http://webofknowledge.com/
- *Zotero*: http://www.zotero.org

REFERENCES

Abstract. (n.d.) *Merriam-Webster.com dictionary*. https://www.merriam-webster.com/dictionary/abstract

American Association of Colleges of Nursing. (2008). *The essentials of baccalaureate education for professional nursing practice*. http://www.aacnnursing.org/Portals/42/Publications/BaccEssentials08.pdf

Association of College and Research Libraries. (2013, October 31). *Information literacy competency standards for nursing*. http://www.ala.org/acrl/standards/nursing

Berger, J., Hardin, H. K., & Topp, R. (2011). Implementing a virtual journal club in a clinical nursing setting. *Journal for Nurses in Staff Development*, 27(3), 116–120. https://doi.org/10.1097/nnd.0b013e318217b3bc

Berkman, N. D., Sheridan, S. L., Donahue, K. E., Halpern, D. J., & Crotty, K. (2011). Low health literacy and health outcomes: An updated systematic review. *Annals of Internal Medicine*, 155(2), 97–107. https://doi.org/10.7326/0003-4819-155-2-201107190-00005

Brockopp, D. Y., Moe, K., Corley, D., & Schreiber, J. (2013). The Baptist Health Lexington evidence-based practice model. *Journal of Nursing Administration*, 43(4), 187–193. https://www.jstor.org/stable/26811567

Broussard, B. S., & Broussard, A. B. (2013). Using electronic communication safely in health care settings. *Nursing for Women's Health*, 17(1), 59–62. https://doi.org/10.1111/1751-486x.12007

Centre for Evidence-Based Medicine. (2013). *Oxford Centre for evidence-based medicine: Levels of evidence*. http://www.cebm.net/index.aspx?o=1025

Childress, D. (2011). Citation tools in academic libraries: Best practices for reference and instruction. *Reference & User Services Quarterly*, 51(2), 143–152. https://www.jstor.org/stable/10.2307/refuseserq.51.2.143

Database. (n.d.). *Merriam-Webster.com dictionary*. https://www.merriam-webster.com/dictionary/database

Drenkard, K. (2013). Change is good. *Journal of Nursing Administration*, 43(10), 489–490. https://www.doi.org/10.1097/NNA.0b013e3182a3e7e7

EBSCO Information Services. (2022). *CINAHL database: Cumulative index to nursing and allied health*. http://www.ebscohost.com/nursing/products/cinahl-databases/the-cinahl-database

Fineout-Overholt, E., & Johnston, L. (2005). Teaching EBP: Asking searchable, answerable clinical questions. *Worldviews on Evidence-Based Nursing*, 2(3), 157–160. https://doi.org/10.1111/j.1741-6787.2005.00032.x

Flood, L. S., Gasiewicz, N., & Delpier, T. (2010). Integrating information literacy across a BSN curriculum. *Journal of Nursing Education*, 49(2), 101–104. https://doi.org/10.3928/01484834-20091023-01

Fox, S., & Duggan, M. (2013, January 15). *Health online 2013*. http://www.pewinternet.org/2013/01/15/health-online-2013/

Glassman, N. R., & Sorensen, K. (2012). Citation management. *Journal of Electronic Resources in Medical Libraries*, 9(3), 223–231. https://doi.org/10.1080/15424065.2012.707097

HealthIT.gov. (2019, October 19). *EHR incentives & certification: Meaningful use definition & objectives*. https://www.healthit.gov/topic/meaningful-use-and-macra/meaningful-use-and-macra

Higgins, J., & Green, S. E. (2011). *Cochrane handbook for systematic reviews of interventions version 5.1.0*. The Cochrane Collaboration. http://handbook-5-1.cochrane.org/

Hoke, L. M., & Papa, A. M. (2014). Increasing the odds, using peer review promotes successful abstract submission. *Clinical Nurse Specialist CNS*, 28(1), 46–55. https://doi.org/10.1097/NUR.0000000000000019

Huang, X., Lin, J., & Demner-Fushman, D. (2006). Evaluation of PICO as a knowledge representation for clinical questions. *AMIA Annual Symposium Proceedings*, 359–363. https://www.ncbi.nlm.nih.gov/pmc/articles/PMC1839740/

Institute of Medicine. (2004). *Health literacy: A prescription to end confusion*. National Academies Press. http://doi.org/10.17226/10883

Institute of Medicine. (2011). *The future of nursing: Leading change, advancing health*. National Academies Press. https://doi.org/10.17226/12956

Koh, H. K., Berwick, D. M., Clancy, C. M., Baur, C., Brach, C., Harris, L. M., & Zerhusen, E. G. (2012). New federal policy initiatives to boost health literacy can help the nation move beyond the cycle of costly "crisis care." *Health Affairs (Project Hope)*, 31(2), 434–443. https://doi.org/10.1377/hlthaff.2011.1169

Levin, R. F., & Feldman, H. R. (2013). *Teaching evidence-based practice in nursing* (2nd ed.). Springer.

LoBiondo-Woods, G., & Haber, J. (2010). *Nursing research* (7th ed.). Mosby.

Melnyk, B. M., & Fineout-Overholt, E. (2011). *Evidence-based practice in nursing & healthcare: A guide to best practice* (2nd ed.). Wolters Kluwer/Lippincott Williams & Wilkins.

Melnyk, B. M., Fineout-Overholt, E., Stillwell, S. B., & Williamson, K. M. (2009). Evidence-based practice: Step by step: Igniting a spirit of inquiry: An essential foundation for evidence-based practice: How nurses can build the knowledge and skills they need to implement ERP. *American Journal of Nursing, 109*(11), 49–52. https://doi.org/10.1097/01.NAJ.0000363354.53883.58

Melnyk, B. M., Fineout-Overholt, E., Stillwell, S. B., & Williamson, K. M. (2010). Evidence-based practice: Step by step: The seven steps of evidence-based practice. *The American Journal of Nursing, 110*(1), 51–53. https://doi.org/10.1097/01.NAJ.0000366056.06605.d2

Noble, J. (2001). *Textbook of primary care medicine* (3rd ed.). Mosby.

Phillippi, J. C., & Wyatt, T. H. (2011). Smartphones in nursing education. *CIN: Computers, Informatics, Nursing, 29*(8), 449–454. https://doi.org/10.1097/NCN.0b013e318fc4aaf

Poe, S., White, K. M., Sigma Theta Tau International, & Johns Hopkins University. (2010). *Johns Hopkins nursing evidence-based practice*. Sigma Theta Tau International.

Ricciardi, L. (2013, September 12). *The blue button movement: Kicking off National Health IT Week with consumer engagement.* http://www.healthit.gov/buzz-blog/electronic-health-and-medical-records/blue-button-movement-kicking-national-health-week-consumer-engagement/

Rosswurm, M. A., & Larrabee, J. H. (1999). A model for change to evidence-based practice. *Image: The Journal of Nursing Scholarship, 31*(4), 317–322. https://doi.org/10.1111/j.1547-5069.1999.tb00510.x

Sackett, D. L. (2000). *Evidence-based medicine: How to practice and teach EBM* (2nd ed.). Churchill Livingstone.

Sewell, J. P., & Thede, L. Q. (2013). *Informatics and nursing: Opportunities and challenges* (4th ed.). Wolters Kluwer Health/Lippincott Williams & Wilkins.

Shaffer, S. T., Zarnowsky, C. D., Green, R., Lim, M. L., Holtzer, B. M., & Ely, E. A. (2013). Strategies from bedside nurse perspectives in conducting evidence-based practice projects to improve care. *Nursing Clinics of North America, 48*(2), 353–361. https://doi.org/10.1016/j.cnur.2013.01.004

The TIGER Initiative. (2008). *The TIGER initiative informatics competencies for every practicing nurse: Recommendations from the TIGER collaborative.* https://www.google.com/url?sa=t&rct=j&q=&esrc=s&source=web&cd=&ved=2ahUKEwjTlZLqwo72AhW1rHIEHf4kAN4QFnoECAYQAQ&url=http%3A%2F%2Fwww.tigersummit.com%2Fuploads%2F3.Tiger.Report_Competencies_final.pdf&usg=AOvVaw0YeRe6sZMspa6JUznznqWWs

Titler, M. G., Kleiber, C., Steelman, V. J., Rakel, B. A., Budreau, G., Everett, L. Q., Buckwalter, K. C., Tripp-Reimer, T., & Goode, C. J. (2001). The Iowa model of evidence-based practice to promote quality care. *Critical Care Nursing Clinics of North America, 13*(4), 497–509. https://doi.org/10.1016/S0899-5885(18)30017-0

U.S. Department of Education. (2006). *Retrieved from the health literacy of America's adults: Results from the 2003 National Assessment of Adult Literacy.* http://nces.ed.gov/pubs2006/2006483.pdf

Weinert, C. (2010). Are all abstracts created equal? *Applied Nursing Research, 23*(2), 106–109. https://doi.org/10.1016/j.apnr.2008.06.003

Wu, R., Rossos, P., Quan, S., Reeves, S., Lo, V., Wong, B., Cheung, M., & Morra, D. (2011). An evaluation of the use of smartphones to communicate between clinicians: A mixed-methods study. *Journal of Medical Internet Research, 13*(3), e59. https://doi.org/10.2196/jmir.1655

14

Diversity, Equity, and Inclusion: Impact on Health Care and Nursing Care Strategies

Malinda L. Whitlow, DNP, FNP-BC, RN, Gretchen Wiersma, DNP, RN, CNE, CHSE, and Elizabeth E. Friberg, DNP, RN

 http://evolve.elsevier.com/Friberg/bridge/

OBJECTIVES

At the completion of this chapter, the reader will be able to:

- Differentiate between the concepts of inclusion, diversity, and equity.
- Identify societal factors affecting the delivery of culturally responsive nursing care in the United States.
- Describe methods used to incorporate cultural humility concepts within clinical practice.
- Explain the role of culture and social determinants of health in the holistic care of the client.

- Identify how social determinants of health impact access to care in the United States.
- Discuss strategies to approach diverse populations in the provision of inclusive care.
- Examine how strategies to approach diverse populations can improve the outcomes for patients, families, communities, and health care organizations.

INTRODUCTION

The United States population becomes more diverse each passing year. It is projected that by 2044 more than half of the U.S. population will belong to a minority group, which is any group other than non-Hispanic White (Colby & Ortman, 2015). These population changes anticipated over the next few decades will directly affect all aspects of our society, including health care delivery. Health care organizations have a growing responsibility to improve diversity, equity, and inclusion (DEI) in employment to serve patients and their families better. Having a diverse workforce within U.S. social systems (i.e., educational, judicial, and health care) will reinforce inclusive and nondiscriminatory beliefs and values in meeting the needs of all. Diversifying the health care workforce to include nursing is one strategy; another approach provides tools for the current and future nursing workforce to render care that is not biased, is equitable, inclusive, and considers the patient's cultural beliefs. To do this, nurses must be aware of the many influencing factors that might impact health and health care delivery.

This chapter provides a list of important DEI terms and definitions (Box 14.1), explores the relationship between diversity and health, and offers frameworks for analyzing culture and care and reducing implicit biases. This chapter also explores specific nursing-related barriers, strategies, and resources for developing cultural humility, as well as provides guidance on how to identify and mitigate implicit cultural biases to promote the highest level of health care delivery for all people.

BOX 14.1   Definition of Terms

Cultural humility: The process of self-reflection and discovery in order to build honest and trustworthy relationships.

Culture: The customary beliefs, social norms, and material traits of racial, religious, or social groups.

Diversity: How people differ, including but not limited to: age, race, ethnicity, national origin, gender, gender identity, sex, sexual orientation, mental or physical abilities, primary language, education, socioeconomic status, religion, work experience, cultural values, geographic location, family status, organizational level, work style, philosophical views, veteran status, and intellectual perspectives.

Equity: Social justice or fairness.

Ethnicity: Membership of persons in a particular cultural group who typically have a sense of shared common origins, distinct history, or collective individuality.

Implicit bias: The ability to find patterns from positive or negative attitudes and stereotypes that develop about certain groups of people that form outside of our own consciousness which promote inconsistent decision-making or systemic errors in judgment.

Inclusion: The act or practice of including and accommodating people who have historically been excluded.

Race: A person's self-identification with one or more social groups (e.g., White, Black or African American, Asian, American Indian and Alaska Native, Native Hawaiian, and Other Pacific Islander, or other race).

CONTEXTUALIZING CULTURE IN THE HEALTH CARE SETTING

Living in a pluralistic society, representative of individuals that may look different, speak differently, and have different values and beliefs from our own, nurses must provide equitable and inclusive care. It is not enough to educate people about cultural and other differences; one must also conform to these competing standards of truth. The 4.2 million nurses will need to manage and provide care to patients from diverse cultural and social backgrounds. This is a significant challenge for the nursing profession, with sources reporting a range of 71.5% to 81% of registered nurses (RNs) being non-Hispanic White (National Academies of Sciences, Engineering, and Medicine, 2021; Smiley et al., 2021).

In a discipline having up to 81% non-Hispanic White nurses, the discipline reflects the values and norms of society. In the United States, these values and norms are predominantly Eurocentric, middle-class, Christian, and androcentric in view. Thus, integrating one's culture and professional nursing experience needs to emphasize value-based education so nurses can apply their professional values of human dignity, altruism, and social justice to a legacy of caring behavior (Parandeh et al., 2015). For example, the concept of a single autonomous decision-maker, the hallmark of a Eurocentric worldview, does not accurately capture the involvement of family members and other significant people in health care decision-making (Stanfield & Browne, 2013). Understanding how one's culture influences the development of professional values is essential for examining the effect of

culture on value-based decision-making by nurses. One's socialization is influenced by culture, affecting one's worldview and ethical decision-making (Parandeh et al., 2015).

THEORIES TO GUIDE CULTURE AND HEALTH CARE

Many theoretical frameworks provide contextual bases for understanding and providing culturally and linguistically appropriate care. Leininger's (1991) classic theoretical framework for transcultural nursing emphasizes the commonalities and differences among worldviews of diverse health systems. The purpose of the theory is to provide culturally congruent, safe, and meaningful care to clients from different or similar cultures. It posits that worldview, as well as cultural and social structures, influences care outcomes related to culturally congruent care, and the three modes for transcultural care actions and decisions (culture preservation and maintenance; cultural care accommodation and/or negotiation; and cultural care repatterning and/or restructuring) provide culturally congruent care (Leininger, 2002). Further discussion of Leininger's framework occurs in Chapter 5 (Theories and Frameworks for Professional Nursing Practice).

Another classic model for examining cultural competence in nursing care is the Campinha-Bacote Model of Cultural Competence (Campinha-Bacote, 2009). In this model, nurses continuously work toward cultural competence by addressing five constructs: cultural awareness, cultural knowledge, cultural skill, cultural encounters, and cultural desire. The model's final and most critical concept is cultural desire or wanting to become culturally competent (Campinha-Bacote, 2009).

The Campinha-Bacote Model of Cultural Competence is a dynamic interactional model of cultural competence that requires the achievement of all five identified constructs. The process of cultural awareness occurs when the nurse can examine their values, biases, and stereotypes. It also requires the nurse to explore the potential cultural biases (systemic racism) that may exist within the health care setting. Cultural knowledge occurs when nurses educate themselves about the worldviews of other cultures and ethnic groups. This cultural knowledge may include learning how disease processes and management may vary depending on the cultural group. Cultural skill occurs when the nurse can conduct a relevant cultural assessment; hence, cultural data is used to develop and implement a culturally appropriate treatment plan. Cultural encounters encourage the nurse to engage directly with patients from different ethnic and cultural backgrounds to modify existing beliefs about a cultural group and prevent potential stereotyping. Finally, cultural desire addresses the motivation of the health care provider (HCP) to acquire new knowledge about different cultures. This last construct is based solely on the nurse's intrinsic need to develop new cultural understanding; it cannot be driven by external regulations or requirements (Kulbok et al., 2012) and is often a lifelong process (Isaacs et al., 2016).

CULTURE AS A SOCIAL DETERMINANT OF HEALTH

In 1980, the U.S. Department of Health and Human Services (USDHHS) created the Healthy People initiative, representing individuals, organizations, and communities across the country with goals focused on Health Promotion and Disease Prevention, and revises the objectives every 10 years based on information gained in previous decades (USDHHS, 2022). The current initiative, Healthy People 2030, contains the highest priority health issues in the United States (https://health.gov/healthypeople). Three concepts within the Healthy People 2030 initiative that have gained momentum in the last few decades are: addressing social determinants of health (SDOH), health equity, and health disparities (USDHHS, n.d.-b).

Although critical to understand for community health nurses, all nurses should be aware of the impact that SDOH has on the management of health. Interventions can be developed that include social services to improve health or reduce costs for individuals (Taylor et al., 2016). There is a strong emphasis on improving the inequitable social and race/ethnicity health disparities, with a closer examination of the individual's available socioeconomic or social resources to best meet their needs. The U.S. Census and Healthy People 2030 reports provide valuable information about how populations have changed over time but rarely have focused on the cultural values, beliefs, practices, or preferences of a particular subgroup. As a result, there is limited evidence to understand one's behavior around health care issues. However, we can learn how the health of our nation is changing by examining the trends over time.

From 2008 to 2018, life expectancy has increased for Hispanic, non-Hispanic White, and non-Hispanic-Black, with Hispanic persons having the longest life expectancy age at birth at 81.8 years and the infant mortality rate showing no clear trend from 2008 to 2018 for all racial/ethnic groups (Arispe et al., 2021). From 2013 to 2017, all racial and ethnic groups experienced improved health coverage, access, and utilization since the implementation of the Affordable Care Act, and, while there was an increase in coverage, people of color remained more likely to be uninsured (Artiga et al., 2020).

Drivers of making health a shared value include the value of health, the role that SDOH plays in influencing health, and a shared sense of community to influence health (Carman et al., 2019). The "value of health" is rising, with more adults indicating they value the importance of health equity and equality of opportunity in general. Adults reporting that our country should do whatever is necessary to ensure everyone has an equal opportunity to be healthy increased from 58% to 62% (Bye & Ghiradelli, 2021).

SOCIETAL TRENDS AND THE HEALTH CARE IMPACT

The values that shape health care and nursing were further put under the radar at the start of 2020 when the nation's resilience was tested during the novel COVID-19 pandemic. The pandemic brought further awareness that Black, Latinx/Hispanic, and Native American communities had disproportionate rates of illness and death related to the COVID-19 virus (Golden, 2020). Those communities shared societal trends even before COVID-19, which consisted of inconsistent access to health care, chronic health conditions, and stress and immunity, which were further strained throughout the pandemic (Golden, 2020). Fighting the racial disparity during the COVID-19 pandemic became a priority due to the health care impact. While the need to address the health impact of the pandemic within underrepresented communities was underway, unprecedented events soon occurred that opened the door wider to increase the priority of developing DEI strategies within organizations.

The George Floyd Case, Black Lives Matter Campaign, and LGBTQ+ and Asian Hate Crimes emphasized that discrimination within the United States is a major problem. Those unfortunate events led to movements resulting in several nursing programs reflecting on how they cover DEI content in the curriculum. Nursing programs also realized that there are several knowledge gaps and unanswered questions on how best to prepare professional nursing students on how to care for diverse patients. The unprecedented events of 2020 reminded national nursing organizations and institutions that societal trends affect the provision of services and health care outcomes, particularly within diverse populations. Nursing education programs helped lead the call to change the curriculum by mapping where DEI content is taught within the program and strategizing how to revise the curriculum to meet national accreditation core competencies and concepts.

NURSING'S CHALLENGES AND BARRIERS

Equitable and Inclusive Care

Nursing is strategically positioned to provide care to diverse groups with diverse expectations, problems, and goals. However, if HCPs continue to exhibit bias, stereotyping, and clinical uncertainty, this may continue to contribute to racial and ethnic disparities in health care (Edgoose et al., 2019). For example, the COVID-19 pandemic also brought challenges to accepting and receiving the emergency use COVID-19 vaccine, particularly within ethnically diverse populations driven by misinformation and the historical mistrust of the health care system. Historical and current interpersonal and systemic racism in the United States resulted in racial differences in vaccine trust and added to the complexity of providing nursing care (Latkin et al., 2021). With the COVID-19 pandemic, evidence suggested disparities and inequities existed for specific groups within the United States regarding illness and health (Sarfraz et al., 2021). See Chapter 1 (A Brief History of the Professionalization of Nursing in the United States) for further discussion on the historical perspective of responding to a public health emergency and/or health care recommendations.

The case study presented in Box 14.2 is based on a true story and provides an example of how biases and stereotypes can influence medical decision-making and lead to barriers for individuals seeking care. If HCPs are not accepting or compassionate as to how individuals identify, loss to follow-up could occur. Despite these perceived difficulties, the integration of patients' beliefs and values, when done, can result in effective nursing care (Farrell et al., 2013). The continued discussion within this chapter will further provide evidence-based strategy tools to HCPs to improve cultural humility and help decrease implicit biases and structural racism.

Cultural Humility

More than 3000 different cultural groups exist in the world. Regardless of their ability to interact with 20 or

---

BOX 14.2   Case Study

Barriers to Care

Crystal is a transgender patient who presents to an outpatient clinic for an annual physical exam. Crystal was born male; however, identifies with the pronouns she, her, and hers. Her electronic medical record has not been updated to reflect this change and she is still listed as Chris of male gender. Upon being called to the exam room, the registered nurse (RN) calls out for Chris in the waiting room. Crystal walks forward and when entering the exam room, Crystal updates another RN with her preferred name and pronouns, and the updates are noted by the RN. While waiting for the health care provider to enter the room, Crystal overhears the health care provider's conversation with the RN outside of the exam room door. "The patient in Room 5 is Crystal who identifies as female; however, Crystal is still listed in the medical record as Chris, a male patient." The provider quickly responds, "Well, until I see a change in the medical record, this patient is a male and that is how I will proceed with the visit. I don't understand this generation, the phases they go through, and what they identify with. He still has male organs, so he is a male no matter what he says." After overhearing the provider, Crystal quickly gets up from the exam table and walks out of the clinic promising that she will never go back to that office again.

1. How should the health care provider respond to Crystal?
2. If you were the RN working within this practice, what evidence-based strategies would you incorporate to ensure Crystal and other LGBTQ+ individuals receive the appropriate support when they are seeking care within this clinical setting?
3. Which strategies would you incorporate to reduce implicit biases within this clinical practice that could promote inclusive care?

200 patients, nurses must be sensitive to recognizing and confronting their own biases that may hinder their ability to provide high-quality patient-centered care. As previously mentioned, to manage diversity effectively, nurses must be sensitive to differences and similarities, be knowledgeable about expected behavior patterns, and be skillful at integrating their sensitivity and knowledge into appropriate assessments and interventions. Information about acceptable behavior patterns and their interpretation should constantly be tested against an individual's perception of a specific situation. Not verifying one's perception with that of the individual may lead to biases and stereotypes.

The health care profession must reflect the diversity of the individuals and communities we serve, provide opportunities to practice and improve *cultural humility* (Box 14.3), and recognize societal trends to help knock down barriers that cause hesitancy of diverse backgrounds to access care. Unlike cultural competence, cultural humility has no endpoint and requires continual self-reflection, self-critique, appreciation of intracultural variations, and the willingness to learn from other lived, diverse experiences (Prasad et al., 2016; Stubbe, 2020).

Decreasing Implicit Biases and Structural Racism

Implicit bias and structural racism can affect the delivery of culturally responsive nursing care due to the attitudes and behaviors of HCPs that contribute to health disparities

(Hall et al., 2015). Outside of conscious awareness, implicit attitudes, thoughts, and feelings exist that often happen automatically and can influence human behaviors (Hall et al., 2015). The field of DEI has created implicit/unconscious bias training that created awareness, but not always a behavioral shift.

Historical and current data demonstrate that discrimination based on race, gender, and LGBTQ+ has an ongoing negative health impact and results in highly emotional and physical health costs (USDHHS, n.d.-a). The Agency for Healthcare Research and Quality indicated that White patients receive better quality of care than 20% of Hispanic patients, 11% of Black patients, 11% of American Indian/Alaska Native patients, and 19% of Asian and Pacific Islander patients (Agency for Healthcare Research and Quality [AHRQ], 2022). Women who experience discrimination are 30% more likely to report unhappiness, loneliness, and depression than women who do not report discrimination (Pavalko et al., 2003; USDHHS, n.d.-a). LGBTQ+ individuals are also exposed to discrimination and report lifetime and day-to-day experiences compared to heterosexual individuals (Mays & Cochran, 2001; USDHHS, n.d.-a). LGBTQ+ adolescents are more likely to exhibit symptoms of emotional distress, suicidal ideation, and self-harm and be in settings where they experience social rejection, isolation, decreased support, and verbal or physical abuse (Hafeez et al., 2017; USDHHS, n.d.-a). Due to the continued health impacts of discrimination on various populations, it is recommended

---

BOX 14.3 Practicing Cultural Humility

- Consider whether politics or laws are adding to the stress on diverse communities
- Reflect on how your implicit biases may affect your practice with diverse patients
- Reflect on office practices (e.g., are there interpreters or is it a welcoming atmosphere)
- Address patients by their preferred pronouns
- Use a journal to write down self-reflections of implicit biases or observations
- Reduce stereotyping by not assuming someone's background, practices, religion, or culture
- Reassure by words that you are interested in understanding the patient
- Ask patients about their health care goals and treatment plan

- Ask patients if they have experienced discrimination, bullying, trauma, or harassment
- Identify strengths, interests, and resilience factors
- Discuss patient-centered care
- Inquire about what the patient feels would be helpful
- During the encounter, ask the patient if clarification is needed
- After the encounter, ask the patient if they felt understood or understood the treatment plan
- Model co-construction of the treatment plan by asking about goals and working together on goal attainment
- Clarify the patient's preference for family involvement

Source: Stubbe, D. E. (2020). Practicing cultural competence and cultural humility in the care of diverse patients. *Focus: The Journal of Lifelong Learning in Psychiatry, 18*(1), 49–51. https://doi.org/10.1176/appi.focus.20190041

that ongoing evidence-based studies examine the impact of discrimination on health outcomes or disparities in care (USDHHS, n.d.-a).

Narayan (2019) provided an overview of addressing implicit bias in nursing. This review pulled literature from several resources to help define a clear picture of why implicit bias has been an issue in health care. The author explains that the Institute of Medicine (IOM, 2003) produced a review of the racial and ethnic health care disparities within the United States. It was discovered that racial and ethnic minorities receive a lower quality of health care than nonminorities. Chapman et al. (2013) explained that if implicit bias among health care workers occurs, this can lead to inadequate patient assessments, inappropriate diagnoses and treatment decisions, less time involved in patient care, and patient discharges without proper follow-up. Narayan (2019) mentioned that we unconsciously categorize and assign good or bad judgments as we get older. Subsequently, suppose nurses categorize people in the health care arena. In that case, they may demonstrate less compassion for specific patients and invest less time and effort in the therapeutic relationship, affecting patient assessment and care (Narayan, 2019). Therefore, it is recommended that nurses adhere to best patient practices by completing self-interventions to mitigate bias, which includes, but is not limited to, nurses being able to reflect on "gut feelings" and negative reactions of vulnerable groups to be more empathetic and compassionate, develop a personal toolkit of self-interventions to replace bad habits of bias thinking, and seek to understand diverse patients as individuals instead of as a stigmatized group (Devine et al., 2012; Institute for Healthcare Improvement [IHI], 2017; Joint Commission, 2016).

CULTURAL ASSESSMENT

A patient should not expect to receive a lower standard of care because of race, ethnicity, or other irrelevant characteristics. However, unconscious associations may influence our judgments and actions, resulting in bias. Awareness of implicit biases and microaggressions and recognition that these phenomena are problematic are the first steps toward cultivating a more equitable and inclusive health care culture.

Project Implicit, released in 1998, is an international collaboration hosted by Harvard University to educate the public about hidden biases (Greenwald et al., 1998). A psychometric test developed for use, known as the **implicit association test** (IAT), enables the measurement of implicit bias via a test of automatic associations between concepts.

Research using the IAT to examine HCP bias was first published in 2007 (Maina et al., 2018). Since then, several research studies to address racial and ethnic bias in HCPs have utilized the implicit bias test. Many social psychologists believe that these cognitive associations lead to "implicit bias," which may influence subtle forms of discrimination (Azar, 2008).

The research focused on implicit bias in health care teams indicates that providers' biases influence their ability to establish a therapeutic relationship, adversely affecting assessment and care (FitzGerald & Hurst, 2017). The implicit biases that most concern health care professionals operate to the disadvantage of those who are already vulnerable. Examples include minority ethnic populations, immigrants, the poor, low health-literacy individuals, sexual minorities, the overweight, and the disabled, but anyone may be vulnerable given a particular context.

Nurses should identify their prejudices and biases because these biases may distort the level of care provided. The IHI recommends strategies to reduce implicit bias that includes identifying stereotype responses and being mindful to change the responses, imagining an individual is of the opposite stereotype, seeing the person as an individual, increasing opportunities to connect with individuals from different groups, and collaborating with others as equals and not as a hierarchical encounter (IHI, 2017). Edgoose et al. (2019) also recommend identifying our own implicit bias by completing an implicit bias association test, practicing stress reduction techniques, considering experiences from the stereotyped person's perspective, pausing and reflecting on potential biases before interacting with individuals, evaluating an individual's characteristics rather than by groups, welcoming and embracing multiculturalism, promoting procedural change at the organizational level, and practicing critical reflection and redressing power imbalances of the clinician-patient relationship.

Self-awareness or cultural awareness is the first step toward becoming culturally competent (Leininger, 2002; Purnell & Paulanka, 2003). Biases can be so intrinsic that the nurse is unaware of them. Research studies have found that HCPs can unknowingly bias the care provided to patients based on race or gender (Zestcott et al., 2016). Nurses who adopt strategies for controlling their own implicit biases could mitigate the health disparities of often stigmatized groups.

Fig. 14.1 illustrates the health outcomes that vary across these various cultural and racial groups that impact nursing care and the health care system and provide an additional example of how to recognize and process biases (Braveman & Gottlieb, 2014).

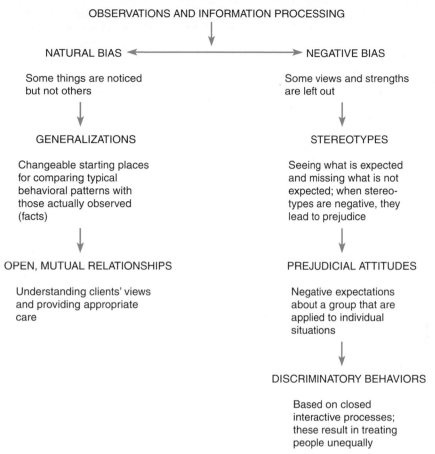

Fig. 14.1 Open Versus Closed Information Processing.

LINKING DIVERSITY, EQUITY, AND INCLUSION TO OUTCOMES FOR PATIENTS, FAMILIES, COMMUNITIES, POPULATIONS, AND ORGANIZATIONS

Over the past 20 years, health care organizations have developed diversity initiatives to seek employees "who looked like people in the community they serve." Although DEI initiatives to date have been started and more awareness was brought to the importance of DEI due to the unprecedented events that started in 2020, the outcomes have not been measurable or sustainable because the DEI initiatives were not fully integrated into an institution's culture, focused on inclusion, or linked directly to patient and family outcomes such as access to quality care, effective patient/family-provider communication, or satisfaction with the care provided (Puritty et al., 2017). As mentioned earlier,

DEI strategies have brought about awareness, but not behavior changes.

If we focus on removing structural racism and systemic biases and create more strategies that promote behavioral changes within our organizations that address the lack of health care or access to care for diverse populations, successful organizations can meet their mission and values by developing a greater understanding and a diversity of thought to transform the health and resilience of the organization. In Davidson's (2011) novel book on understanding difference, he suggests that directors of diversity initiatives should become "chief learning officers" to guide the discovery at all levels of the organization. Rather than focusing on diversity as a nebulous concept, the focus should be on a four-step process: (1) identify strategically relevant differences, (2) develop strategies to learn about the relevant differences, (3) integrate what is salient to the target population into programs and services, and (4) create results from the relevant differences. Once an organization captures relevant differences, services or programs can be integrated into the strategic plan. The outcomes for the patient, family, and health care organization can be evaluated. The process will ensure that an organization integrating diverse values and beliefs of both the nurses and the patients will better equip the health care community and meet the needs of people in its service area, and ultimately have a positive impact on the organization's future (Davidson, 2011; Puritty et al., 2017).

SUMMARY

America is composed of a diverse group of individuals, yet 81% of RNs are non-Hispanic White (Smiley et al., 2021). Racial minorities will represent the population majority by mid-century (Colby & Ortman, 2015), which further validates the great need for nurses to engage in learning experiences that create new avenues of how to implement and evaluate DEI initiatives. Remaining cognizant of personal intrinsic biases and those that permeate throughout the world is vital.

Nurses serve as gatekeepers to the health care system and are in a unique position to help bridge the gap in health disparities that impact diverse patients. As nurses develop cultural humility, they can help address the challenges and barriers that divide the health care system. The unprecedented situational challenges of 2020 brought increased awareness of the diverse population's hesitancy to seek medical care and recognition of the associated and continued discrimination in the United States. The events led to organizations looking internally at their DEI programs, and national accountability to make universal changes, and resulted in national nursing accreditation bodies and institutions recommending that nursing program curricula be mapped and/or revised to address DEI content. Integrating DEI strategies within organizations that also address implicit biases is imperative, needs to be intentional, and needs to reflect an ongoing strategic commitment from institutions and individuals for behavioral changes to occur. Embracing and being compassionate to everyone's unique differences will help build inclusive communities. There is still a lot of work to be done to improve the DEI impact on health care; however, having ongoing DEI conversations is a great start.

SALIENT POINTS

- Recognizing and acknowledging differences among varying populations will provide the best possible care for all patients and help minimize racial disparities.
- Health care organizations and nursing programs have a growing responsibility to improve diversity, equity, and inclusion (DEI) efforts within their workplace and curriculum.
- There is limited diversity in nursing. Diversifying the workforce with recruitment initiatives needs to be intentional and is vital to the communities that we serve.
- Societal factors and the novel COVID-19 pandemic heightened awareness about discrimination and health disparities that exist in the United States.
- Health care professionals and institutions may possess implicit biases against diverse populations; thus, nurses must remain hypervigilant to identify and correct those biases.
- Nurses should be knowledgeable about social determinants of health that could be a barrier to individuals seeking health care.
- Cultural assessment in nursing involves a systematic appraisal of the beliefs, values, and practices of the patient.
- Nurses must remain mindful not to make automatic assumptions about patients based on their unique differences.
- Nurses must remain motivated to learn about different cultural humility strategies and recognize implicit biases, to provide holistic and compassionate care to all.

CRITICAL REFLECTION EXERCISES

1. Discuss strategies that nurses could implement to promote inclusive care.
2. Discuss current challenges and barriers within health care institutions that hinder diversity, equity, and inclusion efforts.
3. How could a nurse develop the requisite balance of cultural humility, knowledge, and skills needed to manage diverse patients effectively?
4. In your experience, what strategies work well for the practice of reducing implicit biases to provide culturally acceptable nursing care?

REFERENCES

Agency for Healthcare Research and Quality. (2022). *2021 National healthcare quality and disparities report.* https://www.ahrq.gov/research/findings/nhqrdr/nhqdr21/index.html

Arispe, I., Gindi, R., & Madans, J. H. (2021). *Health, United States, 2019.* Centers for Disease Control and Prevention (CDC), National Center for Health Statistics (U.S.). https://doi.org/10.15620/cdc:100685

Artiga, S., Orgera, K., & Pham, O. (2020). *Disparities in health and health care: Five key questions and answers.* Kaiser Family Foundation. https://files.kff.org/attachment/Issue-Brief-Disparities-in-Health-and-Health-Care-Five-Key-Questions-and-Answers

Azar, B. (2008). *IAT: Fad or fabulous?* PsycEXTRA Dataset. https://doi.org/10.1037/e517642009-023

Braveman, P., & Gottlieb, L. (2014). The social determinants of health. It's time to consider the causes of the causes. *Public Health Reports, 129*(1 Suppl. 2), 19–31. https://doi.org/10.1177%2F00333549141291S206

Bye, L., & Ghiradelli, A. (2021, May 20). *American health values survey II.* Robert Wood Johnson Foundation. https://www.rwjf.org/en/library/research/2016/06/american-health-values-survey-topline-report.html

Campinha-Bacote, J. (2009). Culture and diversity issues. A culturally competent model of care for African Americans. *Urologic Nursing, 29*(1), 49–54.

Carman, K. G., Chandra, A., Weilant, S., Miller, C., & Tait, M. (2019). *2018 National Survey of Health Attitudes: Description and top-line summary data.* RAND Corporation. https://www.rand.org/pubs/research_reports/RR2876.html

Chapman, E. N., Kaatz, A., & Carnes, M. (2013). Physicians and implicit bias: How doctors may unwittingly perpetuate health care disparities. *Journal of General Internal Medicine, 28*(11), 1504–1510. https://doi.org/10.1007/s11606-013-2441-1

Colby, S. L., & Ortman, J. M. (2015, March 3). *Projections of the size and composition of the U.S. Population: 2014 to 2060.* United States Census Bureau, 25-1143. https://www.census.gov/library/publications/2015/demo/p25-1143.html

Davidson, M. N. (2011). *The end of diversity as we know it by Martin N. Davidson.* Berrett-Koehler.

Devine, P. G., Forscher, P. S., Austin, A. J., & Cox, W. T. L. (2012). Long-term reduction in implicit race bias: A prejudice habit-breaking intervention. *Journal of Experimental Social Psychology, 48*(6), 1267–1278. https://doi.org/10.1016/j.jesp.2012.06.003

Edgoose, J., Quiogue, M., & Sidhar, K. (2019). How to identify, understand, and unlearn implicit bias in patient care. *Family Practice Management, 26*(4), 29–33. https://www.aafp.org/fpm/2019/0700/p29.html

Farrell, B., McCabe, M. S., & Jevit, L. (2013). The Institute of Medicine report on high-quality cancer care: Implications for oncology nursing. *Oncology Nursing Forum, 40*(6), 603–609. https://doi.org/10.1188/13.ONF.603-609

FitzGerald, C., & Hurst, S. (2017). Implicit bias in healthcare professionals: A systematic review. *BMC Medical Ethics, 18*(1), 19. https://doi.org/10.1186/s12910-017-0179-8

Golden, S. H. (2020, April 20). *Coronavirus in African Americans and other people of color.* https://www.hopkinsmedicine.org/health/conditions-and-diseases/coronavirus/covid19-racial-disparities

Greenwald, A. G., McGhee, D. E., & Schwartz, J. L. (1998). Measuring individual differences in implicit cognition: The implicit association test. *Journal of Personality and Social Psychology, 74*(6), 1464. https://doi.org/10.1037/0022-3514.74.6.1464

Hafeez, H., Zeshan, M., Tahir, M., Jahan, N., & Naveed, S. (2017). Health care disparities among lesbians, gay, bisexual, and transgender youth: A literature review. *Cureus, 9*(4), e1184. https://doi:10.7759/cureus.1184

Hall, W. J., Chapman, M.V., Lee, K. M., Merino, T. T., Payne, B. K., Eng, E., Day, S. H., & Coyne-Beasley, T. (2015). Implicit racial/ethnic bias among health care professionals and its influence on health care outcomes: A systemic review. *American Journal of Public Health, 105*(12), e60–e76. https://doi:10.2105/AJPH.2015.302903

Institute for Healthcare Improvement. (2017, September 28). *How to reduce implicit bias: Institute for Healthcare Improvement.* http://ihi.org/communities/blogs/how-to-reduce-implicit-bias

Institute of Medicine. (2003). *Unequal treatment: Confronting racial and ethnic disparities in health care.* The National Academies Press. https://doi:10.17226/12875

Isaacs, A. N., Raymond, A., Jacob, E., Jones, J., McGrail, M., & Drysdale, M. (2016). Cultural desire need not improve with cultural knowledge: A cross-sectional study of student nurses. *Nurse Education in Practice, 19*, 91–96. https://doi.org/10.1016/j.nepr.2016.05.009

Joint Commission. (2016, April). Implicit bias in health care. *Quick Safety: An Advisory on Safety & Quality Issues, 23.* https://www.jointcommission.org/-/media/tjc/documents/newsletters/quick-safety-issue-23-apr-2016-final-rev.pdf

Kulbok, P. A., Mitchell, E. M., Glick, D. F., & Greiner, D. (2012). International experiences in nursing education: A review of the literature. *International Journal of Nursing Education Scholarship, 9*(1). https://doi.org/10.1515/1548-923X.2365

Latkin, C. A., Dayton, L., Yi, G., Konstantopoulos, A., & Boodram, B. (2021). Trust in a COVID-19 vaccine in the U.S.: A social-ecological perspective. *Social Science Medicine, 270.* https://doi.org/10.1016/j.socscimed.2021.113684

Leininger, M. M. (Ed.). (1991). The theory of culture care diversity and universality. In M. M. Leininger (Ed.), *Culture and diversity and universality: A theory of nursing* (pp. 5–68). National League for Nursing.

Leininger, M. (2002). Culture care theory: A major contribution to advance transcultural nursing and practices. *Journal of Transcultural Nursing, 13*(3), 189–192. https://doi.org/10.1177/10459602013003005

Maina, I. W., Belton, T. D., Ginzberg, S., Singh, A., & Johnson, T. J. (2018). A decade of studying implicit racial/ethnic bias in healthcare providers using the Implicit Association Test. *Social Science & Medicine, 199*, 219–229. https://doi.org/10.1016/j.socscimed.2017.05.009

Mays, V. M., & Cochran, S. D. (2001). Mental health correlates of perceived discrimination among lesbian, gay, and bisexual adults in the United States. *American Journal of Public Health*, *91*(11), 1869–1876. https://doi.org/10.2105/AJPH.91.11.1869

Narayan, M. C. (2019). Addressing implicit bias in nursing: A review. *American Journal of Nursing*, *119*(7), 36–43. https://doi:10.1097/01.NAJ.0000569340.27659.5a

National Academies of Sciences, Engineering, and Medicine. (2021). *The future of nursing 2020–2030: Charting a path to achieve health equity*. The National Academies Press. https://doi.org/10.17226/25982

Parandeh, A., Khaghanizade, M., Mohammadi, E., & Nouri, J. M. (2015). Factors influencing the development of professional values among nursing students and instructors: A systematic review. *Global Journal of Health Science*, *7*(2), 284–293. https://doi.org/10.5539/gjhs.v7n2p284

Pavalko, E. K., Mossakowski, K. N., & Hamilton, V. J. (2003). Does perceived discrimination affect health? Longitudinal relationships between work discrimination and women's physical and emotional health. *Journal of Health and Social Behavior*, *44*(1), 18–33. https://pubmed.ncbi.nlm.nih.gov/12751308/

Prasad, S. J., Nair, P., Gadhvi, K., Barai, I., Danish, H. S., & Philip, A. B. (2016). Cultural humility: Treating the patient, not the illness. *Medical Education Online*, *21*(1), 1–2. https://doi.org/10.3402/meo.v21.30908

Puritty, C., Strickland, L. R., Alia, E., Blonder, B., Klein, E., Kohl, T. M., McGee, E., Quintana, M., Ridley, R. E., & Gerber, L. R. (2017). Without inclusion, diversity initiatives may not be enough. *Science*, *357*(6356), 1101–1102. https://www.science.org/doi/10.1126/science.aai9054

Purnell, L. D., & Paulanka, B. J. (2003). *Transcultural health care: A culturally competent approach*. Davis.

Sarfraz, A., Sarfraz, Z., Barrios, A., Agadi, K., Thevuthasan, S., Pandav, K., Manish, K. C., Sarfraz, M., Rad, P., & Michel, G. (2021). Understanding and promoting racial diversity in healthcare: Settings to address disparities in pandemic crisis management. *Journal of Primary Care & Community Health*, *12*, 1–7. https://doi.org/10.1177/21501327211018354

Smiley, R. A., Ruttinger, C., Oliveira, C. M., Hudson, L. R., Allgeyer, R., Reneau, K. A., Silvestre, J. H., & Alexander, M. (2021). The 2020 national nursing workforce survey. *Journal of Nursing Regulation*, *12*(1), S4–S96. https://doi.org/10.1016/S2155-8256(21)00027-2

Stanfield, D., & Browne, A. J. (2013). The relevance of indigenous knowledge for nursing curriculum. *International Journal of Nursing Education Scholarship*, *10*(1), 1–19. https://doi.org/10.1515/ijnes-2012-0041

Stubbe, D. E. (2020). Practicing cultural competence and cultural humility in the care of diverse patients. *Focus: The Journal of Lifelong Learning in Psychiatry*, *18*(1), 49–51. https://doi.org/10.1176/appi.focus.20190041

Taylor, L. A., Tan, A. X., Coyle, C. E., Ndumele, C., Rogan, E., Canavan, M., Curry, L. A., & Bradley, E. H. (2016, August 17). Leveraging the social determinants of health: What works? *PloS One*, *11*(8), 1–20. https://doi.org/10.1371/journal.pone.0160217

U.S. Department of Health and Human Services. (n.d.-a). *Healthy People 2030: Discrimination*. https://health.gov/healthypeople/objectives-and-data/social-determinants-health/literature-summaries/discrimination#cit8

U.S. Department of Health and Human Services. (n.d.-b). *Healthy People 2030: Leading health indicators*. https://health.gov/healthypeople/objectives-and-data/leading-health-indicators

U.S. Department of Health and Human Services. (2022). *Healthy People 2030: Questions & answers*. https://health.gov/our-work/national-health-initiatives/healthy-people/healthy-people-2030/questions-answer

Zestcott, C. A., Blair, I. V., & Stone, J. (2016). Examining the presence, consequences, and reduction of implicit bias in health care: A narrative review. *Group Processes & Intergroup Relations*, *19*(4), 528–542. https://doi.org/10.1177/1368430216642029

PART III

Themes in Professional Nursing Practice

15

Health and Health Promotion

Aliria Muñoz Rascón, PhD, RN, CCRN-K and
Sandra Paul Thomas, PhD, RN, FAAN

 http://evolve.elsevier.com/Friberg/bridge/

OBJECTIVES

At the completion of this chapter, the reader will be able to:

- Describe psychological, behavioral, socioeconomic, and environmental factors related to wellness.
- Apply the stages of change model to a selected health behavior.
- Apply the health belief model (HBM) to a selected health behavior.

- Describe the use of evidence-based interventions to promote behavior change.
- Describe the goals of *Healthy People* 2030.
- Compare several types of community-level health promotion programs.

INTRODUCTION

Monica Trujillo is a 38-year-old mother of three who recently separated from her husband. For the past 4 years, she has worked the night shift in a meat packing facility. On her drive home one morning, she was involved in a motor vehicle crash and subsequently evaluated in the emergency department for neck pain. Upon discharge, the nurse practitioner discusses some health concerns with Monica. Monica's nonfasting blood glucose was 178 mg/dL, weight was 168 pounds (height 5 feet 3 inches), blood pressure 155/87, and heart rate 93. After the nurse recommends that she consult her primary care provider regarding hyperglycemia and hypertension, Monica appears tearful and shares that she does not have a primary care provider or insurance. She mentions that ever since she started working the night shift, she and her children have eaten more fast food and are less active. Before the separation from her husband, Monica was encouraging the family to go on walks together in the evening, but this has stopped with the recent stress of her and her husband's separation.

Like Monica and her family, people all over the United States are experiencing challenges that impact health. Changing health behavior is difficult—and this change intersects with dynamic life events. One family member may initiate efforts to improve family health. Yet, even when successful in the short term, these changes are challenging to sustain. Further, not all individuals have the knowledge or resources to make appropriate behavior changes that last. Monica's efforts to increase walking were commendable; however, identifying more healthful dietary choices and effective stress management strategies were still warranted. Some health professionals have a mistaken notion that the mere provision of didactic information will bring about health-promoting actions. However, to convert knowledge into behavior, environmental and sociocultural factors must be considered. Health care providers need a more sophisticated understanding of the principles of health behavior change to help clients make health-promoting decisions. This chapter explores the concepts of health and health behaviors as well as a variety of evidence-based interventions to change health behavior.

CONCEPT OF HEALTH

Philosophers from Plato to Gadamer have pondered how to capture the essence of health. Gadamer called it "a condition of inner accord, of harmony with oneself … a condition of being involved, of being in the world, of being together with one's fellow human beings, of active and rewarding engagement in one's everyday tasks" (Gadamer, 1996, pp. 108, 113). To the average layperson, it is an *illness* that compels attention, a departure from taken-for-granted smooth functioning. Likewise, traditional medical and nursing curricula have prepared health professionals to care for the acutely ill. Many textbooks still place greater emphasis on morbidity and mortality than on health promotion. Yet nursing, since the time of Nightingale (1859), also has been concerned with preventing disease and keeping people healthy. As articulated by Cowling (2013, p. 121), "the nature of nursing is one of responding to the wholeness of human experience." Various conceptions of health by nurse theorists can be found in Chapter 5.

For this chapter, a broad concept of health was selected, in which separating mind, body, and spirit becomes impossible. Moreover, the patient's embeddedness in family, friendships, culture, and the environment cannot be ignored. Also, the patient's own power for healing is recognized. The role of the nurse is that of *facilitator* of the patient's own innate capabilities for healing and growth. Skilled counseling is as important as technical competence.

HEALTH PROMOTION AND DISEASE PREVENTION

The terms *health promotion* and *disease prevention,* although often used synonymously, have different meanings. Health promotion refers to activities that protect good health and take people beyond their present level of wellness. In contrast, disease prevention emphasizes behaviors of avoidance, deprivation, or restraint. Mortality statistics demonstrate the importance of lifestyle modifications to prevent premature death. The chief causes of death in the United States are strongly related to unhealthy behaviors such as smoking and poor dietary patterns (Box 15.1).

MODIFICATION OF HEALTH ATTITUDES AND BEHAVIORS

Convincing empirical evidence shows that healthy lifestyles can significantly reduce the mortality rate from obesity, diabetes, cancer, and cardiovascular and respiratory diseases. Therefore, the modification of health attitudes and behavior is one of the most important responsibilities of every nurse. As shown in Fig. 15.1, a

---

> **BOX 15.1 The Leading Causes of Death in the United States, 2019**
>
> - Heart disease
> - Cancer
> - Accidents (unintentional injuries)
> - Chronic lower respiratory diseases
> - Stroke (cerebrovascular diseases)
> - Alzheimer disease
> - Diabetes
> - Nephritis, nephrotic syndrome, and nephrosis
> - Influenza and pneumonia
> - Intentional self-harm (suicide)

From National Center for Health Statistics, Centers for Disease Control and Prevention. https://www.cdc.gov/nchs/databriefs/395

comprehensive model of wellness includes interacting factors such as psychological characteristics, health-promoting behaviors, and aspects of the environments in which people live and work. Both attitudes and behaviors are modifiable by health care providers, as well as some (but not all) aspects of environments. The sections that follow examine a number of these modifiable factors as addressed by classical theories and landmark studies. Although a comprehensive wellness model includes organismic variables (e.g., genetic predispositions), social determinants of health (e.g., poverty), and personal demographic characteristics (e.g., age, income, gender), these are not amenable to modification by health care providers. *We emphasize the factors that can be affected by nurses while taking into consideration these important (albeit less modifiable) contextual factors.*

Psychological Attitudes and Characteristics Associated With Wellness

Self-Concept. Many theorists consider a healthy self-concept (and closely related concepts such as self-acceptance or self-esteem) essential for wellness. Persons who feel better about themselves are more inclined to enact self-care behaviors that promote good health, whereas lower self-concept may result in self-destructive habits such as substance misuse. Adverse childhood experiences, racial discrimination, or victimization because of one's sexual orientation can negatively affect self-concept (Scheer et al., 2021; Turner et al., 2017). Although early experiences with parents, teachers, and peers may inhibit the formation of a healthy self-concept, later life experiences offer opportunities to alter it. A client's negative evaluation of the self can be altered in an ongoing, supportive relationship with a nurse. For example, the nurse can guide the client to recall

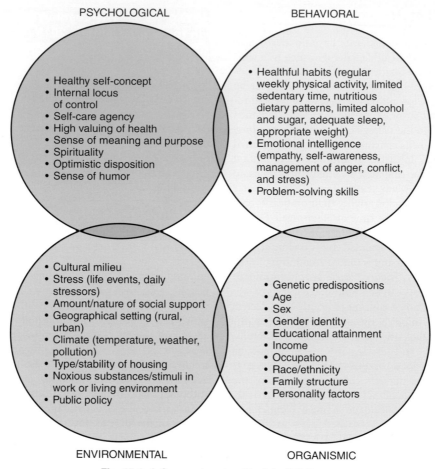

Fig. 15.1 A Comprehensive Model of Wellness.

strengths, such as persistence and resilience in confronting life stressors.

Locus of Control. Psychologists developed the term "health locus of control" to investigate people's beliefs about where control of their health lies: either within themselves (called *internal locus of control*) or mainly influenced by others, fate, or luck (called *external locus of control*). Researchers found that health locus of control beliefs can influence people's preferences about medical decision-making as well as their likelihood of engaging in health-promoting behaviors (Marton et al., 2021). A nurse can easily assess locus of control by asking questions such as the following: "What do you think caused this health problem? Who do you think knows best what you really need? Do you normally follow instructions pretty well, or do you prefer to work things out your own way?" Nursing interventions can

be tailored accordingly. If the person has an internal locus of control, a nurse should allow a high degree of client participation in goal setting and selection of rewards for adherence to goals. If the person has an external locus of control, providing plenty of concrete guidance and support is important. For example, if the goal is weight loss, suggesting involvement in a weight loss accountability group may be beneficial.

Self-Care Agency and Self-Efficacy. *Self-care agency,* a term coined by nurse theorist Dorothea Orem (2001), refers to the ability to care for oneself, for which the person must have knowledge, skills, understanding, and willingness. In working with a client, an assessment of all these factors is necessary. A parallel concept from social cognitive theory called *self-efficacy* (Bandura, 1997, 2012) has generated a sizable body of health psychology and nursing literature. According to Bandura's theory, when people perceive that they have the efficacy to accomplish a specific behavior (e.g., breast self-examination, smoking cessation, exercise), they are predisposed to undertake the behavior. This empirical evidence suggests that a nurse's first step in working with many clients is to enhance their belief in personal capability. Research shows that self-efficacy is modifiable through strategies such as anticipatory guidance and persuasive motivational messages (Bandura, 2012; Resnick, 2018).

Values. Values are elements that show how a person has decided to use their life. Values serve as a basis for decisions and choices. The nurse must assess whether the client's values promote a healthy lifestyle. How important is health to an individual compared with other life values such as pleasure or social recognition? Jackson et al. (2007) found that individuals who place a higher value on health also display greater involvement in a health-promoting lifestyle. Of course, some people declare that they highly value health, but their behaviors contradict this. A value system may contain conflicting values. For example, highly valuing achievement and financial prosperity may result in overwork and neglect of health. Highly valuing their social world may cause adolescents to make unhealthy food choices, such as frequenting fast-food restaurants to be with their friends (Strommer et al., 2021). Assisting a client to clarify conflicting values can be a useful intervention. Chapter 12 on ethics has a further discussion on values.

Sense of Purpose. Having a sense of meaning and purpose for one's life may be an important factor in individuals' responsiveness to health providers' instructions. Purpose in life includes having goals for the future and a sense of directedness. Exploring whether clients aim to follow a particular career trajectory, pursue an enjoyable hobby or avocation, or see their children and grandchildren grow and mature is often helpful. Persons with clear goals may devote more effort to health maintenance because most goals cannot be achieved without good health.

In older adults, greater purpose in life was associated with higher physical activity (Yemiscigil & Vlaev, 2021), and with lower risk for mortality, even when their chronic medical conditions were taken into account (Boyle et al., 2009). When assessing a client, it can be thought-provoking to ask about aims to make a difference or leave a legacy.

Spirituality. Across 7000 years and diverse cultures, spirituality has been integral to the care of the sick, although it received less emphasis as modern care became technologically oriented. Presently, there is renewed interest in spirituality as an essential component of holistic health (Lalani & Chen, 2021). Spirituality is not synonymous with involvement in organized religion, but the sense of connection with a divine wisdom or higher power often motivates practices such as meditation, prayer, and attendance at religious services. Studies have examined the relationship of spirituality and/or religious practice with disease conditions (e.g., heart disease, cancer, mental illness) and health risk behaviors (e.g., smoking, excessive drinking, using illicit drugs) (Burdette et al., 2018; Page et al., 2020). Spiritual practices may also help clients reduce stress (Callen, et al., 2011) and loneliness (Rote et al., 2012).

Optimism. An optimistic disposition has been shown to be important to health in studies conducted for at least 35 years. Optimism includes tendencies to look on the bright side and anticipate good things in the future. Higher levels of optimism have been associated with positive health outcomes such as completion of an alcohol treatment program and faster recovery after coronary bypass surgery, bone marrow transplant, and traumatic injury (Carver et al., 2010). An optimistic outlook can be cultivated if it does not come naturally.

Sense of Humor. Although a sense of humor is a socially appealing trait that elicits pleasure in others, it also conveys health benefits. The physical effects of mirth have been compared with the effects of exercise. For example, laughing 100 times expends the same number of calories as 10 minutes on a rowing machine (Godfrey, 2004). The efficiency of the respiratory system increases and the cardiovascular and muscular systems relax. Humor and laughter have been linked to higher levels of endorphins and immunoglobulin A and lower levels of cortisol (Godfrey, 2004). Laughter is an excellent way to dispel stress and tension. Health-promoting humor styles also positively correlate with mental health (Schneider et al., 2018).

Health Behaviors Associated With Wellness

Behaviors associated with wellness are listed in Fig. 15.1.

Nurse researcher Nola Pender developed a model that predicts health-promoting behaviors (Fig. 15.2). Individual characteristics and prior behavior are theorized to affect perceptions of self-efficacy, benefits and barriers to action, and a factor called *activity-related affect,* which refers to the feelings about the behavior in question. For example, is exercise fun or unpleasant? All these factors, as well as interpersonal and situational variables, can influence commitment to a plan of action. Additionally, competing demands such as work or family care

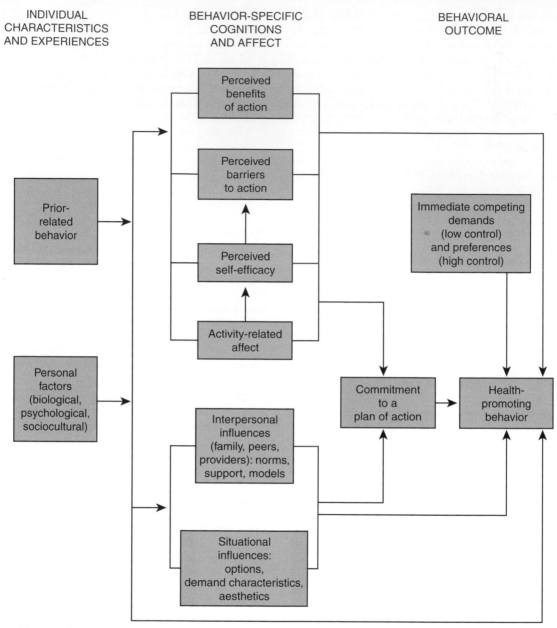

INDIVIDUAL
CHARACTERISTICS
AND EXPERIENCES

BEHAVIOR-SPECIFIC
COGNITIONS
AND AFFECT

BEHAVIORAL
OUTCOME

Fig. 15.2 Pender's Revised Health Promotion Model. (From Pender, N., Murdaugh, C. L., & Parsons, M. A. [2002]. *Health promotion in nursing practice* [4th ed.]. Prentice Hall.)

responsibilities are taken into account in the prediction of health-promoting behavior. Of the individual factors in the model, the best predictors of health-promoting behavior in most studies are perceived self-efficacy, attitude, perceived barriers, and prior behavior (Biasini et al., 2021; Pender et al., 2006). Nurse counseling can directly address the reduction of barriers and strengthen client self-efficacy.

Health Habits. Longitudinal studies have conclusively established that good health habits, such as regular exercise, are correlated with better health status and longevity

(Yoneda et al., 2021). Given that the benefits of healthful habits are well established, the average American's lack of adherence to the recommended wellness lifestyle regimen is discouraging. We focus here on physical activity, dietary patterns, substance misuse, sleep, social engagement, and emotional intelligence.

Physical Activity. Analysis of a massive database showed that exercise is as effective as prescriptive medications for the prevention of diabetes and secondary prevention of heart disease and *more* effective than prescriptive medications during stroke rehabilitation (Naci & Ioannidis, 2013). Yet less than one-quarter of U.S. adults meet governmental guidelines for weekly aerobic and muscle strengthening activity (National Center for Health Statistics, 2021) specifying 150 minutes of moderate activity or 75 minutes of vigorous activity and muscle strengthening activities for two or more days (US Department of Health and Human Services [DHHS], 2018). Physical activity relates to many aspects of health beyond cardiovascular fitness. During stay-at-home orders due to the COVID-19 pandemic, rates of physical activity decreased (Stockwell et al., 2021) and trended with increased anxiety and depression (Puccinelli et al., 2021).

Physical inactivity (e.g., sitting, reclining, lying down), has increased in the United States, with all states reporting at least 15% of adults as physically inactive and some southern states reporting inactivity rates over 30% (Centers for Disease Control and Prevention [CDC], January 2020). It is estimated that children and adults spend approximately 7.7 hours per day being sedentary (DHHS, 2018). Interrupting prolonged sitting with physical activity breaks can reduce blood glucose and insulin levels, especially in overweight and obese individuals (Loh et al., 2020).

Integrating physical activity into one's life requires changing routines. While there are a multitude of options to engage in physical activity, not all options may be feasible, safe, or appealing. Options such as walking outside may appear to be universally available due to the minimal equipment necessary; however, this still requires a safe outdoor area amenable to walking, suitable weather, and the freedom and time to do so. If unsafe neighborhoods or inclement weather preclude outdoor walking, the nurse can recommend visiting safe indoor areas such as a shopping mall. The nurse must assess resources, preferences, and barriers to collaborate with the client in creating a sustainable change (Fig. 15.3). For example, if childcare responsibilities are identified as a barrier to physical activity, recommending activities that involve children (e.g., dancing) could be more feasible. Associating physical activity with a daily routine, such as going for a walk after dinner, can also promote sustainable behavior change.

With the continual expansion of available online videos and social media outlets, videos of at-home workouts are literally at the fingertips of anyone with a smart phone and access to the Internet; however, quality of videos can vary and may not consider the safety of the participant. Concern also exists for "vicarious goal fulfillment," in which watching videos of exercises from social media "influencers" does not lead to any increase in physical activity—and ironically can even increase sedentary behavior (Sokolova & Perez, 2021). When online video exercise programs are evidence based, they are more likely to demonstrate beneficial outcomes such as improvements in physical activity engagement, muscle strength, motivation, and sleep quality (Emberson et al., 2021). Additionally, the use of technology such as mobile phone applications and wearable activity trackers can reduce sedentary behavior and weight- especially in older populations and when used for six months or longer (Emberson et al., 2021).

Because so many clients are completely sedentary, nurses must remember to suggest realistic and achievable goals. Replacing sedentary behaviors with enjoyable more mobile activities may be less intimidating for some clients. Thorough assessment, creating a communication and feedback system, appropriate use of technology, goal setting, and involvement of a multidisciplinary team can contribute to the sustainable incorporation of physical activity into one's lifestyle (Collado-Mateo et al., 2021).

Physical activity recommendations must also be tailored to client preferences and abilities. For example, stationary rowing machines can be a safe and effective option for the visually impaired. As the population ages, nurses should be well-equipped to make evidence-based recommendations for physical activity in older adults. Increasing physical activity in older adults can improve cognitive functioning and reduce frailty (Racey et al., 2021); however, some older adults may find technological approaches to exercise less appealing and may also be concerned about fatigue and pain (Collado-Mateo et al., 2021; Huffman & Amireault, 2021). Educating clients to stop if an activity causes pain or discomfort, identifying activities that are convenient, pleasurable, and social could enhance the benefits of exercise for older adults.

Dietary Patterns. Close to 74% of Americans are overweight or obese, with adults aged 40 to 59 having the highest rates of obesity (43%). Not only is obesity (a body mass index [BMI] greater than 30) rapidly rising, but so is severe obesity (defined as a BMI >40) (CDC, 2021). Cardiovascular disease is the leading cause of death in the US and 48% of adults aged 65 and older have prediabetes. Child and adolescent health is also worsening, with rates of overweight and obesity at about 40%. High cholesterol, formerly

As you just start, the obstacles might seem difficult to overcome. The following examples offer common obstacles and strategies for overcoming them.

Obstacle	Try This
I don't have time to be physically active.	Monitor your daily activities for one week. Identify at least three 30-minute time slots you could use for physical activity.
I don't have anyone to go with me.	Develop new friendships with physically active people. Join a group, such as the YMCA or a hiking club.
I'm so tired when I get home from work.	Schedule physical activity for times in the day or week when you feel energetic.
I have so much on my "to do" list already; how can I do physical activity too?	Plan ahead. Make physical activity a regular part of your daily or weekly schedule by writing it on your calendar. Keep the appointment with yourself.
I'll probably hurt myself if I try to be more physically active.	Consult with a health professional or educational material to learn how to exercise appropriately for your age, fitness level, skill level, and health status.
I'm not coordinated. I can't learn something new at my age!	Skip the dance classes if they require coordination; choose activities such as walking or biking instead.
My job requires me to be on the road; it's impossible for me to exercise.	Stay in places with swimming pools or exercise facilities. Or find an exercise you enjoy and be sure you can access it on a mobile device wherever you are.
I have small children and it's impossible to have time to myself for exercise.	Trade babysitting time with a friend, neighbor, or family member who also has small children. As children get older, family bike rides or walks might be another option.

Adapted from Physical Activity for Everyone: Making Physical Activity Part of Your Life: Overcoming Barriers to Physical Activity.

Fig. 15.3 Strategies for Overcoming Obstacles to Physical Activity. (CDC. [2021]. https://www.cdc.gov/healthyweight/physical_activity/getting_started.html)

considered an adult disease, is now diagnosed in 7% of children and adolescents as well (U.S. Department of Agriculture [USDA] & DDHS, 2010).

Despite efforts to enhance public awareness of these issues and efforts to improve access to useful nutrition information, the adherence of the US population to the USDA dietary guidelines has remained low (USDA & DDHS, 2010). As a country, Americans consumed 11.18 million metric tons of sugar in 2017, with per-capita consumption higher than any other country in the world. A leading source of sugar is sugar-sweetened beverages (e.g., sports drinks, sodas, and coffees). The majority of adults in the US (63%) consume one or more sugar-sweetened beverages per day (Chevinsky et al., 2021), and consumption of sugary drinks by children and adolescents is well above recommended levels (Della Corte et al., 2021).

When counseling clients about dietary modifications, nurses may find the "Dietary Guidelines for Americans 2020–2025" useful (https://www.dietaryguidelines.gov/) because rather than providing a rigid prescription, these guidelines recommend (1) following a healthy eating pattern across the life span; (2) focusing on nutrition density in food and beverages that consider socioeconomic and cultural factors; (3) meeting necessary amounts of each food group while staying within calorie limits; and (4) limiting alcohol, sugary beverages, and foods including those with added saturated fat and sodium.

Food is laden with emotional, social, and cultural significance, complicating attempts at dietary modification. For many clients, foods high in salt, fat, or sugar may be "comfort food." Banishing these foods as "bad" is ineffective and unrealistic- and can even have the opposite of the intended effect. Thus, behavior change interventions should work within sociocultural contexts. While each culture may have foods deemed to be unhealthful, each also has options that enhance health: grilled bison, pico de gallo salsa, and sauteed collard greens, to name a few.

There are many ways in which someone can eat healthfully. The USDA My Plate program (available in English and Spanish) provides useful shopping tips, recipes, and online resources to promote healthful choices while considering cultural and socioeconomic factors (myplate.gov). Dietary patterns are also influenced by the people the client regularly eats with. While a mother may be limiting her carbohydrate intake after a diabetes diagnosis, this could be challenging if her children prefer starchy foods. Preparing two separate menus—especially when one may be less healthy but more appealing, is rarely sustainable. Instead, the nurse can work with the client's family and consider options that are appealing and healthful to all members.

Adult clients could be incentivized to improve their diet by new research findings about the Mediterranean-Dash Intervention for Neurodegenerative Delay (MIND) diet shown to slow cognitive decline and significantly lower the risk of all-cause mortality (Corley, 2020). The diet emphasizes fish, nuts, whole grains, berries, avocados, coffee, dark chocolate, olive oil, and vegetables while discouraging butter, cheese, and fried food.

Substance Misuse. The world is facing a substance misuse crisis. Alcohol, tobacco, cannabinoids, opioids, depressants, stimulants, and hallucinogens have the potential to cause short and/or long-term health and social problems. Individuals over age 12 in the US report binge alcohol behavior at rates of 24.5% and tobacco use at 21.5% (National Center for Health Statistics, 2021). Substance misuse also affects the health of the public (e.g., motor vehicle crashes, domestic violence, child abuse and neglect) and can lead to temporary or chronic substance use disorders, which are diagnosable illnesses characterized by repeated use over time. In 2019, over 70,000 individuals died of a drug overdose, with the vast majority involving opioids (CDC, 2021). The national opioid epidemic declared in 2015 directed increased prescriber training, improved access to Medication-Assisted Treatment (MAT) for those with opioid use disorders, and expanded use of naloxone. Nurses can directly impact the opioid crisis through efficient intervention when pain arises and educating clients and families about non-opioid pain treatment strategies (American Nurses Association [ANA], 2018). Unfortunately, nurses have also fallen victim to the opioid crisis.

With 10% to 15% of nurses estimated to suffer from substance use disorders, the International Nurses Society on Addictions (http://www.intnsa.org/) provides resources and programs to support nurse treatment and recovery.

Smoking is the leading cause of preventable death across the globe (DHHS, 2014). Despite public restrictions on smoking in restaurants and public spaces, smoking prevalence remains high. In 2020, almost 23 of every 100 high school students reported tobacco use—a concerning statistic considering that most tobacco use habits are started during the adolescent years (Gentzke et al., 2020). Thus, public health efforts against tobacco often target younger populations. Electronic cigarettes (e-cigarettes) are increasingly popular among youths. When first introduced, e-cigarettes or "vaping" was perceived to be less harmful than smoked tobacco; however, the U.S. Food and Drug Administration (FDA) banned the sale of e-cigarettes to anyone younger than 18 because of increased concern about long-term consequences (FDA, 2016). While some research suggests that e-cigarettes might help smokers quit (Hartmann-Boyce et al., 2021), they are not harm-free; they have been linked to "E-Cigarette or Vaping Product Use Associated Lung Injury" (EVALI) characterized by fever, fatigue, and respiratory and gastrointestinal symptoms (Smith et al., 2021a). Nurse-delivered nicotine cessation counseling can be effective even when relatively brief; only a few minutes is necessary for a nurse to ask about tobacco use, assess a client's desire to quit, and provide evidence-based advice about tactics (Aveyard et al., 2012). When smoking cessation counseling includes follow-up sessions, educational materials, and nicotine replacement therapy overseen by a provider, clients are more likely to quit (Duangchan & Matthews, 2020).

James Prochaska et al. (1992) studied the stages of change in addictive behaviors and their model is applied to smoking cessation in Table 15.1. Health professionals can promote client movement to subsequent stages through interventions

TABLE 15.1 Prochaska's Transtheoretical Model of Change Applied to Smoking Cessation

Stage 1: Precontemplation	Smokers do not see their smoking as a problem and do not intend to stop within the next 6 months.
Stage 2: Contemplation	Smokers see their smoking as a problem and think about quitting but are not ready to change.
Stage 3: Preparation	Smokers intend to take action in the next month; some have made small changes, such as cutting down on the number smoked or delaying the first smoke of the day.
Stage 4: Action	Smokers adopt a goal of smoking cessation and make an attempt to quit, involving overt behavior change and environmental modification.
Stage 5: Maintenance	Smokers work to prevent relapse and maintain abstinence.

Modified from Prochaska, J. O., DiClemente, C. C., & Norcross, J. C. (1992). In search of how people change: Applications to addictive behaviors. *American Psychologist, 47*, 1102–1114.

TABLE 15.2   Application of the Health Belief Model in Interventions to Promote Smoking Cessation

Factor	Interventions
Perceived susceptibility	Teach about morbidity and mortality statistics of smokers versus nonsmokers.
Perceived severity	Illustrate what happens to lungs and other organs when smoking; show pictures of diseased lungs and wrinkled skin.
Perceived barriers	Identify barriers unique to the individual and counsel regarding common fears about weight gain, greater stress, and irritability.
Perceived benefits	Identify benefits, such as more pleasant breath and body odor; increased energy; decreased cough; improved circulation; enhanced ability to taste; and reduced risk for heart disease, stroke, and cancers of the mouth, throat, esophagus, lungs, bladder, and cervix.
Cues to action	Use telephone calls and postcard reminders. Provide pamphlets about cessation strategies. Organize support groups and buddy systems.

that raise consciousness. Interventions to promote smoking cessation can be guided by the health belief model (HBM), as shown in Table 15.2. Using basic cognitive behavioral therapy (CBT), nurses can help their clients understand the links between smoking and their thoughts, emotions, behavior, and physical sensations (Taylor et al., 2021). Research by Judith Prochaska's team showed that exercise during smoking cessation not only improves mood but also increases the probability of staying smoke-free (Prochaska et al., 2008). Lapses in abstinence are common, and clients must be encouraged to resume the strategies that initially helped them quit. Successful quitters usually make several attempts.

Sleep. Health professionals are gaining an increased appreciation for the relationship between sleep and overall wellbeing as new research emerges. Adults aged 18 to 60 should be sleeping at least 7 hours a night. Less than this recommended amount can affect resistance to infection, ability to concentrate, productivity, and mood. Insufficient sleep is associated with an increased risk of obesity, hypertension, diabetes, cardiovascular disease, anxiety, and depression (Atrooz & Salim, 2020). Even insufficient napping in infants has been found to increase the risk for obesity outcomes within the first 6 months of life (Petrov et al., 2021). Research shows that a good night's sleep improves thinking and memory (Gorman, 2004). Unfortunately, millions of Americans are sleep deprived, with one in three adults reporting insufficient sleep (CDC, 2016). Many people are exposed to excessive light from TV screens and electronic devices during evening hours (Flaskerud, 2015); however, other factors such as chronic disease, smoking, obesity, and physically inactivity can put someone at risk for insufficient sleep (CDC, 2017). The National Sleep Foundation

estimated that about 55% of children and adolescents are also not sleeping enough (Buxton et al., 2015). Many parents are unaware of the recommended amount of sleep for their children and the need to limit their evening use of electronic devices. However, mental health concerns such as anxiety and depression as well as life stressors related to everything from neighborhood safety to school achievement can also keep children up at night. Nurses' can encourage commonly recommended sleep hygiene practices such as having a consistent sleep time with minimized noise, regular physical activity, appropriate stress management, and avoiding naps and substance use (Chung et al., 2018).

Emotional Intelligence. One's ability to identify, understand, regulate, and constructively express emotions is fundamental to wellness, yet this rarely receives sufficient attention from health care professionals. Emotional intelligence describes the knowledge, abilities, and traits to recognize and manage emotions in real-world situations. Appropriately managed emotions can lead to constructive relationships throughout all facets of an individual's life (Sarrionandia & Mikolajczak, 2020). Anger is one of the more obvious emotions to identify and assess in a client. Although anger is a normal human emotion, it is pathogenic when it is too frequent, too intense, too prolonged, or managed ineffectively. Habitual suppression is just as problematic as the tendency to have explosive outbursts because suppression of emotion requires great effort and often results in rumination for hours about the incident (Thomas, 2007).

Emotional intelligence has been found to shape the health of children and adolescents as well. Emotion perception and attention to one's own feelings has been linked to less alcohol consumption in adolescents (González-Yubero et al., 2019) and healthy diet adherence in elementary students (Melguizo-Ibañez et al., 2020). However, emotional intelligence can deteriorate in children of dysfunctional families. Development of emotional intelligence is facilitated by a supportive environment, which nurses are skilled in creating.

Problem Solving. Problem-solving skills must be taught to clients who do not know systematic strategies and techniques for enacting healthful habits or making changes in health behavior. For example, recovering alcoholics need to learn ways to slowly sip on nonalcoholic beverages at a party; parents of a new baby will need to practice asking potential visitors if they have received their influenza, COVID, and pertussis vaccines before visiting. Individuals who lack assertiveness may need to rehearse firm insistence that sex partners use condoms. When giving exercise or diet prescriptions to clients, health care providers should ask what problems or barriers they envision; this will point the way to the skills that need to be taught. The possibility of family or friends undermining nutrition and exercise decisions should always be explored with clients when behavior changes are undertaken, and counseling should be offered about ways of resisting it.

EVIDENCE-BASED INTERVENTIONS TO PROMOTE BEHAVIOR CHANGE

Health professionals often use threats of future disease when urging behavior change. However, when people are frightened, they may use denial to convince themselves that the threatening event (e.g., human immunodeficiency virus/acquired immunodeficiency syndrome [HIV/AIDS], cancer) is not likely to happen to them. Such threats of distant adverse outcomes are not as likely to be as successful as approaches that confer immediate benefits or reduce denial. Motivational interviewing strategies aim to increase client motivation to make behavior changes by focusing on client's thoughts about change rather than delivering provider imperatives. Components of the motivational interviewing approach are provider empathy, a spirit of collaboration with the client, avoidance of lecturing or arguing, and support of client self-efficacy (Modesto-Lowe & Alvarado, 2017; Riegel et al., 2006).

Behavior change recommended by nurses relies upon strong and trusting nurse-client relationships. According to the American Board of Internal Medicine (ABIM, 2021), some ethnic minorities are more likely to feel mistrust of all health care providers. From the rise of eugenics in the early 1900s to forced sterilization of Native American women in the 1970s and Black female inmates as recently as 2014, health care professionals cannot ignore the shameful overt racism in health care and the consequent influence on client interactions with the health care system. The additional strain placed on the health care system during the COVID-19 pandemic juxtaposed with an explosion of misinformation further strained client-provider relationships. Misinformation predominantly shared through social media can seem uncontrollable. However, nurses can review posts for appropriate citations and be alerted when information is sensationalized, has a conspiratorial tone, or is simply incorrect. Crossmatching content with reputable sources, nurses can respectfully correct misinformation by reflecting on any valid concerns, providing reputable sources, and minimizing jargon in responses (Bautista et al., 2021).

Once trust is developed, readiness to change can then be assessed. When promoting behavior change, be aware that "approach goals" (e.g., increasing consumption of vegetables) are easier for clients to work on than "avoidance goals" (e.g., decreasing sweets) (Sullivan & Rothman, 2008). It is also essential to focus on incremental, achievable goals because clients can be overwhelmed by the prospect of drastic change. A nurse could begin by simply asking an adolescent if they would consider drinking carbonated water instead of a soda for lunch. Clients should be taught that slow weight loss achieved through habitual lifestyle changes is preferable to rapid loss from fad diets. Diets, which commonly involve some level of deprivation, frequently result in rebound weight gain—often more than what was lost.

When health care providers write *prescriptions* for physical activity or nutrition changes, adherence improves (Dobson, 2008). Another strategy with proven effectiveness is contracting. This provides an accountability mechanism that is frequently supported in health behavior research. The purpose of writing a contract is to arrange a favorable, positively reinforcing experience when the client performs the desirable health behavior. Elements of a good contract are depicted in Box 15.2. A sample contract for weight loss appears in Fig. 15.4. Keeping a log or diary also contributes to successful behavior change. Combining self-monitoring (e.g., with wearable devices or mobile phone applications) with goal setting and counseling provide an added benefit such as increased daily step count (Vetrovsky et al., 2021).

An impediment to the use of written prescriptions and contracts is the low functional literacy of Americans. Literacy levels are lower among historically marginalized populations, older adults, and those with less education and lower income. If giving written materials to clients, use simple, everyday vocabulary. Ascertain clients' comprehension of the behavior change instructions by asking them to share what they have learned before they leave the clinical area. This strategy is known as the *teach-back method.*

BOX 15.2 Elements of a Good Contract for Behavior Change

- The behavior must be carefully selected and explicitly described.
- The behavior must be measurable (e.g., number of cigarettes smoked, minutes of exercise).
- A data collection plan must be developed (e.g., calendar, log, chart, graph, diary).
- Client and nurse agree on the goals (short-term and long-term) and time frame.
- Client and nurse agree on the reinforcers (extrinsic and intrinsic).
- Reinforcers are specified for step-by-step approximations of the desired behavior.
- Client and nurse sign the written contract and both keep a copy.
- Client and nurse evaluate effectiveness of the plan.
- The plan is revised as needed.

ENVIRONMENTAL FACTORS THAT AFFECT WELLNESS

Nurses must look beyond individual capabilities in the quest to help clients become healthier. The range of health-promoting choices available to individuals may be drastically limited by societal forces, structures, and policies. As depicted in Fig. 15.1, numerous environmental factors affect wellness.

Culture

The cultural milieu in which a person develops and resides has a profound influence on health and health-related behaviors. The term "culture" applies beyond ethnicity; one individual often identifies with multiple cultures. Age groups or generations, genders, and geographic regions also create cultures. The way cultures are grouped and described also has implications. For example, the commonly used terms "Latino" or "Asian American" lump together

Desired outcome:	Weight loss of 10 lb
Long-term goal:	To lose 2½ lb per week for 4 weeks
Short-term goals:	1. Maintain 1200 calorie/day diet.
	2. Increase water consumption to eight glasses per day.
	3. Avoid skipping meals.
	4. Ride exercise machine:
	Week 1: 15 minutes 3 times per week
	Week 2: 20 minutes 3 times per week
	Week 3: 25 minutes 3 times per week
	Week 4: 30 minutes 3 times per week
	5. Weigh self on Monday mornings. Record weight on flow sheet.
Intrinsic rewards:	Increased self-esteem and confidence
	Clothes fit better
	Improved physical fitness and appearance
Extrinsic rewards:	Upon successful completion of each day's regimen, a 20-minute bubble bath
	At end of each week, movie with a friend
	At end of contract, purchase of a new outfit

Signature of nurse _____ Signature of client _____ Date _____

Fig. 15.4 Example of a Health Behavior Change Contract.

multiple unique nationalities, each with distinct historical, geographical, and political influences. *Thus, it is imperative that nurses not assume cultural affiliations based on a patient's demographics.* Although an individual may identify with a specific culture, they may not ascribe to all commonly understood beliefs and practices. Some traditions may also be interpreted differently within a culture. For example, a commonly cited traditional belief in some Latino subpopulations is *susto*, described as an intensely traumatic or emotional event that leads to illness or disease. However, only some Latinos believe *susto* can be cured, description of symptoms and treatment of *susto* vary broadly, as do risks and protective factors, and some do not believe in *susto* at all (Moreira et al., 2018). Regardless of what information is available about *common* norms for a specific cultural group, it is the nurse's responsibility to ask the client about their personal practices, preferences, and beliefs—and tailor care accordingly.

Environmental Hazards

As record-breaking temperatures become the norm, causing a dramatic rise in sea levels, the changing climate will directly impact human health. Premature death due to increasing temperatures and worsening air quality is projected to increase substantially. Some estimates suggest that areas in the western, southern, and southeastern United States could expect to see climate-associated mortality rates as high as 10 per 100,000 by the year 2040 (Fann et al., 2021). Extreme weather, forest fires, droughts, flooding, and other environmental catastrophes also directly impact millions each year. Not only do some families lose their homes and undergo insurmountable stress, but the death, injury, and disease that result from enduring these climate-related disasters make them an undeniable public health issue. Nurses are called to serve during these crises and must be prepared to support individuals and families in dire circumstances. All health care professionals have a responsibility to advocate for the public by communicating with policymakers and urging meaningful change. Professional organizations such as the Alliance of Nurses for Healthy Environments (envirn.org) and Health Care Without Harm (noharm.org) are working together to promote environmental health by engaging hospital leadership, influencing legislation, and educating the public.

Nurses' attention to environmental hazards was heightened when the American Nurses Association adopted the Precautionary Principle in 2004. Thousands of new chemicals have been introduced in recent years, but research regarding their effects on human beings is often lacking. If adverse health effects of chemicals or products are suspected, the Precautionary Principle mandates that nurses take precautionary measures even if cause-effect relationships have not been scientifically demonstrated. Nurses are also urged to include an environmental exposure history in routine health assessments (Buchanan, 2005).

Many people are exposed to noxious substances or stimuli in their daily lives. Asbestos, mercury, radiation, and toxic chemicals such as pesticides are just a few of the hazards workers may encounter. Queries about a client's place of residence may reveal safety concerns such as proximity to polluting industries or hazardous waste sites. Further assessment could identify additional risks such as crime rates or violence as well as limited coping resources.

Social and psychological hazards must be considered as well. Racial and/or sexual discrimination presents known health risks for millions. Structural racism permeates virtually all sectors of society and influences physical and mental states, access to health care, and the type of care received. For example, Black and Latina women receive significantly less pain medication than non-Hispanic White women during the postpartum period (Badreldin et al., 2019), and Black and Latino children are less likely than non-Hispanic White children to undergo diagnostic imaging in the emergency department (Marin et al., 2021). Federal law perpetuates health disparities with a lack of funding for services and outreach for Native American elders and deficient tribal consultation when formulating health policy (Willging et al., 2021).

Stress

What happens when the environment bombards individuals with stressors? Researchers now know that stress is a psychological appraisal that the environmental demands exceed one's coping resources (Lazarus, 1991). Early stress research focused on major life events, such as foreclosure of a mortgage, bereavement, divorce, or job loss, demonstrating that an accumulation of such events could be detrimental to health (Holmes & Rahe, 1967). These major life events are undoubtedly disruptive, but minor daily hassles are disruptive as well (Kanner et al., 1981). Increased stress attributed to the COVID-19 pandemic trended with rises in depression and anxiety but was especially notable in health care workers and pediatric populations (Manchia et al., 2022). This trend is particularly concerning because suicide rates among female nurses were higher than the general female population even before the pandemic (Davis et al., 2021), mandating more attention to effective stress management in our own profession.

Allostasis (the continual adjustment of our bodies to stressors) can slide into health-damaging allostatic load when stress lasts too long or the body's response is too strong. Chronic stress increases vulnerability to cardiovascular disease (Shivpuri et al., 2012) and accelerates the aging process by shortening the life span of cells

(Epel et al., 2004). Research on a nationally representative sample showed that the risk for premature death was increased in individuals who reported high stress (Keller et al., 2012).

Stress can undermine the enactment of health-promoting behavior such as exercise. Fortunately, stress management modalities such as mindfulness, breathing techniques, meditation, and yoga movements can be practiced when other modalities are not feasible (see Chapter 22 for a deeper discussion). However, health care providers must keep environmental contexts in mind. Individuals in highly stressful environments may choose health-damaging behaviors such as smoking or consuming alcohol to help them cope. The over 37 million Americans living in poverty (US Census, 2021) are not likely to perceive that they can master stress. In fact, when poverty is chronic and resources scant, pervasive feelings of powerlessness and a fatalistic outlook about the future are likely (Kaplan et al., 2013).

Social Support

Social support is directly related to physical, mental, and emotional health. Loving relationships with significant others may buffer or moderate stress. Connectedness to others is a central element in health throughout life. Considerable empirical evidence shows that social support produces improved resistance to disease, influences recovery from a health crisis such as myocardial infarction, and predicts longevity (Lett et al., 2007). How does social support result in improved health? Both emotional and instrumental types of support have been identified (Finfgeld-Connett, 2005). Support from relatives and friends can include concrete material help (e.g., money) as well as encouragement. Extrafamilial support groups and health professionals also can play a vital role in promoting health behavior change. The value of a dieting or jogging "buddy" is well known. Stigmatized and marginalized client populations, such as individuals experiencing homelessness, may lack a supportive network. Mobilizing social support can be an essential nursing intervention in such cases. Lockdowns that occurred during the COVID-19 pandemic brought to light the importance of social health and the detrimental effects of social isolation. Older adults, females, and health care workers were found to be at especially high risk for the negative effects of social isolation early in the pandemic (Sepúlveda-Loyola et al., 2020). Social isolation has also been linked to an increased risk of dying from coronary heart disease or stroke (Smith et al., 2021b). Addressing social isolation is challenging because those experiencing it may be less likely to seek support. Nurses can address social isolation by encouraging clients to use video applications to strengthen social connections, identify support groups, encourage regular sleep-wake

times, improve physical activity, and engage in cognitively stimulating activities (Sepúlveda-Loyola et al., 2020). Although social media can open channels of communication that facilitate social connection, there is also the danger of social media misuse which can lead to body and life dissatisfaction, depression, and addictive behaviors (Robinson et al., 2019).

NATIONAL HEALTH PROMOTION GOALS

Nurses' health promotion efforts must be supported and guided by an adequate understanding of U.S. public policy. The *Healthy People* documents published in 1979, 1990, 2000, 2010, and 2020 by the U.S. Public Health Service within the DHHS, have focused on both individual and societal influences on health. These widely disseminated publications have drawn attention to health disparities among Americans and provided guidance to state and local planners of public health programs. Health promotion and disease prevention objectives are precisely stated and measurable. The precisely delineated objectives in the *Healthy People* documents have enabled measurement of the nation's progress.

Healthy People 2030, published in 2020, contained 5 overarching goals promoting healthy, thriving lives; eliminating health disparities; creating environments that foster the attainment of health and well-being; fostering healthy development and behaviors across the life stages; and engaging leadership and the public in the design of policies for health improvement (U.S. Public Health Service [USPHS], 2020). The document delineates 355 core objectives as well as developmental and research objectives. A small subset of high-priority objectives, termed Leading Health Indicators, directs the attention of the nation to urgent concerns such as infant mortality, diabetes, maternal deaths, drug overdose deaths, and suicide. Progress on achievement of the objectives will be reported biennially during the decade 2020–2030. Selected objectives from *Healthy People 2030* are shown in Table 15.3.

COMMUNITY HEALTH PROMOTION

Health professionals are collaborating increasingly with community leaders to design interventions such as youth activity programs, nutrition classes, school-based clinics, and health screenings. Among the indicators of a community's health are communication patterns, ability to take organized action, level of social functioning (work and school attendance), proportion of individuals at the poverty level, crime rates, and traditional morbidity and mortality statistics. One type of community intervention

TABLE 15.3 Selected Examples of National Health Promotion Objectives as Identified in *Healthy People 2030*

Focus Area	Goal	Objective	Target
Health communication	Improve health communication	HC/HIT-02 Decrease the proportion of adults who report poor communication with their health care provider	8% of adults will report poor communication
Nutrition and healthy eating	Improve health by promoting healthy eating and making nutritious foods available	NWS-01 Reduce household food insecurity and in doing so reduce hunger	6% of households will be food insecure
Tobacco use	Reduce illness, disability, and death related to tobacco use and secondhand smoke	TU-05 Reduce current e-cigarette use in adolescents	10.5% of adolescents will use e-cigarettes

is the Healthy Cities initiatives, first developed in Canada and Europe. The first site in the United States, the Indiana Healthy Community Project, was developed by a nurse (Flynn et al., 1992). The Healthy Cities initiatives address a broad range of concerns that are identified by community members, such as gang violence and job creation. Coalitions of community groups are formed to develop programming. For individuals who live in rural areas rather than cities, county-based programs involving county extension agents, such as Walk Kansas, have proven successful (Estabrooks et al., 2008). A randomized intervention trial in 16 rural towns in Montana and New York targeted physical activity and healthy eating among overweight, sedentary women, highlighting the importance of support for behavior change within the rural women's close relationships (Lo et al., 2021). Because a lack of public transportation and childcare presents barriers to participation in health-promoting activities in rural areas, church buses and vans have been recommended (Kruger et al., 2012).

School-based health fairs and health promotion carnivals for elementary, middle, and high schools are frequently conducted by nursing faculty and students (Sims & McFadden, 2021). An innovative approach used by school nurses to engage youth in health promotion initiatives is Photovoice (Lofton & Bergren, 2019). Typically, students are given a few days to take photographs, followed by group discussions and the creation of a photo exhibit for their school and/or community policymakers. Photographs in various projects have vividly depicted tobacco and drug influences, garbage in the streets, and stressful aspects of daily life such as fighting and other forms of violence in the community. These projects often result in beneficial media exposure and community activism.

Increased emphasis is being placed on tailoring preventive interventions to meet the needs of diverse groups that are culturally different from the participants in scientifically rigorous controlled trials. To reach Asian American communities that may not be reached by mainstream health care channels, faith-based organizations (Christian, Muslim, and Sikh) were recruited for a health promotion project in New York City and New Jersey (Kwon et al., 2017). The project implemented healthier food options for congregational communal meals and a blood pressure monitoring program. Bangladeshi, Filipino, Korean, and Asian Indian communities participated.

Willingness to solicit and listen to community input when planning health promotion programs is essential. Programs designed to reduce health disparities or to combat problems such as substance abuse or teenage pregnancy may be evidence-based but mismatched for the particular community (Ramanadhan et al., 2012). Castro et al. (2004, p. 41) quote a Southwestern community leader who asked (in Spanish), "What good is science if it doesn't help us?" Unless programs are adapted in collaboration with the intended audience, people will "vote with their feet" (Crowley et al., 2012, p. 101). The greatest challenge of health promotion in the 21st century may be reaching the more vulnerable and historically marginalized members of society and involving them in strategies to enhance and prolong their lives.

SUMMARY

Health is complex and can be conceptualized differently by diverse populations. When a health behavior change is necessary, the nurse must respect and collaborate with the client considering the dynamic forces that impact health and the ability to change behavior. Changing health behavior is difficult even when doing so would lessen the likelihood of future illness. Although individuals are often aware of the risks associated with poor health behaviors, they may modify their thinking about these risks rather than changing the behaviors. Information is the solution only when ignorance is the sole problem. Nurses who understand the principles of behavior change can help patients make health-promoting decisions. Using a comprehensive model of wellness identifies the behavioral, psychological, environmental, and organismic factors associated with wellness. Pender's Health Promotion Model assists in predicting the likelihood of successful behavior change based on personal factors and prior related behavior. Motivational interventions are more likely to produce health behavior change than threats of future diseases. Environmental factors, including the cultural milieu, climate change, safety hazards, and stressors, also affect wellness. Although not often modifiable, social determinants of health (e.g., related to ethnicity, income, and gender) cannot be ignored when collaborating with clients to achieve health outcomes. National health promotion goals to guide equitable health policy are defined in the *Healthy People* initiative but must be carried out at the community level by strong public-provider partnerships.

SALIENT POINTS

- Conceptualizing health more broadly than "the absence of disease" has significant implications for nursing practice.
- Health promotion and disease prevention have different foci, in that health promotion activities aim to take people beyond their present level of wellness, whereas disease prevention efforts are undertaken to prevent specific diseases.
- The major causes of death in the United States are related to lifestyle.
- A comprehensive model of wellness includes modifiable attitudinal and behavioral variables as well as environmental factors and nonmodifiable organismic characteristics.
- Pender's Health Promotion Model is useful in guiding health promotion research and practice.
- Prochaska's transtheoretical model can be used to assess client readiness to change health behavior.
- Motivational interventions are more likely to produce health behavior change than threats of future disease or distant adverse outcomes.
- Health care providers should make greater use of written prescriptions, contracting, and other evidence-based interventions.
- Nurses' health promotion efforts should be guided by national health promotion goals, such as those articulated in *Healthy People 2030*.
- Health promotion initiatives must target families and communities as well as individuals, with greater attention to culturally diverse community voices and health equity.

CRITICAL REFLECTION EXERCISES

1. Assess your own health behavior, and then select one behavior that you desire to change. It can be something you want to *increase,* such as aerobic exercise, *decrease,* such as drinking sugary beverages, or *stop,* such as smoking. Develop a plan to change the behavior, and then implement the plan for 1 month. Critically assess factors that facilitated or hindered the achievement of your behavior change.

2. Select one detrimental health behavior, such as excessive drinking. Review the research literature regarding evidence-based interventions to change this behavior. Is it clear which interventions are most effective? Is sufficient information available about changing the behavior in people of diverse ages, ethnicity, sexual orientation, and socioeconomic status? Develop at least three questions for future research.

ⓔ EVOLVE WEBSITE/RESOURCES LIST

American Council on Science and Health: https://www.acsh.org
Center for Advancing Health: http://www.cfah.org/
Center for Tobacco Cessation: http://www.centerforcessation.org/

For calculating calories in food and calories burned in activities of daily living: https://www.livestrong.com/myplate/
For nurses who smoke: https://www.tobaccofreenurses.org

For physical activity guidelines: https://health.gov/our-work/nutrition-physical-activity-guidelines

For tips on achieving better sleep: https://www.sleepfoundation.org/

For weight control information: https://niddk.nih.gov/health-information/community-health-outreach/healthy-living-tips

Healthy People 2030: https://health.gov/healthypeople

Nutrition information: https://www.nutrition.gov/

Substance Abuse and Mental Health Services Administration: SAMHSA: https://www.samhsa.gov/

Substance use Disorder in Nursing Resources from the NCSBN: https://www.ncsbn.org/substance-use-in-nursing.htm

USDA/DHHS Dietary Guidelines: https://health.gov/our-work/nutrition-physical-activity/dietary-guidelines

REFERENCES

American Board of Internal Medicine Foundation. (2021). *Surveys of trust in the U.S. health care system.* NORC, University of Chicago. https://www.norc.org/PDFs/ABIM%20Foundation/20210520_NORC_ABIM_Foundation_Trust%20in%20Healthcare_Part%201.pdf

American Nurses Association. (2018). *The opioid epidemic: The evolving role of nursing.* https://www.nursingworld.org/~4a4da5/globalassets/practiceandpolicy/work-environment/health–safety/opioid-epidemic/2018-ana-opioid-issue-brief-vfinal-pdf-2018-08-29.pdf

Atrooz, F., & Salim, S. (2020). Sleep deprivation, oxidative stress and inflammation. *Advances in Protein Chemistry and Structural Biology, 119,* 309–336. https://doi.org/10.1016/bs.apcsb.2019.03.001

Aveyard, P., Begh, R., Parsons, A., & West, R. (2012). Brief opportunistic smoking cessation interventions: A systematic review and meta-analysis to compare advice to quit and offer of assistance. *Addiction, 107*(6), 1066–1073. https://doi.org/10.1111/j.1360-0443.2011.03770.x

Badreldin, N., Grobman, W. A., & Yee, L. M. (2019). Racial disparities in postpartum pain management. *Obstetrics and Gynecology, 134*(6), 1147–1153. https://doi.org/10.1097/AOG.0000000000003561

Bandura, A. (1997). *Self-efficacy: The exercise of control.* W. H. Freeman.

Bandura, A. (2012). On the functional properties of perceived self efficacy revisited. *Journal of Management, 38,* 9–44. https://doi.org/10.1177%2F0149206311410606

Bautista, J. R., Zhang, Y., & Gwizdka, J. (2021). Healthcare professionals' acts of correcting health misinformation on social media. *International Journal of Medical Informatics (Shannon, Ireland), 148,* 104375. https://doi.org/10.1016/j.ijmedinf.2021.104375

Biasini, B., Rosi, A., Giopp, F., Turgut, R., Scazzina, F., & Menozzi, D. (2021). Understanding, promoting and predicting sustainable diets: A systematic review. *Trends in Food Science & Technology, 111,* 191–207. https://doi.org/10.1016/j.tifs.2021.02.062

Boyle, P. A., Barnes, L. L., Buchman, A. S., & Bennett, D. A. (2009). Purpose in life is associated with mortality among community-dwelling older persons. *Psychosomatic Medicine, 71,* 574–579. https://doi.org/10.1097%2FPSY.0b013e3181a5a7c0

Buchanan, M. (2005). Rebuilding the bridge. *American Journal of Nursing, 105*(4), 104.

Burdette, A. M., Hill, T. D., Webb, N., Ford, J., & Haynes, S. (2018). Religious involvement and substance use among urban mothers. *Journal for the Scientific Study of Religion, 57,* 156–172. https://doi.org/10.1111/jssr.12501

Buxton, O. M., Chang, A. M., Spilsbury, J. C., Bos, T., Emsellem, H., & Knutson, K. L. (2015). Sleep in the modern family: Protective family routines for child and adolescent sleep. *Sleep Health, 1*(1), 15–27. https://doi.org/10.1016/j.sleh.2014.12.002

Callen, B. L., Mefford, L., Groer, M., & Thomas, S. P. (2011). Relationships among stress, infectious illness, and religiousness/spirituality in community-dwelling older adults. *Research in Gerontological Nursing, 4*(3), 195–206. https://doi.org/10.3928/19404921-20101001-99

Carver, C. S., Scheier, M. F., & Segerstrom, S. C. (2010). Optimism. *Clinical Psychology Review, 30*(7), 879–889. https://doi.org/10.1016/j.cpr.2010.01.006

Castro, F. G., Barrera, Jr., M., & Martinez, Jr., C. R. (2004). The cultural adaptation of prevention interventions: Resolving tensions between fidelity and fit. *Prevention Science, 5*(1), 41–45. https://doi.org/10.1023/B:PREV.0000013980.12412.cd

Centers for Disease Control and Prevention. (2016). *1 in 3 adults don't get enough sleep.* https://www.cdc.gov/media/releases/2016/p0215-enough-sleep.html

Centers for Disease Control and Prevention. (2017). *Data and statistics: Short sleep duration among US adults.* https://www.cdc.gov/sleep/data_statistics.html

Centers for Disease Control and Prevention. (2020). *Adult physical inactivity prevalence maps by race/ethnicity.* https://www.cdc.gov/physicalactivity/data/inactivity-prevalence-maps/index.html

Centers for Disease Control and Prevention. (2021). *Opioid basics.* https://www.cdc.gov/opioids/basics/epidemic.html

Centers for Disease Control and Prevention. (2021). *Prevalence of overweight, obesity, and severe obesity among adults aged 20 and Over: United States, 1960–1962 through 2017–2018.* https://www.cdc.gov/nchs/data/hestat/obesity-adult-17-18/obesity-adult.htm

Chevinsky, J. R., Lee, S. H., Blanck, H. M., & Park, S. (2021). Prevalence of self-reported intake of sugar-sweetened beverages among US adults in 50 states and the District of Columbia, 2010 and 2015. *Preventing Chronic Disease, 18,* E35. https://doi.org/10.5888/pcd18.200434

Chung, K. F., Lee, C. T., Yeung, W. F., Chan, M. S., Chung, E. W. Y., & Lin, W. L. (2018). Sleep hygiene education as a treatment of insomnia: A systematic review and meta-analysis. *Family Practice, 35*(4), 365–375. https://doi.org/10.1093/fampra/cmx122

Collado-Mateo, D., Lavín-Pérez, A. M., Peñacoba, C., Del Coso, J., Leyton-Román, M., Luque Casado, A., Gasque, P.,

Fernández-Del-Olmo, M. Á., & Amado-Alonso, D. (2021). Key factors associated with adherence to physical exercise in patients with chronic diseases and older adults: An umbrella review. *International Journal of Environmental Research and Public Health, 18*(4), 2023. https://doi.org/10.3390/ijerph18042023

Corley, J. (2020). Adherence to the MIND diet is associated with 12-year all-cause mortality in older adults. *Public Health Nutrition, 25*(2), 358–367. https://doi.org/10.1017/S1368980020002979

Cowling, W. T. (2013). Healing as appreciating wholeness. In W. K. Cody (Ed.), *Philosophical and theoretical perspectives for advanced nursing practice.* Jones & Bartlett.

Crowley, D. M., Greenberg, M. T., Feinberg, M. E., Spoth, R. L., & Redmond, C. R. (2012). The effect of the PROSPER Partnership Model on cultivating local stakeholder knowledge of evidence-based programs: A five-year longitudinal study of 28 communities. *Prevention Science, 13*, 96–105. https://doi.org/10.1007/s11121-011-0250-5

Davis, M. A., Cher, B. A., Friese, C. R., & Bynum, J. P. (2021). Association of US nurse and physician occupation with risk of suicide. *JAMA Psychiatry, 78*(6), 651–658. https://doi.org/10.1001/jamapsychiatry.2021.0154

Della Corte, K., Fife, J., Gardner, A., Murphy, B. L., Kleis, L., Della Corte, D., Schwingshackl, L., LeCheminant, J. D., & Buyken, A. E. (2021). World trends in sugar-sweetened beverage and dietary sugar intakes in children and adolescents: A systematic review. *Nutrition Reviews, 79*(3), 274–288. https://doi.org/10.1093/nutrit/nuaa070

Dobson, R. (2008). Half of patients given exercise prescriptions are more active. *BMJ, 337*, 894–895. https://doi.org/10.1136/bmj.a2084

Duangchan, C., & Matthews, A. K. (2020). The effects of nurse led smoking cessation interventions for patients with cancer: A systematic review. *Pacific Rim International Journal of Nursing Research, 24*(1), 118–139. https://www.ncbi.nlm.nih.gov/pmc/articles/PMC8344177/pdf/nihms-1726864.pdf

Emberson, M. A., Lalande, A., Wang, D., McDonough, D. J., Liu, W., & Gao, Z. (2021). Effectiveness of smartphone-based physical activity interventions on individuals' Health Outcomes: A systematic review. *BioMed Research International, 2021*, 6296896. https://doi.org/10.1155/2021/6296896

Epel, E. S., Blackburn, E. H., Lin, J., Dhabhar, F. S., Adler, N. E., & Morrow, J. D. (2004). Accelerated telomere shortening in response to life stress. *Proceedings of the National Academy of Science, 101*(49), 17312–17315. https://doi.org/10.1073/pnas.0407162101

Estabrooks, P., Bradshaw, M., Dzewaltowski, D., & Smith-Ray, R. (2008). Determining the impact of Walk Kansas: Applying a team-building approach to community physical activity promotion. *Annals of Behavioral Medicine, 36*, 1–12. https://doi.org/10.1007/s12160-008-9040-0

Fann, N. L., Nolte, C. G., Sarofim, M. C., Martinich, J., & Nassikas, N. J. (2021). Associations between simulated future changes in climate, air quality, and human health. *JAMA Network Open, 4*(1), e2032064. https://doi.org/10.1001/jamanetworkopen.2020.32064

Finfgeld-Connett, D. (2005). Clarification of social support. *Journal of Nursing Scholarship, 37*(1), 4–9. https://doi.org/10.1111/j.1547-5069.2005.00004.x

Flaskerud, J. (2015). The cultures of sleep. *Issues in Mental Health Nursing, 36*, 1013–1016. https://doi.org/10.3109/01612840.2014.978960

Flynn, B. C., Rider, M. S., & Bailey, W. W. (1992). Developing community leadership in healthy cities: The Indiana model. *Nursing Outlook, 49*(3), 121–126.

Gadamer, H. G. (1996). *The enigma of health: The art of healing in a scientific age.* Stanford University Press.

Gentzke, A. S., Wang, T. W., Jamal, A., Park-Lee, E., Ren, C., Cullen, K. A., & Neff, L. (2020). Tobacco product use among middle and high school students—United States, 2020. *MMWR Morbidity and Mortality Weekly Report, 69*, 1881–1888. https://doi.org/10.15585/mmwr.mm6950a1

Godfrey, J. R. (2004). Toward optimal health: The experts discuss therapeutic humor. *Journal of Women's Health, 13*, 474–479. https://doi.org/10.1089/1540999041280972

González-Yubero, S., Palomera Martín, R., & Lázaro-Visa, S. (2019). Trait and ability emotional intelligence as predictors of alcohol consumption in adolescents. *Psicothema, 31*(3), 292–297. https://doi.org/10.7334/psicothema2018.315

Gorman, C. (2004). Why we sleep. *Time, 164*(25), 46–56.

Hartmann-Boyce, J., McRobbie, H., Butler, A. R., Lindson, N., Bullen, C., Begh, R., Theodoulou, A., Notley, C., Rigotti, N. A., Turner, T., Fanshawe, T. R., & Hajek, P. (2021). Electronic cigarettes for smoking cessation. *Cochrane Database of Systematic Reviews, 2021*(8), CD010216. https://doi.org/10.1002/14651858.CD010216.pub5

Holmes, T. H., & Rahe, R. H. (1967). The social readjustment rating scale. *Journal of Psychosomatic Research, 11*, 213–218. https://doi.org/10.1016/0022-3999(67)90010-4

Huffman, M. K., & Amireault, S. (2021). What keeps them going, and what gets them back? Older adults' beliefs about physical activity maintenance. *The Gerontologist, 61*(3), 392–402. https://doi.org/10.1093/geront/gnaa087

Jackson, E. S., Tucker, C. M., & Herman, K. C. (2007). Health value, perceived social support, and health self-efficacy as factors in a health-promoting lifestyle. *Journal of American College Health, 56*(1), 69–74. https://doi.org/10.3200/JACH.56.1.69-74

Kanner, A., Coyne, J., Schaefer, C., & Lazarus, R. (1981). Comparison of two modes of stress measurement: Daily hassles and uplifts versus major life events. *Journal of Behavioral Medicine, 4*, 1–39. https://doi.org/10.1007/bf00844845

Kaplan, S., Madden, V., Mijanovich, T., & Pucaro, E. (2013). The perception of stress and its impact on health in poor communities. *Journey of Community Health, 38*, 142–149. https://doi.org/10.1007/s10900-012-9593-5

Keller, A., Litzelman, K., Wisk, L. E., Maddox, T., Cheng, E. R., Crewswell, P. D., & Witt, W. P. (2012). Does the perception that stress affects health matter? The association with health and mortality. *Health Psychology, 31*(5), 677. https://doi.org/10.1037/a0026743

Kruger, T. M., Howell, B. M., & Haney, A. (2012). Perceptions of smoking cessation programs in rural Appalachia. *American*

Journal of Health Behavior, 36, 373–384. https://doi.org/10.5993/AJHB.36.3.8

Kwon, S. C., Patel, S., Choy, C., Zanowiak, J., Rideout, C., & Islam, N. S. (2017). Implementing health promotion activities using community-engaged approaches in Asian American faith-based organizations in New York City and New Jersey. *Translational Behavioral Medicine, 7*, 444–466. https://doi.org/10.1007/s13142-017-0506-0

Lalani, N., & Chen, A. (2021). Spirituality in nursing and health: A historical context, challenges, and way forward. *Holistic Nursing Practice, 35*(4), 206–210. https://doi.org/10.1097/HNP.0000000000000454

Lazarus, R. (1991). *Emotion and adaptation.* Oxford University Press.

Lett, H. S., Blumenthal, J. A., Babyak, M. A., Catellier, D. J., Carney, R. M., Berkman, L. F., Burg, M. M., Mitchell, P., Jaffe, A. S., & Schneiderman, N. (2007). Social support and prognosis in patients at increased psychosocial risk recovering from myocardial infarction. *Health Psychology, 26*(4), 418–427. https://doi.org/10.1037/0278-6133.26.4.418

Lo, B. K., Graham, M. L., Folta, S. C., Strogatz, D., Parry, S. A., & Seguin-Fowler, R. A. (2021). Physical activity and healthy eating behavior changes among rural women: An exploratory mediation analysis of a randomized multilevel intervention trial. *Translational Behavioral Medicine, 11*(10), 1839–1848. https://doi.org/10.1093/tbm/ibaa138

Lofton, S., & Bergren, M. (2019). Collaborating with youth in school health promotion initiatives with photovoice. *NASN School Nurse, 34*(1), 55–56. https://journals.sagepub.com/doi/epub/10.1177/1942602X18779424

Loh, R., Stamatakis, E., Folkerts, D., Allgrove, J. E., & Moir, H. J. (2020). Effects of interrupting prolonged sitting with physical activity breaks on blood glucose, insulin and triacylglycerol measures: A systematic review and meta-analysis. *Sports Medicine (Auckland, N.Z.), 50*(2), 295–330. https://doi.org/10.1007/s40279-019-01183-w

Manchia, M., Gathier, A. W., Yapici-Eser, H., Schmidt, M. V., de Quervain, D., van Amelsvoort, T., Bisson, J. I., Cryan, J. F., Howes, O. D., Pinto, L., van der Wee, N. J., Domschke, K., Branchi, I., & Vinkers, C. H. (2022). The impact of the prolonged COVID-19 pandemic on stress resilience and mental health: A critical review across waves. *European Neuropsychopharmacology: The Journal of the European College of Neuropsychopharmacology, 55*, 22–83. https://doi.org/10.1016/j.euroneuro.2021.10.864

Marin, J. R., Rodean, J., Hall, M., Alpern, E. R., Aronson, P. L., Chaudhari, P. P., Cohen, E., Freedman, S. B., Morse, R. B., Peltz, A., Samuels-Kalow, M., Shah, S. S., Simon, H. K., & Neuman, M. I. (2021). Racial and ethnic differences in emergency department diagnostic imaging at US children's hospitals, 2016–2019. *JAMA Network Open, 4*(1), e2033710. https://doi.org/10.1001/jamanetworkopen.2020.33710

Marton, G., Pizzoli, S., Vergani, L., Mazzocco, K., Monzani, D., Bailo, L., Pancani, L., & Pravettoni, G. (2021). Patients' health locus of control and preferences about the role that they want to play in the medical decision-making process. *Psychology,*

Health & Medicine, 26(2), 260–266. https://doi.org/10.1080/13548506.2020.1748211

Melguizo-Ibañez, E., Viciana-Garófano, V., Curita-Ortega, F., Ubago-Jiménez, J. L., & González-Valero, G. (2020). Physical activity level, Mediterranean diet adherence, and emotional intelligence as a function of family functioning in elementary school students. *Children, 8*(1), 6. https://doi.org/10.3390/children8010006

Modesto-Lowe, V., & Alvarado, C. (2017). E-cigs: Are they cool? Talking to teens about e cigarettes. *Clinical Pediatrics, 56*, 947–952. https://doi.org/10.1177/0009922817705188

Moreira, T., Hernandez, D. C., Scott, C. W., Murillo, R., Vaughan, E. M., & Johnston, C. A. (2018). Susto, Coraje, y Fatalismo: Cultural-bound beliefs and the treatment of diabetes among socioeconomically disadvantaged Hispanics. *American Journal of Lifestyle Medicine, 12*(1), 30–33. https://doi.org/10.1177/1559827617736506

Naci, H., & Ioannidis, J. P. A. (2013). Comparative effectiveness of exercise and drug interventions on mortality outcomes: Metaepidemiological study. *BMJ (Online), 22*(1), f55–f5577. https://doi.org/10.1136/bmj.f5577

National Center for Health Statistics. (2021). *Health, United States, 2019.* https://doi.org/10.15620/cdc:100685

Nightingale, F. (1859). *Notes on nursing: What it is and what it is not.* Harrison & Sons.

Orem, D. E. (2001). *Nursing: Concepts of practice* (6th ed.). Mosby.

Page, R. L., Peltzer, J., Burdette, A., & Hill, T. (2020). Religiosity and health: A holistic biopsychosocial perspective. *Journal of Holistic Nursing, 38*(1), 89–101. https://doi.org/10.1177/0898010118783502

Pender, N., Murdaugh, C. L., & Parsons, M. A. (2006). *Health promotion in nursing practice* (5th ed.). Prentice-Hall.

Petrov, M. E., Whisner, C. M., McCormick, D., Todd, M., Reyna, L., & Reifsnider, E. (2021). Sleep-wake patterns in newborns are associated with infant rapid weight gain and incident adiposity in toddlerhood. *Pediatric Obesity, 16*(3), e12726. https://www.ncbi.nlm.nih.gov/pmc/articles/PMC8344177/pdf/nihms-1726864.pdf

Prochaska, J. O., DiClemente, C. C., & Norcross, J. C. (1992). In search of how people change: Applications to addictive behaviors. *American Psychology, 47*, 1102–1114.

Prochaska, J. J., Hall, S. M., Humfleet, G., Muñoz, R., Reus, V., Gorecki, J., & Hu, D. (2008). Physical activity as a strategy for maintaining tobacco abstinence: A randomized controlled trial. *Preventive Medicine, 47*(2), 215–220. https://doi.org/10.1016%2Fj.ypmed.2008.05.006

Puccinelli, P. J., da Costa, T. S., Seffrin, A., de Lira, C. A. B., Vancini, R. L., Nikolaidis, P. T., Knechtle, B., Rosemann, T., Hill, L., & Andrade, M. S. (2021). Reduced level of physical activity during COVID-19 pandemic is associated with depression and anxiety levels: An internet-based survey. *BMC Public Health, 21*(1), 425. https://doi.org/10.1186/s12889-021-10470-z

Racey, M., Ali, M. U., Sherifali, D., Fitzpatrick-Lewis, D., Lewis, R., Jovkovic, M., Bouchard, D. R., Giguère, A., Holroyd-Leduc, J., Tang, A., Gramlich, L., Keller, H., Prorok, J., Kim, P.,

Lorbergs, A., & Muscedere, J. (2021). Effectiveness of physical activity interventions in older adults with frailty or prefrailty: A systematic review and meta-analysis. *CMAJ Open, 9*(3), E728–E743. https://doi.org/10.9778/cmajo.20200222

Ramanadhan, S., Crisostomo, J., Alexander-Molloy, J., Gandelman, E., Grullon, M., Lora, V., Reeves, C., Savage, C., & Viswanath, K. (2012). Perceptions of evidence-based programs among community-based organizations tackling health disparities: A qualitative study. *Health Education Research, 27*(4), 717–728. https://doi.org/10.1093/her/cyr088

Resnick, B. (2018). Theory of self-efficacy. In M. J. Smith & P. R. Liehr (Eds.), *Middle range theory for nursing* (4th ed., pp. 215–240). Springer Publishing.

Riegel, B., Dickson, V. V., Hoke, L., McMahon, J., Reis, B., & Sayers, S. (2006). A motivational counseling approach to improving heart failure self-care: Mechanisms of effectiveness. *Journal of Cardiovascular Nursing, 21*, 232–241. https://doi.org/10.1097/00005082-200605000-00012

Robinson, A., Bonnette, A., Howard, K., Ceballos, N., Dailey, S., Lu, Y., & Grimes, T. (2019). Social comparisons, social media addiction, and social interaction: An examination of specific social media behaviors related to major depressive disorder in a millennial population. *Journal of Applied Biobehavioral Research, 24*(1), e12158. https://doi.org/10.1111/jabr.12158

Rote, S., Hill, T. D., & Ellison, C. G. (2012). Religious attendance and loneliness in later life. *The Gerontologist, 53*, 39–50. https://doi.org/10.1093/geront/gns063

Sarrionandia, A., & Mikolajczak, M. (2020). A meta-analysis of the possible behavioural and biological variables linking trait emotional intelligence to health. *Health Psychology Review, 14*(2), 220–244. https://doi.org.10.1080/17437199.2019.1641423

Scheer, J. R., Edwards, K. M., Sheinfil, A. Z., Dalton, M. R., Firkey, M., & Watson, R. J. (2021). Interpersonal victimization, substance use, and mental health among sexual and gender minority youth: The role of self-concept factors. Published online ahead of print. *Journal of Interpersonal Violence, 37*(19–20), NP18104–NP18129. https://doi.org/10.1177/08862605211035868

Schneider, M., Voracek, M., & Tran, U. S. (2018). "A joke a day keeps the doctor away?" Meta-analytical evidence of differential associations of habitual humor styles with mental health. *Scandinavian Journal of Psychology, 59*(3), 289–300. https://doi.org/10.1111/sjop.12432

Sepúlveda-Loyola, W., Rodríguez-Sánchez, I., Pérez-Rodríguez, P., Ganz, F., Torralba, R., Oliveira, D. V., & Rodríguez-Mañas, L. (2020). Impact of social isolation due to COVID-19 on health in older people: Mental and physical effects and recommendations. *The Journal of Nutrition, Health & Aging, 24*(9), 938–947. http://doi.org/10.1007/s12603-020-1469-2

Shivpuri, S., Gallo, L., Crouse, J. R., & Allison, M. A. (2012). The association between chronic stress type and C-reactive protein in the multi-ethnic study of atherosclerosis: Does gender make a difference? *Journal of Behavioral Medicine, 35*, 74–85. https://doi.org/10.1007/s10865-011-9345-5

Sims, T., & McFadden, P. (2021). Peanuts, popcorn, and pediatrics: School-based carnival for health promotion. *Teaching and Learning in Nursing, 16*(4), 401–403. https://doi.org/10.1016/j.teln.2021.03.008

Smith, R. W., Barnes, I., Green, J., Reeves, G. K., Beral, V., & Floud, S. (2021b). Social isolation and risk of heart disease and stroke: Analysis of two large UK prospective studies. *Lancet Public Health, 6*, e232–e239. https://doi.org/10.1016/S2468-2667(20)30291-7

Smith, M. L., Gotway, M. B., Crotty Alexander, L. E., & Hariri, L. P. (2021a). Vaping-related lung injury. *Virchows Archiv: An International Journal of Pathology, 478*(1), 81–88. https://doi.org/10.1007/s00428-020-02943-0

Sokolova, K., & Perez, C. (2021). You follow fitness influencers on YouTube. But do you actually exercise? How parasocial relationships, and watching fitness influencers relate to intentions to exercise. *Journal of Retailing and Consumer Services, 58*, 102276. https://doi.org/10.1016/j.jretconser.2020.102276

Stockwell, S., Trott, M., Tully, M., Shin, J., Barnett, Y., Butler, L., McDermott, D., Schuch, F., & Smith, L. (2021). Changes in physical activity and sedentary behaviours from before to during the COVID-19 pandemic lockdown: A systematic review. *BMJ Open Sport & Exercise Medicine, 7*(1), e000960. https://doi.org/10.1136/bmjsem-2020-000960

Strommer, S., Shaw, S., Jenner, S., Vogel, C., Lawrence, W., Woods-Townsend, K., Farrell, D., Inskip, H., Baird, J., Morrison, L., & Barker, M. (2021). How do we harness adolescent values in designing health behavior change interventions? A qualitative study. *British Journal of Health Psychology, 26*, 1176–1193. https://doi.org/10.1111/bjhp.12526

Sullivan, H. W., & Rothman, A. J. (2008). When planning is needed: Implementation intentions and attainment of approach versus avoidance health goals. *Health Psychology, 27*, 438–444. https://doi.org/10.1037/0278-6133.27.4.438

Taylor, G. M., Baker, A. L., Fox, N., Kessler, D. S., Aveyard, P., & Munafo, M. R. (2021). Addressing concerns about smoking cessation and mental health: Theoretical review and practical guide for healthcare professionals. *BJPsych Advances, 27*(2), 85–95. https://doi.org/10.1192/bja.2020.52

Thomas, S. P. (2007). Trait anger, anger expression, and themes of anger incidents in contemporary undergraduate students. In E. I. Clausen (Ed.), *Psychology of anger* (pp. 23–69). Nova Science Publishers.

Turner, H., Shattuck, A., Finkelhor, D., & Hamby, S. (2017). Effects of poly-victimization on adolescent social support, self-concept, and psychological distress. *Journal of Interpersonal Violence, 32*(5), 755–780. https://doi.org/10.1177/0886260515586376

U.S. Census. (2021). *Income and poverty in the United States: 2020.* https://www.census.gov/library/publications/2021/demo/p60-273.html

U.S. Department of Agriculture, & U.S. Department of Health and Human Services. (2010). *Dietary guidelines for Americans 2010* (7th ed.). U.S. Government Printing Office. https://health.gov/sites/default/files/2020-01/DietaryGuidelines2010.pdf

U.S. Department of Health and Human Services. (2014). *Healthy people 2020 leading health indicators: Progress report.* http://www.health.gov/healthypeople

U.S. Department of Health and Human Services. (2018). *Physical activity guidelines for Americans* (2nd ed.). Department of Health and Human Services. https://health.gov/sites/default/files/2019-09/Physical_Activity_Guidelines_2nd_edition.pdf

U.S. Food and Drug Administration (FDA). (2016). *FDA news release: FDA takes significant steps to protect Americans from dangers of tobacco through new regulation.* http://www.fda.gov/NewsEvents/Newsroom/PressAnnouncements/ucm499234.htm

U.S. Public Health Service. (2020). *Healthy People 2030.* U.S. Department of Health and Human Services. http://health.gov/healthypeople

Vetrovsky, T., Wahlich, C., Borowiec, A., Jurik, R., Smigielski, W., Steffl, M., Tufano, J., Drygas, W., Stastny, P., Malek, L., & Harris, T. (2021). Benefits of physical activity interventions combining self-monitoring with other components versus self-monitoring alone: A systematic review and meta-analysis. *The Lancet (British Edition), 398,* S87–S87. https://doi.org/10.1016/S0140-6736(21)02630-1

Willging, C. E., Jaramillo, E. T., Haozous, E., Sommerfeld, D. H., & Verney, S. P. (2021). Macro- and meso-level contextual influences on health care inequities among American Indian elders. *BMC Public Health, 21*(1), 1–14. https://doi.org/10.1186/s12889-021-10616-z

Yemiscigil, A., & Vlaev, I. (2021). The bidirectional relationship between sense of purpose in life and physical activity: A longitudinal study. *Journal of Behavioral Medicine, 44,* 715–725. https://doi.org.10.1007/s10865-021-00220-2

Yoneda, T., Lewis, N. A., Knight, J. E., Rush, J., Vendittelli, R., Kleineidam, L., Hyun, J., Piccinin, A. M., Hofer, S. M., Hoogendijk, E. O., Derby, C. A., Scherer, M., Riedel-Heller, S., Wagner, M., van den Hout, A., Wang, W., Bennett, D. A., & Muniz-Terrera, G. (2021). The importance of engaging in physical activity in older adulthood for transitions between cognitive status categories and death: A coordinated analysis of 14 longitudinal studies. *The Journals of Gerontology. Series A, Biological Sciences and Medical Sciences, 76*(9), 1661–1667. https://doi.org/10.1093/gerona/glaa268

16

Genetics and Genomics in Professional Nursing

Donna L. Schiminkey, PhD, MPH, RN, CNM

 http://evolve.elsevier.com/Friberg/bridge/

OBJECTIVES

After completion of this chapter, the reader will be able to:
- Define genomic health care.
- Discuss the effect of the human microbiome on human health and disease.
- Discuss the usefulness of the *Essentials of Genetic and Genomic Nursing* to nursing practice.
- Discuss the nursing role in family history assessment.
- Describe nursing roles in genetic testing.
- Explain the nursing role in the referral of individuals and families for specialized genetic and genomic services.
- List two ways genetic testing is being used in clinical practice.
- List two ways genomic testing is being used in clinical practice.
- Differentiate between genetic and genomic testing methodologies.
- Describe basic gene therapy techniques.
- Identify ethical issues of concern about genomic health care.

INTRODUCTION

Why should nurses learn about genetics and genomics? Health care increasingly relies on genetic and genomic explanations combined with an understanding of environmental influences on behavior to understand the spectrum of health, well-being, and disease, which in turn drives both health care policy and practice. The increasing number of direct-to-consumer genetic tests available prompts people to seek nurses and other health care providers to help interpret their results. Consumers also bring nurses questions about new treatments involving the manipulation of genes that are being tested and brought to market. Nurses need to be knowledgeable to communicate with and educate individuals, families, and communities about the roles that genetics and genomics have in their health care. This involves ensuring access to the genetic and genomic testing and interventions that can optimize health care in all settings in their role as patient advocates in today's health care environment. In addition, nursing leaders in public health increasingly use genomic information to guide efficient and effective strategies that prevent or mitigate specific disease burdens within communities.

In the past several decades our understanding of how genes function has expanded. It still holds true that genotype establishes phenotype, that is, that the genes a person possesses determine their observable characteristics. But what we understand now is that it is often groups of genes relating to one another in multiple ways that create variety in phenotype and health outcomes. A lot more is happening than simply protein transcription; genes make other things that work to produce and regulate protein manufacturing by genes. As our understanding has expanded, it may be helpful to use language from computer science to describe genes and the genome. If you think of the genome as being the body's operating system, then individual genes and groups of genes perform like subroutines in that program (Gerstein et al., 2007). Those subroutines can be affected by changed, extra, or missing code, as well as by interactions involving other subroutines.

The first reference human genomes were completely mapped and sequenced in 2003, and since 2007 researchers have been exploring the human microbiome (Collins et al., 2021). As costs decreased, more genomes, both human and nonhuman, have been sequenced. This has allowed scientists to begin assembling a record of all the variations of deoxyribonucleic acid (DNA) sequences that occur in our species and, indeed, in all of nature. Although this task is vast and ongoing, it has uncovered relationships between disease risk and specific genetic variants (Sherman & Salzberg, 2020). For instance, studying a group of Icelanders has revealed that the insertion of "extra" base pairs of DNA on Chromosome 17 decreases a person's risk of having a myocardial infarction (Kehr et al., 2017). Such discoveries from ongoing research endeavors are increasing our understanding of the role genes play in health and rare and common diseases. A new era of health care—termed alternatively *precision health* or *genomic medicine*—is rapidly advancing. *Precision health* means that health care providers now have access to new tools for *tailoring* health care to the individual by combining a person's or microbe's unique genomic information with other environmental and behavioral considerations to diagnose, design, and prescribe the most effective treatment for each patient (Kurnat-Thoma et al., 2021; National Human Genome Research Institute [NHGRI], 2020a). These advances are ushering in new directions in the provision of health care and already have a significant effect on nursing and all other health care. Nurses in all practice settings are increasingly expected to use genetic- and genomic-based approaches and technologies in their patient care.

This chapter is grounded in the *Essentials of Genetic and Genomic Nursing* (Consensus Panel on Genetic/Genomic Nursing Competencies, 2008) and presents genetic and genomic discoveries and applications from yesterday to today and for tomorrow. Applications of genetics and genomics to nursing and health care are addressed, including family history assessment, genetic screening and testing, pharmacogenetics and pharmacogenomics, the human microbiome, direct-to-consumer genetic testing, gene therapies, and public health. Ethical and social issues related to genetics and genomics are also described. Genetics and genomics educational and clinical resources are provided to support the needs of all nurses wanting to learn more about and provide competent genomic health care, as noted in the *Essentials of Genetic and Genomic Nursing.*

Because essentially all diseases and conditions have a genetic or genomic component, options for prevention, screening, diagnostics, prognostics, selection of treatments, and monitoring of treatment effectiveness will soon be commonplace in clinical practice. These are key components of the National Institutes of Health (NIH)

initiative on precision medicine (Sabatello & Appelbaum, 2017). The clinical application of genetic and genomic knowledge may not have been an explicit part of the nursing curriculum for more experienced nurses, but family history taking, for instance, is an indispensable competency for all nurses regardless of academic preparation, role, or practice setting (Consensus Panel on Genetic/Genomic Nursing Competencies, 2008). Because this is a rapidly developing field, ongoing continuing education is essential to develop and maintain these competencies (Kurnat-Thoma et al., 2021).

Box 16.1 provides a list of basic genetic and genomic terms and their definitions as a beginning step for nurses to become familiar with and knowledgeable about genetics and genomics.

Yesterday's Genetics

It was not until the late 1800s that scientists first began to discover chromosomes, the threadlike structures inside of cells that contain genes. In the early 1900s, people first linked inherited diseases to chromosomes. Scientific research and discoveries from the 1950s through the 1980s helped scientists develop tests for genetic conditions such as Down syndrome, cystic fibrosis (CF), and Duchenne muscular dystrophy. During those years, genetic testing was used to confirm a diagnosis of disorders involving mutations in the DNA sequences of single genes—for example, screening newborns for conditions such as phenylketonuria (PKU) so that early treatments and interventions could be administered (Sumaily & Mujamammi, 2017). Therefore, nurses practicing in neonatal and pediatric settings were the first nurses to become informed about and involved with genetics in their practice with the advent of genetic testing for newborns and children and their families. But were those nurses prepared with genetics knowledge so that they could competently provide informed patient care? Not necessarily. The recognition that nurses did not have adequate knowledge of genetics to practice genetics health care was first documented in the nursing literature in 1979 (Cohen, 1979).

Although planning for the Human Genome Project began in the 1980s, it took 15 years for the first human genome to be mapped and sequenced. It was an expensive undertaking, costing 2.7 billion dollars (NHGRI, 2021). This project led the way for new tools and pathways for understanding the role of genes in health and disease. As an example, genetic discoveries have led to the development of an increasing number of genetic tests that can be used to identify a trait, diagnose a genetic disorder, and/or identify individuals who have a genetic predisposition to diseases such as cancer or heart disease. Our

BOX 16.1   Common Genetic and Genomic Terms

Allele—One of the two or more forms of a gene at a particular location on a chromosome. Human genes and noncoding areas on the chromosome each have two alleles, one inherited from each parent. Variations in the alleles create different characteristics in inherited characteristics such as hair color or blood type. If the two alleles are the same, the individual is homozygous for that gene. If they are not identical, the individual is heterozygous for that gene.

Big data—Refers to large and complex data sets that cannot be analyzed with traditional software. Parallel computing methods are used to analyze this type of data.

Bioinformatics—Is the science that deals with collection, classification, and analysis of complex biological data such as genomic data.

Chromosome—One of the threadlike "packages" of genes and other DNA that are located in the nucleus of a cell. Humans have 23 pairs of chromosomes, 46 in total: 44 autosomes and 2 sex chromosomes.

Deoxynucleic acid (DNA)—The main constituent of chromosomes and the heritable carrier of genetic information that is arranged in a double helix of the nucleic acids: adenine, cytosine, guanine, and thymine; joined by hydrogen bonds.

DNA sequencing—This laboratory technique is used to map the precise sequence of nucleic acids in a DNA molecule.

Double helix—The structural arrangement of DNA. It looks something like an immensely long ladder twisted into a helix or coil. The sides of the ladder are formed by a backbone of sugar and phosphate molecules and the "rungs" are comprised of nucleotide bases joined weakly in the middle by hydrogen bonds.

Epigenetics—The field that deals with the biological mechanisms that control the level of gene activity or to what degree the gene is expressed.

Epigenome—The chemical compounds that modify the genome affecting the way that genes are expressed.

Gene—The functional and physical unit of heredity passed from parent to offspring. Genes are pieces of DNA and most genes contain the information for making a specific protein. There are approximately 20,000–21,000 genes in the human genome.

Genetic disorders—A disease or syndrome caused in whole or in part by a variation (polymorphism or mutation) of a gene.

Gene expression—The process through which genetic information made of DNA is used to guide the RNA to assemble proteins. Each group of three bases, called a codon, can make one of the twenty different amino acids that when put together form various proteins.

Genetics—A term that refers to the study of individual genes and their role in inheritance; this includes how certain traits or conditions are passed down from one generation to another.

Genome—The complete set of genes that is present in a cell or in an organism.

Genomics—The study of the entire genome.

Karyotype—The laboratory technique that creates a picture of an individual's chromosomes to determine if there are abnormalities in number or structure.

Mendelian inheritance—The way in which genes and traits are passed from parents to children. Examples of Mendelian inheritance include autosomal dominant, autosomal recessive, and sex-linked genes.

Human microbiome—The genes of the microbes that live in human skin, tissues, and fluids. These microbial genes influence the human immune system, and the constituents of a person's microbiome influence the person's health.

Pharmacogenomics—The science that uses data from genomes to guide the application of drug development, testing, and prescribing.

Polymerase chain reaction—This laboratory technique is used to amplify DNA sequences. The technique can produce a billion copies of the DNA sequence of interest in just a few hours.

Protein—A large complex molecule comprised of one or more chains of amino acids. Proteins are essential building blocks and cell signals in the human body.

Ribonucleic acid (RNA)—Is a chemical similar to DNA. It only contains one strand, and it has a single difference in the nucleotide code that comprises the strand. Instead of thymines, RNA contains uracil.

Data from National Human Genome Research Institute. (2014b). *Talking glossary of genetic terms.* https://www.genome.gov/glossary/

understanding of genes and their roles in health and disease expanded beyond *genetics,* which involves the study of individual genes and their effect on relatively rare, single-gene disorders, to the field of *genomics.* When we study the human genome in its entirety—that is, how genes interact with each other and the environment, including the cultural and psychosocial phenomena and alterations in regulation and production of proteins manufactured by those genes—we are studying *genomics* (NHGRI, 2020b).

GENETICS AND GENOMICS TODAY

The challenges of nursing practice during the COVID-19 pandemic era present an extraordinary opportunity to utilize genomic information in our attempts to both protect populations and provide optimal care for individual patients. At this time, advances in genomics have fully entered the world of public health and clinical practice. Although the human genome was sequenced more than 20 years ago and the annotation of the genome is ongoing, now there is an urgent and ongoing need for surveillance and annotation of the ever-evolving SARS-CoV-2 (the cause of COVID-19) viral genome. *Genome annotation* is the process by which coding sequences and their functions are identified, answering the question, "What do these genes do?."

The viral genome of SARS-CoV-2 evolves rapidly and new lineages, or variants, circulate swiftly across the globe. Real-time population surveillance with genomic sequencing techniques is being used to track viral variants, identifying those that are more transmissible or associated with more severe clinical diseases (Park et al., 2021). Sentinel surveillance of SARS-CoV-2 in wastewater has become routine in some areas. This is the process by which variants can be detected in sewage up to a month before clinical cases of COVID-19 are identified, thus allowing the emergence and transmission of variant genotypes to be tracked (Thompson et al., 2020). This provides critical lead-time to organize resources and operationalize mitigation strategies such as increased use of personal protective equipment, physical distancing, availability of testing, and conservation of other health care resources (i.e., canceling elective medical procedures in local hospitals when the viral load detected in wastewater increases).

Beyond the COVID-19 pandemic, the use of genomic tools allows us to predict susceptibility to diseases and counsel individuals and communities about their options for screening and risk reduction and treatment. The "one size fits all" approach of pregenomic treatment regimens has been rapidly transformed, as genomic sequencing and data analysis alter the diagnosis and treatment of diseases ranging from cancer (Dienstmann & Tabernero, 2017), type 2 diabetes (Brunkwall & Orho-Melander, 2017), and heart disease (Lempiäinen et al., 2018) in addition to infectious diseases (Liu et al., 2017). For example, genomic testing of tumors in breast cancer can both identify specific mutations belonging to tumor types that are susceptible to treatment by particular chemotherapy regimens and predict the likelihood of cancer recurrence in the presence or absence of specific treatments. Such testing now guides disease management for these patients (Grill & Kline, 2021). For the past two decades, genomic testing has been used to monitor the risk of rejection in transplant recipients by measuring levels of gene expression in nearby white blood cells (Collins et al., 2021).

One of the major barriers to this transformation is health care practitioners themselves. Lack of awareness and understanding about available testing and responsive treatment plans along with a lack of good strategies to manage genomic data all contribute to hesitation by clinicians to fully utilize this technology (Snir et al., 2021). Nurses at all levels of practice need to stay abreast of developing genomic technologies; this will foster their ability to incorporate these assessment and treatment tools into their practice. Nurses play crucial clinical and leadership roles in identifying high-risk patients and educating them about available testing and treatment options. These genomic advances are changing health care, becoming an integral part of health care for people across the life span, from preconception through older adulthood. Many genomic interventions involve altering a person's environment or behavior by teaching strategies to address modifiable risks by way of avoiding toxins, eating, drinking, and sleeping appropriately. This was the foundational strategy in Florence Nightingale's *Notes on Nursing* (1859) and remains fundamental to the profession today. Genomic interventions enhance our ability to care for individuals, families, and entire populations.

Other aspects of this transformation include the expanding understanding and clinical application of *epigenetics* and *the microbiome* (discussed later) in both research and clinical practice. These two fields are changing our understanding of the human environment and the approaches we take to treating clients.

EPIGENETICS

Epigenetics refers to how the expression of genes is controlled, in other words, which genes are active, which are inactive, and to what degree. If you think of the DNA in the human genome as a recipe, then the epigenetic changes that occur might resemble the small or large changes that cooks make when preparing the dishes. One time the cook might use a level teaspoon of baking powder and salt and another time the cook might use heaping tablespoons of both. Room temperature and oven speed also affect the final product. In this way, environmental exposures from embryonic life throughout the life span affect which of a cell's genes are being read to make proteins and other functional elements in our metabolism and which ones are silenced. Not only is the DNA, or the recipe, inheritable, but a person might also inherit parts of the epigenome, in the same way cooks may have learned from their parents to use a particular technique to whip the eggs or grease the pan to make a particular dish. Thus, a person's *epigenome* is both heritable and flexible; what is silenced can be turned on and turned up, and what is active can be turned down or off again. What and how much we eat and drink, what we breathe, where we live, how much we sleep, how active we are, and the stresses we encounter all can influence the epigenetics in our genome. As you can see, many, if not all, nursing interventions have the potential to influence gene expression. Areas of active research include trying to quantify how and to what extent our interventions may alter a person's epigenome to improve the person's health and what will be passed on to future generations.

By studying the epigenome of identical twins, it is possible to see how environment and experiences change the epigenome. As twins age, there is a greater difference in their epigenomes than was present in early childhood. Epigenetic molecular changes can include DNA methylation, which is like putting a cap on top of the DNA so that it cannot be transcribed, and histone changes, which determine the way strands of DNA are packed, which areas of DNA are exposed to be read, and which are packed too densely to be transcribed. Other epigenetic mechanisms include changes to various types of ribonucleic acid (RNA) that affect the degree of gene expression.

THE MICROBIOME

There are diverse communities of microbes that live in and on our bodies. The collection of these microbes is called the *human microbiome*. There is typically a symbiotic relationship that occurs between these microbes and their human hosts. As the technology to sequence DNA advances, the more we discover about that relationship. The human body contains at least as many microbial cells as human cells, with microbial genes outnumbering human genes (Pederzoli et al., 2022). A microbiome that is highly diverse with beneficial microbes that can respond to change under physiological stress is said to be "healthy." An "unhealthy" microbiome conversely is susceptible to disease and has a lower diversity of species and fewer beneficial microbes. In extreme, an "unhealthy" microbiome is said to be in a state of *dysbiosis*, a situation in which the populations of microbes in a body have been altered in ways that interrupt the normal microbe/host interactions leading to disease or dysfunction (Illiano et al., 2020). Microbes exist on every available surface in and on the body, including the gut, skin, reproductive tract, and lungs.

The goal of NIH's Human Microbiome Project is to characterize the human microbiome and analyze its role in human health and disease. Since the impetus of the Human Microbiome Project, a multitude of studies have shown that alterations in the microbiome are associated with numerous disease states. The findings reported in these studies support the possibility of manipulating the various communities of microorganisms that make up the microbiome to treat a wide range of disease processes.

The most common method for identifying bacterial strains in the human microbiome is 16S ribosomal RNA (16S rRNA) gene profiling. The marker 16S rRNA is present in almost all bacteria; therefore, an entire bacterial community from a specific site (i.e., gut, skin, lung) can be explored (McElroy et al., 2017). In addition, bacterial DNA can be isolated from human, viral, and fungal DNA. Databases are available from published gene sequences, and researchers match bacterial DNA isolated from a given specimen to those published gene sequences. More than 660,000 bacterial genomes have been sequenced and are available in the public domain (Blackwell et al., 2021).

When nurses bathe a patient, change the patient's bedding, provide hydration and nourishment, or care for wounds and catheters, they are performing acts that influence a person's microbiome. Understanding the microbiome and how this understanding guides care is an important aspect of nursing. There are modifiable factors that can promote dysbiosis of the various microbiomes. Diet, environmental toxins, and medications such as antibiotics are examples of these factors. Gastrointestinal diseases such as inflammatory bowel disease, irritable bowel disease, and colorectal cancer have been implicated in states of gut dysbiosis, as well as obesity, diabetes, atherosclerosis, and nonalcoholic fatty liver disease. Nurses can educate high-risk populations to decrease potentially harmful behaviors. Maintenance or restoration of a healthy microbiome can be accomplished through exercise (Wosinska et al., 2019), the administration of underrepresented live microbes, ingestion of prebiotics or probiotics that encourage the growth of healthy microbes, or a combination of both (Corbett et al., 2021; Parida & Sharma, 2021).

PHARMACOGENOMICS

Pharmacogenomics brings together the fields of pharmacology and genomics, to study how a person's genomic makeup affects their response to medications. It has been the practice in health care to prescribe common doses to everyone. Although some people respond well to a particular drug, others may not respond at all. Adverse medication reactions do not occur in everyone. Pharmacogenomics can address these issues, using genomics to understand why a particular person reacts to medication, anesthesia, or chemotherapy in a particular way. We are already examining the genomes of cancer cells to help tailor chemotherapy that will destroy particular cancer cells. It is already possible to modify not only doses but also actual drugs to treat a variety of disease processes in a precise individualized way (Brandl et al., 2021; Harris et al., 2021).

For most of the history of modern medicine, treatments have been prescribed based on how a population of people with the disease responded to the therapy. As we learn more about the role of genetics and genomics, we have begun to practice *precision health care* or *personalized health care.* This approach allows us to first study the pathophysiological process involved in an individual's health, studying how their gene expression and protein metabolism respond on a molecular level to both disease and certain therapies. The goal is to provide individuals with the (precise) correct therapy to treat the disorder while minimizing side effects. Thus, personalized or precision care may involve designing a novel treatment for an individual based on the person's genotype, phenotype, and particular environment, or it may consist of prescribing medications that are going to have the most benefit with the least side effects. Gene therapies will be discussed in a separate section, but ultimately these will provide definitive and precise treatments for a variety of conditions. Currently, gene editing techniques, which allow us to replace mutated genes or less desirable variants with normal genes, are in clinical trials or already being used to treat primary immunodeficiencies and β-thalassemias (Ferrari et al., 2021) and many previously incurable heritable disorders.

ESSENTIALS OF GENETIC AND GENOMIC NURSING FOR NURSES

In recognition of the need for all nurses to become proficient in incorporating genetics and genomics into their practice, nursing leaders from clinical, research, and academic settings came together to create "the minimum basis by which to prepare the nursing workforce to deliver competent genetic- and genomic-focused nursing care," the *Essentials of Genetic and Genomic Nursing* (American Nurses Association (ANA), 2009). This document was designed to apply to all nurses regardless of their academic preparation, practice setting, role, or specialty. Again in 2011, a consensus panel was convened that built on the previously published competencies for nurses, to produce the *Essential Competencies in Genetics and Genomics for Nurses with Graduate Degrees* (Greco et al., 2011). Competencies outlined in both documents are broken down into two categories: professional responsibilities and professional practice domain. The professional responsibilities in the 2008 document are consistent with the nursing scope and standards of practice developed by the American Nurses Association (ANA, 2021). They include the incorporation of genetic and genomic technologies and information into registered nursing assessment practice

and the ability to tailor genetic and genomic information and services to clients based on their knowledge level, literacy, culture, religion, and preferred language in the planning, implementation, care coordination, and health teaching aspects of practice. The professional practice domain includes competencies in nursing assessment (applying and integrating genetic and genomic knowledge); identification of clients who could benefit from genetic and genomic information and services as well as reliable genetic and genomic resources; referral activities; and provision of education, care, and support, such as using genetic- and genomic-based interventions and information to improve client outcomes (ANA, 2009).

Box 16.2 provides examples of currently available genetics and genomics educational resources for nurses.

FAMILY HISTORY

Knowing the role of family history in common and rare genetic conditions and disorders is an important first step in genetic and genomic risk assessment and early intervention. Nurses need to be able to gather a minimum of three generations of family health history information and assist families in learning about their family health history. Individuals and families can be informed about the *My Family Health Portrait Web Tool* (Centers for Disease Control and Prevention [CDC], 2021) to begin this process. Following the *Essentials of Genetic and Genomic Competencies for Nurses,* and using the standardized symbols and terminology, nurses also need to be prepared to construct *pedigrees* from the collected family history information (Greco et al., 2011).

Individuals who have a family history of chronic diseases such as heart disease, diabetes, and cancer in close relatives are more likely to have a higher risk of developing these diseases. Having a first-degree relative with any one of these diseases has been shown to increase a person's risk for developing the disease, with the risk increasing, even more, when there are more affected relatives or if the disease was diagnosed at an early age. All health care providers, including nurses, have a responsibility to collect family history information and to use this information to provide specific clinical prevention and management interventions for those diseases that run in the patient's family (NHGRI, 2014a).

Family medical history is a nonmodifiable risk factor that can direct genetic or genomic screening and create an opportunity for the nurse to educate and provide strategies for decreasing modifiable risk behaviors and avoiding high-risk environments. Upon discovering such a risk in an individual's family history, the nurse should assess and educate the person about modifying diet, activity level,

---

BOX 16.2   Genetics and Genomics Educational Resources for Nurses

- The American Society of Human Genetics—A wide range of resources accessible at: https://www.ashg.org/discover-genetics/
- The Centers for Disease Control and Prevention, Office of Public Health Genomics Offers online resources for credible health information and training programs related to genomics and precision health, genetic counseling and testing, family health histories, and other related reports and publications including the Public Health Genomics and Precision Health Knowledge Base.
  - https://www.cdc.gov/genomics/
  - https://www.cdc.gov/genomics/training/index.htm
- The Global Genomics Nursing Alliance (G2NA): https://www.g2na.org/index.php
- The International Society of Nurses in Genetics (ISONG): http://www.isong.org/
- The National Health Service, United Kingdom:
  - *Genomics Education Programme:* https://www.genomicseducation.hee.nhs.uk/
  - *National Genetics and Genomics Education Centre:* http://www.tellingstories.nhs.uk/
- The National Human Genome Research Institute:
  - *All About the Human Genome Project:* https://www.genome.gov/human-genome-project
  - *Genetic Education Modules for Teachers:* https://www.genome.gov/about-genomics/teaching-tools

- *Genomics Education Websites:* https://www.genome.gov/about-genomics/teaching-tools/Genomics-Education-Websites
- *About Genomics:* https://www.genome.gov/about-genomics
- *Talking Glossary of Genetic Terms:* https://www.genome.gov/genetics-glossary
- *Healthcare Provider Genomics Education Resources:* https://www.genome.gov/For-Health-Professionals/Provider-Genomics-Education-Resources
- *Online Education Kit: Understanding the Human Genome Project:* https://www.genome.gov/25019879/online-education-kit-understanding-the-human-genome-project
- The National Institute of Health Precision Medicine Initiative website: https://allofus.nih.gov/
- The National Library of Medicine maintains MedlinePlus: *Genetics Home Reference: Your Guide to Understanding Genetic Conditions:* http://ghr.nlm.nih.gov
- The *Wellcome Genome Campus* offers a website that explains deoxynucleic acid (DNA), genes, and genomes. This organization supports a comprehensive website with extensive videos and interactive tutorials ranging from basic concepts to methods, technology, personalized health care, and ethics. This is an outstanding starting point for nurses who want to learn more about these topics. https://www.yourgenome.org/

---

occupational exposures to toxins, air pollution, sleep hygiene, and drug and alcohol use, which may decrease their risks for developing a disease and be essential to disease management.

Fig. 16.1 provides an example of a pedigree and standardized symbols. Nurses need to be alert for clients who present with family histories with multiple generations affected with a particular disorder (e.g., autosomal dominant inheritance), those with multiple siblings who have a genetic disorder (e.g., autosomal recessive inheritance), and those affected with a disease or condition at an early age (e.g., multiple generations with early-onset breast or ovarian cancer). When a client is identified as having a family history of a possible inherited genetic disorder, the nurse should inform the health care practitioner, to assist in targeting the physical examination appropriately. When a nurse discovers there is a risk for a genetic/genomic disorder or predisposition to such a disorder, it is appropriate to provide education and counseling

and ensure the appropriate genetic/genomic tests are ordered that can further illuminate the patient's situation. In some cases, it may be important to refer not only the individual but also other family members for further assessment by specialized genetic and genomic services.

While family history may not be something that can be modified, there are treatment options for families with some genetic diseases that exist entirely because of our advances in genetics and genomics. Carriers and people living with CF, for instance, have preimplantation genetic screening available to help identify unaffected embryos. There are now specific medications that target a particular mutation of the cystic fibrosis transmembrane conductance regulator (*CFTR*) gene that is present in 90% of cases of people living with CF. For the remaining ten percent of people with CF, gene therapy clinical trials are now underway. These three strategies of screening, targeted drug therapy, and gene editing completely

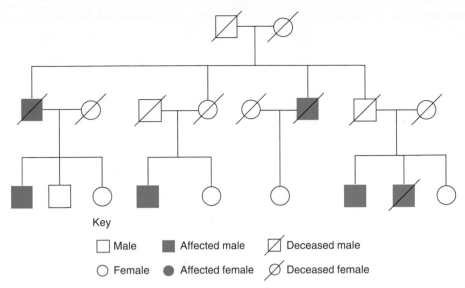

Key

☐ Male   ◼ Affected male   �«▨ Deceased male

○ Female   ● Affected female   ⊘ Deceased female

Fig. 16.1 Example of Pedigree and Standardized Symbol. Note: A pedigree is a diagram of a family history that shows family members' relationships to each other and how a particular disease or trait is being passed on (inherited) in that family. For more information about how to construct a family history pedigree, go to the National Human Genome Research Institute, Your Family History, http://www.genome.gov/Pages/Education/Modules/YourFamilyHealthHistory.pdf (From National Human Genome Research Institute. *Talking glossary of genetic terms.* https://www.genome.gov/glossary/)

transform the future for affected individuals and their families.

GENETIC TESTING: WHAT IS IT, AND HOW IS IT USED IN CLINICAL PRACTICE?

One of the most significant and rapidly expanding applications of genomics to health care since the mapping of the human genome is genetic testing. Genetic testing involves the use of a laboratory test to find genetic variations that are associated with a disease. Genetic testing results are used to confirm or rule out a genetic disorder or to determine the chance of a person passing a mutation on to his or her children. When more than 1% of the population has a particular genetic variation, we no longer refer to it as a *mutation* but rather call it a *polymorphism.* Variations in human ABO blood types, taste preferences, lactose tolerance/intolerance, and human hair color differences are examples of phenotypic differences because of polymorphisms. Susceptibility or protection from particular diseases also can be attributed to polymorphisms (e.g., sickle cell anemia, some hearing impairments, dementias, cardiovascular diseases, osteoarthritis, and our responses to some medications).

Genetic testing can be done prenatally or after birth. Genetic screening involves the testing of a population for a particular genetic variation (a polymorphism) to identify a subgroup of individuals that may have a disease or that indicates the potential exists to pass the disease on to their children. Some genetic polymorphisms can protect against a particular disease, whereas others may increase a person's risk of developing that disease.

TYPES OF GENETIC TESTING

Genetic testing to determine whether a person has a particular polymorphism on a particular gene can be done in several different ways. These tests may involve the collection of a hair follicle, epithelial cells, amniotic fluid, saliva, blood, or bone marrow. DNA remains stable over time, so it even can be used to test ancient human remains. Genetic testing is now available for more than 77,000 genetic disorders ranging from single-gene disorders, such as CF, to complex disorders, such as diabetes, cancer, and heart disease (MedlinePlus, 2022a). There are many situations in which genetic tests may be used in health care today.

Carrier testing is a type of genetic testing that identifies people who have one copy of a polymorphism that can cause disease when two copies are present. Carriers of one copy do not usually show any signs of the disorder because they carry one normal version of the gene. However, carriers can pass on the genetic variation to their children, who may develop the disorder or be carriers themselves. Thus, testing may be offered or sought when couples are considering pregnancy or during early pregnancy. Carrier testing is offered to couples who have a family history or are from ethnic or racial backgrounds that indicate they may have an increased risk of being carriers of an autosomal recessive gene for specific genetic disorders. Examples include African American couples who have an increased chance to carry a gene for sickle cell anemia and couples of Ashkenazi Jewish ancestry who have an increased chance of being carriers of a gene for Tay-Sachs disease (NHGRI, 2019).

Preimplantation testing, sometimes referred to as *preimplantation genetic diagnosis,* can be done in conjunction with assisted reproductive techniques such as in-vitro fertilization to detect more than 175 genetic disorders. To conduct these types of tests, a small number of cells are taken from the embryo before implantation in a uterus. This is a way to avoid passing on some significant hereditary diseases to the next generation.

Prenatal testing detects abnormalities in the fetus's genes or chromosomes before birth. There are screening tests that use the mother's blood, often combined with ultrasound, to detect signs of aneuploidy (an abnormal number of chromosomes). These may be done in the first or second trimester, depending on the test. For couples who have a known risk for trisomies, such as Down syndrome, or abnormal sex chromosomes, cell-free DNA tests that evaluate small amounts of fetal DNA that have passed into the mother's bloodstream can be done as early as 9 weeks gestation. If a prenatal screening test is positive, diagnostic testing such as amniocentesis or chorionic villi sampling is recommended.

Newborn screening tests are population-based testing within the first few days after birth to identify genetic disorders that are not clinically apparent at birth for which treatment is available. Early treatment will greatly increase the chance of these children living full and healthy lives. Examples of conditions screened for include congenital hypothyroidism, PKU, sickle cell disease, CF, maple syrup urine disease, congenital adrenal hyperplasia, and fatty acid oxidation disorders.

Predictive or presymptomatic testing can be done on asymptomatic family members of people who have developed diseases that are related to genetic mutations. *BRCA* testing is perhaps the most widely known type of predictive test; it looks for tumor suppressor gene mutations associated with breast, ovarian, and other types of cancers. Increasingly there are susceptibility screening tests that can be done by employers to determine who may be at risk for developing cancers because of exposure to carcinogens that may be present in the workplace. Presymptomatic testing, such as for Duchenne muscular dystrophy or Huntington disease, can determine whether someone is at particular risk. Negative test results indicate that a person's risk falls back to the risk of the general population for developing a disease.

Diagnostic testing identifies a particular genetic variation that is causing specific symptoms or a disease that is related to a genetic variation. Many diseases have multiple genes that can be responsible for a particular phenotype presentation. Identifying which variation a person has can guide treatment decisions and management of the disorder. One example of this type of testing is in people who have rheumatoid arthritis. The presence or absence of genetic variations associated with the production of anti-citrullinated protein antibodies guides pharmacological treatment. Diagnostic testing is also being used to guide therapies in many cancers.

Research testing helps scientists learn more about how particular genes or groups of genes contribute to health and disease. In the past two decades, research testing has evolved from a mapping project into a study of function. The genomic tools described in the next section provide a vast amount of data, allowing us to thoroughly explore the genomic regions that are associated with various diseases, which provides us with new targets for treatments (Collins et al., 2021).

Nurses at all levels of practice are increasingly involved in the genetic testing process and need to become knowledgeable about the different types of genetic tests in their field of specialization to provide competent genetic- and genomic-based care. This is a vital service to provide for individuals and families who need guidance and interpretation of selective genetic and genomic information such as genetic testing results.

How the Testing Is Done

Genetic and genomic testing can be done using several different technologies. Genetic and genomic testing involves analyzing the DNA of an individual. The type of DNA alteration that is being tested determines the method of testing that should be done.

Cytogenetic testing is sometimes referred to as *karyotyping* or *chromosome analysis.* This type of testing involves the study of the number, shape, and staining patterns of chromosomes to detect genetic abnormalities. It can identify missing chromosomes, extra chromosomes, or rearranged chromosomes. This technique involves extracting chromosomes from the nuclei of cells during mitosis. Blood, amniotic fluid, chorionic villi tissue, bone marrow, and other tissues can be studied in this manner. Traditionally the chromosomes have been manually interpreted even after computers increased the efficiency of the chromosome reconstruction process. Recently the field of tumor biology has fueled the development of *next-generation sequencing* (NGS) *techniques* (discussed later under "Genome Testing") for chromosome analysis, thus making this a much more efficient and accurate process (Bai et al., 2021).

DNA testing can be done on any cellular matter. In the laboratory, DNA can be extracted from these cells and examined for polymorphisms that are responsible for disease or an abnormal condition. It might be done by cutting the DNA into small segments that are faster to work with than longer strands of DNA. These fragments can then be amplified and sequenced to determine whether they contain a potentially harmful variation of a gene.

Protein truncation testing is a highly sensitive method for detecting genetic mutations and polymorphisms in large coding sequences of genes. This method uses polymerase chain reaction (PCR) and then allows the amplified sample of DNA to be transcribed into RNA. It is often used to examine variations in tumor suppressor genes and in screening for single-gene inherited disorders. A few current uses for protein truncation techniques include *BRCA* testing, mentioned above, and identifying people at risk for passing polycystic kidney disease or neurofibromatosis on to their children. These techniques are highly sensitive and specific for detecting mutations.

Genomic testing, unlike genetic testing, examines either large parts of the genome or the entire genome at once, in contrast to genetic testing, which looks at only a very small number of genes. Currently, nurses are most likely to encounter genomic testing when working with cancer patients or with newborns who have complex birth defects or potential rare diseases. However, these tests are increasingly being used in other clinical situations, including diagnosing neuropsychiatric and neurodevelopmental disorders and making treatment decisions for cardiovascular diseases and endocrine disorders.

NGS is sometimes referred to as *high-throughput sequencing.* Several techniques fall under these umbrella terms. All of them involve methods that have increased the speed and decreased the cost compared with traditional sequencing methods. NGS breaks the DNA into fragments that are then sequenced all at the same time. The downside of these techniques is that they provide a massive amount of information to explore. Some of these tests essentially take more than 250 million pictures of different parts of the genome, which can then be pieced together (sequenced) in less than a day. It is like taking many, many pictures of people standing in a long line, and then piecing all these pictures together to come up with a panoramic view of the line. The tests that are described in the following section all use some form of NGS.

Whole genome sequencing maps an entire DNA sequence from cells, including DNA from both the cell nucleus and the cell mitochondria. This originally took years and billions of dollars, yet it can now be done in as few as 4 hours and for under $600 (Collins et al., 2021). In the last decade, these methods have been used to help diagnose many individuals who have rare diseases. It is also a useful way to profile tumors to aid clinical decision-making around cancer therapies. Another application for whole genome sequencing occurs when an infectious agent cannot be cultured in a laboratory; in these cases, sequencing a bacterial or viral genome can help researchers understand mutations that may lead to drug resistance (Deurenberg et al., 2017). And perhaps the most well-known application for this testing, as mentioned earlier, is in managing infectious disease outbreaks as microbial variants are tracked across the globe.

Exome sequencing is a type of NGS that looks only at protein-coding genes (known as the *exome*). This is used to identify mutations in single-gene disorders as wide-ranging as familial amyotrophic lateral sclerosis, Charcot-Marie-Tooth disease, and neonatal diabetes mellitus, or to predict prognosis or best treatments in cancer treatments (Sastre, 2014). In cases involving suspected single-gene disorders often several family members may need to have their exomes sequenced, along with the individual who is affected by a disorder. This is a particularly useful technique when a patient presents with multiple birth defects, musculoskeletal issues, neurological/neurodevelopmental issues, and immunological, metabolic, or connective tissue disorders of unknown origin (Retterer et al., 2016).

Multiple-gene panels, as their name implies, can sequence multiple genes at once. This type of testing has most commonly been used to screen people who, based on family history, may be at risk for developing inherited cancers. It is often favored over whole exome sequencing and whole genome sequencing because there are less data to be evaluated and less cost to perform (sometimes costing even less than $30). Several of these tests look at gene variants associated with the risk of developing multiple cancers, (e.g., Lynch syndrome). These multigene panels are also commonly used for preconception or prenatal screening (e.g., CF, Tay Sachs, or Canavan disease screening) in people who have presumptive risks for these rare diseases. Increasingly these panels are used to guide clinical treatment decisions in people already diagnosed with a disease or syndrome (Krier et al., 2016).

DNA microarrays, also referred to as *DNA chips* or *bead arrays,* are used to evaluate thousands of genes with one test. These tests compare a reference DNA sample containing the most common variants of genes present, with an unknown sample (from an individual). These microarrays are an excellent tool for evaluating epigenetic activity. Results can tell you whether a gene is active in either of the two samples. Even more interesting, it can tell us degrees of upregulation (increased production of gene products such as proteins or RNA), downregulation (decreased production of gene products), and whether a gene in the individual is being continually transcribed when it is only transcribed under specific circumstances in the referent sample (NHGRI, 2020c).

RNA sequencing (RNA seq) is another form of NGS that is an alternative to microarray technology for sequencing whole genomes. RNA seq uses technologies that allow the analysis of the entire *transcriptome* to evaluate levels of gene expression. The transcriptome includes all the RNA being produced by the organism or person. Unlike DNA microarrays, RNA seq does not require a referent sample to sequence an entire genome and it appears capable of detecting very low levels of gene expression (Merrick et al., 2018). Clinical uses include identifying specific rare diseases, autoimmune diseases, unusual skin lesions, and cancer management.

REFERRAL FOR GENETIC COUNSELING AND SUPPORT SERVICES

Genetic counselors and other genetics professionals are wonderful resources for both nurses and their clients. Nurses will benefit from knowing these professionals because they can help nurses stay up to date on changing test methodologies and options available for clients. Equally important, knowing the available local counselors will help the nurse facilitate genetic referrals for clients. It is appropriate to refer individuals or families who may have a genetic risk factor, abnormal genetic test result, or questions about a genetic or genomic condition or disorder that are beyond the nurse's skill set. Genetics specialists are health care professionals who have specialized degrees and experience in medical genetics and counseling. Genetics professionals include medical geneticists, genetic counselors, and genetics nurses.

Genetics professionals work as members of health care teams to provide information and support to individuals and families who have a genetic disorder or may be at risk for inherited conditions. Genetic professionals conduct the following activities during a *genetic consultation* (NHGRI, 2013):

- Assess the risk for a genetic disorder by evaluating and researching a family's history and evaluating medical records.
- Consider the medical, social, and ethical decisions surrounding genetic testing.

- Provide support and information to help a person decide about genetic testing.
- Help interpret the results of genetic tests and medical data.
- Provide counseling and refer individuals and families to support services as needed.
- Act as patient advocates.
- Discuss and explain the possible treatments or preventive measures.
- Review and discuss reproductive options.

Box 16.3 lists resources that provide genetics and genomics clinical services that nurses can use to locate genetics professionals and services in their practice locality.

Direct-to-Consumer Testing

Several companies now market genetic tests directly to consumers. People can order test kits that are sent to their homes where they can, for instance, swab the inside of their cheek to collect the sample and then return it to the company for processing. Results may be provided to the customer by mail, phone, or the Internet. Cost varies for these tests from less than a hundred up to a thousand dollars. The support these companies provide to help customers interpret the results also varies (NHGRI, 2022a).

In a health care setting, nurses, other health care providers, and genetics professionals spend a significant amount of time explaining the risks, limitations, and benefits of genetic and genomic testing to their clients. It is the role of these professionals to verify that the information is understood so a person can give fully informed consent. Companies that offer these tests may not have a rigorous process to validate whether consumers understand the risks, limitations, and benefits of direct-to-consumer testing (MedlinePlus, 2022b).

Companies that provide these tests usually suggest that their customers consult their health care provider or a genetics counselor when interpreting these tests. This is important because nurses and other providers can help interpret an individual's genetic test results in the context of other known risks, health behaviors, past health history, and family history. As it has become more common for people to order at-home genetics or genomics tests, it is appropriate to inquire about this when obtaining a health history.

These direct-to-consumer tests create new responsibilities for health care professionals, who may be called on to interpret dense, complex data to assist their patients in making health care decisions. In the same way that nurses and primary care providers are not usually equipped to read and interpret a CD of a full-body magnetic resonance imaging scan their patient may have obtained because of an imaging center's direct-to-consumer marketing, the amount of information a person may receive from direct-to-consumer genetics or genomics tests can be overwhelming. Complete

BOX 16.3 Genetics and Genomics Clinical Resources

- *Genetic Alliance*—Provides individuals and organizations with dynamic resources that emphasize expanded access to quality, vetted information, including information about specific diseases, support groups for specific diseases, family history, and other resources: http://www.geneticalliance.org
- *Genomics and Medicine*—Created by the National Human Genome Research Institute; provides detailed information about genetic disorders, background on genetic and genomic science, the new science of pharmacogenomics, tools to create your own family health history, and a list of online health resources: http://www.genome.gov/19016903
- *Genetics and Rare Diseases Information Center (GARD)*—Established by the National Human Genome Research Institute (NHGR) and the Office of Rare Diseases (ORD) to help members of the general public, including patients and their families, health professionals, and biomedical researchers find useful information about genetic and rare diseases. GARD has a website (http://rarediseases.info.nih.gov) and also provides immediate, virtually round-the-clock access to experienced information specialists who can furnish current and accurate information (in both English and Spanish) about genetic and rare diseases: https://www.genome.gov/For-Patients-and-Families/Genetic-and-Rare-Diseases-Information-Center
- *Genetics Home Reference*—Provides consumer-friendly information about the effects of genetic variations on human health on MedlinePlus: https://medlineplus.gov/genetics/
- *Genes in Life*—Genes in Life is a website where people can learn about all the ways genetics is a part of their life. This site provides information about how genetics affects individuals and their families, why they should talk to their health care providers about genetics, how to get involved in genetics research, and much more: http://www.genesinlife.org/
- *GeneReviews*—Features expert-authored, peer-reviewed, current disease descriptions that apply genetic testing to the diagnosis, management, and genetic counseling of patients and families with specific inherited conditions. https://www.ncbi.nlm.nih.gov/books/NBK279899/ GeneReviews also provides a directory of resources for Genetics Professional: https://www.ncbi.nlm.nih.gov/books/NBK481802/#resource_mats.Resources_for_Genetics_Pro
- *National Institutes of Mental Health (NIMH)*—Looking at my genes: What can they tell me? Frequently asked questions about genome scans and genetic testing: https://www.nimh.nih.gov/health/publications/looking-at-my-genes
- *National Society of Genetic Counselors (NSGC)*—The NSGC has a resource link to assist individuals and health professionals in locating genetic counseling services. Genetic counselors can be searched by state, city, counselor's name, institution, or areas of practice or specialization: https://findageneticcounselor.nsgc.org/
- *Personalized Medicine*—Provides up-to-date information about a new era in health care, personalized medicine, which is creating new methods for earlier diagnoses and individualized interventions: http://www.ageofpersonalizedmedicine.org
- *U.S. Surgeon General's Family History Initiative, Family History Tool*—This web-based tool helps users organize family history information and then print it out for presentation to the family doctor. In addition, the tool helps users save their family history information to their own computer and even share family history information with other family members: http://kahuna.clayton.edu/jqu/FHH/html/index.html

and competent interpretation of these results is likely beyond the scope of practice for many health care professionals. Referrals to genetics professionals may be appropriate, and in some cases, it will likely create the need for additional testing to clarify vague or incomplete results.

Microbiome Direct-to-Consumer Testing

A variety of start-up companies are offering to analyze an individual's gut microbiome. Whereas some must be ordered by medical professionals and are covered by most health insurance, others can be purchased as a subscription service to test the microbiome monthly. These companies suggest the ability to predict risk for certain diseases based on the microbial composition of the gut and provide dietary recommendations. Diagnosis cannot be made with the currently available technology, and the reliability of the tests is unknown. Nurses must familiarize themselves with the microbiome and the types of results people are receiving from these companies.

Gene Therapies

There are currently at least eight approved gene therapies available in the United States (US FDA, 2021) with many more in development and clinical trials. Gene therapies can either replace a disease-causing gene with one that is normal, add a gene into the genome that can perform a function that the original genome could not perform, or downregulate a gene that is causing disease. The first gene-addition therapy was approved for use in the United States in 2017 for patients with a rare inherited form of blindness (Prado et al., 2020). This therapy works by inserting the desired gene into an adenovirus that can then deliver the new gene into cells. The therapy in this case is delivered via sub-retinal injection directly into the patient. In other cases of gene therapy, such as the chimeric antigen receptor (CAR)-T cells therapies, this process occurs in a laboratory using a person's blood or tissue, which, after a period of time, allows the newly modified cells to replicate, and then be transferred back into the body. In CAR-T therapies, it is a person's T-cells that are genetically modified to create a receptor specific to a diseased target-cell. When these cells are reintroduced to the person's body, the T-cells coordinate, attack, and initiate the processes that lead to the destruction of the targeted cells. Since 2012, the CRISPR (clustered regularly interspaced short palindromic repeats) technologies have become increasingly available to change a person's genome. In the United States, the first human clinical trials of these CRISPR technologies targeting sickle cell disease began in 2021. A CRISPR-based treatment for beta thalassemia began human clinical trials in Germany 2 years prior. These are both still gene-addition strategies. Genome editing strategies are currently in human clinical trials (Ledford, 2021). Gene therapies are being evaluated for diseases ranging from relatively common diseases such as Alzheimer and Parkinson to many rare diseases such as Canavan and aromatic L-amino acid decarboxylase deficiency (Mendell et al., 2021). When the technology is mastered to consistently produce successful gene therapies, the next big challenge will be to scale these therapies so that they can be available to large numbers of people. That will be the moment when hopes for personalized and precision health care can be realized. However, solving issues of access and affordability may be a bigger challenge than the development of gene therapy technologies.

ETHICAL ISSUES IN GENETICS AND GENOMICS

The nursing profession has long recognized the importance of ethics as an integral component of professional nursing practice. In recognition of the importance of an ethical foundation in nursing practice, the ANA created the *Code of Ethics for Nurses.* The Code of Ethics "makes explicit the primary goals, values, and obligations of the profession" (ANA, 2015, p. vii). Genetics, genomics, and gene therapies raise many ethical issues of concern for nurses. These include accessibility, informed decision-making, and consent; privacy and confidentiality of genetic and genomic information; social, cultural, and religious issues in genomic research; data-sharing; and the regulation of biorepositories and concerns about insurance and employment discrimination based on a person's genetic and genomic information. Nurses have a responsibility to help individuals, families, and society navigate the complex issues that arise surrounding genomic health care. The Code of Ethics for Nurses (ANA, 2015) serves as a foundation and guide for nurses when confronted with ethical issues relating to genetics and genomics. Readers are directed to Chapter 12 for an overview of ethical issues for nurses, including more information on informed decision-making and consent, as well as privacy and confidentiality of medical information, and further resources can be found in Box 16.3.

PROTECTIONS AGAINST DISCRIMINATION BASED ON GENETIC AND GENOMIC INFORMATION

When offering genetic or genomic tests, in addition to explaining the testing procedure, what might be learned, and what cannot be answered, it is also important for the nurse to explain the possible consequences of obtaining this kind of test result. To protect people who avail themselves of genetic testing, technologies, and therapies from discrimination surrounding the acquisition of health insurance or employment, the Genetic Information Nondiscrimination Act (GINA) became law in the United States in 2008 (NHGRI, 2022b). Although this was an important step for providing privacy to people who have single-gene disorders, over time, GINA may become increasingly inadequate. Now that we understand that everyone carries gene variants that may influence their risk of developing a disease, and that environment, lifestyle modification, and pharmacogenomics and gene editing technologies may mitigate these risks, we need to advocate for more broad legislation to protect rights to nondiscrimination in health care (Green et al., 2015).

In the meantime, erosion of GINA has been occurring through employee assistance programs that require genetic testing for risk assessment. Many employers have penalized people who opt out of their employee wellness programs (and the concomitant laboratory tests) by charging higher premiums to nonparticipants (Zhang, 2017). It will be important to watch federal legislation related to GINA and the Americans with Disabilities Act of 1990 (ADA, 1990) because current proposals will exempt employers from some GINA restrictions.

Furthermore, GINA protections have never applied to health care entities administered by the United States government: the military, Veterans Administration, and Indian Health Service. GINA also does not protect people against discrimination as they seek disability insurance, long-term care insurance, or life insurance. Nor does it protect people against housing discrimination or discrimination by schools. However, some states, such as California, have enacted legislation to address these gaps. These protections are becoming more important as genetic and genomic screening and diagnostic tests become the standard of care in many settings.

Nurses must have the capacity to guide and assist clients' ethical choices related to genetic/genomic screening, risk reduction, and treatment in a manner that is consistent with the clients' sociocultural and religious beliefs and long-term goals. Educating individuals and families about the ethical issues related to genetic or genomic testing is essential to fulfilling obligations as patient and family advocates. In addition, nurses must be equipped to help people effectively navigate and manage information that is acquired through genetic/genomic testing (Greco et al., 2011). Nurses must be able to accurately explain the protections afforded by and limits of protection through GINA. This sort of advocacy and education will possibly circumvent the subsequent development of ethical dilemmas.

SOCIAL, CULTURAL, AND RELIGIOUS ISSUES IN GENOMIC RESEARCH AND PRECISION HEALTH CARE

Using the human genome for research, testing, and treatment raises some difficult questions related to scientific, biomedical, and legal issues. Some of the most difficult questions, however, are related to social, cultural, or religious implications of new genetic knowledge and technology. Emerging knowledge about the history of our evolution and the small variations within an individual's genomes now informs our concepts and discourse around race, ethnicity, and even gender (Guttinger & Dupré, 2016; Nielsen et al., 2017). To address the challenges associated with the relationships among genomics, race, and ethnicity, researchers have now moved into the areas of social science and psychology to learn about genetic effects on behavior, as well as explore new dimensions of religious or philosophical concepts about identity, potentially redefining what it means to be human.

As genetics and genomics become more commonplace in health care, more attention needs to be paid to potential misuse and equitable access to treatments. Ethical, legal, and social issues (ELSI) research and education have become increasingly important. This work is multidisciplinary and often brings in consumers, policymakers, ethicists, and many other stakeholders beyond health care providers. ELSI-funded activities have included multiple research and education projects, books, articles, newsletters, websites, and television and radio programs, as well as conferences and other activities that focus on translating ELSI research into clinical and public health practices (McEwen et al., 2014).

SUMMARY

Genetic and genomic applications in clinical and population health settings are evolving at a fast pace. The era of personalized precision health care has arrived, though it is still in its infancy. Genomic tools are being used to track disease across populations and to tailor health care at the individual level by using a person's unique genetic and genomic information to guide care and treat disease. These methods are being transformed into increasingly common screening, diagnostic, and treatment tools. Nurses in all practice settings must acquire the essential knowledge and skills outlined in the *Essentials of Genetic and Genomic Nursing: Competencies, Curriculum and Outline Indicators* (ANA, 2009). As our understanding of disease is reshaped in this era of genomics, nurses are called upon to communicate these understandings, advocate for our patients, and provide care that is effective and meaningful.

REFERENCES

Americans With Disabilities Act of 1990, Pub. L. No. 101-336, 104 Stat. 328 (1990). https://www.ada.gov/pubs/ada.htm

American Nurses Association. (2009). *Essentials of genetic and genomic nursing: Competencies, curricula guidelines, and outcome indicators*. American Nurses Association. Accessed January 20, 2023. https://www.genome.gov/Pages/Careers/HealthProfessionalEducation/geneticscompetency.pdf

American Nurses Association. (2015). *Code of ethics for nurses with interpretive statements*. American Nurses Association. Available for purchase at https://www.nursingworld.org/practice-policy/nursing-excellence/ethics/code-of-ethics-for-nurses/coe-view-only/

American Nurses Association. (2021). *Nursing scope and standards of practice* (4th ed.). American Nurses Association.

Bai, X., Li, Y., Zeng, X., Zhao, Q., & Zhang, Z. (2021). Single-cell sequencing technology in tumor research. *Clinica*

Chimica Acta, 518, 101–109. https://doi.org/10.1016/j.cca.2021.03.013

Blackwell, G. A., Hunt, M., Malone, K. M., Lima, L., Horesh, G., Alako, B. T., Thompson, N. R., & Iqbal, Z. (2021). Exploring bacterial diversity via a curated and searchable snapshot of archived DNA sequences. PLoS Biology, 19(11), e3001421. https://doi.org/10.1371/journal.pbio.3001421

Brandl, E., Halford, Z., Clark, M. D., & Herndon, C. (2021). Pharmacogenomics in pain management: A review of relevant gene-drug associations and clinical considerations. Annals of Pharmacotherapy, 55(12), 1486–1501. https://doi.org/10.1177/10600280211003875

Brunkwall, L., & Orho-Melander, M. (2017). The gut microbiome as a target for prevention and treatment of hyperglycaemia in type 2 diabetes: From current human evidence to future possibilities. Diabetologia, 60(6), 943–951. https://doi.org/10.1007/s00125-017-4278-3

Centers for Disease Control and Prevention. (2021, November 5). Knowing is not enough—Act on your family health history. https://www.hhs.gov/programs/prevention-and-wellness/family-health-history/family-health-portrait-tool/index.html

Cohen, F. L. (1979). Genetic knowledge possessed by American nurses and nursing students. Journal of Advanced Nursing, 4(5), 493–501. https://doi.org/10.1111/j.1365-2648.1979.tb00883.x

Collins, F. S., Doudna, J. A., Lander, E. S., & Rotimi, C. N. (2021). Human molecular genetics and genomics—important advances and exciting possibilities. New England Journal of Medicine, 384(1), 1–4. https://doi.org/10.1056/NEJMp2030694

Consensus Panel on Genetic/Genomic Nursing Competencies. (2008). Essentials of genetic and genomic nursing: Competencies, curricula guidelines, and outcome indicators. American Nurses Association.

Corbett, G. A., Crosby, D. A., & McAuliffe, F. M. (2021). Probiotic therapy in couples with infertility: A systematic review. European Journal of Obstetrics & Gynecology and Reproductive Biology, 256, 95–100. https://doi.org/10.1016/j.ejogrb.2020.10.054

Deurenberg, R. H., Bathoorn, E., Chlebowicz, M. A., Couto, N., Ferdous, M., García-Cobos, S., & Rossen, J. W. A. (2017). Application of next generation sequencing in clinical microbiology and infection prevention. Journal of Biotechnology, 243, 16–24. https://doi.org/10.1016/j.jbiotec.2016.12.022

Dienstmann, R., & Tabernero, J. (2017). Cancer: A precision approach to tumour treatment. Nature, 548(7665), 40–41. https://doi.org/10.1038/nature23101

Ferrari, G., Thrasher, A. J., & Aiuti, A. (2021). Gene therapy using haematopoietic stem and progenitor cells. Nature Reviews Genetics, 22(4), 216–234. https://doi.org/10.1038/s41576-020-00298-5

Gerstein, M. B., Bruce, C., Rozowsky, J. S., Zheng, D., Du, J., Korbel, J. O., & Snyder, M. (2007). What is a gene, post-ENCODE? History and updated definition. Genome Research, 17(6), 669–681. https://doi.org/10.1101/gr.6339607

Greco, K. E., Tinley, S., & Seibert, D. (2011). Essential genetic and genomic competencies for nurses with graduate degrees. American Nurses Association & International Society of Nurses in Genetics. https://www.genome.gov/Pages/Health/HealthCareProvidersInfo/Grad_Gen_Comp.pdf

Green, R. C., Lautenbach, D., & McGuire, A. L. (2015). GINA: Genetic discrimination and genomic medicine. New England Journal of Medicine, 372(5), 397–399. https://doi.org/10.1056/NEJMp1404776

Grill, S., & Klein, E. (2021). Incorporating genomic and genetic testing into the treatment of metastatic luminal breast cancer. Breast Care, 16(2), 101–107. https://doi.org/10.1159/000513800

Guttinger, S., & Dupré, J. (2016). Genomics and postgenomics. In E. N. Zalta (Ed.), Stanford Encyclopedia of Philosophy (2016 Winter ed.). https://plato.stanford.edu/archives/win2016/entries/genomics/

Harris, D. M., Stancampiano, F. F., Burton, M. C., Moyer, A. M., Schuh, M. J., Valery, J. R., & Bi, Y. (2021). Use of pharmacogenomics to guide proton pump inhibitor therapy in clinical practice. Digestive Diseases and Sciences, 66(12), 4120–4127. https://doi.org/10.1007/s10620-020-06814-1

Illiano, P., Brambilla, R., & Parolini, C. (2020). The mutual interplay of gut microbiota, diet and human disease. The FEBS Journal, 287(5), 833–855. https://doi.org/10.1111/febs.15217

Kehr, B., Helgadottir, A., Melsted, P., Jonsson, H., Helgason, H., Jonasdottir, A., Sigurdsson, A., Gylfason, A., Halldorsson, G. H., Kristmundsdottir, S., Thorgerisson, G., Olafsson, I., Holm, H., Thorsteinsdottir, U., Sulem, P., Helgason, A., Gudbjartsson, D. F., Halldorsson, B. V., & Stefansson, K. (2017). Diversity in non-repetitive human sequences not found in the reference genome. Nature Genetics, 49(4), 588–593. https://doi.org/10.1038/ng.3801

Krier, J. B., Kalia, S. S., & Green, R. C. (2016). Genomic sequencing in clinical practice: Applications, challenges, and opportunities. Dialogues in Clinical Neuroscience, 18(3), 299–312. https://doi.org/10.31887/DCNS.2016.18.3/jkrier

Kurnat-Thoma, E., Fu, M. R., Henderson, W. A., Voss, J. G., Hammer, M. J., Williams, J. K., Calzone, K., Conley, Y. P., Starkweather, A., Weaver, M. T., Shiao, P. K., & Coleman, B. (2021). Current status and future directions of US genomic nursing health care policy. Nursing Outlook, 69(3), 471–488. https://doi.org/10.1016/j.outlook.2020.12.006

Ledford, H. (2021). Landmark CRISPR trial shows promise against deadly disease. Nature. https://doi.org/10.1038/d41586-021-01776-4

Lempiäinen, H., Brænne, I., Michoel, T., Tragante, V., Vilne, B., Webb, T. R., & Björkegren, J. L. M. (2018). Network analysis of coronary artery disease risk genes elucidates disease mechanisms and druggable targets. Scientific Reports, 8(1), 3434. https://doi.org/10.1038/s41598-018-20721-6

Liu, X., Speranza, E., Muñoz-Fontela, C., Haldenby, S., Rickett, N. Y., & Garcia-Dorival, I. (2017). Transcriptomic signatures differentiate survival from fatal outcomes in humans infected with Ebola virus. Genome Biology, 18, 4. https://doi.org/10.1186/s13059-016-1137-3

McElroy, K. G., Chung, S. Y., & Regan, M. (2017). CE: Health and the human microbiome—a primer for nurses. AJN The American Journal of Nursing, 117(7), 24. https://doi.org/10.1097/01.NAJ.0000520917.73358.99

McEwen, J. E., Boyer, J. T., Sun, K. Y., Rothenberg, K. H., Lockhart, N. C., & Guyer, M. S. (2014). The Ethical, Legal, and Social Implications Program of the National Human Genome Research

Institute: Reflections on an ongoing experiment. *Annual Review of Genomics and Human Genetics, 15*, 481–505. https://doi.org/10.1146/annurev-genom-090413-025327

MedlinePlus [Internet]. (2022a, February 7). *What is genetic testing? Genetics home reference.* National Library of Medicine (US). Accessed January 27, 2023. https://medlineplus.gov/genetics/understanding/testing/genetictesting/

MedlinePlus [Internet]. (2022b, June 21). *What is direct-to-consumer genetic testing? Genetics home reference.* National Library of Medicine (US). Accessed January 27, 2023. https://medlineplus.gov/genetics/understanding/dtcgenetictesting/directtoconsumer/

Mendell, J. R., Al-Zaidy, S. A., Rodino-Klapac, L. R., Goodspeed, K., Gray, S. J., Kay, C. N., Boye, S. L., Boye, S. E., George, L. A., Salabarria, S., Corti, M., Byrne, B. J., & Tremblay, J. P. (2021). Current clinical applications of in vivo gene therapy with AAVs. *Molecular Therapy: The Journal of the American Society of Gene Therapy, 29*(2), 464–488. https://doi.org/10.1016/j.ymthe.2020.12.007

Merrick, B. A., Chang, J. S., Phadke, D. P., Bostrom, M. A., Shah, R. R., Wang, X., & Wright, G. M. (2018). HAfTs are novel lncRNA transcripts from aflatoxin exposure. *PLOS ONE, 13*(1), e0190992. https://doi.org/10.1371/journal.pone.0190992

National Human Genome Research Institute. (2013). *Genetic counseling FAQ.* https://www.genome.gov/19016905/faq-about-genetic-counseling/

National Human Genome Research Institute. (2014a). *Guidelines and tools to assess history of common diseases.* https://www.genome.gov/27527602/guidelines-and-tools-to-assess-history-of-common-diseases/

National Human Genome Research Institute. (2014b, April 4). *Talking glossary of genetic terms.* Accessed January 27, 2023. https://www.genome.gov/glossary/

National Human Genome Research Institute. (2019). *Genetic testing FAQ.* https://www.genome.gov/FAQ/Genetic-Testing

National Human Genome Research Institute. (2020a). *A brief guide to genomics.* https://www.genome.gov/about-genomics/fact-sheets/A-Brief-Guide-to-Genomics

National Human Genome Research Institute. (2020b). *Human genome project FAQ.* https://www.genome.gov/human-genome-project/Completion-FAQ

National Human Genome Research Institute. (2020c). *DNA microarray technology fact sheet.* https://www.genome.gov/about-genomics/fact-sheets/DNA-Microarray-Technology

National Human Genome Research Institute. (2021). *The cost of sequencing a human genome.* https://www.genome.gov/about-genomics/fact-sheets/Sequencing-Human-Genome-cost

National Human Genome Research Institute. (2022a). *Direct-to-consumer genomic testing.* https://www.genome.gov/dna-day/15-ways/direct-to-consumer-genomic-testing

National Human Genome Research Institute. (2022b). *Genetic discrimination.* https://www.genome.gov/about-genomics/policy-issues/Genetic-Discrimination

Nielsen, R., Akey, J. M., Jakobsson, M., Pritchard, J. K., Tishkoff, S., & Willerslev, E. (2017). Tracing the peopling of the world through genomics. *Nature, 541*(7637), 302–310. https://doi.org/10.1038/nature21347

Nightingale, F. (1859). *Notes on nursing.* Appleton and Company.

Parida, S., & Sharma, D. (2021). The microbiome and cancer: Creating friendly neighborhoods and removing the foes within. *Cancer Research, 81*(4), 790–800. https://doi.org/10.1158/0008-5472.CAN-20-2629

Park, S. Y., Faraci, G., Ward, P. M., Emerson, J. F., & Lee, H. Y. (2021). High-precision and cost-efficient sequencing for real-time COVID-19 surveillance. *Scientific Reports, 11*(1), 1–10. https://doi.org/10.1038/s41598-021-93145-4

Pederzoli, F., Murdica, V., Salonia, A., & Alfano, M. (2022). The gut and urinary microbiota: A rising biomarker in genitourinary malignancies. In *Neoadjuvant immunotherapy treatment of localized genitourinary cancers* (pp. 247–261). Springer. https://doi.org/10.1007/978-3-030-80546-3_19

Prado, D. A., Acosta-Acero, M., & Maldonado, R. S. (2020). Gene therapy beyond luxturna: A new horizon of the treatment for inherited retinal disease. *Current Opinion in Ophthalmology, 31*(3), 147–154. https://doi.org/10.1097/ICU.0000000000000660

Retterer, K., Juusola, J., Cho, M. T., Vitazka, P., Millan, F., Gibellini, F., & Bale, S. (2016). Clinical application of whole-exome sequencing across clinical indications. *Genetics in Medicine, 18*(7), 696–704. http://dx.doi.org/10.1038/gim.2015.148

Sabatello, M., & Appelbaum, P. S. (2017). The precision medicine nation. *Hastings Center Report, 47*(4), 19–29. http://dx.doi.org/10.1002/hast.736

Sastre, L. (2014). Exome sequencing: What clinicians need to know. *Advances in Genomics and Genetics, 4*, 15–27. https://doi.org/10.2147/AGG.S39108

Sherman, R. M., & Salzberg, S. L. (2020). Pan-genomics in the human genome era. *Nature Reviews. Genetics, 21*(4), 243–254. https://doi.org/10.1038/s41576-020-0210-7

Snir, M., Nazareth, S., Simmons, E., Hayward, L., Ashcraft, K., Bristow, S. L., Esplin, E. D., & Aradhya, S. (2021). Democratizing genomics: Leveraging software to make genetics an integral part of routine care. *American Journal of Medical Genetics. Part C, Seminars in Medical Genetics, 187*(1), 14–27. https://doi.org/10.1002/ajmg.c.31866

Sumaily, K. M., & Mujamammi, A. H. (2017). Phenylketonuria: A new look at an old topic, advances in laboratory diagnosis, and therapeutic strategies. *International Journal of Health Sciences, 11*(5), 63–70. https://www.ncbi.nlm.nih.gov/pmc/articles/PMC5669513/

Thompson, J. R., Nancharaiah, Y. V., Gu, X., Lee, W. L., Rajal, V. B., Haines, M. B., Girones, R., Ng, L. C., Alm, E. J., & Wuertz, S. (2020). Making waves: Wastewater surveillance of SARS-CoV-2 for population-based health management. *Water Research, 184*, 116181. https://doi.org/10.1016/j.watres.2020.116181

United States Food and Drug Administration. (2021). *Approved cellular and gene therapy products.* https://www.fda.gov/vaccines-blood-biologics/cellular-gene-therapy-products/approved-cellular-and-gene-therapy-products

Wosinska, L., Cotter, P. D., O'Sullivan, O., & Guinane, C. (2019). The potential impact of probiotics on the gut microbiome of athletes. *Nutrients, 11*(10), 2270. https://doi.org/10.3390/nu11102270

Zhang, S. (2017, March 13). *The loopholes in the law prohibiting genetic discrimination.* The Atlantic. https://www.theatlantic.com/health/archive/2017/03/genetic-discrimination-law-gina/519216/

17

Global Rural Nursing Practice

Marianne Baernholdt, PhD, MPH, RN, FAAN, Barbara Shellian, RN MN, and Victoria Petermann, RN, BSN, PhD(c)

 http://evolve.elsevier.com/Friberg/bridge/

OBJECTIVES

After completion of this chapter, the reader will be able to:

- Discuss the social determinants of health for global rural populations.
- Identify major health issues impacting global rural areas.
- Discuss the scope of global rural nursing practice.

- Identify common professional practice issues for nurses working in global rural areas.
- Apply knowledge of factors, including social determinants of health, that impact rural health to develop the provision of health care to global rural populations.

INTRODUCTION

About half of the world's population (44%) or 3.402 billion people live in rural areas (World Bank, 2020a). In the United States, about 14% of the population, or 46 million people, reside in the 97% of the U.S. land mass considered rural (U.S. Census Bureau, 2017; U.S. Department of Agriculture [USDA], Economic Research Service [ERS], 2021a). In Canada according to the 2016 Census, 18% of the population of more than 6.3 million Canadians were living in rural areas (Statistics Canada, 2016). Nurses are often the first point of health care and, in some instances, the only one. Recognizing that rural or remote, resource-poor areas are similar across the world, this chapter focuses on nursing practice in global rural areas. We define global rural nursing practice as practice in *both* local and international rural contexts. To practice in these areas and be strong advocates for health promotion, nurses need knowledge, skills, and attitudes that enable them to understand world cultures and events, analyze global systems, recognize the impact of social determinants of health (SDOH), appreciate cultural differences, and apply this knowledge and appreciation to their practice (Canadian Association for Rural and Remote Nursing [CARRN], 2020; MacKinnon & Moffat, 2014).

Global rural nursing practice encompasses learning and employment opportunities in rural and international areas. Currently, there are 27.9 million nurses in the world, but their distribution is uneven (World Health Organization [WHO], 2020). Over 80% of nurses are in countries that account for only half of the world's population. Further, it is estimated that there is a global shortage of 5.9 million nurses, of which 89% (5.3 million) are missing in low- and middle-income countries, including countries with large rural populations such as Africa, South-East Asia, and countries in Latin America. Recruitment and retention of nurses in rural and remote areas is a growing concern in many countries (WHO, 2020).

Resource-poor (often rural) communities benefit from much-needed access to care when nurses are aware of power dynamics between health care organizations or professionals and rural communities and are mindful of actions or interventions that may further stigmatize the community in which they work (Jones et al., 2020). Rural communities and the people that comprise them must be equal partners in addressing gaps in health care services and considered experts in the needs of their community (Jones et al., 2020). A community-engaged approach results in long-term sustainable relationships that can develop appropriate and relevant changes in health and health care for the community (Jones et al., 2020). In turn, the global rural practicing nurse learns from the community and builds invaluable skills in effective community engagement and clinical care. This perspective is a key building block for developing an understanding of global rural nursing practice.

DEFINITION OF RURAL

There are several definitions for rural or remoteness, all contingent on geographic location and sociocultural differences (Farmer et al., 2010). In the United States, there are more than 15 definitions of rural used in federal programs using county, zip code, or census tract data (Coburn et al., 2007). According to the 2010 U.S. Census definition, Maine, Vermont, West Virginia, and Mississippi had more than 50% of their residents living in rural areas (World Population Review, 2021). In Canada, an often-used definition considers areas outside the commuting zone of centers with a population of 10,000 or more as rural (MacLeod et al., 2017). Globally, the spread among countries is from 0% (Singapore and Kuwait) to 87% (Papua New Guinea) (World Bank, 2020a). While Africa and Asia are urbanizing rapidly, these regions are still home to most of the world's rural population. South Asia has the largest rural population at 1209 billion people, including India with the largest rural population at 898 million, followed by sub-Saharan Africa at 667 million and China with 544 million.

The global rural population is expected to decline to 3.1 billion by 2050 (Our World in Data, n.d.). In the United States, from 2010 to 2020, the rural areas had a 0.6% decline in population compared to an increase of 8.8% in urban areas (USDA ERS, 2021a). However, changes varied greatly, often depending on local economic differences; for example, North Dakota saw an increase of 12.5% in its rural population because of its booming energy sector during the 2010s, while West Virginia had a decrease of 6.6% because of lower rates of extraction of coal, gas, oil, and other natural resources. Other Western states have a positive net migration to rural areas caused by the attraction of abundant recreational features and retirement-based economies. The retirees often tend to make up the largest and most financially well-off social group in the rural area (USDA ERS, 2016). Migration patterns can have a considerable effect in terms of "watering down" the collective rural culture.

GLOBAL RURAL NURSING PRACTICE

Some argue rural nursing practice requires unique competencies as an "expert generalist" who needs knowledge in many areas of nursing practice (Baernholdt et al., 2010; Scharff, 2013). Rural nursing practice has characteristics of isolation from health care specialists; limited access to communication connectivity, resources, and facilities; coping and planning for unpredictable weather and travel conditions; high burden of mental health and substance abuse disorders; and working with an extended scope of practice but with a limited number of nurses (CARRN, 2020). Rural nursing practice requires skills and knowledge about development across the life span and adaptability to a variety of health care settings. The rural nurse needs to be ready for the not-uncommon shift that begins in the emergency room (ER), moves by noon to assist in a delivery, and ends by providing nursing care for a child with a severe asthmatic episode.

A commitment to ongoing professional development is essential in rural areas, as nurses may not perform a task or procedure more than once a year yet, must maintain proficiency in a variety of competencies. Further, rural nurses are expected to work with a high degree of independence and function more autonomously in expanded nursing roles. Additionally, rural nurses often work with limited or delayed access to resources.

Practicing in global rural areas involves a high degree of community visibility, including a unique interconnectedness between nurses and their communities (Baernholdt et al., 2010), described as "permeability between the rural workplace and the community setting." Experienced rural nurses use knowledge of their patients outside of the health care system to better plan for their care within the health care system (Baernholdt et al., 2010; CARRN, 2020). Besides having strong clinical knowledge, the nurse in the rural setting also needs to understand community capacity, community assets, politics, and intersectoral collaboration to practice effectively.

SOCIAL DETERMINANTS OF HEALTH

Nurses have to consider the SDOH, which is often responsible for health and health care inequities between urban and rural populations. SDOH are the conditions in which people are born, grow, live, work, and age and are shaped by the distribution of money, power, and resources at global, national, and local levels (WHO, 2022). Globally, efforts to improve living conditions in the world's least-resourced areas have been guided by the United Nations

---

BOX 17.1   Sustainable Development Goals

Goal 1. End poverty in all its forms everywhere

Goal 2. End hunger, achieve food security and improved nutrition and promote sustainable agriculture

Goal 3. Ensure healthy lives and promote well-being for all at all ages

Goal 4. Ensure inclusive and equitable quality education and promote lifelong learning opportunities for all

Goal 5. Achieve gender equality and empower all women and girls

Goal 6. Ensure availability and sustainable management of water and sanitation for all

Goal 7. Ensure access to affordable, reliable, sustainable, and modern energy for all

Goal 8. Promote sustained, inclusive, and sustainable economic growth, full and productive employment, and decent work for all

Goal 9. Build resilient infrastructure, promote inclusive and sustainable industrialization, and foster innovation

Goal 10. Reduce inequality within and among countries

Goal 11. Make cities and human settlements inclusive, safe, resilient, and sustainable

Goal 12. Ensure sustainable consumption and production patterns

Goal 13. Take urgent action to combat climate change and its impacts

Goal 14. Conserve and sustainably use the oceans, seas, and marine resources for sustainable development

Goal 15. Protect, restore, and promote sustainable use of terrestrial ecosystems, sustainably manage forests, combat desertification, and halt and reverse land degradation and halt biodiversity loss

Goal 16. Promote peaceful and inclusive societies for sustainable development, provide access to justice for all and build effective, accountable, and inclusive institutions at all levels

Goal 17. Strengthen the means of implementation and revitalize the Global Partnership for Sustainable Development

Data from United Nations. (2015). *Transforming our world: The 2030 agenda for sustainable development.* Retrieved from http://www.un.org/ga/search/view_doc.asp?symbol=A/RES/70/1&Lang=E

Sustainable Development Goals since 2015 (UN, 2015). These 17 goals aim to end poverty, protect the planet, ensure prosperity for all, and address the SDOH outcomes (Box 17.1). Because rural nurses are most successful if they consider the SDOH, this chapter addresses how eight determinants of health (rural culture, structural racism, physical environment, social support, economic factors, education, personal characteristics, and access to health care) impact rural health and shape global rural nursing practice (see Fig. 17.1).

Rural Culture

I know I've had difficulty not being from here. I've had difficulty communicating with some of my patients, but [as you] work closely with the nurses that are from here, you're able to learn what the best way is to go about educating the patients.

Baernholdt et al., 2010, p. 1351

Culture is a specific set of beliefs and attributes for a group, region, or nation (Hofstede, 2001) that determines how a group thinks, feels, and acts and is important to individuals' health and how health care is delivered (Baernholdt et al., 2010; Leipert & George, 2008). The values and beliefs of a rural culture not only influence how rural people

define health but also from whom they seek advice, treatment, and care. Rural populations value and embrace "their" nurses, and they believe rural nurses have a strong sense of accountability. Nurses in rural areas have to be viewed as part of the community to be able to practice (Baernholdt et al., 2010; Bushy, 2012). While knowledge of the rural culture is a basic requirement for nurses, community connectedness, in which nurses and patients know one another outside the health care setting, can create boundary-related ethical conflicts (Brooks et al., 2012). Delivering care consistent with local customs and beliefs yet understanding how to set limits to avoid ethical conflicts is essential for successful nursing practice in a rural area (Baernholdt et al., 2010).

Structural Racism

I have been a nurse for 12 years and have experienced and witnessed overt racism—of patients toward clinicians, but also clinicians toward patients. I have felt the systemic racism permeating through our health care system.

Danda, 2020

Discrimination by race creates patterns of structural racism (differential access to services and opportunities,

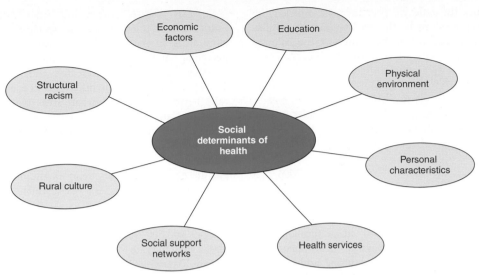

Fig. 17.1 Social Determinants of Health in Global Rural Communities.

such as health care or education), interpersonal racism (personally mediated racism that manifests as prejudice or discrimination), and internalized racism (internal negative messages about one's abilities and worth based on race or ethnicity) (Jones, 2000). For this chapter, we will address structural racism, though the other two forms are relevant to understanding dynamics within rural communities. Structural or systemic racism against marginalized communities in rural areas manifests through policies around housing, economic structures, and environments that have effects on health outcomes.

Historical systemic racism in the United States and other countries has impacted the health outcomes of populations of marginalized racial or ethnic groups in rural areas. Residential segregation limited the transportation, employment, and education opportunities of majority Black communities. Such practices were codified into law during the Jim Crow era (Hswen et al., 2020). South Africa also has a long history of segregation policies (Coovadia et al., 2009).

Segregation in rural areas has affected access to quality health care (Hswen et al., 2020).

Individuals of racial or ethnic identities who live in more segregated rural areas are more likely to experience poorer health outcomes (e.g., overall mortality, poor health behaviors, and receipt of appropriate cancer treatment) (Landrine et al., 2017; Logan & Parman, 2018). (See Chapter 14 for a further discussion on diversity, equity, and inclusion.) Marginalized rural populations in the United States tend to live further from health care services,

which increases the burden and cost of accessing those services. Economic and educational opportunities are limited, reducing health literacy, access to quality foods, and the ability to pay for health insurance. Similarly, in South Africa, access to health care is scarce in rural areas (Neely & Ponshunmugam, 2019).

Indigenous populations have faced historic and present-day discrimination and oppression (e.g., forced sterilization, assimilation, funding of health care resources, etc.) that impact health quality and access to care (Allan & Smylie, 2015; Allen et al., 2020; Jones, 2006). Additionally, traditional healing practices that are integral to these communities are disregarded, and individuals face aggression, discrimination, and lack of trauma-informed care (Anderson & Brodkin, 2013). Such experiences are rooted in histories of oppression and colonialism. (See Chapter 18 for a further discussion on trauma-informed care.) Well into the 1980s, Canada's residential school system for Aboriginal children was sanctioned, and systematic tools used to force the assimilation and elimination of Aboriginal culture, governments, and rights (Truth and Reconciliation Commission of Canada [TRC], 2015). The TRC, established out of the Indian Residential Schools Settlement Agreement, demands multi-level action by institutions at multiple levels of influence and power to address the repercussions of historic legacies of colonial oppression (TRC, 2015).

Rural practicing nurses must be aware of the legacies of colonial power that have shaped the histories and present-day realities of rural areas in which they practice. To be effective, rural nurses have to embrace decolonization, which combines the reflexive practice of acknowledging how colonial legacies impact the lived realities of populations with the practice of actively undoing the colonial legacy in partnership with affected communities.

Physical Environment

You go out here and get back in these mountains and just look at the scenery. … Makes you wonder why people want to leave and everything like this. You know it's God's creation and our mountains are ours—and we love them.

Coyne et al., 2006, p. 3

People's health is determined largely by the physical environment in which they live, learn, and work. A natural physical environment with clean water and air, fertile soil, and thriving green spaces; and a built physical environment with healthy workplaces, good roads, safe housing, and communities that promote good health (WHO, 2022). Deficiencies in these elements negatively affect psychological and physical health (Centers for Disease Control [CDC], 2013).

The term *rural* brings to mind isolated, quaint small towns, sparsely populated farmland, remote Arctic communities accessible only by air or ice road, mountains, forests, and open ranges, where successive generations have engaged in farming, ranching, mining, or logging. Quiet rural areas with abundant natural beauty, clean air, and closeness to nature are seen as the antithesis of crowded, noisy, and polluted cities. Unfortunately, these health-promoting features are offset by negative factors disproportionally affecting rural populations.

Rural regions in Europe, Australia, New Zealand, Canada, and the United States have higher rates of injuries related to occupational hazards (Smith et al., 2008). Rural industries (e.g., fishing, forestry, agriculture, and mining) are the most dangerous occupations in the world and are associated with higher frequencies of fatal accidents (Smith et al., 2008). Agriculture has the highest rate of injuries (Ravi & Joseph, 2019; The National Institute for Occupational Safety and Health [NIOSH], 2022). In the United States, unintentional injuries (e.g., traffic accidents) are highest in rural areas (County Health Ranking and Roadmap [CHRR], 2016). Rural children are at higher risk of unintentional injury compared to urban children at 12.4 versus 6.3/100,000, respectively (Garnett et al., 2021). The isolated and remote rural physical environment requires longer emergency response times that contribute to higher rural accident-related death rates.

Though the effect of the rural physical environment as a single determinant of health is unclear (Smith et al., 2008), rural populations have poorer health than their urban counterparts. In 2019, the 10 leading causes of death (i.e., heart disease, cancer, and other chronic diseases, influenza and pneumonia, and suicide) were higher in rural areas. In the United States, rural areas have a high percentage of older adults and people with chronic diseases (Agency for Healthcare Research and Quality [AHRQ], 2021, p. 5) increasing the difference in age-adjusted death rates between rural and urban areas (Curtin & Spencer, 2021). In Canada, the difference in life expectancy between urban and rural populations varies by as much as 16 years in favor of urban areas (Canadian Institute for Health Information [CIHI], 2009; Government of Canada, 2022). For the Aboriginal Inuits living in the northern rural regions, life expectancy is 70.8 years, which is well below the Canadian average of 80.6 years (Statistics Canada, 2020). In the Canadian Inuit communities, the suicide rate was 135 per 100,000 from 1999 to 2003, which was 11 times higher than the rate for all Canadians (11.8/100,000) (Inuit Tapiriit Kanatami [ITK], 2007). Inuit children and teenagers were more than 30 times as likely to die from suicide as were those in the rest of Canada; half of all deaths of young people in the Nunavut Territory (the largest Inuit community) were suicides, compared with approximately 10% in the rest of Canada (Statistics Canada, 2012). Similarly, rates for behavioral health conditions are higher in rural areas in North America, Europe, Australia, and New Zealand (Bolin et al., 2015; Smith et al., 2008).

For most of the COVID-19 pandemic, the U.S. rural mortality rates have been higher than urban mortality rates (Ullrich & Muller, 2022). In Canada, the COVID-19 incidence and mortality are not significantly different between rural and urban areas, but the differences noted for rural areas are access to resources such as vaccines, testing, and medical care (Statistics Canada, 2022). Many rural/urban health differentials are mitigated, when socioeconomic variables such as age, gender, income, education, and race/ethnicity are controlled, suggesting a complex multifactorial and interrelated association among health, the rural environment, and other determinants of health (CIHI, 2009; Smith et al., 2008; Statistics Canada, 2020).

Social Support

When a disease is so rare and there are no folks in your town, and few in your state who are going through what you are going through, you need a support group that encompasses people from all over the world. Getting to know people through the disorder has been an amazing experience and has created incredibly wonderful friendships and ties.

Fox, 2011, p. 11

Social support is *support* from families, friends, and communities. Greater social support is linked to better health

(WHO, 2022) and is associated with lower rates of depression (Mechakra-Tahiri et al., 2009). Conversely, social isolation is an independent risk factor for mortality (Pantell et al., 2013). In rural areas, social isolation has been linked to higher mortality rates in Botswana (Clausen et al., 2007), poorer cardiovascular health in Ecuador (Del Brutto et al., 2013), and depression in Japanese elderly and U.S. elderly women (Buys et al., 2009; Kimura et al., 2012). It is often the sense of belonging to a community that draws people to rural areas (Baernholdt, 2017). Not surprisingly, data from Canada and the United States indicate rural individuals participate in community groups at a higher level than their urban counterparts (Keating et al., 2011; Stern et al., 2011). Yet others have reported that, compared with older adults in urban areas, rural elders have less social support (Baernholdt et al., 2012).

For nurses and other health care providers, rural practice settings can present challenges and professional isolation. The dense social networks present in small, rural communities may challenge confidentiality (Brooks et al., 2012). Limited access to other providers, peer support, and clinical mentorship factor prominently in rural nurses' negative descriptions of professional isolation (Williams, 2012).

For both rural dwellers and their nurses, the Internet offers an alternative approach to creating and maintaining social support across geographically isolated areas (Stern et al., 2011). For rural nurses who lack access to traditional resources and support, online forums and social media can provide opportunities to share ideas and practice challenges with colleagues (Barry & Hardiker, 2012). However, in the United States, 22.3% of rural people and 27.7% of people living in tribal lands (also rural) lack access to broadband compared to 1.5% in urban areas (Federal Communications Commission, 2020). Globally, only about 35% of the population in developing countries has access to the Internet (vs. about 80% in advanced economies), with rural populations having less access to the Internet services within countries (World Bank, 2022a). While the COVID-19 pandemic increased the use of virtual options for health care for rural and remote people, it exposed limitations related to access to broadband to facilitate online work and school (Canadian Rural Revitalization Foundation, 2021; USDA ERS, 2021a).

Economic Factors

Take the death of this small boy this morning, for example. The boy died of measles. We all know he could have been cured at the hospital. But the parents had no money and so the boy died a slow and painful death, not of measles, but out of poverty.

Narayan et al., 2000, p. 36

Economic factors include income, employment, and occupation (WHO, 2022). Higher incomes are associated with improved health, and conversely, poverty contributes significantly to ill health. Despite differing societal norms across the globe, there is agreement that poverty is a state that results in social and material deprivation (Halseth & Ryseth, 2010). Social deprivation includes a lack of access to resources that could alleviate poverty and a lack of power to make decisions that could enhance quality of life. Material deprivation encompasses hunger, insufficient housing, inadequate income, and lacking other goods that would be considered necessities (Halseth & Ryseth, 2010). The World Bank (2022b) defines poverty as the percentage of a country's population living on less than the extreme poor, quantified as those living on less than $1.90 a day. Following the COVID-19 pandemic, poverty increased from 655 million to 732 million people living in poverty globally (Mahler et al., 2021).

About 70% of the world's very poor populations reside in rural regions (International Fund for Agricultural Development [IFAD], 2011). Rural poverty, although more prevalent in low-income countries, also disproportionately affects rural populations in affluent countries. In the United States, the poverty rate was higher in rural areas (15.4%) than in urban areas (11.9%) in 2019 (USDA ERS, 2021b). However, regional differences are wide. From 2015 to 2019, out of the 138 counties in the United States with child poverty rates of 40% or higher, 127 were rural, primarily in the south (84.3%) with concentrations in Mississippi, Georgia, Kentucky, and Texas, with persistently high rates among the Black or African American population. In Canada, the income earnings of rural people are about 25% lower than those in large metropolitan areas (Beckstead et al., 2010). Rural poverty is widely dispersed and might have pockets in marginalized areas with low agricultural or other economic potential and subsequently lacking in public or private investment (IFAD, 2011).

The path out of poverty is very complex, yet its importance is underscored in UNSDG-1, which aims to end all poverty (see Box 17.1). In subsequent target goal 1.4, solutions include: ensuring rights to economic resources and access to basic services; ownership and control over land and other forms of property; inheritance; natural resources; appropriate new technology; and financial services, including microfinance (UN, 2015). Emergence from poverty requires diversification of income sources to alleviate the risks associated with relying solely on crop production or livestock management. Income source diversity is seen across all income levels, and higher household incomes are associated with higher rates of nonfarm employment (Brown & Weber, 2013; IFAD, 2011). In a sample of rural households in 15 Asian, Latin American, and sub-Saharan African countries, 30% to 60% derived significant amounts of their annual incomes from non-farm activities. These are highly variable, for example, trade, manufacturing, construction, agricultural-related businesses, and service industries (IFAD, 2011).

In the United States, rural employment is also diversified. For example, in farming households, 91% had one or more family members working off the farm for pay. Off-farm employment for farm operators was in construction followed by various agricultural-related businesses, mining, and manufacturing, whereas employment for women was in health care or education (Brown & Weber, 2013). In Canada, rural communities have significant economic activity and job creation (Flanagan, 2015). Rural Canada is the site of food production, resource extraction, energy generation, and clean water and air and of increasing importance for carbon sequestration. As global society transitions to alternative energy sources, other opportunities exist for rural areas, particularly in the clean energy sector.

In the United States, rural areas had a decade of decline in unemployment rates prior to the COVID-19 pandemic, reaching a low of 3.5% in September 2019. However, in early 2020, unemployment rates reached levels not seen since the Great Depression in the 1930s, peaking in April 2020 at 13.6% in rural areas, 14.6% in urban areas, and 14.4% nationally. While this increase was similar for both rural and urban counties, it varied by a county's persistent poverty status, so both poor rural and urban counties were hit the hardest (USDA ERS, 2021b).

Education

… if I had been to school, I could have had a good job in town. I could be in a nice office … But you see, I am illiterate and I got married too early. That is precisely the problem of being illiterate. You have no way of knowing what the possibilities are out there. I can't know. All I know is farming.

IFAD, 2011, p. 63

The level of education is a major correlate of the variation in earnings between rural and urban workers (Beckstead et al., 2010), with low education levels linked with poor health, more stress, and lower self-confidence (WHO, 2022). In both low- and high-income countries, those with greater levels of education are more likely to be healthier and live longer (Cutler & Lleras-Muney, 2006). For both low- and high-income countries, rural children are nearly twice as likely to be out of school as urban children (United Nations Educational, Scientific, and Cultural Organization [UNESCO], 2013). In Canada, rural communities have higher high school dropout rates (16.4%) relative to urban communities (9.2%) and less than 50% of

adults with post secondary education compared to more than 60% in urban communities (Canada Council on Learning, 2006).

Literacy statistics provide a common measure of educational attainment. Globally, more than 750 million adults lack basic reading and writing skills (UNESCO, 2017a) and more than two-thirds are women. Further, 6 out of 10 children and adolescents (more than 617 million) are not achieving minimum proficiency levels in reading and mathematics (UNESCO, 2017b). Adult literacy rates range from 5% in Somalia to greater than 99% in high-income countries (World Bank, 2020a). The relationship between education and health is at least partly explained by health literacy, or "the degree to which individuals have the capacity to obtain, process, and understand basic health information and services needed to make appropriate health decisions" (Institute of Medicine [IOM], 2004, p. 2). Health literacy is influenced by individual factors such as language and reading skills, as well as characteristics of health care systems. Lower health literacy is associated with poorer health, poorer adherence to prescribed medical treatments, and higher rates of hospital admission (Kanj & Mitic, 2009). Rural areas have lower health literacy levels compared with urban areas. In Taiwan, 30% of adults had inadequate or marginal health literacy and tended to be older with lower household income, and live in rural areas (Lee et al., 2010). In the United States, 7.7% of rural adults have proficient health literacy skills compared with 12% of the overall adult U.S. population, and more than 39% of rural adults with basic or below basic health literacy skills compared to 35% in urban areas (Zahnd et al., 2009).

The ability of health care providers, including nurses, to provide easily understood health information is critical to improving health literacy across settings. Indeed, the AHRQ (2017) provides a health literacy toolkit with evidence-based guidance on the implementation of simplified communication about health information and accessing health services. The toolkit is in its second edition and has been used in many settings in the United States and New Zealand.

Personal Characteristics

Personal characteristics influencing health include age, race/ethnicity, and gender (WHO, 2022). The makeup of global rural populations is somewhat different than urban populations.

Age

Most people's biggest fear as you get older … you start to think well you know I don't want to be cared for, I don't want to be unable to look after myself.

Terrill & Gullifer, 2010, p. 713

By international standards, a society is aging when more than 10% of the population is 60 years of age and older. In both rural and urban areas, the growth of the population, 60 years of age and older, is outpacing total population growth in almost all of the world's regions (United Nations Population Fund and Help Age International, 2012). Population aging in rural areas is happening more rapidly (Cai et al., 2012) due to declining fertility rates, increasing life expectancy, and population migration (Berry & Kirschner, 2013; Glascow & Brown, 2012). In 2005, the proportion of the Chinese population 60 years of age and older was 13.7% in rural areas compared with 12.1% in urban areas (Cai et al., 2012). Similar trends are seen in the United States, where, in 2010, 15.5% of rural residents were 65 years of age and older and comprised more than 25% of all U.S. seniors (Housing Assistance Council, 2014).

The increased rural population aging increases the prevalence of chronic diseases and noncommunicable diseases in rural communities. Ischemic heart disease, stroke, and chronic lung disease are the greatest causes of mortality worldwide, although hearing and visual impairments, dementia, and osteoarthritis contribute to the largest burden of disability (United Nations Population Fund and Help Age International, 2012).

Race/Ethnicity

My mother has brown skin; she is from the Philippines. My father had white skin; he was from Czechoslovakia. I look racially ambiguous. I have personal experiences of overt racism, like the kids on the playground calling me racial slurs, and covert racism, like people openly asking me, "where are you really from?" When I responded that I was from Canada, some people assumed my mom was my nanny, others complimented me on my "great tan" in the middle of winter.

Danda, 2020

Racial/ethnic distributions vary in rural areas within and across countries. Low-income countries have more ethnic diversity, including in rural areas. Most notable is Uganda, which is ranked as the world's most ethnically diverse country (Alesina et al., 2003), with more than three-quarters of its population living in rural areas (Baker, 2001). In high-income countries, minorities tend to be underrepresented in rural areas when compared with urban areas. However, the share of racial and ethnic minorities in persistently poor rural counties is more than double the share in other rural counties (USDA ERS, 2021a). In the United States, in 153 rural persistent poverty counties located in the southeastern Coastal Plains, Blacks make up 43.3% of the population. In Texas, New Mexico, and Colorado, 63.1% of the population in the 39 rural

persistent poverty counties are Hispanics. American Indians make up 45.5% of residents in the 34 rural persistent poverty counties in Alaska, Arizona, Oklahoma, Utah, and the northern Great Plains.

Gender and Sexuality

For the women that are having children, we have a really good group ... but the older women don't get out to talk about issues like menopause and breast cancer.

Leipart & George, 2008, p. 214

The politics of the region, it makes it difficult ... for myself and friends of mine who are trans to find affirming care ... or going to medical providers that would be able to treat us in the way we needed to be treated without making it some sort of traumatizing experience.

Joudeh et al., 2021, p. 9

Gender and sexuality are also important determinants of health and well-being for individuals in rural areas. In this section, *gender* refers to a person's socially constructed identity—different from biological sex, though the two are often congruent; *gender minority* refers to an individual whose gender identity is different from their assigned gender or sex at birth and/or does not fall strictly into a gender binary; and *sexual minority* refers to an individual whose sexual orientation is not heterosexual (VandenBos & American Psychological Association, 2015). It is important to note that an individual's gender identity does not determine their sexuality, and vice versa.

Rural areas have higher rates of women, especially in rural communities with high rates of older adults, reflecting the greater life expectancies for women (Inter-Agency Task Force on Rural Women, 2012). Globally, rural women spend more time than urban women and men on reproductive and household work, obtaining water and fuel, caring for children and the sick, and processing food (Inter-Agency Task Force on Rural Women, 2012). In developing regions with large rural populations, about 1 in 3 to 1 in 10 married women had no control over spending on major purchases or their cash earnings (UN Statistics Division, 2017) and had limited employment opportunities (Inter-Agency Task Force on Rural Women, 2012).

Additionally, women in rural areas have limited obstetrics–gynecology (OB/GYN) services (Bennet et al., 2013) and unique problems with intimate partner violence (IPV). Although rural women experience IPV at similar rates as urban women (Breiding et al., 2009), rural IPV may be harder to report (Burholdt & Dobbs, 2012). In rural Canada, women attributed this to the dense social relationships common in rural communities. Rural health providers and police may have familial or other relationships with abusers and their families, presenting challenges to confidentiality in the reporting of abuse (Leipert & George, 2008). Fewer resources exist in rural areas for preventing IPV (Breiding et al., 2009).

Sexual and gender minority persons also face barriers to accessing quality, affirming care in both rural and urban areas; however, those challenges may be particularly pronounced in rural areas (Joudeh et al., 2021; Price-Feeney et al., 2019), leading to negative health outcomes (Joudeh et al., 2021). Harassment, abuse, and discrimination (White Hughto et al., 2015) can contribute to higher rates of increased anxiety, depression, and suicide among sexual and gender minorities youth in rural settings (Price-Feeney et al., 2019; Smith et al., 2018).

Access to Health Care

Not long ago we had … a baby, small for gestational age, and … we got two ambulances 5 minutes apart, and they were both cardiac with chest pain. While that was happening there was surgery going on, and there was somebody in the unit. I don't know if God is watching you or what, but for the most part, things seem to come out ok in the end.

Scharff, 2013, p. 253

Access to health care includes access to services and the quality of those services, both of which contribute to a person's health status (CDC, 2013). Compared with urban areas, health care providers, specialized services, and facilities are in shorter supply in rural areas (IOM, 2005), along with limited transport options, and medical resources (Strasser, 2003). Access to quality health care is the top concern of rural residents in the United States (Bolin et al., 2015) and rural people in Canada have expressed similar concerns (Government of Canada, 2022).

While nearly half of the world's population lives in rural areas, only 38% of the world's nurses and less than 25% of doctors work in rural areas (WHO, 2010). WHO has identified four areas for increasing recruitment and retention: education, financial incentives, regulations, and personal and professional support tailored to a specific country's circumstances (WHO, 2010). In Kenya and South Africa, better educational opportunities or rural allowances would be most effective in increasing nurses in rural areas, whereas in Thailand better health insurance coverage would have the greatest impact (Blaauw et al., 2010). Several U.S. rural nurse residency programs are in place (Bratt et al., 2014), but limited continuing education for rural nurses is a major concern (Baernholdt et al., 2010; Bushy, 2012).

Specialized services and facilities are sparse in rural areas. Two-thirds of Canadian residents in the northern and remote regions live more than 100 km from health

services (Browne, 2008), which have limited or no rehabilitation, palliative care, home care, counseling, respite, and long-term care (Ministerial Advisory Council on Rural Health, 2002). In the United States, the typical rural hospital offers outpatient surgical services and mammography but does not offer hospice, home health, chemotherapy and dental services, or outpatient drug/alcohol abuse care (Freeman et al., 2015). Increasing services without community input may not be beneficial. In rural Australia, services were provided because of available funding, bypassing community needs (Allan et al., 2007). Rural patients in Costa Rica and Panama traveled significant distances to urban hospitals where they felt they would get better care, whereas in Central America, small rural hospitals have been preferable to rural residents in Honduras (Leon, 2003). For some rural areas, access may be improved by partnering with urban hospitals and using telehealth technologies (Arora et al., 2011).

Rural hospital closings have created a rise in access problems. From 2010 to 2016, 76 U.S. rural hospitals closed, and more than 200 hospitals were on the brink of closure due to loss of market share, lower patient volumes, and decreases in reimbursements (IVantage Health Analytics, 2016). Moreover, hospital closures have a negative economic impact on rural communities since hospitals are not only majority employers but they also generate other economic spin-offs (Liuui et al., 2001).

IMPLICATIONS FOR NURSING PRACTICE

Nurses practicing in global rural areas must adopt the expert generalist role. Preparation necessitates broad-based education and clinical experience that are best achieved in rural nurse residency programs in which essential knowledge and skills can be attained within the local cultural context. However, nursing programs often lack content about rural nursing practice. A survey found that 55.7% of programs did not offer rural-specific content in their curricula, and only 5.5% offered a specific course in rural health (Rural Health Research Gateway, 2021).

Rural connectedness is an important aspect of rural living. To connect and integrate with the rural community, a nurse will likely face challenges related to confidentiality, trust, and various roles associated with being a community member, neighbor, and health care professional. In 2020, the CARRN introduced a framework for practice that is centered on knowing the community as an essential component of practice (CARRN, 2020). Experienced rural nurses advise nurses new to rural practice to know what they are getting into, consider whether their personal qualities are suited for rural practice, learn to listen and listen to learn, expect a steep learning curve, and take action to prevent burnout (Martin-Misener et al., 2008).

Rural nurses will be highly visible in their communities and thus will be well-positioned for leadership in rural health advocacy initiatives targeted at removing negative determinants of health. Although local circumstances dictate the rural nurse's activities, Healthy People 2030's five foundational health measures (health conditions, health behaviors, populations, settings and systems, and SDOH) provide an excellent start for examining rural communities' needs (U.S. Department of Health and Human Services [USDHHS], 2021). Evaluating community needs can be facilitated through a community needs assessment that engages both other professionals and community members. Valuing the input and priorities of community members and adopting an informed advocacy perspective helps nurses make an important contribution toward improving the health of people living in rural communities and can help tailor interventions to better meet their needs (MacKinnon & Moffat, 2014).

Nurses must also recognize the multilevel nature of structural determinants of health, including structural racism and historical colonial oppression, that not only impact the health and well-being, education, and economic opportunities of a community but may also impact trust with health care professionals. Understanding the history and context of the rural area in which one practices is a critical first step in building a decolonization approach to rural nursing practice in a community.

Another challenge for rural practicing nurses is building up their resources to support their practice and professional development. They must be adept at accessing Internet-based patient and professional development resources, including telehealth services, information for clinical decision support, and continuing education. Memberships in rural nursing and other organizations help network and form coalitions to address both local and global rural health issues. Nurses can also advocate and lobby for policy changes to address determinants of health, including policies around education, employment, and poverty.

SUMMARY

Practicing in global rural areas is a unique experience sought by many nurses (CARRN, 2020; Macleod et al., 2017). Whether for short-term or more permanent assignments, nurses have to prepare to practice in a rural area just as they would for any other specialty position. In addition to multiple clinical and cultural competencies, nurses need a deep understanding and appreciation for the complex interrelated SDOH in rural settings. Nonetheless, although rural areas may differ from country to country and even within a country, lessons learned in one country can be useful information for rural nurses in other countries.

SALIENT POINTS

- Global rural nursing practice is practiced in both local and international rural contexts.
- A global rural nurse is an expert generalist with a broad knowledge base and skill set that can be applied within rural contexts.
- Definitions of "rural" vary across the globe.
- The social determinants of health are the conditions in which people are born, grow, live, work, and age. In this chapter, rural culture, structural racism, physical environment, social support, economic factors, education, personal characteristics, and access to health care as social determinants of rural health were considered.
- Rural culture is a separate entity comprised of a set of beliefs and attributes differing from those generally held in urban settings.
- Structural or systemic racism against marginalized communities in rural areas can manifest through policies around housing, economic structures, and the environment that all have immediate or downstream effects on health outcomes for those rural populations.

- The effect of the rural physical environment as a single determinant of health is unclear, but statistically, rural populations have poorer health than urban dwellers.
- Lack of social support or social isolation is associated with poor health throughout the world. However, social connectedness is an important characteristic of rural communities that nurses practicing in rural regions need to embrace. Education and health literacy levels are lower in rural areas and associated with poor health.
- Personal characteristics such as age, race/ethnicity, gender, and sexuality affect health. Globally, rural populations are disproportionately older and female. Rural ethnic and racial distributions vary greatly worldwide.
- Limited communications, transport options, and medical resources are common barriers to health care access in rural regions worldwide.
- Professional isolation is an important barrier to the recruitment, retention, and competency of rural nurses.

CRITICAL REFLECTION EXERCISES

1. Discuss factors that influence a rural nurse's success in improving health in their community.
2. In what ways can the strengths of rural communities offset factors causing poorer health outcomes?
3. For nurses in rural and remote settings, discuss the advantages and disadvantages of online resources for clinical support and continuing education.
4. You have decided to participate in a humanitarian medical mission in a medically underserved region of rural El Salvador. You have all the necessary information concerning personal health and safety. What are some of the challenges you might encounter in providing health care in that setting? Discuss how you might prepare for clinical practice in that region.

Ⓔ WEBSITE RESOURCES

Canadian Association of Rural and Remote Nursing. https://www.carrn.com/

Canadian Rural Health Research Society. https://crhrs-scrsr.usask.ca

Canadian Rural Revitalization Foundation (2021). https://sorc.crrf.ca/

CMS Toolkit for Making Written Material Clear and Effective. https://www.cms.gov/Outreach-and-Education/Outreach/WrittenMaterialsToolkit/index.html?redirect=/WrittenMaterialsToolkit/

Global Health Council. https://www.globalhealth.org/

International Council of Nurses. https://www.icn.ch/

National Rural Health Association. https://www.ruralhealthweb.org

Office of Rural Health Policy. https://www.hrsa.gov/ruralhealth/

Our World in Data. https://ourworldindata.org/

Partners in Health. https://www.pih.org/

Rural Health Information Hub. https://www.ruralhealthinfo.org/

Rural Health Research Institute. https://www.gatewayresearch.ca/

Rural Nurse Organization. https://www.rno.org/

Things you can do to fight poverty. https://billmoyers.com/2013/05/12/twelve-things-you-can-do-to-fight-poverty-now/

United States Department of Agriculture. https://www.usda.gov/wps/portal/usda/usdahome

United States Department of Health and Human Services. https://www.globalhealth.gov/

World Health Organization. https://www.who.int/

REFERENCES

Agency for Healthcare Research and Quality. (2017). *AHRQ health literacy universal precautions toolkit.* https://www.ahrq.gov/health-literacy/improve/precautions/index.html

Agency for Healthcare Research and Quality. (2021, November). *2014 National healthcare quality and disparities report chartbook on rural health care.* Agency for Healthcare Research and Quality. AHRQ Pub. No. 22-0010. https://www.ahrq.gov/sites/default/files/wysiwyg/research/findings/nhqrdr/chartbooks/2019-qdr-rural-chartbook.pdf

Alesina, A. F., Devleeschauwer, A., Easterly, W., Kurlat, S., & Wacziarg, R. (2003). Fractionalization. *Journal of Economic Growth*, 8(2), 155–194. http://link.springer.com/article/10.1023%2FA%3A1024471506938#page-1

Allan, J., Ball, P., & Alston, M. (2007). Developing sustainable models of rural health care: A community development approach. *Rural and Remote Health*, 7(4), 818. http://www.rrh.org.au/articles/subviewnew.asp?ArticleID=818

Allan, B., & Smylie, J. (2015). *First peoples, second class treatment: The role of racism in the health and well-being of indigenous peoples in Canada, discussion paper.* Wellesley Institute. https://www.wellesleyinstitute.com/wp-content/uploads/2015/02/Summary-First-Peoples-Second-Class-Treatment-Final.pdf

Allen, L., Hatala, A., Ijaz, S., Courchene, E. D., & Bushie, E. B. (2020). Indigenous-led health care partnerships in Canada. *CMAJ: Canadian Medical Association Journal*, 192(9), E208–E216. https://doi.org/10.1503/cmaj.190728

Anderson, J. F., & Brodkin, P. (2013). *Sts'ailes primary health care project: Report.* Health Integration Project Planning Committee (HIPP), Centre for Addictions Research of BC. https://www.uvic.ca/research/centres/cisur/assets/docs/report-stsailes-primary-healthcare-project.pdf

Arora, S., Kalishman, S., Dion, D., Som, D., Thornton, K., Bankhurst, A., Boyle, J., Harkins, M., Moseley, K., Murata, G., Komaramy, M., Katzman, J., Colleran, K., Deming, P., & Yutzu, S. (2011). Partnering urban academic medical centers and rural primary care clinicians to provide complex chronic disease care. *Health Affairs*, 30(6), 1176–1184. https://doi.org/10.1377/hlthaff.2011.0278

Baernholdt, M. (2017). Rural health. In J. Fitzpatrick & M. W. Kazer (Eds.), *Encyclopedia of nursing research* (4th ed., pp. 454–457). Springer.

Baernholdt, M., Hinton, I., Yan, G., Rose, K., & Mattos, M. (2012). Factors associated with quality of life in older adults in the United States. *Quality of Life Research*, 21(3), 527. https://doi.org/10.1007/s11136-011-9954-z

Baernholdt, M., Jennings, B. M., Merwin, E., & Thornlow, D. (2010). What does quality care mean to nurses in rural hospitals? *Journal of Advanced Nursing, 66*(6), 1346–1355. https://doi.org/10.1111/j.1365-2648.2010.05290.x

Baker, W. G. (2001). *Uganda: The marginalization of minorities.* Minority Rights Group International. http://www.minorityrights.org/1042/reports/uganda-the-marginalization-of-minorities.html

Barry, J., & Hardiker, N. (2012). Advancing nursing practice through social media: A global perspective. *The Online Journal of Issues in Nursing, 17*(3), Manuscript 5. https://doi.org/10.3912/OJIN.Vol17No03Man05

Beckstead, D., Brown, W. M., Guo, Y., & Newbold, K. B. (2010). *Cities and growth: Earning levels across urban and rural areas: The role of human capital.* Statistics Canada. https://www150.statcan.gc.ca/n1/pub/11-622-m/11-622-m2010020-eng.pdf

Bennet, K., Lopes, Jr., J. E., Spencer K., & van Heck, S. (2013). *Rural women's health [Policy Brief].* https://www.ruralhealth.us/getattachment/Advocate/Policy-Documents/RuralWomensHealth-(1).pdf.aspx?lang=en-US

Berry, E. H., & Kirschner, A. (2013). Demography of rural aging. In N. Glascow & E. H. Berry (Eds.), *Rural aging in 21st century America: Understanding population trends and processes* Vol. 7, pp. 17–36. Springer. https://doi.org/10.1007/978-94-007-5567-3_2

Blaauw, D., Erasmus, E., Pagaiya, N., Tangcharoensathien, V., Mullei, K., Mudhune, S., & Lagarde, M. (2010). Policy interventions that attract nurses to rural areas: A multicountry discrete choice experiment. *Bulletin of the World Health Organization, 88*(5), 350–356. https://doi.org/10.2471/BLT.09.072918

Bolin, J. N., Bellamy, G. R., Ferdinand, A. O., Vuong, A. M., Kash, B. A., Schulze, A., & Helduser, J. W. (2015). Rural Healthy People 2020: New decade, same challenges. *The Journal of Rural Health, 31*, 326–333. https://doi.org/10.1111/jrh.12116

Bratt, M. M., Baernholdt, M., & Pruszynski, J. (2014). Are rural and urban newly licensed nurses different? Results from a nurse residency program. *Journal of Nursing Management, 22*(6), 779–791. https://doi.org/10.1111/j.1365-2834.2012.01483.x

Breiding, M. J., Ziembroski, J. S., & Black, M. C. (2009). Prevalence of rural intimate partner violence in 16 US states, 2005. *Journal of Rural Health, 25*(3), 240–245. https://doi.org/10.1111/j.1748-0361.2009.00225.x

Brooks, K. D., Eley, D. S., Pratt, R., & Zink, T. (2012). Management of professional boundaries in rural practice. *Academic Medicine, 87*(8), 1091–1095. https://journals.lww.com/academicmedicine/Fulltext/2012/08000/Management_of_Professional_Boundaries_in_Rural.24.aspx

Brown, J., & Weber, J. (2013). *The off-farm occupations of U.S. farm operators and their spouses.* https://www.ers.usda.gov/webdocs/publications/43789/40009_eib-117.pdf

Browne, A. (2008). *Issues affecting access to health services in northern, rural and remote regions of Canada.* University of Northern British Columbia, Prince George. Northern Articles Series. https://www2.unbc.ca/sites/default/files/sections/northern-studies/issuesaffectingaccesstohealthservicesinnorthern.pdf

Burholdt, V., & Dobbs, C. (2012). Research on rural ageing: Where have we got to go and where are we going in Europe? *Journal of Rural Studies, 28*, 432–446. https://doi.org/10.1016/j.jrurstud.2012.01.009

Buys, L., Roberto, K. A., Miller, E., & Blieszner, R. (2009). Prevalence and predictors of depressive symptoms among rural older Australians and Americans. *International Journal of Geriatric Psychiatry, 24*(11), 1226–1236. https://doi.org/10.1111/j.1440-1584.2007.00948.x

Cai, F., Giles, J., O'Keefe, P., & Wang, D. (2012). *The elderly and old age support in rural China: Challenges and prospects. (No. 67522).* World Bank. https://doi.org/10.1596/978-0-8213-8685-9

Canada Council on Learning. (2006). *The rural-urban gap in education.* http://en.copian.ca/library/research/ccl/rural_urban_gap_ed/rural_urban_gap_ed.pdf

Canadian Association for Rural and Remote Nursing. (2020). *Knowing the rural community: A framework for nursing practice in rural and remote Canada.* CARRN. https://www.carrn.com/images/pdf/CARRN_RR_framework_doc_final_LR-2_1.pdf

Canadian Institute for Health Information. (2009). *Health care in Canada 2009: A decade in review.* https://secure.cihi.ca/free_products/Healthindicators2009_en.pdf

Canadian Rural Revitalization Foundation. (2021). *State of rural Canada 2021: Opportunities, recovery, and resiliency in changing times.* https://sorc.crrf.ca/fullreport2021/

Centers for Disease Control. (2013). *Social determinants of health [FAQs].* http://www.cdc.gov/socialdeterminants/FAQ.html

Clausen, T., Wilson, A. O., Molebatsi, R. M., & Holmboe-Ottesen, G. (2007). Diminished mental- and physical function and lack of social support are associated with shorter survival in community dwelling older persons of Botswana. *BMC Public Health, 7*(1), 144. https://doi.org/10.1186/1471-2458-7-144

Coburn, A. F., MacKinney, A. C., McBride, T. D., Mueller, K. J., Slifkin, R. T., & Wakefield, M. K. (2007). *Choosing rural definitions: Implications for health policy* [Issue Brief No. 2]. Rural Policy Research Institute. https://digitalcommons.usm.maine.edu/insurance/60/

Coovadia, H., Jewkes, R., Barron, P., Sanders, D., & McIntyre, D. (2009). The health and health system of South Africa: Historical roots of current public health challenges. *The Lancet, 374*(9692), 817–834. https://doi.org/10.1016/S0140-6736(09)60951-X

County Health Rankings and Roadmap. (2016). *What works? Strategies to improve rural health.* https://www.county-healthrankings.org/sites/default/files/media/document/key_measures_report/CHRR_WhatWorks_RuralReport.pdf

Coyne, C. A., Demian-Popescu, C., & Friend, D. (2006). Social and cultural factors influencing health in southern West Virginia: A qualitative study. *Preventing Chronic Disease, 3*(4), A124. https://www.ncbi.nlm.nih.gov/pmc/articles/PMC1779288/pdf/PCD34A124.pdf

Curtin, S. C., & Spencer, M. R. (2021). *Trends in death rates in urban and rural areas: United States, 1999–2019* [NCHS Data

Brief, No. 417]. National Center for Health Statistics. https://stacks.cdc.gov/view/cdc/109049

Cutler, D. M., & Lleras-Muney, A. (2006, July). *Education and health: Evaluating theories and evidence* [Working Paper No. 12352]. https://www.nber.org/system/files/working_papers/w12352/w12352.pdf

Danda, M. (2020, August 23). *Where are you really from? Why nurses must confront the racism in health care.* Canadian Nurse: Opinion. https://www.canadian-nurse.com/blogs/cn-content/2020/08/13/where-are-you-really-from-why-nurses-must-confront

Del Brutto, O. H., Tettamanti, D., Del Brutto, V. J., Zambrano, M., & Montalvan, M. (2013). Living alone and cardiovascular health status in residents of a rural village of coastal Ecuador (the Atahualpa Project). *Environmental Health & Preventive Medicine*, 18(5), 422–425. https://doi.org/10.1007/s12199-013-0344-8

Farmer, J., Clark, A., & Munoz, S. (2010). Is a global rural and remote health research agenda desirable or is context supreme? *The Australian Journal of Rural Health*, 18(3), 96–101. https://doi.org/10.1111/j.1440-1584.2010.01140.x

Federal Communications Commission. (2020, June). *2020 Broadband Progress Report.* https://www.fcc.gov/reports-research/reports/broadband-progress-reports/2020-broadband-deployment-report

Flanagan, E. (2015, April). *Crafting an effective Canadian energy strategy.* Pembina Institute. http://www.pembina.org/pub/crafting-an-effective-canadian-energy-strategy

Fox, S. (2011). *Peer-to-peer healthcare: Many people—especially those living with chronic or rare diseases—use online connections to supplement professional medical advice.* Pew Research Center's Internet & American Life Project. https://www.pewresearch.org/internet/wp-content/uploads/sites/9/media/Files/Reports/2011/Pew_P2PHealthcare_2011.pdf

Freeman, V. A., Thompson, K., Howard, H. A., Randolph, R., & Holmes, G. M. (2015, March). *The 21st century rural hospital: A chartbook.* http://www.shepscenter.unc.edu/wp-content/uploads/2015/02/21stCenturyRuralHospitalsChartBook.pdf

Garnett, M. F., Spencer, M. R., & Hedegaard, H. (2021). *Urban-rural differences in unintentional injury death rates among children aged 0–17 years: United States, 2018–2019* [NCHS Data Brief, No. 421]. National Center for Health Statistics. https://www.cdc.gov/nchs/data/databriefs/db421.pdf

Glascow, N., & Brown, D. L. (2012). Rural ageing in the United States: Trends and contexts. *Journal of Rural Studies*, 28(4), 422–431. https://doi.org/10.1016/j.jrurstud.2012.01.002

Government of Canada. (2022, June 14). *Social determinants of health and health inequalities.* Accessed January 14, 2023. https://www.canada.ca/en/public-health/services/health-promotion/population-health/what-determines-health.html

Halseth, G., & Ryseth, L. (2010). *A primer for understanding issues around rural poverty.* University of Northern British Columbia, The Community Development Institute at UNBC. https://www2.unbc.ca/sites/default/files/sections/community-development-institute/a_primer_for_understanding_issues_around_rural_poverty.pdf

Hofstede, G. (2001). *Culture's consequences* (2nd ed.). Sage.

Housing Assistance Council. (2014). *Housing an aging rural America: Rural seniors and their homes.* https://ruralhome.org/wp-content/uploads/storage/documents/publications/rrreports/ruralseniors2014.pdf

Hswen, Y., Qin, Q., Williams, D. R., Viswanath, K., Brownstein, J. S., & Subramanian, S. V. (2020, October). The relationship between Jim Crow laws and social capital from 1997–2014: A 3-level multilevel hierarchical analysis across time, county and state. *Social Science of Medicine*, 262, 113142. https://doi.org/10.1016/j.socscimed.2020.113142

Institute of Medicine. (2004). *Health literacy: A prescription to end confusion.* National Academies Press. https://doi.org/10.17226/10883

Institute of Medicine. (2005). *Quality through collaboration. The future of rural health.* National Academies Press. https://doi.org/10.17226/11140

Inter-Agency Task Force on Rural Women. (2012). *Facts & figures: Rural women and the millennium development goals.* http://www.un.org/womenwatch/feature/ruralwomen/facts-figures.html

International Fund for Agricultural Development. (2011). *Rural poverty report.* https://www.ifad.org/documents/38714170/39315751/annual+report+2011+english.pdf/397a0cf9-e4e1-49cc-9fee-3449e56f2d61?t=1505483114000

Inuit Tapiriit Kanatami. (2007, May). *Alianait Inuit Mental Wellness Action Plan* [Report]. https://www.itk.ca/wp-content/uploads/2009/12/Alianait-Inuit-Mental-Wellness-Action-Plan-2009.pdf

IVantage Health Analytics. (2016). *What's the state of rural healthcare in America in 2016?* https://cdn2.hubspot.net/hubfs/333498/2016_INDEX_Rural_Relevance/INDEX_2016_Rural_Relevance_Study_FINAL_Formatted_02_01_16.pdf?__hssc=31316192.1.1454600056802&__hstc=31316192.3bbce70cf2ffd8de05aebc94589dc17e.1454600056802.1454600056802.1454600056802.1&__hsfp=&hsCtaTracking=518d16d3-8af6-40cb-85a9-6802175ad7d0%7C38fb6460-e237-4dbd-b7e6-94ec137b5f45

Jones, C. P. (2000, October 10). Levels of racism: A theoretic framework and a gardener's tale. *American Journal of Public Health*, 90(8), 1212–1215. https://doi.org/10.2105/AJPH.90.8.1212

Jones, D. S. (2006, December). The persistence of American Indian health disparities. *American Journal of Public Health*, 96(12), 2122–2134. https://doi.org/10.2105/AJPH.2004.054262

Jones, D., Lyle, D., McAllister, L., Randall, S., Dyson, R., White, D., Smith, A., Hampton, D., Goldsworthy, M., & Rowe, A. (2020). The case for integrated health and community literacy to achieve transformational community engagement and improved health outcomes: An inclusive approach to addressing rural and remote health inequities and community healthcare expectations. *Primary Health Care Research & Development*, 21, e57. https://doi.org/10.1017/S1463423620000481

Joudeh, L., Harris, O. O., Johnstone, E., Heavner-Sullivan, S., & Propst, S. K. (2021, July–August). "Little Red Flags": Barriers to accessing health care as a sexual or gender minority individual in the rural Southern United States—a qualitative intersectional approach. *Journal of the Association of Nurses in AIDS Care*, 32(4), 467–480. https://europepmc.org/backend/ptpmcrender.fcgi?accid=PMC8238829&blobtype=pdf

Kanj, M., & Mitic, W. (2009). *Health literacy and health promotion*. World Health Organization. https://www.dors.it/documentazione/testo/201409/02_2009_OMS%20Nairobi_Health%20Literacy.pdf

Keating, N., Swindle, J., & Fletcher, S. (2011). Aging in rural Canada: A retrospective and review. *Canadian Journal on Aging*, 30(3), 323–338. http://dx.doi.org/10.1017/S0714980811000250

Kimura, Y., Wada, T., Okumiya, K., Ishimoto, Y., Fukutomi, E., Kasahara, Y., & Matsubayashi, K. (2012). Eating alone among community-dwelling Japanese elderly: Association with depression and food diversity. *Journal of Nutrition, Health & Aging*, 16(8), 728–731. https://doi.org/10.1007/s12603-012-0067-3

Landrine, H., Corral, I., Lee, J., Efird, J. T., Hall, M. B., & Bess, J. J. (2017). Residential segregation and racial cancer disparities: A systematic review. *Journal of Racial and Ethnic Health Disparities*, 4(6), 1195–1205. https://doi.org/10.1007/s40615-016-0326-9

Lee, S., Tsai, Y., & Ku, K. N. (2010). Health literacy, health status, and healthcare utilization of Taiwanese adults: Results from a national survey. *BMC Public Health*, 10, 614. https://doi.org/10.1186/1471-2458-10-614

Leipert, B. D., & George, J. A. (2008). Determinants of rural women's health: A qualitative study in southwest Ontario. *Journal of Rural Health*, 24(2), 210–218. https://doi.org/10.1111/j.1748-0361.2008.00160.x

Leon, M. (2003). Perceptions of health care quality in Central America. *International Journal in Health Care*, 15(1), 67–71. https://doi.org/10.1093/intqhc/15.1.67

Liu, L., Hader, J., Brossart, B., & White, R. (2001). Impact of rural hospital closures in Saskatchewan, Canada. *Social Science & Medicine*, 52(12), 1793–1804. https://doi.org/10.1016/s0277-9536(00)00298-7

Logan, T. D., & Parman, J. M. (2018). Segregation and mortality over time and space. *Social Science & Medicine*, 199, 77–86. https://doi.org/10.1016/j.socscimed.2017.07.006

MacKinnon, K., & Moffat, P. (2014). Informed advocacy: Rural, remote and northern nursing praxis. *Advances in Nursing Science*, 37(2), 161–173. https://doi.org/10.1097/ANS.0000000000000025

MacLeod, L. P. M., Stewart, J. N., Kulig, J. C., Anguish, P., Andrews, M. E., Banner, D., Garraway, L., Hanlon, N., Karunanayake, C., Kilpatrick, K., Koren, I., Kosteniuk, J., Martin-Misener, R., Mix, N., Moffitt, P., Olynick, J., Penz, K., Sluggett, L., Van Pelt, L., & Zimmer, L. (2017). Nurses who work in rural and remote communities in Canada: A national survey. *Human Resources for Health*, 15(34). https://doi.org/10.1186/s12960-017-0209-0

Mahler, D. G., Yonzan, N., Lakner, C., Aguilar, A., & Wu, H. (2021). *Updated estimates of the impact of COVID-19 on global poverty: Turning the corner on the pandemic in 2021?* [Data Blog]. World Bank. https://blogs.worldbank.org/opendata/updated-estimates-impact-covid-19-global-poverty-turning-corner-pandemic-2021

Martin-Misener, R., MacLeod, M. L. P., Vogt, C., Morton, M., Banks, C., & Bentham, D. (2008). "There's rural and then there's rural": Advice from nurses providing primary health care in rural communities. *Nursing Leadership*, 21(3), 54–63. https://doi.org/10.12927/cjnl.2008.20062

Mechakra-Tahiri, S., Zunzunegui, M. V., Preville, M., & Dube, M. (2009). Social relationships and depression among people 65 years and over living in rural and urban areas of Quebec. *International Journal of Geriatric Psychiatry*, 24(11), 1226–1236. https://doi.org/10.1002/gps.2250

Ministerial Advisory Council on Rural Health. (2002). *Rural health in rural hands: Strategic directions for rural, remote, northern and aboriginal communities*. Health Canada. https://publications.gc.ca/collections/Collection/H39-657-2002E.pdf

Narayan, D., Patel, R., Schafft, K., Rademacher, A., & Koch-Schulte, S. (2000). The definitions of poverty. In: *Can anyone hear us? Voices from 47 countries*. Oxford University Press.

National Institute for Occupational Safety and Health. (2022, September 21). *Agricultural safety*. https://www.cdc.gov/niosh/topics/aginjury/default.html

Neely, A. H., & Ponshunmugam, A. (2019). A qualitative approach to examining health care access in rural South Africa. *Social Science & Medicine*, 230, 214–221. https://doi.org/10.1016/j.socscimed.2019.04.025

Our World in Data. (n.d.). *Urban and Rural Population projected to 2050, World, 1500 to 2050*. https://ourworldindata.org/grapher/urban-and-rural-population-2050?country=~OWID_WRL

Pantell, M., Rehkopf, D., Jutte, D., Syme, S. L., Balmes, J., & Adler, N. (2013). Social isolation: A predictor of mortality comparable to traditional clinical risk factors. *American Journal of Public Health*, 103(11), 2056–2062. https://doi.org/10.2105/AJPH.2013.301261

Price-Feeney, M., Ybarra, M. L., & Mitchell, K. J. (2019). Health indicators of lesbian, gay, bisexual, and other sexual minority (LGB+) youth living in rural communities. *The Journal of Pediatrics*, 205, 236–243. https://doi.org/10.1016/j.jpeds.2018.09.059

Ravi, S., & Joseph, B. (2019). Incidence of occupational injuries among adults residing in a selected rural area of India: A cross sectional study. *Pakistan Journal of Medical Sciences*, 35(3), 737–742. https://doi.org/10.12669/pjms.35.3.293

Rural Health Research Gateway. (2021). *Rural nursing workforce*. https://www.ruralhealthresearch.org/assets/4556-20071/rural-nursing-workforce-recap.pdf

Scharff, J. E. (2013). The distinctive nature and scope of rural nursing practice: Philosophical bases. In C. A. Winters (Ed.), *Rural nursing: Concepts, theory, and practice* (4th ed., pp. 241–258). Springer.

Smith, A. J., Hallum-Montes, R., Nevin, K., Zenker, R., Sutherland, B., Reagor, S., Ortiz, M. E., Woods, C., Frost, M., Cochran, B., Oost, K., Gleason, H., & Brennan, J. M. (2018). Determinants of transgender individuals' well-being, mental health, and suicidality in a rural state. *Rural Mental Health*, 42(2), 116–132. https://doi.org/10.1037/rmh0000089

Smith, K. B., Humphreys, J. S., & Wilson, M. G. A. (2008). Addressing the health disadvantage of rural populations: How does epidemiological evidence inform rural health policies and research? *The Australian Journal of Rural Health*, *16*(2), 56–66. https://doi.org/10.1111/j.1440-1584.2008.00953.x

Statistics Canada. (2012, July). *Mortality rates among children and teenagers living in Inuit Nunavut* [Report No. 82-003-X]. https://www150.statcan.gc.ca/n1/en/pub/82-003-x/2012003/article/11695-eng.pdf?st=MpuQnaSx

Statistics Canada. (2016). *2016 Census Dictionary*. Statistics Canada [Database]. http://www12.statcan.gc.ca/census-recensement/2016/ref/98-304/index-eng.cfm

Statistics Canada. (2020). *2016 Census Aboriginal community portraits*. Statistics Canada [Database]. https://www150.statcan.gc.ca/n1/en/catalogue/41260001

Statistics Canada. (2022). *Covid-19 data trends*. [Database]. https://www.canada.ca/en/public-health/services/diseases/coronavirus-disease-covid-19/epidemiological-economic-research-data.html

Stern, M. J., Adams, A. E., & Boase, J. (2011). Rural community participation, social networks, and broadband use: Examples from localized and national survey data [Adobe file]. *Agricultural and Resource Economics Review*, *40*(2), 158–171. http://ageconsearch.umn.edu/bitstream/117769/2/ARER%2040-2%20pp%20158-171%20Stern%20Adams%20Boase.pdf

Strasser, R. (2003). Rural health around the world: Challenges and solutions. *Family Practice*, *20*(4), 457–463. https://doi.org/10.1093/fampra/cmg422

Terrill, L., & Gullifer, J. (2010). Growing older: A qualitative inquiry into the textured narratives of older. https://doi.org/10.1177%2F1359105310368180

Truth and Reconciliation Commission of Canada. (2015). *Honouring the truth, reconciling for the future: Summary of the final report of the Truth and Reconciliation Commission of Canada*. National Centre for Truth and Reconciliation. https://ehprnh2mwo3.exactdn.com/wp-content/uploads/2021/01/Executive_Summary_English_Web.pdf

Ullrich, F., & Muller, K. (2022). *COVID-19 cases and deaths, metropolitan and nonmetropolitan counties over time (update)*. RUPRI Center for Rural Health Policy Analysis [Rural Data Brief]. https://rupri.public-health.uiowa.edu/publications/policybriefs/2020/COVID%20Longitudinal%20Data.pdf

United Nations. (2015, October 21). *Transforming our world: the 2030 agenda for sustainable development*. https://sdgs.un.org/2030agenda

United Nations Educational, Scientific, and Cultural Organization. (2013, September). *Adult and youth literacy: UIS fact sheet (No. 26)*. UNESCO Institute for Statistics. http://uis.unesco.org/sites/default/files/documents/fs26-adult-and-youth-literacy-2013-en_1.pdf

United Nations Educational, Scientific and Cultural Organization. (2017a, September). *Literacy rates continue to rise from one generation to the next*. Fact sheet No. 45. http://uis.unesco.org/sites/default/files/documents/fs45-literacy-rates-continue-rise-generation-to-next-en-2017.pdf

United Nations Educational, Scientific and Cultural Organization. (2017b, September). *More than one-half of children and adolescents are not learning worldwide*. Fact sheet No. 46. http://uis.unesco.org/sites/default/files/documents/fs46-more-than-half-children-not-learning-en-2017.pdf

United Nations Population Fund and Help Age International. (2012). *Ageing in the twenty-first century*.

United Nations Statistics Division Demographic and Social Statistics. (2017). *Population density and urbanization*. https://unstats.un.org/unsd/demographic/sconcerns/densurb/densurbmethods.htm

U.S. Census Bureau. (2017, August 9). *What is rural America?* https://www.census.gov/library/stories/2017/08/rural-america.html

U.S. Department of Agriculture, Economic Research Service. (2016, January). *Rural America at a glance, 2015 Edition*. https://www.ers.usda.gov/webdocs/publications/44015/55581_eib145.pdf

U.S. Department of Agriculture, Economic Research Service. (2021a, November). *Rural America at a glance*. 2021 Edition EIB-230. USDA, Economic Research Service. https://www.ers.usda.gov/webdocs/publications/102576/eib-230.pdf?v=2220.6

U.S. Department of Agriculture, Economic Research Service. (2021b). *Rural poverty and well-being*. https://www.ers.usda.gov/topics/rural-economy-population/rural-poverty-well-being/

U.S. Department of Health and Human Services. (2021). *Healthy people 2030: Building a healthier future for all*. https://health.gov/healthypeople

VandenBos, G. R., & American Psychological Association. (2015). *APA dictionary of psychology* (2nd ed.). American Psychological Association.

White Hughto, J. M., Reisner, S. L., & Pachankis, J. E. (2015). Transgender stigma and health: A critical review of stigma determinants, mechanisms, and interventions. *Social Science & Medicine (1982)*, *147*, 222–231. https://doi.org/10.1016/j.socscimed.2015.11.010

Williams, M. A. (2012). Rural professional isolation: An integrative review. *Journal of Rural Nursing and Health Care*, *12*(2). https://doi.org/10.14574/OJRNHC.V12I2.51

World Bank. (2020a). *Rural Population (% of total population)*. https://data.worldbank.org/indicator/SP.RUR.TOTL.ZS

World Bank. (2020b). *Literacy rate, adult total (% of people ages 15 and above)*. https://data.worldbank.org/indicator/SE.ADT.LITR.ZS

World Bank. (2022a). *Connecting for inclusion: Broadband access for all*. https://www.worldbank.org/en/topic/digitaldevelopment/brief/connecting-for-inclusion-broadband-access-for-all

World Bank. (2022b). *Poverty & equity data portal* [Database]. https://povertydata.worldbank.org/poverty/home/

World Health Organization. (2010). *Increasing access to health workers in remote and rural areas through improved retention*. Global policy recommendations. https://www.who.int/publications/i/item/increasing-access-to-health-workers-in-remote-and-rural-areas-through-improved-retention

World Health Organization. (2020). *State of the world's nursing 2020: Investing in education, jobs and leadership*. World Health Organization. https://www.who.int/publications/i/item/9789240003279

World Health Organization. (2022). *Social determinants of health*. https://www.who.int/health-topics/social-determinants-of-health#tab=tab_1

World Population Review. (2021). *Most rural states 2021*. https://worldpopulationreview.com/state-rankings/most-rural-states

Zahnd, W. E., Scaife, S. L., & Francis, M. L. (2009). Health literacy skills in rural and urban populations. *American Journal of Health Behavior*, 33(5), 550–557. https://doi.org/10.5993/AJHB.33.5.8

18

Trauma-Informed Care

Susan Elizabeth Harrell, DNP, RN, PMHNP-BC and
Karen J. Saewert, PhD, RN, CPHQ, ANEF

 http://evolve.elsevier.com/Friberg/bridge/

OBJECTIVES

At the completion of this chapter, the reader will be able to:

1. Differentiate trauma, trauma-informed care, and trauma-specific services.
2. Identify etiology and manifestations related to trauma.
3. Discuss trauma-informed care assumptions, concepts, and principles.
4. Identify trauma-informed care practices.
5. Make connections between adverse childhood experiences, social determinants of health, and health and health care disparities.
6. Describe an awareness of social and political activism to prevent and reduce the manifestations of trauma across the lifespan.

INTRODUCTION

Acquiring practice competencies (knowledge, skills, and attitudes/values) needed to recognize trauma and its effects—physically, emotionally, and behaviorally—enables nurses and other health care providers to respond with a strengths-based *trauma-informed care* (TIC) approach, not only for those they serve but also for self-preservation.

TRAUMA

The Substance Abuse and Mental Health Services Administration (SAMHSA) is the agency within the U.S. Department of Health and Human Services (DHHS) that leads national public health efforts to advance behavioral health, including the identification of trauma and subsequent best care practices. SAMHSA (2022, para. 2) describes *individual trauma* as resulting from: "an event, series of events, or set of circumstances that is experienced by an individual as physically or emotionally harmful or life-threatening." Trauma can occur as a result of violence, abuse, neglect, loss, disaster, war, and emotionally harmful experiences

(SAMHSA, 2014a) and can have "lasting adverse effects on the individual's functioning and mental, physical, social, emotional, or spiritual well-being" (SAMHSA, 2014a, p. 1). Further, trauma is widespread, costly, and can be experienced by individuals no matter their "age, gender, socioeconomic status, race, ethnicity, geography, and sexual orientation diversity" and is an "almost universal experience of people with mental and substance disorders" (SAMHSA, 2014b, p. 1).

The experience of trauma also impacts health care providers who care for those who are traumatized. *Secondary trauma* is defined as "the emotional duress that results when an individual hears about the firsthand trauma experiences of another" (National Child Traumatic Stress Network [NCTSN], n.d.-a, para. 1). Secondary trauma contributes to *burnout* or compassion fatigue, and is now understood to be an occupational consequence, not an individual problem, for nurses, especially those at risk (Kelly, 2020).

The COVID-19 pandemic and its associated health, social, and economic challenges; the national conversation on racial inequality, systemic racism, and injustice; and the increase in children arriving unaccompanied at the border have created a heightened need for attention to the adversities faced by children, youth, families, and communities (SAMHSA, n.d., para. 4).

COVID-19 brought national attention to the increase in the burnout that nurses and other health care professionals are experiencing caring for individuals, even before the recent pandemic crises (Hospital IQ, 2021).

A paradigm shift in care delivery strategies is needed for children, families, communities, and those that care for them. This includes clinical-level and system-level stress reduction and resilience building solutions that address root causes and must be used (Kelly, 2020). Understanding trauma's attributes is critical in building an effective health service delivery system. An effective health care system will:

- require a multipronged, multiagency public health approach;
- include public education and awareness;
- incorporate prevention and early identification; and
- offer effective trauma-specific assessment and treatment (SAMHSA, 2014a).

Etiology and Manifestations

Stress, a layman's term, refers to the body's response to harmful or threatening events or situations. Hormones produced in reaction to normal stressors systematically affect almost every tissue and organ. Edley and Morsey (2019) emphasized that while small amounts of periodic stress can enhance performance due to hyperarousal (fight or flight response), threatening situations that occur too often, too intensely, or in the absence of protective factors produce harmful hormonal changes. These toxic changes affect brain development, immune and hormonal systems, and gene expression. In turn, behavior, cognitive ability, and emotional and/or physical health are negatively impacted.

A quick Google search for trauma synonyms produces a powerful list of descriptors that includes: torment, agony, suffering, anguish, misery, distress, heartbreak, wretchedness, hell, purgatory, and excruciation. Trauma was once considered infrequent and characterized as an abnormal military experience (World War I, *shell shock*; World War II, *battle fatigue*) associated with either the individual's inability to recover or moral fault. This led to classifying trauma-related symptoms as *neuroses* best identified and treated by mental health specialists (SAMHSA, 2014a).

However, trauma is not uncommon and is consistently reported. Six of every ten men (60%) and five of every ten women (50%) experience at least one trauma in their lives (U.S. Department of Veterans Affairs, 2022). Of those reporting trauma, one in four (25%) cite exposure to multiple traumatic events, and individuals exposed to repeated trauma, on average, experience a 20-year decrease in longevity if they do not receive treatment (SAMHSA, 2020).

Given the depth of pain associated with trauma, it seems naïve to have once thought of trauma only as a mental affliction. The link between trauma, mental health, and physical health was explicitly made in the Felitti et al. (1998) classic study on adverse childhood experiences (ACEs). In this classic study, researchers mailed a questionnaire about ACEs to 13,494 adults who received a standardized medical evaluation at a large HMO; over 70% responded. The questionnaire asked about childhood experiences in seven categories: psychological or physical or sexual abuse; violence against mother; or living with household members who were substance abusers, mentally ill or suicidal, or ever imprisoned. These categories were then compared to adult risk behaviors, health status, and disease. Over one-half of the participants reported experiencing at least one category of childhood exposure.

Researchers reported that respondents who experienced four or more categories of childhood exposure, compared to those who reported no exposures, had a:

- 4- to 12-fold increase in health risks for alcoholism, drug abuse, depression, and suicide attempt;
- 2- to 4-fold increase in smoking, poor self-rated health, 50 or more sexual intercourse partners, and sexually transmitted disease; and
- 1.4- to 1.6-fold increase in physical inactivity and severe obesity.

The seven categories of ACEs were strongly interrelated, and persons with multiple categories of childhood exposure were likely to have multiple health risk factors (comorbidities or multimorbidities) later in life, including ischemic heart disease, cancer, chronic lung disease, skeletal fractures, and liver disease (Felitti et al., 1998).

Complex Trauma

"*Complex trauma* can arise in any situation where one feels an ongoing sense of fear, horror, helplessness, or powerlessness over time, with the perceived or actual inability to escape" (Lebow, 2021, para. 1) stemming from trauma experienced in childhood (although it can also develop from trauma experienced in adulthood). The emotional and physical dysregulation and loss of safety, direction, and the inability to detect or respond to danger cues appropriately leads to future trauma exposure later in life (NCTSN, n.d.-b, 2022). Trauma-related symptoms and behaviors originate from the adaptation to these traumatic experiences as survival mechanisms (SAMHSA, 2014a).

In addition to later life comorbidities, children with complex trauma often have difficulty forming attachments, controlling and expressing emotion, and may struggle with authority figures, romantic relationships, and developing friendships throughout their life. Physically, children with complex trauma may have increased somatic complaints, hypersensitivity to sounds, smells, or physical touch, or be unaware of pain, touch, and injuries. Emotionally, children with complex trauma may dissociate from their surroundings and lose memories. Children who use dissociation as a protective mechanism have difficulty with learning and social behavior (e.g., problems with attention, judgment, reasoning, and goal setting). Traumatized children often do not view the world as a safe place or one in which they can succeed and, therefore, dreaming of the future is considered futile. Learned helplessness, caused by the inability to control or improve one's circumstances, leads to a loss of productivity. The cumulative economic and social burden of complex trauma is significant. The NCTSN estimates these costs at $103.8 billion annually ($294.3 million per day). The average lifetime cost per survivor of child abuse is estimated at $210,012 and includes costs related to health care across their lifetime (NCTSN, n.d.-c).

Children can be protected, or the effects of toxic stress diminished, by their psychosocial context. "Protective factors are conditions or attributes that, when present in families and communities, increase the well-being of children and families" (Children's Bureau, n.d., para. 2). Protective factors include relationship bonds and social connections for both children and parents, understanding of child development, and the capacity for both parental and child resilience.

On the other hand, children's experiences of trauma can be worsened or complicated due to community and/or environmental factors. Safe, nurturing neighborhoods and/or communities, family and/or other adult role models, and school environments allow for the development of resilience. Social influences, when positive, help children constructively manage emotions and develop positive coping skills and other adaptive measures such as effective self-regulation and resiliency (Centers for Disease Control and Prevention [CDC], Risk and Protective Factors, 2022).

Resilience: Beyond Victim and Survivor

Resiliency is the ability to bounce back or rise above adversity as an individual, family, community, or provider by using available resources to negotiate hardship and/or the consequences of adverse events (SAMHSA, 2014a). Resilience (mental, emotional, and behavioral flexibility and adjustment to external and internal demands) depends on how individuals view and engage with the world, coping skills and strategies, and the availability and quality of social resources. "Psychological research demonstrates that the resources and skills associated with more positive

adaptation (i.e., greater resilience) can be cultivated and practiced" (American Psychological Association [APA], 2020, para. 1).

Additionally, health care organizations can support nurses and other health care providers by encouraging and managing health care team function. High-performing health care teams have been shown to share mental models of how care will be delivered, believe they collectively make a difference, recognize all members of the health care delivery team's effort (even those not on the front lines), monitor their team performance, work to develop a sense of psychological safety, proactively attend to the team member's family situation and support the supporters of the team (Tannenbaum et al., 2021). High-performing health care teams also support individual team member resilience through the development of team coping skills, the shared view of the health care delivery environment, and readily available social support and resources.

MAKING CONNECTIONS

Social determinants of health are the "conditions in the places where people live, learn, work, and play that affect a wide range of health and quality-of-life risks and outcomes" (CDC, 2021, para. 1). Combined with individual toxic stress and subsequent complex trauma, they magnify poor health outcomes at the micro-, meso- and macro-levels. Increasing data on the health of communities determined by zip code (i.e., where people live, learn, work, and play) have shed light on the connections between individual and environmental factors that create and perpetuate trauma and trauma sequelae. Individuals (micro-level), families and communities (meso-level), and geographical areas (macro-level) that lack environmental protective factors experience greater disease burdens. Trauma, viewed through an environmental lens, can explain generational trauma and violence. Community and population subgroups exposed to generational neglect, discrimination, and trauma give context to health disparities. Health disparities, the preventable differences in the burden of disease, injury, violence, or opportunities to achieve optimal health, are experienced by socially disadvantaged populations (CDC, 2020). Nurses and health care providers must be competent in identifying and addressing trauma to improve the overall health and well-being of individuals, families, communities, subpopulations, and populations (Fig. 18.1).

TRAUMA-INFORMED CARE

To improve the overall health and well-being of those we serve, a trauma-informed approach is needed. A "trauma-informed approach incorporates three key elements: (1) *realizing* the

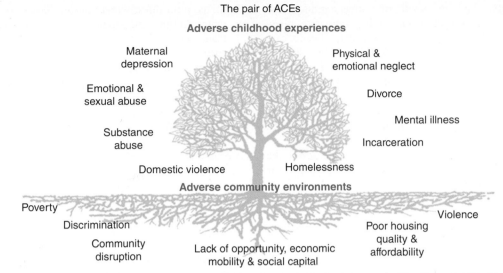

Fig. 18.1 Adverse Childhood Experiences (ACEs) Community Environments. The Pair of ACEs Tree indicating multiple types of ACEs and the relationship to adverse community environments. (Ellis, W., & Deitz, W. [2017]. A new framework for addressing adverse childhood and community experiences: The building community resilience (BCR) model. *Academic Pediatrics, 17*[7S], S86–S93. https//doi.org/10.1016/j.acap.2016.12.011.)

prevalence of trauma; (2) *recognizing* how trauma affects all individuals involved with the program, organization, or system, including its own workforce; and (3) *responding* by putting this knowledge into practice" (SAMHSA, 2014b, p. 4).

Definition

Trauma-informed care (TIC) is a strengths-based service delivery approach, "grounded in an understanding of and responsiveness to the impact of trauma, that emphasizes physical, psychological, and emotional safety for both providers and survivors, and that creates opportunities for survivors to rebuild a sense of control and empowerment" (Hopper et al., 2010, p. 82).

TIC can refer to either evidence-based trauma interventions (e.g., trauma-focused cognitive behavioral therapy) or to a broader systems-level approach that integrates trauma-informed practices (acknowledging that potentially traumatic exposures have taken place) throughout a service delivery system (e.g., health care system, educational system, law enforcement) (SAMHSA, n.d., p. 3).

TIC aims to help nurses and health care professionals become aware of screening and assessment strategies and evidence-based interventions to provide *trauma-specific services* and avoid *retraumatization*, that is, the occurrence of traumatic symptoms in response to current stimuli that replicate past experiences (Duckworth & Follette,

2011). *Trauma-specific services* represent prevention, intervention, or treatment services that address traumatic stress and any cooccurring disorders (e.g., substance use, mental disorders) that develop during or after trauma (SAMHSA, 2014a).

Primary and pediatric care is best suited for the early identification of trauma. Processes for the identification of trauma and its sequelae are a necessity to diminish or prevent further health deterioration. The identification of trauma and its effects (physical, emotional, and behavioral) allows nurses, health care providers, and organizations to respond effectively with *trauma-informed* and *trauma-specific* care and services. These services include evidence-based strategies (assessment, prevention, intervention, and treatment) to address traumatic stress and comorbidities (during or after trauma) across health care and community settings.

Key Assumptions, Concepts, and Principles

Nurses and other health care providers can facilitate TIC by incorporating key assumptions, concepts, and principles into their daily practice. Approaching all patients and their families using TIC guiding principles creates the opportunity for patients and families to recognize and address their own lived experiences and how those experiences impact their health and well-being.

Assumptions. TIC is based on understanding and responding to the impact of trauma that emphasizes physical, psychological, and emotional safety for health care providers and trauma survivors (SAMHSA, 2014a). Feeling safe creates the metaphorical space needed for trauma survivors to rebuild a sense of control and empowerment.

Concepts. SAMHSA's (2014a, p. 5) treatment improvement protocol presents fundamental concepts that health service providers can use to:

- Become trauma aware and knowledgeable about the impact and consequences of traumatic experiences for individuals, families, and communities.
- Evaluate and initiate use of appropriate trauma-related screening and assessment tools.
- Implement interventions from a collaborative, strengths-based approach, appreciating the resilience of trauma survivors.
- Learn the core principles and practices that reflect TIC.
- Anticipate the need for specific trauma-informed treatment planning strategies that support the individual's recovery.
- Decrease the inadvertent retraumatization that can occur from implementing standard organizational policies, procedures, and interventions with individuals, including clients and staff, who have experienced trauma or are exposed to secondary trauma.
- Evaluate and build a trauma-informed organization and workforce.

Principles. The six guiding principles of TIC are: (1) safety; (2) trustworthiness and transparency; (3) peer support and mutual self-help; (4) collaboration and mutuality; (5) empowerment, voice, and choice; and (6) cultural, historical, and gender issues. These principles are described in Table 18.1.

Identification starts with screening. Many individuals, including nurses and health care providers, do not recognize how trauma affects them or their families in the short and long term. Due to the sheer number of individuals who have experienced trauma, a general screening approach is indicated with studies that have shown that increased screening leads to better health outcomes (Oral et al., 2020). Screening supports essential functions, such as:

- for individuals, screening increases insight into health-associated behaviors and provides a launching point for further assessment, education, referral, and behavioral change interventions;
- for organizations, screening increases the identification of system gaps and provides focused feedback on how to improve health care delivery; and

- for communities, screening provides information on which to build infrastructure, capacity, and interventions across the micro-, meso-, and macro-levels of society.

Validated screening tools are readily accessible for use by nurses, other health care providers, and organizations to assess trauma at the micro- (individual), meso- (families and organizations), and macro- (communities, geographical areas) levels.

Definitions of TIC care can vary greatly among stakeholders, but all agree that being *trauma-informed* falls on a spectrum ranging from basic knowledge (where care providers, organizations, and communities engage in education to increase their intellectual knowledge and skills) to taking action (where organizations and communities implement broad, system-level interventions that include the evaluation of practices, procedures, and health policy) (SAMHSA, n.d.).

Nurses and other health professionals need self-awareness and a working understanding of their own trauma experiences to be able to effectively provide TIC. This allows for mindful approaches to working with individuals experiencing and/or recovering from trauma. When ready, there are numerous resources available for assessing one's ACEs. One such tool is the ACE Quiz (https://www.npr.org/sections/health-shots/2015/03/02/387007941/take-the-ace-quiz-and-learn-what-it-does-and-doesnt-mean) (Starecheski, 2015). Take a look at the many resources available and learn more. Note the significant number of supportive resources also made available at these and other sites for dealing with one's own or another's trauma.

SOCIAL AND POLITICAL ACTIVISM

Nurses consistently are viewed as the most trusted health profession (Stone, 2022). In large part, this is due to the nursing *Code of Ethics* which guides the ethical obligations and duties of practice. The nursing *Code of Ethics* (particularly the moral principles of nonmaleficence, fidelity, and veracity) demands that nurses provide care that avoids or minimizes risk to the patient, health care team, or organization, honors the responsibility of providing safe, competent, high-quality nursing care, and that nurses are honest in their interactions with patients and colleagues (Faubion, 2022). The public's trust, the nursing *Code of Ethics*, and increased evidence in the extant literature demonstrating the intersectionality between trauma and poor health outcomes emphasize the need for action. Individual nurses and the nursing profession as a whole must lead the charge for change. So how can a nurse and/or the nursing profession do this?

TABLE 18.1   Principles of Trauma-Informed Care

Guiding Principle	Description
Safety	• Throughout the organization, staff and the people they serve feel physically and psychologically safe.
Trustworthiness and transparency	• Organizational operations and decisions are conducted with transparency and the goal of building and maintaining trust among staff, clients, and family members of those receiving services.
Peer support and mutual self-help	• These are integral to the organizational and service delivery approach and are understood as a key vehicle for building trust, establishing safety, and empowerment.
Collaboration and mutuality	• There is recognition that healing happens in relationships and in the meaningful sharing of power and decision-making. • The organization recognizes that everyone has a role to play in a trauma-informed approach. • One does not have to be a therapist to be therapeutic.
Empowerment, voice, and choice	• Organization aims to strengthen the staff, client, and family members' experience of choice and recognizes that every person's experience is unique and requires an individualized approach. • This builds on what clients, staff, and communities have to offer rather than responding to perceived deficits.
Cultural, historical, and gender issues	• The organization actively moves past cultural stereotypes and biases, offers culturally responsive services, leverages the healing value of traditional cultural connections, and recognizes and addresses historical trauma.

Substance Abuse and Mental Health Services Administration. (2014). SAMHSA's concept of trauma and guidance for a trauma-informed approach. HHS Publication No. (SMA) 14-4884. Substance Abuse and Mental Health Services Administration.

Activism

Micro-Level. Nurses must advocate for increased education and training. Nurses need to increase competency and comfort level in implementing TIC language and approaches (Oral et al., 2020). Studies that report health care providers' gaps in knowledge and confidence in addressing trauma in their patients also report a strong desire for training in trauma approaches to address clients' psychological distress. Oral et al. (2020) found that despite surveyed trauma survivors consistently wanting trauma-specific assessment and intervention because they felt it improved care, they also feared asking about trauma would offend clients.

Nurses are formally and informally recognized as educators and are obligated to self-advocate for education and training to increase TIC knowledge and skills needed to model and impact practice and health care outcomes across all health care delivery settings. Additionally, Oral et al. (2020) found providers with their own trauma history and need to self-protect may create barriers to asking about trauma.

Meso- and Macro-Level. There is a "great potential to reduce the burden of ACEs with policies that address the social determinants of health inequity, such as programs that reduce poverty, improve housing, or increase access to services such as healthcare and/or education" (Oral et al.,

2020, p. 913). Yet, there is a paucity of environmental and/or policy strategies to reduce ACEs in the literature and there are no published studies that have examined ACEs as outcomes of larger policy approaches to date (Oral et al., 2020). Community health, primary care, and pediatric nurses have a huge opportunity to help connect national policy changes to "on the ground" outcomes.

One such policy, The SUPPORT for Patients Substance Use-Disorder Prevention that Promotes Opioid Recovery and Communities (SUPPORT for Patients and Communities) Act (P.L. 115-271) became law on October 24, 2018 (Act, S. N.–o., 2018). The SUPPORT Act was created in recognition and response to the sequelae of trauma. The act addresses substance use and the opioid epidemic by bringing much-needed resources to "supporting children and families who experience trauma and adverse childhood experiences (ACEs), including trauma from substance misuse" (SAMHSA, n.d., para. 1).

Understanding the political national conversation revolving around social policy affecting health and health care delivery is especially important for nurses. Registered nurses are the largest segment of the nation's health care profession, and growing, as "employment of registered nurses is projected to grow 15% from 2016 to 2026, much faster than the average for all occupations" (American Association of Colleges of Nursing [AACN], 2019, para. 5). Collectively, nurses have the potential to enact major change.

SUMMARY

The plasticity of the human brain allows for all individuals to adapt and grow. An individual can move from a trauma victim to a trauma survivor capable of achieving resilience. The health care system is positioned to choose its responses, or nonresponses, to micro-, meso-, and macro-level trauma. Although prevention is the goal, patient- and family-centered, trauma-informed, resiliency-focused health care has the greatest potential for improving health outcomes, reducing social and health care costs, improving the experience of receiving care, and improving the experience of providing care now and into the future.

The need for TIC is urgent. At the micro-level, learning about ACEs and subsequent sequelae helps nurses and other health care providers understand behaviors and gauge whether existing coping strategies are adequate. Understanding protective factors and how to promote resilience-building provides a roadmap to improved health and well-being while also providing hope. At the meso-level, nurses and health care providers can use existing evidence-based tools and strategies to create and maintain organizations and environments. These efforts are needed to support individuals, families, organizations, communities, and the health care workforce as well as to encourage connection and healing. At the macro-level, nurses can advocate for broader public education, interagency collaboration across multisectoral fields, and support policies that prevent trauma, respond appropriately to those impacted, and build individual, group, and community resilience.

SALIENT POINTS

- The ability of nurses and other health care providers to recognize trauma and its effects on self and others and to respond with a strengths-based approach reflects essential practice competencies (knowledge, skills, and attitudes/values).
- Trauma is widespread, costly, and can be experienced by individuals across all diversity spectrums and is almost universally experienced by individuals with mental health and substance use disorders.
- TIC increases focus on nurses and other health care providers' self-care and awareness of one's needs, compassion, satisfaction, and the need for peer support; thus, it may mitigate secondary traumatization and contribute to resilience.
- The majority of trauma survivors desire screening and TIC. Even so, health care provider behaviors (e.g., fear of offending their patients by asking about trauma and/ or their personal need to self-protect) serve as major barriers.
- The greatest potential for reducing the burden of ACEs lies with policies and programs that address social determinants of health inequity, such as programs that reduce poverty, improve housing, or increase access to health care, education, and other needed services.
- A coordinated strategy to build community capacity to identify trauma, implement evidence-based best practices, and disseminate outcomes on the micro-, meso-, and macro-levels can be led by the nursing profession. System change is needed to improve care for families with exposure to substance misuse, enhance recognition of and response to trauma, and strengthen resilience.

Resilience (mental, emotional, and behavioral flexibility and adjustment to external and internal demands) depends on how individuals view and engage with the world, their coping skills and strategies, and the availability and quality of social resources.

CRITICAL THINKING EXERCISES

- Summarize the role and importance of trauma-informed care (and related concepts) knowledge and skills in your nursing practice. Provide examples to illustrate the implications and impact.
- Discuss how the guiding principles of trauma-informed care support the empowerment of individuals, families, health care workers, and communities. What opportunities and/or barriers to modeling these principles in your practice have you already encountered and/or do you anticipate? What ideas do you have that may increase opportunities and/or reduce barriers?
- Connections between adverse childhood experiences, social determinants of health, and health and health care disparities are well-documented in the literature. Do any connections surprise you? Provide a rationale for your response.
- A national conversation during the COVID-19 pandemic uncovered deep divisions in how individuals

view health care delivery through a social and political lens. How do you think this division might help or hinder trauma prevention and mitigation advocacy?

• Examine the alignment of the TIC guiding principles with a health care teams' need to be high functioning. Describe how this alignment supports individual caregiver and team resilience.

REFERENCES

Act, S. N.–o. (2018). *Interagency Task Force on trauma-informed care.* Substance Abuse and Mental Health Services Administration. https://www.samhsa.gov/sites/default/files/programs_campaigns/trauma_informed_care/support-act-section-n.pdf

American Association of Colleges of Nursing. (2019). *Nursing fact sheet.* https://www.aacnnursing.org/news-Information/fact-sheets/nursing-fact-sheet

American Psychological Association. (2020). *Building your resilience.* https://www.apa.org/topics/resilience/building-your-resilience

Centers for Disease Control and Prevention. (2020, November 24). *Health disparities.* https://www.cdc.gov/healthyyouth/disparities/index.htm#:~:text=Health%20disparities%20are%20preventable%20differences,experienced%20by%20socially%20disadvantaged%20populations

Centers for Disease Control and Prevention. (2021, September 30). *Social determinants of health.* https://www.cdc.gov/socialdeterminants/index.htm

Centers for Disease Control and Prevention. (2022, January 20). *Risk and protective factors.* https://www.cdc.gov/violenceprevention/aces/riskprotectivefactors.html#

Children's Bureau. (n.d.). *Protective factors and adverse childhood experiences.* U.S. Department of Health and Human Services. https://www.childwelfare.gov/topics/preventing/preventionmonth/about/protective-factors-aces/

Duckworth, M. P., & Follette, V. M. (Eds.). (2011). *Retraumatization: Assessment, treatment, and prevention* (1st ed.). Routledge. https://doi.org/10.4324/9780203866320

Edley, Jr., C., & Morsey, L. (2019, May 1). *Toxic stress and children's outcomes.* Economic Policy Institute [Blog]. https://www.epi.org/blog/toxic-stress-and-childrens-outcomes/

Ellis, W. R., & Dietz, W. H. (2017). A new framework for addressing adverse childhood and community experiences: The building community resilience model. *Academic Pediatrics, 17*(7s), S86–S93. https://doi.org/10.1016/j.acap.2016.12.011

Faubion, D. (2022). *The 9 nursing code of ethics (provisions + interpretive statements)—every nurse must adhere to.* https://www.nursingprocess.org/nursing-code-of-ethics-and-interpretive-statements.html

Felitti, V. J., Anda, R. F., Nordenberg, D., Williamson, D. F., Spitz, A. M., Edwards, V., Koss, M. P., & Marks, J. S. (1998). Relationship of childhood abuse and household dysfunction to many of the leading causes of death in adults: The adverse childhood experiences (ACE) study. *American Journal of Preventive Medicine, 14*(4), 245–258. https://doi.org/10.1016/S0749-3797(98)00017-8

Hopper, E. K., Bassuk, E. L., & Olivet, J. (2010). Shelter from the storm: Trauma-informed care in homeless service settings. *The Open Health Services and Policy Journal, 3,* 80–100. https://www.homelesshub.ca/sites/default/files/cenfdthy.pdf

Hospital IQ. (2021, November 17). *Nursing in crisis: Hospital IQ survey highlights significant patient care challenges due to hospital staffing shortages* [Press release]. https://www.hospiq.com/about-us/press-releases/nursing-in-crisis-hospital-iq-survey-highlights-significant-patient-care-challenges-due-to-hospital-staffing-shortages/#:~:text=Impact%20to%20patient%20care%3A%20Due,in%20medication%20errors%20or%20delay

Kelly, L. (2020, Jan/Mar). Burnout, compassion fatigue, and secondary trauma in nurses: Recognizing the occupational phenomenon and personal consequences of caregiving. *Critical Care Nursing Quarterly, 43*(1), 73–80. https://doi.org/10.1097/CNQ.0000000000000293

Lebow, H. (2021). *Can you recover from trauma? 5 therapy options.* PsychCentral. [On-line Newsletter]. https://psychcentral.com/health/trauma-therapy

National Child Traumatic Stress Network. (n.d.-a). *Secondary traumatic stress.* https://www.nctsn.org/trauma-informed-care/secondary-traumatic-stress#:~:text=Secondary%20traumatic%20stress%20is%20the,disasters%2C%20and%20other%20adverse%20events

National Child Traumatic Stress Network. (n.d.-b). *Trauma types.* https://www.nctsn.org/what-is-child-trauma/trauma-types

National Child Traumatic Stress Network. (n.d.-c). *Effects.* https://www.nctsn.org/what-child-trauma/trauma-types/sex-trafficking/effects

Oral, R., Coohey, C., Zarei, K., Conrad, A., Nielsen, A., Wibbenmeyer, W., Segal, R., Wojciak, A., Jennissen, C., & Peek-Asa, C. (2020). Nationwide efforts for trauma-informed care implementation and workforce development in healthcare and related fields: A systematic review. *The Turkish Journal of Pediatrics, 62,* 906–920. https://doi.org/10.24953/turkjped.2020.06.002

Starecheski, S. (2015). *Take the ACE quiz-and learn what it means and doesn't mean.* https://www.npr.org/sections/health-shots/2015/03/02/387007941/take-the-ace-quiz-and-learn-what-it-does-and-doesnt-mean

Stone, A. (2022, January 24). *Gallup poll ranks nurses most honest and ethical profession for 20th consecutive year.* Oncology Nursing Society [News article]. https://voice.ons.org/advocacy/gallup-poll-ranks-nurses-most-honest-and-ethical-profession-for-20th-consecutive-year#:~:text=In%20results%20released%20in%20January,%2C%20pharmacists%2C%20and%20other%20professions

Substance Abuse and Mental Health Services Administration. (2014a). Trauma-informed care in behavioral health services, Historical Account of Trauma, Appendix C. Substance Abuse and Mental Health Services Administration. Treatment Improvement Protocol (TIP) Series 57. HHS Publication No. (SMA) 14-4816. https://store.samhsa.gov/sites/default/files/d7/priv/sma14-4816.pdf

Substance Abuse and Mental Health Services Administration. (2014b). *Concept of trauma and guidance for a trauma-informed approach*. SAMHSA's Trauma and Justice Strategic Initiative. https://ncsacw.acf.hhs.gov/userfiles/files/SAMHSA_Trauma.pdf

Substance Abuse and Mental Health Services Administration. Substance. (n.d.). *National Strategy for trauma informed care operating plan*. https://www.samhsa.gov/sites/default/files/trauma-informed-care-operating-plan.pdf

Substance Abuse and Mental Health Services Administration. (2020, April 22). *Understanding child trauma*. https://www.samhsa.gov/child-trauma/understanding-child-trauma

Substance Abuse and Mental Health Services Administration. (2022, April 27). *Resources for child trauma-informed care*. https://www.samhsa.gov/childrens-awareness-day/past-events/2018/child-traumatic-stress-resources

Tannenbaum, S. I., Traylor, A. M., Thomas, E. J., & Salas, E. (2021). Managing teamwork in the face of pandemic: Evidence-based tips. *British Medical Journal Quality & Safety*, *30*, 59–63. https://qualitysafety.bmj.com/content/qhc/30/1/59.full.pdf

U.S. Department of Veterans Affairs. PTSD: National Center for PTSD. (2022, April 8). *How common is PTSD in adults?* https://www.ptsd.va.gov/understand/common/common_adults.asp#:~:text=A%20trauma%20is%20a%20shocking,one%20trauma%20in%20their%20lives

U.S. Department of Veterans Affairs. PTSD: National Center for PTSD. (2022, June). *Trauma exposure measures*. https://www.ptsd.va.gov/professional/assessment/te-measures/index.asp

19

Telehealth

*Audrey E. Snyder, PhD, RN, ACNP-BC, FAANP, FAEN, FAAN and
Tammy Hall, MSN, RN, RDMS*

e http://evolve.elsevier.com/Friberg/bridge/

OBJECTIVES

At the completion of this chapter, the reader will be able to:
- Define telemedicine and telehealth.
- Describe the components of telehealth technology.
- Discuss the implications of telehealth for nursing practice.
- Articulate the advantages and challenges of telehealth technology.
- Identify health policy implications for telehealth.
- Evaluate local telehealth capabilities.

INTRODUCTION

Telehealth provides the opportunity for health care providers to meet the challenges facing health care delivery. It is often considered an alternative method of health care delivery. It is not a specialty in and of itself but has the potential to facilitate care provided by various specialties. It has been marketed as a tool for providing care in rural areas, for underserved populations, and when patients may have transportation difficulties. The COVID-19 pandemic has highlighted the benefits of telehealth technology use in acute care, clinics, and home settings in both rural and urban environments. Many innovative programs using telehealth have evolved during the pandemic. Nurses can use telehealth technologies to assess patients, make clinical decisions, and support or intervene with patients and families.

The American Telemedicine Association (ATA) now advocates for the term *telehealth* as opposed to earlier use of *telemedicine* terminology (ATA, 2022). This definition has evolved as health care specialties, and not just medicine, use telemedicine. The term *telehealth* is used for the remainder of this chapter to discuss the remote delivery of health care using technology.

Telehealth technology has evolved over the past three decades in response to the need for access to high-quality health care. In the acute-care high-technology environment, monitors transmit physiological parameters directly into medical records. Many pumps are electronic and can be programmed to adjust dose based on imputed patient data. Tele-intensive care units (Tele-ICUs) have evolved to support nurses at the bedside. Electronic medical records for the retrieval of patient data are a standard today. Information technology improves patient care access and reduces health care costs.

Videoconferencing has been used for distance learning in education, especially in rural or underserved areas. Virtual classrooms have existed for the past two decades. Nursing curriculums may now employ virtual clinical practicums as well. When students were excluded from clinical sites as the coronavirus pandemic ramped up in the United States, nursing faculty pivoted to virtual simulations for clinical experience at the same time classes were offered using remote technology. Nurses have adopted electronic health records and videoconferencing as avenues for education, and now they are adopting technology such as telehealth for the evaluation of patients. This chapter provides an overview of telehealth technology and case examples of its use in the health care arena.

MODES OF TELEHEALTH

There are multiple modes of telehealth technology transmission. The first and oldest is the use of voice-only via telephone; for example, to perform telephone triage or management of disease in specific populations, such as the use of telephone triage protocols with pregnant patients. This has evolved into videoconferencing technology in which there is virtual contact with the patient to assess, manage, treat, or educate and counsel patients, including online consultations. The second is to store and forward video images, in which data are collected and then sent to a specialist. Historically radiology has used store and forward methods of evaluation, such as the picture archiving and communications systems (PACS) and teleradiology. An example of this is the forwarding of radiographs from a rural hospital to a radiologist at a distant tertiary center for reading. The third mode is remote patient monitoring using sensors to monitor physiological data from a home unit to a hospital electronic medical record—for example, oxygen saturation monitoring for a patient with chronic obstructive pulmonary disease (COPD) or falls in a patient with Parkinson disease. The fourth is mHealth which uses mobile phones and wearable devices, including watches, to access information at any time. Telehealth can be done with low or high bandwidth, although images and data transfer require higher bandwidth.

TELEHEALTH CENTERS

Because of the rapid explosion of demand and use of telehealth technology, Telehealth Resource Centers (TRCs) were developed. TRCs are funded by the U.S. Department of Health and Human Services (USDHHS) Administration Health Resources and Services Administration (HRSA) Office for the Advancement of Telehealth, which is a division of the Office of Rural Health Policy. There are two national and 12 regional TRCs in the United States. In 2017, a consortium of TRCs was formed to build sustainable telehealth programs and to improve health outcomes for those in rural and medically underserved communities (National Consortium of Telehealth Resource Centers [NCTRC], 2022). For example, the Mid-Atlantic TRC was established in September 2011, and currently covers the states of Delaware, Kentucky, Maryland, New Jersey, North Carolina, Pennsylvania, Virginia, West Virginia, and the District of Columbia. Their website has many resources for nurses and other health care providers and systems (http://www.MATRC.org).

EQUIPMENT

To operate, telehealth technology requires a computer platform, network protocol, and network. The computing platform is the hardware and software framework that together allows the software to run. A network protocol is a set of digital rules for the exchange of data between computers. A network can be a local area network (LAN) for a small geographical area (e.g., in a hospital building) or a wide area network (WAN) that encompasses a larger geographical area and includes leased telecommunication lines.

ADVANTAGES OF TELEHEALTH TECHNOLOGY

Telehealth reaches patients in their home or home community. Encounters via telehealth technology can empower patients to participate actively in their care from home and promote independence. Maintaining a level of independence translates into improved health status and quality of life for older adult patients experiencing chronic health problems. Increased patient satisfaction also may be an outcome of telehealth. In the managed care environment, telehealth can increase patient contact without the expense of a hands-on visit. Access to a specialist who may not be readily available in a rural community is an advantage. Demonstration studies have documented cost savings in travel expense and time for patients, care providers, and health care providers. Patients with chronic illnesses, such as congestive heart failure (CHF), COPD, or diabetes, can be managed using a telehealth system. Patients can connect home monitoring systems to a modem, phone line, or computer and upload their data to be reviewed by clinicians. The Montana Diabetes Program uses telehealth to reach persons with prediabetes in rural and frontier areas (https://dphhs.mt.gov/publichealth/Diabetes). Alternating weekly telehealth and office visits for pregnant women with newly diagnosed gestational diabetes helped them achieve American Diabetes Association targeted fasting postprandial glucose levels (Sacks et al., 2017).

USE OF TELEHEALTH

Televisits can be used to assess, monitor, support, coach, and provide medical care. More than one of these intervention types may occur in the same visit. Chronic care management through remote monitoring has grown rapidly. It allows nurses to monitor and assess for complications early. It lends itself to patients with heart disease, diabetes, asthma, psychiatric illness, and wounds. Home monitoring programs are using equipment for physiological measurements of heart rate, blood pressure, pulse oximetry, weight, spirometry, glucose level, electrocardiogram tracing, and temperature. Stethoscopes, cameras, otoscopes, ophthalmoscopes, and videophones can be used for assessment. Video with magnifying capability can assess wounds and monitor healing. Nurses also can use the camera to view labels on medication bottles. Electronic medication dispensing devices that are controlled remotely can increase medication regimen adherence. Home telehealth should be integrated with hospital electronic medical records so nurses and other care providers can access patient medical information to help make care decisions. Physiological data transmitted via telehealth with warning messages sent for threshold parameters may allow clinicians to manage higher caseloads while identifying parameters outside the reference range.

Monitoring at home has evolved to prevent readmissions and potential Medicare penalties. At hospital discharge, nurses identify at-risk patients and coordinate patient transitions to home with activation of daily provider monitoring and clinical coordination using clinical review software and reporting while documenting outcomes of readmission, population health, costs, and satisfaction. Early during the coronavirus pandemic, persons with chronic illness, like CHF, COPD, and diabetes, as well as obstetrical patients, were monitored at home to avoid COVID-19 exposure. One bright spot in the coronavirus pandemic has been the acceleration of telehealth use for many conditions including its use for evaluating chronic neurologic conditions through remote home visits and the use of remote sensor monitoring for tremors, gait, and falls (Bhaskar et al., 2020). One emergency department (ED) implemented a telehealth-enabled drive-through and walk-in garage care system to evaluate and triage patients and treat, via telehealth, lower-acuity patients. This innovation demonstrated a 17% reduction in ED length of stay and an estimated 25% to 41% reduction in PPE used during COVID-19 surges (Callagy, 2021).

During the coronavirus pandemic, 49 states issued waivers allowing the use of telemedicine via audio-only and/or practice of practitioners across state lines. After year 2 of the pandemic, the number of states with waivers decreased to 23. There are currently 19 states with permanent interstate waivers. The Federation of State Medical Boards maintains an updated directory of telehealth waivers (https://www.fsmb.org/advocacy/covid-19). Insurance coverage of telehealth services by the Centers for Medical and Medicaid Services (CMS) was expanded during the COVID-19 pandemic. Many of these service allowances have expired. In November 2021, CMS announced the expansion of telehealth for mental and behavioral health to include audio-only in person's homes and to cover telepsychiatry at Rural Health Clinics (RHCs) and Federally Qualified Health Centers (FQHCs) to improve access to care for rural and vulnerable populations (https://www.cms.gov/newsroom/press-releases/cms-physician-payment-rule-promotes-greater-access-telehealth-services-diabetes-prevention-programs).

Experienced intensive care unit (ICU) nurses and advanced practice providers can use Tele-ICUs to help monitor and treat intensive care patients at a remote location. They assess the patient by video and have access to the patient's medical records and electronic monitoring results. They speak directly to the patient and providers in the room. In some hospitals, tele-ICU support evolved or was started as a means of protecting vulnerable health care providers, as well as extending experienced ICU nurses' support to bedside nurses without ICU experience when ICU bed capacity was increased during surges (Arneson et al., 2020). The use of telehealth platforms also allowed nurses to connect isolated patients with their family. Another innovative use of telehealth is the telestroke program that assists in the evaluation of individuals experiencing symptoms of a cerebrovascular accident living in rural areas. Upon arrival of a patient to the ED with symptoms of a potential ischemic cerebrovascular accident, a neurologist can remotely examine a patient, obtain the medical history, and review computed tomography studies. Patients can receive alteplase (tPA) within 3 hours of symptom onset to dissolve the clot (Bartlett, 2016). Physicians can make clinical decisions based on data rather than using the telephone alone. Both of these telestroke interventions allow the patient to be treated faster, enhancing outcomes for cerebrovascular accident patients. Another use of telehealth is neuropsychological testing to evaluate cognition in ICU survivors (Han et al., 2020).

Before the pandemic, an innovative Emergency Department Telehealth Express Care Service program started at New York Presbyterian and Weill Cornell Medicine in 2016 has demonstrated a decrease in ED length of stay, increased patient satisfaction, and decreased 72-hour ED return visit rates (Sharma et al., 2017). Nurses triage the patient as they would in a walk-in ED, and then the patient is seen by the provider in a virtual patient room. Another innovative use of telehealth for emergency care is in the prehospital emergency services arena in which the prehospital providers have a telehealth consultation with a provider and nonurgent patients are scheduled and transported to a primary care provider versus the ED, reducing unnecessary ED visits and demonstrating a cost savings (Langabeer et al., 2016).

With the national shortage of health care providers in psychiatry, telepsychiatry has blossomed. Even in urban areas, smaller hospitals may not have a specialist on call to evaluate for suicidal or homicidal risk. Instead of risking transport of the patient to a hospital with a mental health specialist, the assessment can be made through Health Insurance Portability and Accountability Act (HIPAA) secure videoconferencing. The USDHHS strategic plan for 2022 to 2026 objective 1.4 (USDHHS, 2022) addresses the use of telehealth to improve access to mental health and substance abuse care for rural and underserved populations. In 2017, the HRSA awarded more than $200 million to health centers and rural health organizations to increase access to substance abuse and mental health services, with an additional $3.3 million to support 13 rural health organizations under the Rural Health Opioid Program and Substance Abuse Treatment Telehealth Network Grant Program to overcome challenges of emergency response times and lack of access to substance abuse treatment providers in rural, frontier, and underserved areas.

Cameras support, store, and forward capabilities and direct videoconferencing. With teleophthalmology, rural clinic staff can be taught to use a retinal camera to complete the yearly diabetic retinopathy screening. The images can be forwarded to a distant ophthalmologist, who reads the images and provides consultation back to the clinic. During videoconferencing, an enterostomal nurse can observe new ostomies. In the past, if the patient called the specialty clinic with a concern, the patient may have been instructed to travel to the specialty clinic, which may have been a long distance away and incurred cost for the patient. Now when there is a concern, the patient can go to a nearby clinic and connect remotely through videoconferencing with a specialist, who can use the camera to zoom in on the ostomy and evaluate the concern.

Keeping patients close to home is a goal of many evolving telehealth programs. Telehealth allows high-risk obstetrical patients to have their appointments with a high-risk obstetrician via telehealth at a clinic closer to home until they are near their delivery date. The Virginia Department of Corrections is using telehealth sites in prisons to decrease the cost and risks associated with the transport of prisoners to distant sites for health care appointments. For patients who have an abnormal Pap smear, the next step is a colposcopy procedure in which a camera or colposcope is used to examine the vagina and cervix and perform a biopsy of any areas of concern. Video colposcopy is an intervention to help overcome the shortage of specialty providers and expand the role of the nurse practitioner in rural southwest Virginia.

Improving access to specialty care in rural and remote sites can be a telehealth outcome. The neonatology telemedicine program at the Mayo Clinic improves access to neonatology expertise, which improves patient safety and quality of care and prevents unnecessary transfers to a higher level of care (Fang et al., 2016). Telehealth technology may provide the opportunity for a second opinion on a case without the cost of travel or transfer for a patient. In developing nations, there is often limited access to specialists for both natives and visitors. With worldwide travel today, visitors to remote locations may experience medical or trauma concerns in which a specialist consultation

could impact outcomes. The Swinfen Charitable Trust (https://www.swinfentelmed.org) is an organization that assists the poor, sick, and disabled in developing countries by establishing telemedicine links between medical practitioners in the developing world and expert medical and surgical specialists.

As telehealth evolves, there will be an expansion to other environments of care. The use of telehealth in nursing facilities to evaluate acute complaints may help prevent transfer to the ED, and early recognition of a change in patient condition may prevent readmission. One of the current recommendations includes the education of staff and residents in long-term care facilities on telehealth equipment and integrating its use into the daily workflow (Seifert et al., 2020). This will likely increase knowledge and usability when telehealth is needed. A pilot project using a mobile platform for the evaluation of patients in the prehospital arena for cerebrovascular accident symptoms may allow ischemic cerebrovascular accident patients to receive tPA faster (Swensen, 2014). With an aging population, and with cerebrovascular accidents currently being the fourth leading cause of death (Centers for Disease Control and Prevention [CDC], 2021), the use of this technology may reduce cerebrovascular accident morbidity and mortality. Another use of telehealth in the field of neurology is delivering interventions to patients with dementia and their families (Cuffaro et al., 2020).

IMPACT OF COVID-19 PANDEMIC ON TELEHEALTH IMPLEMENTATION

The use of telehealth during the COVID-19 pandemic allowed providers to evaluate patients in their home, limit exposure to COVID-19 for patients, and allow those who were ill to maintain their self-quarantine (Colbert et al., 2020). In long-term care facilities, the use of telemedicine helped with the diagnosis, treatment, and quarantine of patients (Cormi et al., 2020). Challenges included health care providers and patients not having the knowledge or experience to use it. With the COVID-19 pandemic, telehealth utilization increased globally and in the United States. As an example, Vanderbilt Medical Center saw telehealth visits for pediatric and adolescent patients increase from an average of 6.4 visits per week to 1104.8 visits per week after March 16, 2020 (Patel et al., 2020). Much of the recent literature related to telehealth focuses on process change. Patel et al. (2020) describe the security challenges of enrolling pediatric patients in the telehealth portal My Health at Vanderbilt and the need to redesign a system to "identity verification, parentage documentation, and adolescent assent for enrollment." The orthopedic surgeons of Johns Hopkins University School of Medicine designed a comprehensive program to introduce telehealth to their practice following COVID-19 (Loeb et al., 2020). Recognizing this was a significant process change for practitioners and patients, this practice initially limited the number of virtual visits and sent out a letter of intent to patients via the electronic portal, including information explaining what to expect from the visit to promote success (Loeb et al., 2020). Following the implementation of the program, the ongoing challenge became "managing the cameras, microphones, and software on patients' devices to allow HIPAA-compliant video communication" (Loeb et al., 2020, Scheduling section). Mehrotra et al. (2020) identified "training clinicians, explaining arrival procedures to patients, using interpreter services, and getting video equipment to clinician's homes" as challenges encountered with telehealth services. Technology challenges during visits include lag time and image quality, virtual etiquette (as in what is seen in the background and heard during video visits), documentation, and changing regulations (Mehrotra et al., 2020). Cleaning and disinfection of telehealth equipment, when used with multiple patients, is paramount to infection control.

The issues of privacy and technology, specifically broadband connectivity, and patients' inability to use technology are identified by the Center for Connected Health Policy (2020) as issues needing resolution after the COVID-19 pandemic. The digital divide is highlighted as problematic and defined as patients who are not able to use technology, whatever the reason (Center for Connected Health Policy, 2020). Lack of social support, lack of technology access, and technology issues on the day of telehealth visits were considered by Calton et al. (2020) when setting up a telehealth program.

TELE-EDUCATION

Tele-education is a viable means for providing educational content to nursing students, practicing nurses, and patients and their families. The advent of COVID-19 and the necessity to convert many nursing courses to an online format confirmed that tele-education is an effective platform (Kalanlar, 2022). Multiple technologies are available to health care professionals to provide patient education. For instance, videoconferencing is an effective means of diabetes education as it is transmitted by one educator to multiple sites at one time providing a vehicle for group support and management of this chronic illness. The videoconferencing platform offers social bonding while allowing participants to share personal experiences, skills, and insights (Banbury et al., 2018). The use of applications on mobile devices (e.g., mHealth) enables patients to both receive education and record data reflecting the efficacy of education. Other technologies for patient education include self-paced programs obtained through a website, phone calls, and email (Doorenbos et al., 2020). Tele-education has positively impacted global health. Physicians and other health care providers working in remote areas can benefit from continuing medical education when paired with an academic institution. Surgical grand rounds are teleconferenced quarterly to Rwanda from the University of Virginia. Surgeons in both countries present patients (Cattell-Gordon, personal communication, 2018). In addition, nurses can receive training via telehealth. Today it is common for education to occur via online webinars. The use of telehealth hubs for dissemination can reach across miles and continents—for example, the monthly training of midwives in the Democratic Republic of Congo (Cattell-Gordon, personnel communication, 2018). Tele-education is a valid method for providing continuing education to nurses in rural and remote areas. The Project ECHO model at the University of New Mexico teaches primary care providers to provide specialty care in their communities through virtual clinics, increasing specialty care and improving outcomes (Project ECHO, 2018).

CHALLENGES

Challenges to the use of telehealth include the quality of technology, cost, confidentiality and security, physical distancing from patients, licensure across state lines, and lack of reimbursement. As nursing education aligns itself with the social determinants of health, instruction in the use of telehealth platforms will become integral in curriculum design and delivery. This alignment will magnify the presence of the *digital divide* (Gleason & Suen, 2022) or the demarcation between those who have access to health care or learning through technology and those who do not, whether through cost or location.

Telehealth equipment can vary based on the type of services provided. There is a lack of broadband networks in many rural areas, which limits access to telehealth. The initial cost to establish a telemedicine network is high, usually requiring capital investment. The "Broadband Internet Connections for Rural America" (H.R. 4374, 2021) proposes the appropriation of $43.2 billion toward critically needed infrastructure for rural broadband, including $150 million earmarked for distance learning and telemedicine loans and grants.

Confidentiality of patient data is paramount. The potential exists for hackers, but security systems are evolving to prevent access to patient data. The use of third-party health websites poses the risk of having private health information collected and shared with other entities (Chaet et al., 2017). Patients are encouraged to read the privacy policies of health-related websites and mobile applications to determine if their personal information is being shared with other companies or vendors.

Telehealth technology creates a physical distance between the nurse and the patient and a perception of interpersonal disengagement on the part of the provider or patient (Ladin et al., 2021). Distance is a challenge in the use of telemedicine platforms such as eICU, in which the patient is observed, and providers are consulted via technology from a remote location. Although this method of care increases adherence to evidence-based practice and the following of care standards, nurses must be responsive and have confidence in their assessment and nursing skills (Kaplow & Zellinger, 2021). The role of the nurse in telehealth and telemedicine is evolving. Advanced practice nurses are developing ways to be with the patient before, during, and after their virtual visits by reading about their patients before the visit, transmitting information to the patient in advance, listening and communicating, using verbal and nonverbal messaging, and following up with phone calls or monitoring of physiological parameters using telehealth (Nagel et al., 2017). In one study of patient perceptions, patients stated they prefer to hear serious news via video versus face-to-face, so they could be in their own supportive environment (Powell et al., 2017). Rural health innovators who have implemented telehealth visits to monitor patients believe it improved patient outcomes and saved travel costs even though Medicare did not reimburse for the telehealth visit (Knudson et al., 2017).

Standards of practice still apply to care provided remotely. State boards of nursing and medicine may have specific regulations related to the provision of care via telehealth. Staff must be trained and licensed to practice; the appropriate examination must be available to evaluate, diagnose, and treat the patient; and medical records must be maintained. Practicing across state lines is a concern because the practitioner must be licensed in the state in which he or she practices. Nurses may have a compact state agreement that allows them to be licensed in one state and practice in another state, but this model has not been adopted for medicine. A physician, nurse practitioner, or physician assistant is required to be licensed in both the state in which he or she practices and the state in which the patient is receiving care. Telehealth's expansion of care has been a major driver of the advanced practice nurse interstate compact, similar to the enhanced nurse licensure compact for registered nurses, which allows nurses to practice in multiple states with one license. An Advanced Practice Registered Nurse Compact was adopted in 2018 by the National Council of State Boards of Nursing, but as of early 2022, only one state has passed legislation and one state has pending legislation (https://www.ncsbn.org/aprn-compact.htm). Further discussion of the nurse interstate compact occurs in Chapter 11.

A lack of reimbursement exists for remote patient monitoring. Medicare reimbursement is limited by the type of services provided, geographical location, type of institution delivering the services, and type of health care provider, and requires the use of a real-time audiovisual platform. There is a need for federal telehealth legislation and reimbursement by Medicare and other payers to improve access to care by remote monitoring (Butcher, 2021). Medicare does not reimburse for telehealth services in a patient's home except for telepsych, which is a hindrance to remote monitoring programs. The CMS has produced and distributed the "Telehealth Services" Medicare Learning Network Booklet to providers with information on coverage of services, including current procedural terminology (CPT) codes and website resources (CMS, 2018). Medicaid and private insurance payer reimbursement varies by state. The Center for Connected Health Policy's (2017) State Telehealth Laws and Reimbursement Policies Report provides comprehensive information on telehealth laws, regulations, and Medicaid policies for all states and is a resource for clinicians.

The annual 2020 U.S. Telehealth Benchmark Survey, an industry snapshot of virtual care, showed the strongest growth in the use of telehealth programs to be in clinics and private practices (92%) (ATA, n.d.). While the COVID-19 pandemic had a tremendous impact on the rise of virtual care strategy, most organizations have a long-term virtual care strategy beyond the pandemic.

NURSES' ROLE

The role of the nurse in telehealth is evolving. Education and training are important to any telehealth program. Nurses need to learn how to use and troubleshoot the technology and should be aware of the resources available to them. Undergraduate and graduate education should include telehealth technology and simulation experiences to facilitate the transition to practice and comfort with the technology. Rutledge et al. (2021) developed the Four P's of Telehealth competency framework for advanced practice nurses. The competencies include *planning, preparing, providing, and performance.* In addition, Nagel et al. (2017) developed the *Getting a Picture* theory of nursing in the virtual environment. This theory champions the nurse's ability to visualize the patient through a seven-step process: entering in, connecting, sharing and reviewing information, recognizing trends and patterns, recording and reflecting, putting pieces together over time, and transitioning out. Telehealth has great potential to expand the roles of advanced practice nurses. To prepare nurse practitioners for the current health care environment, clinical practicum experiences incorporating telehealth applications must be integrated into the curriculum (Rutledge et al., 2021). The National Organization of Nurse Practitioner Faculty [NONPF] (2018) recognizes telehealth as a consistent form of health care and advocates both telehealth instruction for students and the use of telehealth for faculty to conduct distant site visits and meet with preceptors.

Practicing nurses also need education on telehealth applications. Training needs to meet the needs of the nurse, while simulation offers hands-on experience and the development of competencies before interaction with actual patients. Nurses are active participants in the delivery of health care interventions by telehealth, but more research related to the specific activities, roles, frequency, or dosage of the nursing interventions performed is needed. This is an area for growth of outcomes evaluation and evidence-based research in telehealth. Nurses practicing in critical access hospitals may use telehealth to access distance-based personnel to verify medication dosing or assess a potential stroke patient. Nurses may be involved in diabetic retinal screenings by taking photos of the fundus of the eye and transmitting them for remote interpretation. In one study, diabetic retinal screenings increased after implementation of a telemedicine screening program (Jani et al., 2017).

Quality In Telehealth Delivery

The quality of telehealth delivery is as important as care provided in person. The National Committee for Quality Assurance National Quality Forum (2017) report "Creating a Framework to Support Measure Development for Telehealth" provides guidance for advancing health technology to be safe and effective and identifies areas in which measurement can assess the quality and impact of telehealth services through a framework of four domains: access to care, financial impact/cost, experience, and effectiveness. This report provides guidance for the initiation of telehealth programs and quality improvement in existing programs. In 2018, the National Committee for Quality Assurance updated the Healthcare Effectiveness Data and Information Set (HEDIS) scores to include telehealth for behavioral health.

SUMMARY

Telehealth is revolutionizing health care delivery. The greatest use is in the management of chronic health conditions through remote assessment or monitoring, education, and support in keeping patients at home or in their communities. Telehealth empowers patients to self-manage their disease and improves quality of life. The advent of the COVID-19 pandemic catapulted telehealth technologies from platforms used mainly for primary care to invaluable resources used successfully by many providers and medical specialties (Colbert et al., 2020). Nurses need to understand the technology, equipment, and language used. Nursing and other health professions students in undergraduate and graduate programs should be educated in the use of telehealth as an avenue of patient care. As more patients are cared for in their home environment, telehealth can be increasingly leveraged to improve patient outcomes.

SALIENT POINTS

- Telehealth is medical information exchanged from one site to another via electronic communications to improve a patient's clinical health status.
- Telehealth may not involve clinical services.
- Nurses use telehealth to provide comprehensive care to patients.
- Nurses use telehealth technologies to assess patients, make clinical decisions, and support or intervene with patients.
- Telehealth Resource Centers exist to improve the understanding of telehealth and how it can be used to improve access to care and quality of care in rural and other medically underserved areas and to help develop telehealth programs that match the needs of a practice or community.
- Encounters via telehealth technology can empower patients to participate actively in their care from home and promote independence.
- Telehealth saves travel time for patients, care providers, and specialists and reduces cost for insurance companies and client out-of-pocket expenses.
- Electronic intensive care units can prevent untoward outcomes, such as reintubation or unplanned extubation, and improve patient outcomes by recognizing changes in trends in patient condition.
- Telestroke programs provide more rapid evaluation of cerebrovascular accident patients and allow alteplase (tPA) to be administered sooner.
- Telehealth is a valid method for providing continuing education to nurses in rural areas.

- Challenges to telehealth include the quality of technology, cost, confidentiality and security, physical distancing from patients, patients' health and digital literacy, licensure across state lines, lack of reimbursement, and broadband access.

- Nurses need to integrate telehealth technologies into their nursing practice.
- Telehealth education must be integrated into nursing and other health professions' undergraduate and graduate curriculums.

CRITICAL REFLECTION EXERCISES

1. Identify a telehealth center in your area. What resources are available through this center? What types of specialty services are available for patient consultation?
2. Conduct a literature review to identify studies that provide outcomes data associated with the use of telehealth with a specific patient population or patient

disease. Focus on your current specialty area and practice setting. How might the use of telehealth affect your practice?
3. Consider strategies to use when using telehealth with patients to promote presence, encourage engagement, and convey support.

REFERENCES

American Telemedicine Association. (2023). *About telehealth.* Accessed January 16, 2023. https://www.npr.org/sections/health-shots/2015/03/02/387007941/take-the-ace-quiz-and-learn-what-it-does-and-doesnt-mean

American Telemedicine Association. (n.d.). *2020 US Telehealth benchmark survey results.* Accessed January 16, 2023. https://business.teladochealth.com/resources/white-paper/2020-telehealth-benchmark-survey-results/

Arneson, S. L., Tucker, S. J., Mercier, M., & Singh, J. (2020). Answering the call: Impact of tele-ICU nurses during the COVID-19 pandemic. *Critical Care Nurse, 40*(4), 25–31. https://doi.org/10.4037/ccn2020126

Banbury, A., Nancarrow, S., Dart, J., Gray, L., & Parkinson, L. (2018). Telehealth interventions delivering home-based support group videoconferencing: Systematic review. *Journal of Medical Internet Research, 20*(2), e25. https://doi.org/10.2196/jmir.8090

Bartlett, G. (2016). *For patients, a telestroke of luck.* ENA Connection.

Bhaskar, S., Bradley, S., Chattu, V. K., Adisesh, A., Nurtazina, A., Kyrykbayeva, S., Sakhamuri, S., Yaya, S., Sunil, T., Thomas, P., Mucci, V., Moguilner, S., Israel-Korn, S., Alacapa, J., Mishra, A., Pandya, S., Schroeder, S., Atreja, A., Banach, M., & Ray, D. (2020). Telemedicine across the globe-position paper from the COVID-19 pandemic health system resilience program (REPROGRAM) International Consortium (part 1). *Frontiers in Public Health, 8,* 1–15. https://doi.org/10.3389/fpubh.2020.556720

Butcher, L. (2021). Support for telehealth remains, but reimbursement policies vary state to state. *Neurology Today, 21*(13), 12–16. https://journals.lww.com/neurotodayonline/Fulltext/2021/07080/Support_for_Telehealth_Remains,_but_Reimbursement.6.aspx

Callagy, P., Ravi, S., Khan, S., Yiadom, M. Y., McClellen, H., Snell, S., Major, T. W., & Yefimova, M. (2021). Operationalizing a pandemic-ready, telemedicine-enabled drive-through and walk-in coronavirus disease garage care system as an alternative care area: A novel approach in pandemic

management. *Journal of Emergency Nursing, 47*(5), 721–732. https://doi.org/10.1016/j.jen.2021.05.010

Calton, B., Abedini, N., & Fratkin, M. (2020). Telemedicine in the time of coronavirus. *Journal of Pain and Symptom Management, 60*(1), e12–e14. https://doi.org/10.1016/j.jpainsymman.2020.03.019

Center for Connected Health Policy. (2017). *State telehealth laws and reimbursement policies: A comprehensive scan of the 50 states and District of Columbia.*

Center for Connected Health Policy. (2020, May 14). *After COVID-19: What stays, what goes?* [Video]. YouTube. https://www.youtube.com/watch?reload59&v5xjLsGyhHZC0&feature5youtu.be

Centers for Disease Control and Prevention. (2021). *Underlying cause of death; 1999–2020 results: Deaths occurring through 2020.* https://wonder.cdc.gov/controller/datarequest/D76;jsessionid52CC6E20B8DEDB038D5CBAC0A1063#Citation

Centers for Medicare and Medicaid Services. (2018). *Telehealth Services, Medicare Learning Network Booklet, ICN 901705.*

Chaet, D., Clearfield, R., Sabin, J., Skimming, K., & Sabin, J. E. (2017). Ethical practice in telehealth and telemedicine. *JGIM: Journal of General Internal Medicine, 32*(10), 1136–1140. https://doi-org.unh.idm.oclc.org/10.1007/s11606-017-4082-2

Colbert, G. B., Lerma, E. V., & Venegas-Vera, A. V. (2020). Utility of telemedicine in the COVID-19 era. *Reviews in Cardiovascular Medicine, 21*(4), 583. https://doi.org/10.31083/j.rcm.2020.04.188

Cormi, C., Chrusciel, J., Laplanche, D., Dramé, M., & Sanchez, S. (2020). Telemedicine in nursing homes during the COVID-19 outbreak: A star is born (again). *Geriatrics & Gerontology International, 20*(6), 646–647. https://doi.org/10.1111/ggi.13934

Cuffaro, L., Di Lorenzo, F., Bonavita, S., Tedeschi, G., Leocani, L., & Lavorgna, L. (2020). Dementia care and covid-19 pandemic: A necessary digital revolution. *Neurological Sciences, 41*(8), 1977–1979. https://doi.org/10.1007/s10072-020-04512-4

Doorenbos, A., Jang Min, K., Li, H., & Lally, R. (2020). eHealth education. *Clinical Journal of Oncology Nursing, 24*(3), 42–48. https://doi.org/10.29271/jcpsp.2020.12.1243

Fang, J. L., Collura, C. A., Johnson, R. V., Assay, G. F., Cary, W. A., Derleth, D. P., Lang, T. R., Kroefsky, B. L., & Colby, C. E. (2016). Emergency video telemedicine consultation for newborn resuscitations. *Mayo Clinic Proceedings, 91*(12), 1735–1743. https://doi.org/10.1016/j.mayocp.2016.08.006

Gleason, K., & Suen, J. J. (2022). Going beyond affordability for digital equity: Closing the "digital divide" through outreach and training programs for older adults. *Journal of the American Geriatrics Society, 70*(1), 75–77. https://doi.org/10.1111/jgs.17511

Han, J. H., Collar, E. M., Lassen-Greene, C., Self, W. H., Langford, R. W., & Jackson, J. C. (2020). Feasibility of videophone-assisted neuropsychological testing for intensive care unit survivors. *American Journal of Critical Care, 29*(5), 398–402. https://doi.org/10.4037/ajcc2020492

H.R. 4374—117th Congress (2021–2022): Broadband Internet Connections for Rural America Act. (January 21, 2022). https://www.congress.gov/bill/117th-congress/house-bill/4374

Jani, P. D., Forbes, L., Choudhury, A., Preisser, J. S., Viera, A. J., & Garg, S. (2017). Evaluation of diabetic retinal screening factors for ophthalmology referral in a telemedicine network. *JAMA Ophthalmology, 135*(7), 706–714. https://doi.org/10.1001/jamaophthalmol.2017.1150

Kalanlar, B. (2022). Nursing education in the pandemic: A cross-sectional international study. *Nurse Education Today, 108,* 105213. https://doi.org/10.1016/j.nedt.2021.105213

Kaplow, R., & Zellinger, M. (2021). Nurses' perceptions of telemedicine adoption in the intensive care unit. *American Journal of Critical Care, 30*(2), 122–127. https://doi.org/10.4037/ajcc2021205

Knudson, A., Anderson, B., Schieler, K., & Arsen, E. (2017). *Home is where the heart is—insights on the coordination and delivery of home health services in rural America* (pp. 1–9) [Policy Brief]. Rural Health Reform Policy Research Center. https://ruralhealth.und.edu/assets/480-1335/home-is-where-the-heart-is.pdf

Ladin, K., Porteny, T., Perugini, J. M., Gonzales, K. M., Aufort, K. E., Levine, S. K., Wong, J. B., Isakova, T., Rifkin, D., Gordon, E. J., Rossi, A., Koch-Weser, S., & Weiner, D. E. (2021). Perceptions of telehealth vs. in-person visits among older adults with advanced kidney disease, care partners, and clinicians. *JAMA Network Open, 4*(12), e2137193. https://doi.org/10.1001/jamanetworkopen.2021.37193

Langabeer, J. R., II., Gonzales, M., Alqusairi, D., Champagne-Langabeer, T., Jackson, A., Mikail, J., & Persee, D. (2016). Telehealth-enabled emergency medical services program reduces ambulance transport to urban emergency departments. *Western Journal of Emergency Medicine, 17*(6), 713–720. https://doi.org/10.5811/westjem.2016.8.30660

Loeb, A., Rao, S., Ficke, J., Morris, C., Riley, L., & Levin, A. (2020). Departmental experience and lessons learned with accelerated introduction of telemedicine during the COVID-19 crisis. *The Journal of the American Academy of Orthopaedic Surgeons, 28*(11), e469–e476. https://doi.org/10.5435/JAAOS-D-20-00380

Mehrotra, A., Ray, K., Brockmeyer, D., Barnett, M., & Bender, J. (2020, April 1). Rapidly converting to "virtual practices": Outpatient care in the era of Covid-19. *NEJM Catalyst.* https://catalyst.nejm.org/doi/full/10.1056/CAT.20.0091

Nagel, D. A., Stacey, D., Momtahan, K., Gifford, W., Doucet, S., & Etowa, J. B. (2017). Getting a picture: A grounded theory of nurses knowing the person in a virtual environment. *Journal of Holistic Nursing, 35*(1), 67–85. https://doi.org/10.1177/0898010116645422

National Committee for Quality Assurance National Quality Forum. (2017). *Creating a framework to support measure for telehealth.* National Quality Forum. https://www.ncqa.org/newsroom/details/ncqa-updates-quality-measures-for-hedis-2018?ArtMID511280&ArticleID585&tabid52659

National Consortium of Telehealth Resource Centers. (2022). *About us.* https://telehealthresourcecenter.org/about-us/

National Organization of Nurse Practitioner Faculty. (2018). *Position paper: NONPF supports telehealth in nurse practitioner education. Position paper: NONPF supports telehealth in nurse practitioner education.* http://www.nonpf.org/news/388719/NONPF-Statement-in-Support-of-Telehealth-in-NP-Education.htm

Patel, P., Cobb, J., Wright, D., Turer, R., Jordan, T., Humphrey, A., Kepner, A., Smith, G., & Rosenbloom, T. (2020). Rapid development of telehealth capabilities within pediatric patient portal infrastructure for COVID-19 care: Barriers, solutions, results. *Journal of the American Medical Informatics Association, 27*(7), 1116–1120. https://doi.org/10.1093/jamia/ocaa065

Powell, R. E., Henstenburg, B. S., Cooper, G., Hollander, J. E., & Rising, K. L. (2017). Patient perceptions of telehealth primary care video visits. *Annals of Family Medicine, 15*(3), 225–229. https://doi.org/10.2196/15682

Project ECHO. (2018). *Project ECHO: A revolution in medical education and care delivery.* https://echo.unm.edu/

Reach Health. (2018). *2018 U.S. Telemedicine industry benchmark survey.* https://reachhealth.com/resources/telemedicine-industry-survey/

Rutledge, C. M., O'Rourke, J., Mason, A. M., Chike-Harris, K., Behnke, L., Melhado, L., Downes, L., & Gustin, T. (2021). Telehealth competencies for nursing education and practice: The four P's of telehealth. *Nurse Educator, 46*(5), 300–305. https://doi.org/10.1097/NNE.0000000000000988

Sacks, D. A., Grant, D. L., Macias, M., Xia, L., & Lawrence, J. M. (2017). The virtual office visit for women with gestational diabetes mellitus. *Diabetes Care, 40*(3), e34–e35. https://doi.org/10.2337/dc16-2569

Seifert, A., Batsis, J. A., & Smith, A. C. (2020). Telemedicine in long-term care facilities during and beyond Covid-19: Challenges caused by the digital divide. *Frontiers in Public Health, 8,* 1–5. https://doi.org/10.3389/fpubh.2020.601595

Sharma, R., Gordon, J., Greenwald, P., Hsu, H., Coyne, S., Deland, E. L., & Fleischut, P. (2017). *Revolutionizing the delivery of care for ED patients.* NEJM Catalyst. https://catalyst.nejm.org/telehealth-express-care-service-revolutionizing-ed-care/

Swensen, E. (2014, January 6). *Using tablets, telemedicine to speed stroke treatment.* UVA Today. http://news.virginia.edu/content/using-tablets-telemedicine-speed-stroke-treatment

U.S. Department of Health and Human Services. (2022). *Strategic plan FY 2022–2026.* https://www.hhs.gov/about/strategic-plan/index.html

20

Health Care Quality and Safety

Andrew Kopolow, MPA, MSW, CPHQ, PMP, CLSSMBB, FNAHQ,
Rebeca M. Almanza, MBA, LPN, CPHQ, and
Karen J. Saewert, PhD, RN, CPHQ, ANEF

 http://evolve.elsevier.com/Friberg/bridge/

OBJECTIVES

After completion of this chapter, the reader will be able to:
1. Recognize the predominant health care quality and safety (HCQS) principles and models.
2. Reflect on how culture can play a pivotal role in communication and change management to optimize the quality and safety of health care delivery and outcomes.
3. Examine the relationship between organizational structure and culture.
4. Summarize the purpose and use of select HCQS tools.
5. Discuss the relationship between the concepts, practices, and principles of HCQS and multilevel health care outcomes.

INTRODUCTION

In the two decades since the Institute of Medicine (IOM) released its shocking estimate that between 44,000 and 98,000 hospitalized patients die each year due to error (St. Pierre et al., 2022), the health care industry has taken dramatic and far-reaching steps to improve quality and reduce risk. Legislation was enacted, regulatory agencies created, safety campaigns launched. Technological advancements have reduced risk to safety. At the same time, health care has become more complicated. New specialties, care models, and treatment modalities have presented a challenge for health care quality and safety (HCQS) to keep pace. Yet wrong-site surgeries continue to occur. Medication errors continue to fester. Patients continue to die as a result of the very thing they hoped would heal them. Health care costs continue to rise, as has the inherent waste associated with poor quality. About a trillion dollars each year is estimated to come from waste in our health care system (Bueno et al., 2019; Shrank et al., 2019). This particular point is salient as health care organizations are filing for bankruptcy at alarming rates (Enumah & Chang, 2021) with the effect of increasing access to care difficulties for those communities.

Bleak as this may seem, the drive toward improving quality and safety in health care continues. And for nurses operating in today's health care environment, it is particularly important to understand the principles, tools, and implications of HCQS which we will briefly cover in the following pages.

Framework

This chapter uses the Donabedian model, a predominant and time-honored conceptual model, to discuss HCQS concepts, principles, and practices (models) relevant to present-day nursing and collaborative team-based health professions' practice and care delivery. The Donabedian model draws connections between the manner in which care is delivered (structure), interactions between patients and providers (process), and the effects of health care on the health status of patients and populations (outcomes). Although its conceptual origins can be traced back to the 1960s (Donabedian, 2005), it not only remains highly relevant but is far more appreciated now than at the time of its inception (Berwick & Fox, 2016).

The health care industry has long understood the connection between process and outcomes (i.e., what we do to help patients and how they respond), but less consideration is given to the organizational structure on which processes are built (Singer, 2021). Developing awareness and knowledge about the interconnectivity between structure, process, and outcome enhances your ability to impact multilevel outcomes (e.g., micro [individual-level], meso [group-level], macro [society-level]), directly and indirectly.

The *Structure* section examines HCQS from the perspective of organizational structure. The *Process* section builds on this foundation by reviewing select tools used to understand and improve systems and outcomes alike. As this chapter concludes, the *Outcomes* section explores expanding the scope of responsibilities for practitioners and how HCQS practices improve the quality of care. As you progress through the following pages, reflect on your time in health care and the many risks to safety and health care quality you have undoubtedly observed (Box 20.1). Then ask yourself: what could have been improved, and how?

STRUCTURE

From the HCQS perspective, *structure* (or *organizational structure*) refers to the individual components that influence, enable, or detract from effective processes and desired outcomes. Everything from whom we hire to how we communicate to the technologies we adopt to the cultures we permit or promote falls into this space. Broad as it may be, the two specific elements that merit attention are culture and communication.

Culture

Consider for a moment a time when you spotted an ongoing safety risk or improvement opportunity. Reflect on what you did at the time and why. Did you feel empowered to give it visibility? If you brought it up, was it addressed in a meaningful way? Did you feel like you would get into trouble if you brought it up or, perhaps worse, did you feel like you would be ignored? Your answers speak to that organization's culture.

Culture can be thought of as the manifestation of an organization's values. It influences everything we do and how we do it. Our behaviors (e.g., the way we communicate) and our beliefs (e.g., why we communicate the way we do) stem from the importance or apathy organizations place on a given concept. Think of your organization's mission and/or vision statements. Do your observations of coworkers and extended team members match these ideals, or is there a stark contrast between the values the

---

BOX 20.1 Case Illustration

In 2017, a nurse at Vanderbilt University Medical Center in Nashville, Tennessee, administered what would turn out to be a fatal dose of the wrong medication (Sofer, 2019). An investigation by the Centers for Medicare and Medicaid Services (CMS) found multiple significant deficiencies in the institution's policies and practices related to the incident. From a patient safety perspective, this event—though tragic—is not surprising. Medication errors, even those resulting in patient mortality, are unfortunately common. The significant public attention this case has garnered prompted inclusion of this case illustration in this chapter due to the unusual step taken by prosecutors to file criminal charges against the nurse (i.e., reckless homicide and impaired adult abuse). Apart from the nurse's individual role, the premise that the institution could have taken steps to prevent the patient's death seems largely unimpeachable, although system failures in this case have been readily identified. The Tri-Council for Nursing, comprised of the American Association of Colleges of Nursing (AACN), American Nurses Association (ANA), American Organization of Nurse Executives (AONE), and the National League for Nursing (NLN), stated:

Rarely are errors the fault of an individual; rather, they are the culmination of characteristics of systems of care. Rather than attach blame to individuals for errors committed, organizations must design nonpunitive approaches to error and look well beyond individual providers to understand and redesign system-level processes for error prevention (American Association of Colleges of Nursing [AACN], 2020, para. 1).

The nurse's 2022 conviction spurred renewed outcry over how the situation was handled. The ANA stated that, given the complexity of health care delivery, it is inevitable that mistakes will happen and systems will fail (ANA, 2022). This complexity is reflected in the sophisticated, dynamic, high technology-driven environment that includes high-stakes decisions and levels of risk. The American Hospital Association (AHA) voiced that nurses and other health care providers must be encouraged to report errors (AHA, 2022). The NLN reaffirmed their belief that it is vital to support a just culture that emphasizes individual accountability for misconduct or gross negligence within an environment where individuals can report errors and organizations can improve processes to promote HCQS (NLN, 2022).

HCQS, Health care quality and safety.

organization espouses and the behaviors you observe? A strong culture will *walk the walk* in terms of alignment with stated principles. Though the difficulty in engineering this type of culture cannot be understated, it is recognized as a meaningful step toward achieving HCQS objectives of reducing waste, improving safety, and driving outcomes (Braun et al., 2020; Mannion & Smith, 2018).

Just Cultures and High Reliability

The *Just Culture* model was created to overcome the *culture of blame* and fear-based action, widely recognized as drivers for underreporting of safety risks and health care errors. A focus on learning from mistakes—coupled with an orientation toward future improvement—replaces punitive-oriented behavior. In other words, *just cultures* shift away from the individual and toward failures in systems design. Employees have the psychological safety needed to freely report risks and errors, with the intent of ultimately improving the system (Churruca et al., 2021; Foslien-Nash & Reed, 2020).

High Reliability Organizations (HROs) build on *just culture* principles with a framework that integrates continuous improvement practices and full-throated commitment from its leadership (Oster & Braaten, 2021). HROs are known for their *preoccupation with failure, reluctance to simplify, situation awareness, deference to frontline expertise,* and *commitment to resilience* (Agency for Healthcare Research and Quality [AHRQ], 2019a, 2019b). Not only do organizations that commit to high reliability principles demonstrably improve quality and safety (Cruz & Mick, 2020), but research suggests they also reduce workplace burnout (Isaacks et al., 2021). Of course, it is far easier to declare your organization has high reliability or a just culture than it is to demonstrate it. Table 20.1 offers a few examples of how nurses operating within an HRO framework might behave. As you look over the scenarios, think about how the situation might be handled in your own organization. The goal is not to judge. No organization perfectly emulates HRO ideals. Instead, this exercise offers an opportunity to understand where an organization falls in relation to HRO archetype (i.e., pattern or model) behavior.

Teamwork and Communication

Nurses are part of an expansive clinical team responsible for the provision and coordination of care. As the definition of what constitutes a clinical team has evolved to include individuals well beyond one's organizational structure, so has demand for effective communication and collaboration across professional disciplines, teams, departments, and organizations. Your nursing background is one of several factors that influences how you communicate and whether your communication has the desired effect. The modern-day workplace has up to five generations working together, spanning globally diverse socioeconomic and cultural backgrounds with wide-ranging practices that can significantly influence how we send and interpret information, verbal and nonverbal alike. Communication can prevent or contribute to medical errors, it can bolster or undermine clinical pathways, it can reaffirm or damage relationships, and it can strengthen or degrade organizational culture, which, in turn, can impact quality improvement initiatives and, by extension, patient and population outcomes (Kumra et al. 2020; Walter et al., 2019). See Chapter 8 for further discussion on interprofessional collaboration, teamwork, and communication.

Emails, instant messages, group chats, team meetings, kanban boards, committee meetings, intranet sites, and even clinical documentation are among the many ways in which we communicate. Each has a specific or desired purpose, requiring as much, if not greater, sensitivity to the inherent complexities of nurse-to-nurse or nurse-to-patient verbal interactions. And like any tool, these carry risk if used improperly. Imagine receiving an email notifying you that your clinical team was being disbanded and redeployed. How would you react to seeing a group chat that included a link to a series of major changes to several critical care transition protocols?

To effectively manage its impact on processes and desired outcomes, organizations have leveraged *structured communication* practices. Two of the more common examples are SBAR and team huddles. SBAR (*S*ituation, *B*ackground, *A*ssessment, *R*ecommendation) is a well-established communication approach used to deliver a succinct burst of information regarding a decision that needs to be made. As illustrated in Box 20.2, this formulaic approach is a method for conveying only the most critical information succinctly, comprehensively, and predictably. Though it is compatible with a variety of communication approaches (e.g., email, face to face) and contexts (e.g., patient care and change management), its value as a communication tool is best realized when adopted uniformly across a team. Instead of relying on the recipient to interpret a message, the onus is on the sender to construct a message without ambiguity. Adoption of the SBAR structured approach to communication has repeatedly demonstrated improvement in quality, safety, and outcomes measures (Abbaszade et al., 2021; Choi & Chang, 2021; Lee et al., 2016; Shahid & Sumesh, 2018; Uhm et al., 2019).

Setting and cadence are also components of structured communication practices worthy of discussion, both of which are illustrated in *team huddles*. The term "huddle" is derived from a term used in sports and signifies a very brief meeting period where an entire team gathers together to coordinate the next "play." In a health care setting, huddles,

TABLE 20.1 High Reliability Organization Scenarios

Situation	HRO Behavior	Explanation
A nurse observes a surgeon about to enter the operating theater and is not sure if the surgeon has washed their hands.	The nurse stops the surgeon from entering the operating theater to ask if they had washed their hands. The surgeon replies that they have and thanks the nurse for checking.	Historical power differentials between surgeons and nurses may create a barrier to ensuring patient safety during high-risk situations. A nurse may not feel as if it is their "place" to question a surgeon on hand hygiene. In an HRO, such questions are not only permitted, but expected. Whether the question is coming from a nurse, surgeon, or environmental services staff, there is no hierarchy when it comes to safety.
A primary care physician orders immunizations for a 6-month-old child using an electronic health record system. A nurse believes that a standard immunization may have been overlooked.	The nurse asks the primary care physician if the immunization in question should be included. The physician acknowledges the error (i.e., near miss) and amends the order. The clinical team leader later conducts an RCA to identify how the near miss could have happened. After further discussion with other teams, the organization implements a standardized bundled immunization ordering process in their electronic health record system.	HRO staff are empowered to speak up in the name of quality care. HROs are not just focused on preventing patient harm, but ensuring a positive patient experience of care. Quality improvement tools (e.g., RCAs, FMEAs) are routinely used by HROs to identify and prioritize safety improvement opportunities.
An emergency room physician orders a CT with contrast. A nurse conducts a medication review in the electronic health record system and notes that the patient is prescribed to take metformin on a daily basis, contraindicated in CT with contrast procedures.	The nurse asks the emergency tool physician if they are aware that the patient takes metformin on a daily basis. The physician responds, indicating the medication was not listed on the intake form and thanks the nurse for conducting the medication review. The physician wants to make sure that his, or a similar situation, does not occur again. The physician and nurse use the 5 Whys tool to uncover what went wrong and discover that there is a lag time between when medications are recorded manually during the intake process and when they are entered into the electronic health record system.	Instinctive as it may be to breathe a sigh of relief when patient harm is prevented through the diligence of nurses and other health care professionals, HROs treat such situations far differently. Their preoccupation with failure ensures that a "good catch" such as the one in this example is addressed no differently than if the event had resulted in patient harm. Quality improvement tools (e.g., 5 Whys) are routinely used by HROs to understand the underlying risk factors, with the hope of preventing a similar event from occurring in the future.

FMEA, Failure modes and effects analysis; *HRO,* high reliability organizations; *RCA,* root cause analysis.

similar to surgical *time outs,* are often used to address highly localized topics such as transitions of care (referred to as *transition huddles*) or safety concerns (safety huddles). Similar to SBAR, huddles are designed for succinct yet comprehensive and predictable communication patterns.

Though we have seen proliferation of use and scope of huddles in recent years, their utility as a mechanism for clear, predictable pathways of communication across team members remains intact (Croke, 2020; Lamming et al., 2021; Robertson-Malt et al., 2020; Walter et al., 2019).

BOX 20.2   Structured Versus Unstructured Communication

Nurse to Physician Verbal Communication: Unstructured

I was chatting with the patient in Room 1254 and I noticed some bumps around her lower neck.

I don't think it was there until about 15 minutes ago when I checked on her.

I asked her about it and she said she hadn't noticed, but she started scratching at her chest.

I asked if I could take a look and noticed she had hives all over her chest and back.

It might have something to do with the antibiotics we gave her for strep about half an hour ago.

Nurse to Physician Verbal Communication: SBAR

Situation: The patient in Room 1254 has hives all over her chest and back. She confirms that she has no known medication allergies.

Background: She tested positive for strep this morning and was given oral antibiotics 30 minutes ago.

Assessment: She may be having an allergic reaction to one or more of the antibiotics or the strep-related infection.

Recommendation: I recommend we administer an antihistamine immediately.

Huddles and SBAR are not the only forms of structured communication. Other methods, such as *closed-loop communication*, repeating back what someone just said (the same process as in your local coffee shops and restaurants), are taught and used throughout health care to reduce the risk of miscommunication (Blankenship, 2020). Collectively, their consistent use can reduce risk while reinforcing teamwork, organizational culture, and underlying values. There is little doubt you have experienced situations in which communication was unclear or entirely absent. How could a structured communication have helped? Was your organizational structure similar to an HRO's structure? What opportunity areas can you think of to support nurses in your organization through adoption of the principles outlined in this section?

PROCESS

Improving Health Care Processes

In this section, we examine a few tools commonly used to identify and prioritize risk, to understand cause and effect, and to organize improvement strategies. As a member of multidisciplinary and interprofessional teams, nurses are integral to both understanding why quality and safety risks exist and identifying ways in which the organization can improve and ultimately deliver quality patient care.

Key Tools. *What can go wrong will go wrong* is Murphy's Law in a nutshell. At first glance, it seems pessimistic, but in actuality this statement highlights possibility. Possibility to:

- analyze data and processes or to reflect on near misses, never events, or even the mere chance of a never event; and
- identify and plan for improvement.

Possibility is exciting, and coming up with improvement ideas can be fun, but there is a major difference between an improvement idea and its implementation. Each carries a cost and a benefit, both of which can be difficult to understand, which is why making sure you have a formal process for gathering information is essential. Information on size and scope of a future risk (or a solution), the organizational investment, and the time and resource commitment are all elements of a preliminary data and information collection process. Quality tools give you the foundation to begin to build your structure. As you utilize these tools and formulate ideas or make decisions, the structure starts to come together and turns into something you can act on. Regardless of which tool is used, they all lead down a pathway of comprehension, communication, and improvement of processes.

Review Table 20.2 to learn about some key quality tools and visit the internet addresses provided with each tool to explore examples or templates. While you review this table, think about your own clinical experience. Was there a time one of these tools would have been beneficial to use? If so, how would you have applied it?

Do any of these tools sound familiar? If so, what was your experience using these tools? If you have never used them before, can you think of how you can begin using these? There are a multitude of quality tools available (Healthy Simulation, 2020). The beauty of these tools is the ability to adapt them to fit your needs. Fig. 20.1 provides a sample template that might be used to determine *which* quality tool in *what* specific setting, given *what* specific scenario, could address *what* desired outcome. This sample template can be used to address Critical Thinking Exercise #7 found at the end of this chapter. Whether you use the tools in Table 20.2 or one of the many other tools available to you, what matters is a structured approach to improvement. Take a look at your organization and see what tools they encourage you to use.

TABLE 20.2 Quality Improvement Tools

Tool	Description	Internet Address
Plan-Do-Study-Act (PDSA)	The Agency for Healthcare Research and Quality describes PDSA as "a method to test a change that is implemented" (Agency for Healthcare Research and Quality [AHRQ], 2020). The reason PDSA is a great tool to test change is that a PDSA is a continuous cycle. Once you know what your initiative will be, you can start the cycle. You will plan, do, and study your initiative and then do it all over again by acting on any changes needed or by implementing your initiative in your entire organization.	https://www.ahrq.gov/health-literacy/improve/precautions/tool2b.html
Failure Modes and Effects Analysis (FMEA)	FMEA is a tool used to proactively identify how a process might fail. It asks: What can go wrong, how often can it go wrong, how severe are the consequences if it goes wrong, and how easy is it to know when it goes wrong (Institute for Healthcare Improvement [IHI], 2017a)? The FMEA is a form of organized brainstorming that allows you to prioritize potential risks with the intent of mitigating or eliminating them before patient harm occurs.	http://www.ihi.org/resources/Pages/Tools/FailureModesandEffectsAnalysisTool.aspx
Root Cause Analysis (RCA)	This tool is used to understand why an event occurred. It asks: what were the contributing factors and circumstances that resulted in an error and/or harm (VHA National Center for Patient Safety, 2021)? RCAs are important not to place blame, but to understand.	https://www.patientsafety.va.gov/docs/RCA-Guidebook_02052021.pdf
Fishbone Diagram	Assists with brainstorming to identify possible causes of a problem and sorts ideas into categories (Center for Medicare and Medicaid Services [CMS], 2022), also referred to as a cause-and-effect diagram. This tool aims to get a better understanding of contributing factors or drivers of problems/issues.	https://www.cms.gov/medicare/provider-enrollment-and-certification/qapi/downloads/fishbonerevised.pdf
5 Whys	This is a simple tool, with the sole purpose of *better understanding why a problem exists*. It assumes the most visible reason for a problem is actually a symptom of something else. It asks for a deeper understanding of a given situation instead of taking action on the most visible reason. Ask "why" five times to identify the underlying cause (Institute of Healthcare Improvement [IHI], 2018).	https://mssic.org/wp-content/uploads/2020/04/5-Whys-Tool.pdf
Run Chart	Run Charts are used to visualize process behavior trends over time (Institute for Healthcare Improvement [IHI], 2017b). They allow us to more easily identify patterns (e.g., increases in emergency department average length of stay over the past 6 months) or significant outliers (e.g., a "spike" in reported medical errors). They can be used as a precursor or "trigger" for conducting a Root Cause Analysis and PDCA improvement project.	

For information on additional health care quality tools, we encourage you to explore the Institute for Healthcare Improvement's QI Toolkit (n.d.) available via this link: http://www.ihi.org/resources/Pages/Tools/Quality-Improvement-Essentials-Toolkit.aspx

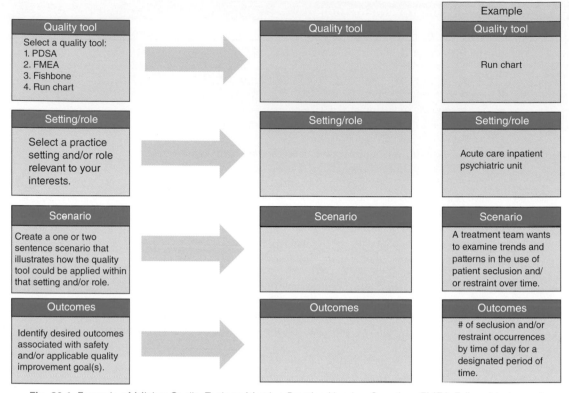

Fig. 20.1 Example of Mixing Quality Tools to Match a Practice Need or Question. *FMEA*, Failure Modes and Effects Analysis; *PDSA*, Plan-Do-Study-Act.

Value of Reporting

As discussed earlier, *To Err Is Human* was published nearly a quarter-century ago, yet it continues to inspire a shift in mindset away from individual fault for most medical errors, replacing it with one oriented toward systems and processes (St. Pierre et al., 2022). It is the system that failed, not the individual. Yet visibility of risks and incident reporting remain a concern. The World Health Organization (WHO) estimates each year about 134 million adverse events occur worldwide (World Health Organization, 2019). High as this is, it only takes into consideration the adverse events, but what about near misses? What about the time someone accidentally almost administered a medication because the bottle looked the same? Reporting something as seemingly inconsequential as that can yield the insight needed to move from a reactive stance (taking action only when a safety event occurs) to a proactive one (taking action to prevent a safety event from occurring). We can learn and grow without a trigger event.

Let's take a medication scenario mentioned earlier in this chapter. If someone almost accidentally administered a medication (i.e., a near miss) because it looked like the bottle of another medication, chances are others could do the same, and there is no guarantee the next time it happens, it will be prevented. If the risk isn't visible, a near miss can turn into an actual event.

Adverse events, though unwanted, are still opportunities to review the process and see where it went wrong so that it will not happen again. This is where those handy quality tools meet organizational culture. Reporting systems allow clinical teams to identify and assess risk. Yet just like structured communication practices, their value is only realized if used routinely (Birkeli et al., 2021). Many times we utilize these quality tools to review our processes and superficially determine where we went wrong, but we stop at the surface. We fail to get to the root of the problem because the answer may lie in deeply rooted processes (Schiff & Shojania, 2021). We need to ask ourselves, would we rather learn from a *near miss* that was reported, or a *never event* that resulted in a patient's death?

Health Data

Health care data are collections of patient information including, but not limited to, demographics, diagnoses, past medical history, medical visit/billing information, and results (NEJM Catalyst, 2018). Health data is stored in an electronic health record; some can be found in registries, third-party repositories, and payor systems, to name a few (Sylvia & Vigil, 2021). Some of the most critical health care data are generated from nurses, like you. Make no mistake, your documentation plays a pivotal role in the process of making informed decisions about health care, quality, safety, and improvement opportunities. As a nurse, you have likely often heard the saying, "If it wasn't documented, it wasn't done." To take this a step further, if you don't document it, health care providers and leaders are making decisions based on incomplete information. Cumbersome and time-consuming as it can feel in the moment, your documentation may have profoundly significant consequences stretching well beyond seemingly mundane tasks such as capturing an accurate blood pressure. A few examples of where your documentation might be present include:

- Malpractice case chart audits
- Billing validations closing care gaps (e.g., diabetic eye exam)
- Communication between providers
- Information sharing with public health entities (e.g., state vaccination registries)

Can you think of other reasons why your documentation may be used or reviewed? Next time you feel overwhelmed with documenting, take a moment to reflect on the impact your documentation can have in the health care industry.

Human Factors Engineering

According to the AHRQ, *Human Factors Engineering* (HFE attempts to identify human strengths and limitations in their interactions with systems, tools, and technology to ensure patient safety (AHRQ, 2019b). In other words, HFE seeks to understand how a person could make a mistake and then takes steps to eliminate the possibility. It is used in a variety of ways such as

- Usability testing of systems or equipment under real-world conditions or to see if there are potential workarounds.
- Forcing functions aimed at preventing unintended or undesirable actions, or allowing actions only after something is performed first (e.g., password).
- Standardization for ensuring standard process exists across organizations (e.g., policies, regulations).
- Resiliency efforts designed to anticipate and manage unexpected risk events.

BOX 20.3   Hypothetical Case Scenario

At Bing Health care, you must go to the medication room on the other side of the unit to gather patient medications before administration. To save time, you decide to gather the medications needed from the medication room for all your patients. You are not the only nurse who does this, and recently the organization has seen an increase in medication administration errors. There is an issue with the process: It is not feasible to have nurses walk back and forth to the medication room between patients. To solve this issue, the hospital purchases a medication scanning system equipped with a rolling medication cart. You now can get your medications ready for your patients on the cart and scan the wristband of the patient against the medications to ensure medications are being administered to the correct patient.

When you think of HFE, consider the hypothetical example in Box 20.3 on medication administration.

Considering human factors and following some of the principles outlined above to review human factors leads to better patient outcomes. Can you think of a workaround developed in your current workplace? If so, consider reviewing this workaround and perhaps using a quality tool to see how you can solve the issue. Remember, it is not about placing blame but about working as a team to improve the process. As frontline staff, giving attention to the concept of HFE is important. Organizations rely on your insights to be able to learn from them and act on them. HFE is everyone's responsibility and your expertise can help engineer better processes that take human factors into account, even when advances in technology (e.g., new medical devices) do not.

In the past 15 years, a concept built on the foundation of HFE has been developed and is known as the *Systems Engineering Initiative for Patient Safety* (SEIPS). This model takes into account systems engineering, HFE, and quality engineering and provides seven simple tools to apply and adapt for specific projects (Holden & Carayon, 2021). As time evolves—so do concepts—but the aim of these concepts is the same, figuring out a way to increase HCQS.

OUTCOME

Organizational structure (e.g., culture, communication, colleagues, committees) can provide a sense of purpose, an orientation toward learning, and a direction toward improvement. Quality tools and effective change management can leverage these three attributes to gain a holistic understanding of why our emergency departments have long wait times, or why patients are readmitted, or why wrong-site surgeries are still a threat to patient well-being. Your awareness of these issues and concerted effort to understand their underlying causes are the first steps toward improving how care is provided and, ultimately, health outcomes. As critically important as internal process improvement might be toward this end, HCQS has taken on an ever-expanding, macro-level view that has augmented patient health with population health.

Population Health is defined by Thomas Jefferson University's College of Population Health as "the large-scale social, economic, and environmental issues that impact health outcomes of groups of people. Population health can also be defined more narrowly as specific interventions to address the health needs of attributed and discretely defined subpopulations" (2023, para. 3). Our ability to further drive health outcomes is no longer solely dependent upon understanding our own processes and the data generated within our own organizations. With the shift toward value-based care, organizations are incentivized to explore the impacts of social determinants of health

and specialized treatment approaches for targeted sub-populations (Djukic et al., 2021).

Historically, we may rely on approved clinical pathways for patients with a given diagnosis, but this added layer demands further understanding of how individuals with unique attributes benefit from a treatment approach. Today's health care industry expects a far more individualized treatment approach based not only on guidance for patients with that condition but also on patients with that condition and living in that zip code, with that type of job and social support network, etc. In other words, a holistic perspective—focused on value and personalized care—is necessary (Jasemi et al., 2017).

The dominance of nurses in clinical care places them, places you, in a position to support the kind of change that allows the structure needed to not only drive internal process improvements to improve quality and safety but also leverage the kind of macro-level data to drive patient and population health outcomes (Tschannen et al., 2021). Your first steps are awareness and understanding (what is happening and why?).

SUMMARY

In this chapter's introduction, we encouraged you to consider your experience and/or current employment and ask yourself: What could have been improved, and how? How did you respond? What came to mind?

The goal of this chapter is twofold: knowledge and empowerment. It is critical for you to understand the important role you play in HCQS and feel empowered to make conscious efforts to apply the concepts and practices discussed. Enhancing your HCQS knowledge and skill contributes to improved safety, quality care, and health outcomes. You can start by seeking a better understanding of your organizational structures and processes. How do they compare to ideals outlined in preceding chapters?

Reflecting on the highly visible event at Vanderbilt University Medical Center outlined in Box 20.1, how do you imagine an organization with a just culture might have handled the situation? How might you handle a similar situation if your colleague was involved? How would you want to talk about it? What if it was you?

Together, we can drive improvement and conversations to: examine errors, take corrective action about near misses and never events, increase conversations about health care system contributions to HCQS, and establish effective and just system improvement mechanisms to improve health and health care outcomes.

SALIENT POINTS

- Communication, teamwork, and culture are intertwined at a fundamental level and a part of the organization's structure.
- A strong organizational culture can strengthen quality and ultimately improve health outcomes.
- Improvement begins with understanding. Quality tools can aid this process and build on it to support effective change management.
- We can't prevent an error if the risk isn't reported. We can't make informed decisions based on incomplete

data sets. Nurses can make a difference in both through documentation.
- HFE anticipates how people can make a mistake and builds protections against those possibilities into the design.
- Holistic care requires a holistic perspective. Social determinant data and population data can help drive individual outcomes and, in turn, population outcomes.

CRITICAL THINKING EXERCISES

1. Reflect on the concepts of a just and high-reliability culture and compare these concepts with your current culture.
2. Think about a misunderstanding you have recently encountered in the workplace and apply SBAR to the situation.
3. Given the simplicity of the 5 Whys tool, consider a problem you have recently had and apply the 5 Whys concept to it. What did you take away from it? Did you get to the root of your problem?
4. Consider your clinical experience and think of an example when HFE could have been used to improve patient safety. How was patient care impacted? Was the improvement proactive, to avoid patient harm or a reactive result of patient harm? How might you use human factors knowledge to influence and lessen risk?
5. What does holistic perspective mean to you in terms of HCQS? What are some examples of leveraging a holistic perspective?
6. Discuss the interrelationship between structure, process, and outcome.
7. Mix and Match: Using the examples provided in Fig. 20.1 as a guide, select one of the listed quality tools and designate a practice setting/role of relevance to your practice. Create a one- or two-sentence scenario that illustrates how the quality tool could be applied within that setting. Identify desirable outcomes associated with the safety and/or quality improvement goal(s) of interest.

REFERENCES

Abbaszade, A., Assarroudi, A., Armat, M. R., Stewart, J. J., Rakhshani, M. H., Sefidi, N., & Sahebkar, M. (2021). Evaluation of the impact of handoff based on the SBAR technique on quality of nursing care. *Journal of Nursing Care Quality*, 36(3), E38–E43. https://doi.org/10.1097/NCQ.0000000000000498

Agency for Healthcare Research and Quality. (2019a, September 7). *High reliability*. https://psnet.ahrq.gov/primer/high-reliability

Agency for Healthcare Research and Quality. (2019b, September 7). *Human factors engineering*. https://psnet.ahrq.gov/primer/human-factors-engineering

Agency for Healthcare Research and Quality. (2020, September 20). *Plan-Do-Study-Act (PDSA) directions and examples*. https://www.ahrq.gov/health-literacy/improve/precautions/tool2b.html

American Association of College of Nursing. (2020). *Response to the Institute of Medicine's Report to err is human: Building a safer health system*. https://www.aacnnursing.org/News-Information/Position-Statements-White-Papers/Tri-Council-Sept-2000

American Hospital Association. (2022). *Statement in response to the conviction of nurse RaDonda Vaught*. https://www.aha.org/public-comments/2022-03-29-aonl-statement-response-conviction-nurse-radonda-vaught

American Nurses Association. (2022). *Statement in response to the conviction of nurse RaDonda Vaught*. https://www.nursingworld.org/news/news-releases/2022-news-releases/statement-in-response-to-the-conviction-of-nurse-radonda-vaught/

Berwick, D., & Fox, D. M. (2016). Evaluating the quality of medical care: Donabedian's classic article 50 years later. *The Milbank Quarterly*, 94(2), 237–241. https://doi.org/10.1111/1468-0009.12189

Birkeli, G. H., Jacobsen, H. K., & Ballangrud, R. (2021). Nurses' experience of the incident reporting culture before and after implementing the green cross method: A quality improvement project. *Intensive & Critical Care Nursing*, 69, 103166. https://doi.org/10.1016/j.iccn.2021.103166

Blankenship, J. C. (2020). Communication to cure cath chaos. *Catheterization and Cardiovascular Interventions*, 95(5), E154–E155. https://doi.org/10.1002/ccd.28687

Braun, B. I., Chitavi, S. O., Suzuki H., Soyemi C. A., & Puig-Asensio M. (2020). Impact on improvement in infection prevention process and outcomes. *Current Infectious Disease Reports*, 22(12), 34. https://doi.org/10.1007/s11908-020-00741-y

Bueno, B., Leo, J. D., Macfie, H., & IHI Leadership Alliance. (2019). *Trillion dollar checkbook: Reduce waste and cost in the U.S. health care system*. Institute for Healthcare Improvement. http://www.ihi.org/Engage/collaboratives/LeadershipAlliance/Documents/IHILeadershipAlliance_TrillionDollarCheckbook_ReduceWaste.pdf

Center for Medicare and Medicaid Services. (2022). *How to use the fishbone tool for root cause analysis*. https://www.cms.gov/medicare/provider-enrollment-and-certification/qapi/downloads/fishbonerevised.pdf

Choi, Y. R., & Chang, S. O. (2021). Exploring interprofessional communication during nursing home emergencies using the SBAR framework. *Journal of Interprofessional Care*, 1–8. https://doi.org/10.1080/13561820.2021.1985985

Churruca, K., Ellis, L. A., Pomare, C., Hogden, A., Bierbaum, M., Long, J. C., Olekalns, A., & Braithwaite, J. (2021). Dimensions of safety culture: A systematic review of quantitative, qualitative and mixed methods for assessing safety culture in hospitals. *BMJ Open*, 11(7), e043982. https://doi.org/10.1136/bmjopen-2020-043982

Croke, L. (2020). Safety huddles improve patient safety and quality of care. *AORN Journal*, 112(5), P11–P13. https://doi.org/10.1002/aorn.13259

Cruz, S. S., & Mick, J. (2020). A high reliability organization's use of the evidence-based practice process to eliminate an identified potential for wrong-site surgery. *AORN Journal*, *112*(5), 520–523. https://doi.org/10.1002/aorn.13219

Djukic, M., Mola, A., Keating, S., Melnyk, H., & Haber, J. (2021). E-learning for population health management: An educational innovation to prepare student and practicing nurses for value-based care. *Nursing Education Perspectives*, *42*(6), E117–E119. https://doi.org/10.1097/01.NEP.0000000000000857

Donabedian, A. (2005). Evaluating the quality of medical care. *The Milbank Quarterly*, *83*(4), 691–729. https://doi.org/10.1111/j.1468-0009.2005.00397.x

Enumah, S. J., & Chang, D. C. (2021). Predictors of financial distress among private U.S. hospitals. *The Journal of Surgical Research*, *267*, 251–259. https://doi.org/10.1016/j.jss.2021.05.025

Foslien-Nash, C., & Reed, B. (2020). Just culture is not "just" culture—It's shifting mindset. *Military Medicine*, *185*(Suppl 3), 52–57. https://doi.org/10.1093/milmed/usaa143

Healthy Simulation. (2020, December 23). *IHI quality improvement essentials toolkit helps optimize outcomes.* https://www.healthysimulation.com/29412/ihi-quality-improvement-essentials-toolkit/

Holden, R., & Carayon, P. (2021). SEIPS 101 and seven simple SEIPS tools. *BMJ Quality & Safety*, *30*(11), 901–910. https://dx.doi.org/10.1136/bmjqs-2020-012538

Institute for Healthcare Improvement. (2017a). *Failure modes and effects analysis (FMEA) tool.* http://www.ihi.org/resources/Pages/Tools/FailureModesandEffectsAnalysisTool.aspx

Institute for Healthcare Improvement. (2017b). *QI essentials toolkit: Run chart and control chart.* http://www.ihi.org/resources/Pages/Tools/RunChart.aspx?PostAuthRed=/resources/_layouts/download.aspx?SourceURL=/resources/Knowledge%20Center%20Assets/Tools%20-%20RunChartTool_35cea96e-7360-4db3-94db-9c4640ab759b/QIToolkit_RunChartControlChart.pdf

Institute for Healthcare Improvement. (2018). *5 Whys: Finding the root cause.* https://mssic.org/wp-content/uploads/2020/04/5-Whys-Tool.pdf

Institute for Healthcare Improvement. (n.d.). *Quality improvement essentials toolkit.* http://www.ihi.org/resources/Pages/Tools/Quality-Improvement-Essentials-Toolkit.aspx

Isaacks, D. B., Anderson, T. M., Moore, S. C., Patterson, W., & Govindan, S. (2021). High reliability organization principles improve VA workplace burnout. *American Journal of Medical Quality*, *36*(6), 422–428. https://doi.org/10.1097/01.JMQ.0000735516.35323.97

Jasemi, M., Valizadeh, L., Zamanzadeh, V., & Keogh, B. (2017). A concept analysis of holistic care by hybrid model. *Indian Journal of Palliative Care*, *23*(1), 71–80. https://doi.org/10.4103/0973-1075.197960

Kumra, T., Hsu, Y.-J., Cheng, T. L., Marsteller, J. A., McGuire, M., & Cooper, L. A. (2020). The association between organizational cultural competence and teamwork climate in a network of primary care practices. *Health Care Management Review*,

45(2), 106–116. https://doi.org/10.1097/HMR.0000000000000205

Lamming, L., Montague, J., Crosswaite, K., Faisal, M., McDonach, E., Mohammed, M. A., Cracknell, A., Lovatt, A., & Slater, B. (2021). Fidelity and the impact of patient safety huddles on teamwork and safety culture: An evaluation of the huddle up for safer healthcare (HUSH) project. *BMC Health Services Research*, *21*(1), 1–11. https://doi.org/10.1186/s12913-021-07080-1

Lee, S. Y., Dong, L., Lim, Y. H., Poh, C. L., & Lim, W. S. (2016). SBAR: Towards a common interprofessional team-based communication tool. *Medical Education*, *50*(11), 1167–1168. https://doi.org/10.1111/medu.13171

Mannion, R., & Smith, J. (2018). Hospital culture and clinical performance: Where next? *BMJ Quality & Safety*, *27*(3), 179–181. https://doi.org/10.1136/bmjqs-2017-007668

National League for Nursing. (2022, March 30). *NLN promotes a just culture approach with health care errors.* https://www.nln.org/detail-pages/news/2022/03/30/nln-promotes-a-just-culture-approach-with-health-care-errors

NEJM Catalyst. (2018, January 1). *Healthcare big data and the promise of value-based care.* https://catalyst.nejm.org/doi/full/10.1056/CAT.18.0290

Oster, C. A., & Braaten, J. S. (Eds.). (2021). *High reliability organizations: A healthcare handbook for patient safety & quality* (2nd ed.). Sigma Theta Tau International.

Robertson-Malt, S., Gaddi, F., & Hamilton, A. (2020). Learning huddles: An innovative teaching method. *Nurse Education in Practice*, *47*, 102830. https://doi.org/10.1016/j.nepr.2020.102830

Schiff, G., & Shojania K. G. (2021). Looking back on the history of patient safety: An opportunity to reflect and ponder future challenges. *BMJ Quality & Safety*, *31*(2), 148–152. https://doi.org/10.1136/bmjqs-2021-014163

Shahid, S., & Sumesh, T. (2018). Situation, background, assessment, recommendation (SBAR) communication tool for hand-off in health care: A narrative review. *Safety in Health*, *4*(1). https://doi.org/10.1186/s40886-018-0073-1

Shrank, W. H., Rogstad, T. L., & Parekh, N. H. (2019). Waste in the U.S. health care system: Estimated costs and potential for savings. *JAMA*, *322*(15), 1501–1509. https://doi.org/10.1001/jama.2019.13978

Singer, S. J. (2021). Value of a value culture survey for improving healthcare quality. *BMJ Quality & Safety*, *31*(7), 479–482. https://doi.org/10.1136/bmjqs-2021-014048

Sofer, D. (2019). Is a medical mistake an error or a crime? *AJN, American Journal of Nursing*, *119*(5), 12. https://doi.org/10.1097/01.NAJ.0000557895.82994.81

St. Pierre, M., Grawe, P., Bergstrom, J., & Neuhaus, C. (2022). 20 years after To Err is Human: A bibliometric analysis of "the IOM report's" impact on research on patient safety. *Safety Science*, *147*, 105593. https://doi.org/10.1016/j.ssci.2021.105593

Sylvia, M. L., & Vigil, I. M. (2021). *Population health analytics.* Jones & Bartlett.

Thomas Jefferson University. (2023). *College of Population Health.* Accessed January 18, 2023. https://www.jefferson.edu/academics/colleges-schools-institutes/population-health.html

Tschannen, D., Alexander, C., Taylor, S., Tovar, E. G., Ghosh, B., Zellefrow, C., & Milner, K. A. (2021). Quality improvement engagement and competence: A comparison between frontline nurses and nurse leaders. *Nursing Outlook, 69*(5), 836–847. https://doi.org/10.1016/j.outlook.2021.02.008

Uhm, J., Ko, Y., & Kim, S. (2019). Implementation of an SBAR communication program based on experiential learning theory in a pediatric nursing practicum: A quasi-experimental study. *Nurse Education Today, 80*, 78–84. https://doi.org/10.1016/j.nedt.2019.05.034

VHA National Center for Patient Safety. (2021, February 5). *Guide to performing a root cause analysis.* https://www.patientsafety.va.gov/docs/RCA-Guidebook_02052021.pdf

Walter, J. K., Schall, T. E., DeWitt, A. G., Faerber, J., Griffis, H., Galligan, M., Miller, V., Arnold, R. M., & Feudtner, C. (2019). Interprofessional team member communication patterns, teamwork, and collaboration in pre–family meeting huddles in a pediatric cardiac intensive care unit. *Journal of Pain and Symptom Management, 58*(1), 11–18. https://doi.org/10.1016/j.jpainsymman.2019.04.009

World Health Organization. (2019, August 26). *10 facts on patient safety.* https://www.who.int/news-room/photo-story/photo-story-detail/10-facts-on-patient-safety

21

Palliative Care: Compassionate Care Across Settings of Care

Cathy Campbell, PhD, RN

 http://evolve.elsevier.com/Friberg/bridge/

OBJECTIVES

At the completion of this chapter, the reader will be able to:
- Define the terms *palliative care* and *hospice*.
- Discuss the role of the nurse as a member of the interprofessional team in palliative care.
- Describe the benefits of palliative care and hospice.
- Describe barriers to palliative care and hospice.
- Identify best practices to increase capacity for hospice and palliative care.

INTRODUCTION

Definition of Palliative Care and Hospice

Palliative care is an interprofessional approach that improves the quality of life of patients and their families facing the problems associated with life-threatening illnesses, through the prevention and relief of suffering by means of early identification and impeccable assessment and treatment of pain and other problems, physical, psychosocial, and spiritual (Connor, 2020). In this chapter, we intentionally use a broad definition of palliative care to describe an interprofessional model of care used to guide care for people in the advanced stages of a life-limiting illness and their care partners.

Palliative care access is limited internationally. The WHO estimates globally that of 56.8 million people, 31.1 million are in the early stages of disease and 25.7 million are in the advanced stages of disease. As our population ages, it is important to note that of the people who have palliative care needs, 67.1% of them are adults 50 years of age or older (Connor, 2020). The unit of care is the person with advanced serious illness and the people that person considers partners or a constellation of support. Palliative care is appropriate across the life span with a life-threatening or debilitating condition, regardless of the patient's age or health care delivery setting.

Palliative care is delivered by an interprofessional team. Health care providers within the interprofessional team have interventions to guide the patient and caregivers during an advanced illness and in the bereavement period. Using a framework by Chochinov and colleagues (Chochinov et al., 2002; Doorenbos et al., 2017), the International Council of Nurses (ICN) has developed a catalog of palliative care interventions to support care for adults. The work of the interprofessional team is described in three domains: illness-related concerns, dignity-conserving concerns, and social dignity concerns (Fig. 21.1).

The first domain within the model is the *illness-related concerns* domain. In this domain, interventions and outcomes are focused on physical, cognitive, and psychological symptom management. In the second domain, the *dignity-conserving repertoire,* the interventions are focused on supporting self-care and building capacity for psychological and spiritual well-being. Finally, in the third domain, the *social dignity inventory,* the interventions are focused on maintaining social support, providing care for the caregivers, and planning for the bereavement period. The major outcomes in this model are dignified dying and bereavement (Chochinov et al., 2002; Doorenbos et al., 2017).

Nursing Role Within the Interprofessional Team

Professional nurses use critical thinking in all aspects of the nursing process to deliver palliative care. Nursing interventions focus primarily on the illness-related domain such as giving direct hands-on care, managing physical symptoms,

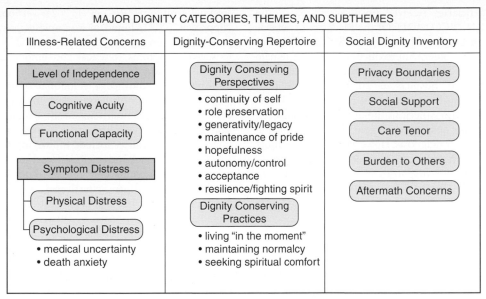

Fig. 21.1 Dignity Framework.

and teaching patients and their care circle. As a member of the interprofessional team, the nurse collaborates with colleagues using interventions in all domains, providing emotional support and facilitating spiritual guidance for the person who is dying and those close to the dying person. The creativity inherent in the art of nursing is more important than ever as nurses work with members of the interprofessional team to create a unique plan of care for each person and the caregivers (Schroeder & Lorenz, 2018).

The American Academy of Nursing's Expert Panel on Universal Access to Palliative Care (AANEP) published a consensus statement in 2021 (Rosa et al., 2021). The 43 authors who participated had extensive international health care experience. They represented eight countries (Australia, Canada, the United Kingdom, Kenya, Lebanon, Liberia, South Africa, and the United States of America). The task force was able to begin to bring a global context to the discussion of palliative care. The work of the AANEP is to be applauded; however, there are multiple global contexts guiding any discussion of palliative care. Their work is only one example of recommendations to guide palliative care nursing practice.

The consensus statement argues that current models of palliative care are not adequately addressing the palliative care needs of people across the lifespan who are nearing the end of life and their circles of support, especially for those who are marginalized or at-risk for not having access to high-quality palliative care partners (Rosa et al., 2021). Without access to compassionate palliative care, patients

and their caregivers are suffering needlessly and experiencing what Dame Cicely Saunders, founder of the modern hospice movement, calls "total pain," suffering that goes beyond the physical to emotional, psychological, and transcendent aspects of a person (Richmond, 2005; Schroeder & Lorenz, 2018).

HOSPICE: A SPECIAL KIND OF PALLIATIVE CARE

The current model of palliative care has its roots in the modern hospice movement and began in London in the late 1960s, first at St. Joseph's and later at St. Christopher's hospice under the leadership of Dame Cicely Saunders (Buck, 2011). The grassroots movement was sparked by a desire to transform the cold, institutionalized, unskilled care of the dying into a compassionate, loving experience at home or in a home-like setting guided by trained staff and volunteers (Buck, 2011). The early founders of the U.S. palliative care movement spoke of being inspired by the work of not only Dr. Saunders but also the public talks and writings of Elisabeth Kübler-Ross. The patient population served by hospice providers in the early days of the movement were primarily white females with cancer (Buck, 2011).

Hospice is an interprofessional model of care that places emphasis on symptom management, psychosocial support, advance care planning, and coordination of care across settings of care (National Hospice and Palliative Care Organization [NHPCO], 2021). In 2019, 1.61 million

Medicare beneficiaries received hospice services in the United States (NHPCO, 2021). Of the Medicare beneficiaries enrolled in hospice in the United States, 62.7% are 85 years of age or older. Approximately 55% are female and 44% are male. The percentages of Medicare recipients by race that used hospice in 2019 are as follows: 53.8% White, 42.7% Hispanic, 40.8% Black, 39.8% Asian-American, and 38.5% American Indian/Alaskan Native. In the early days of the hospice movement, most of the people enrolled had a cancer diagnosis. However, at this time, most people enrolled in hospice care have noncancer diagnoses. The five most common diagnoses are dementia/Alzheimer disease (20.9%), cancer (4.9%), respiratory disease (7.1%), circulatory/heart disorders (6.4%), and CVA/stroke (5.4%) (NHPCO, 2021).

The hospice model of care was the foundation for the development of a significant health policy, the Medicare Hospice Benefit (MHB), in 1984 (Buck, 2011). For the first time in the United States, end-of-life (EOL) care was a covered benefit under Medicare. An interprofessional model of care was described and hospice eligibility was defined as having a life expectancy of 6 months or less (Buck, 2011). The MHB covers care for hospice illness and related conditions (NHPCO, 2021). The per diem payment covers the services of the interprofessional team, medications, durable medical equipment, and supplies related to hospice care. Patients and families who can access hospice services are very satisfied with the pain management, the level of emotional support, and communication from the hospice staff about the plan of care (Vernon et al., 2022).

BENEFITS OF PALLIATIVE CARE

Community-based physician practices have limited ability to provide the intensive psychoeducational, emotional, spiritual, and instrumental support that is needed by families throughout all phases of an illness (Vernon et al., 2022). Two of the major benefits of palliative care for patients and their families are expertise in symptom management and the availability of palliative care across settings of care. In palliative care, the unit of care is the patient and family (as defined by the patient). Palliative care interventions also support the caregivers (Vernon et al., 2022). Caregivers meet the physical and emotional needs of patients such as advocating for patient needs (e.g., bathing, toileting, skin care, spiritual care). The needs of the caregiver also evolve over the course of the illness.

Expertise in Pain and Symptom Management for Patients and Caregivers

People seek palliative care for expertise in safe, effective modalities to manage pain and other physical, emotional, and spiritual symptoms (Rosa et al., 2021; Vernon et al., 2022). Nipp et al. (2022) found in a sample of advanced cancer patients that on average each person had 3.31 moderate to severe symptoms (physical and emotional). Although physical symptom management may take precedence, it is important to acknowledge emotional symptoms as well. More than one-fifth of the sample from the work of Nipp et al. (2022) had clinically significant symptoms of depression and anxiety. Comprehensive symptom management interventions by nurses include multisymptom assessment (physical, emotional, and spiritual), teaching about pharmacological and nonpharmacological modalities, and the evaluation of treatment effectiveness (Doorenbos et al., 2017; Rosa et al., 2021). In collaboration with other team members, such as physicians, psychiatric nurse practitioners, clinical psychologists, and spiritual care providers, emotional symptoms and spiritual distress are also addressed in the plan of care.

Early palliative care intervention improves patient quality of life, lowers depression, and increases the likelihood that patients will discuss EOL wishes with a physician (Temel et al., 2017). A nurse-led telephone-delivered palliative care intervention realized similar patient outcomes. Findings included improved quality of life, decreased depression, and decreased trends in symptom intensity (Bakitas et al., 2009). Interestingly, early palliative care has been found to extend life. Temel and colleagues found that although their intervention did not increase the length of stay in hospice, the people who received the palliative care intervention survived longer (median survival of 11.6 months for the experimental group vs. 8.9 months for the group receiving usual care) (Temel et al., 2010).

Caregivers often experience great psychological distress (El-Jawahri et al., 2021) and decreased well-being (Unsar et al., 2021) in their role as caregivers. In addition, palliative care improves outcomes for family caregivers (Dionne-Odom et al., 2021). Early involvement in palliative care leads to improvements in family caregiver depression, anxiety, and other aspects of quality of life (Dionne-Odom et al., 2021).

Care Across Settings of Care: Hospice is Not a Place

As a response to the aging baby boomer generation, hospice is provided across settings of care. Even at the end of life, symptoms are dynamic, the plan of care changes, and therefore patients may have care transitions (NHPCO, 2021; Rosa et al., 2021). The definition of *place of residence* has been expanded to include not only a private residence but also a nursing home or residential facility. The majority of hospice care is provided in a private residence. The median length of stay in days by location of care is 27 days (private residence), 22 days (nursing facilities), and 56 days (assisted living facility). The remainder of the care is provided in inpatient settings (hospice inpatient unit or acute care hospital) (NHPCO, 2021). A nurse coordinator or case manager supports families in this transition across settings of care. Patients and families have options to receive hospice care across many settings, including home-based care to meet their needs. Optimally, with the support of the interprofessional team, patients can live their last days in the place of their choice and the patient/family will be highly satisfied with the care received.

BARRIERS TO PALLIATIVE CARE AND HOSPICE

Challenges in Accessing Palliative Care and Hospice

The American Academy of Nursing's Expert Panel on Universal Access to Palliative Care (Rosa et al., 2021) concluded that current models of palliative care are not adequately addressing the needs of people who are nearing the end of life and their care partners. Although there are national and global initiatives intended to increase the number of people who receive palliative care (Doorenbos et al., 2017; NHPCO, 2021; Rosa et al., 2021), significant barriers exist to palliative care across settings of care. The four most common barriers identified are the lack of an educated palliative care workforce, inadequate social support and services for home-based care, late referrals, and limited diversity in the people who receive hospice services.

Regarding an educated palliative care workforce, the WHO affirms the importance of the interprofessional palliative care model, yet in clinical practice, health professionals are not always adequately educated to deliver "basic" or "primary" palliative care to patients, especially in rural settings (Connor, 2020; Rosa et al., 2021). Nurses have unique roles to play in the provision of palliative care, regardless of diagnosis, because of their role as direct care providers, educators, and patient/family advocates, but their capacity to do so is limited by a lack of training and education. As the baby boomer population ages, an educated palliative workforce will become imperative to manage the complex needs of this cohort and their families (Ferrell et al., 2016; Rosa et al., 2021).

Late Referrals

A key indicator within the health care system is the length of stay. The length of stay is the mean number of days a person is enrolled in or receiving services from a health care facility or agency. A *late referral* is defined as when a person is admitted to a hospice program, 7 days or less

before death. Wang and colleagues argue that late referrals are a marker of poor-quality care and family dissatisfaction with EOL care (Wang et al., 2017). The data we have about the length of stay from palliative care providers comes from the hospice sector. In the United States, the calculated median length of stay across all settings of care is 18 days, with approximately 25% dying within 5 days of admission (NHPCO, 2021). In some settings, a length of stay of 5 days may appear to be very long. However, the patient and family may not be able to fully benefit from palliative care services in that period or learn the skills needed to provide care, especially skills related to medication administration or other treatments.

The reasons for late referrals are multifactorial (Diamond et al., 2016). People may be referred, but the actual admission or enrollment with the hospice or palliative care provider may be delayed. Three major categories for late referrals to hospice and palliative care have been identified, namely patient/family-related, health system-related, and health care provider-related. Patient/family-related factors include lack of knowledge about palliative care, fear of loss of hope (Kennard, 2016), and mistrust of the medical system (Siegel et al., 2021). Health system-related factors include hospice enrollment policies that preclude concomitant use of cancer therapies (chemotherapy, radiation therapy, and blood products) (Duff & Thomas, 2017) and the availability of a hospice or palliative care provider.

Finally, other health care provider–related reasons for late referrals are not including key patient/family decision-makers in goals of care conversations (Sloan et al., 2016; Sloan et al., 2021) failure to recognize signs and symptoms of approaching death, and health care providers' lack of skill to communicate with patients and families when goals of care change from cure to palliation (Rosa et al., 2021). When palliative care is provided at its optimum, it is a life-affirming community treasure for patients with advanced disease, their constellations of support, and their communities.

Lack of Community Resources to Support Care at Home

A "good death" at home is often set as an outcome for patients, their support systems, and the palliative care team (Rosa et al., 2021; Vernon et al., 2022). However, many people do not have the support network to provide care in the home (Campbell et al., 2021)

Hospice and palliative care staff are only present in the home for regularly scheduled intermittent visits. Therefore, most of the home care must be provided by informal caregivers such as biological family, chosen family, neighbors, or friends (Lee et al., 2019). While many caregivers do find great meaning, triumph, and reward in their role as caregivers (Horsfall et al., 2017) this work requires physical, emotional, and spiritual resources from caregivers that may not be readily available through local social services or acknowledged by the medical treatment team (Campbell et al., 2017; Lee et al., 2019).

Five factors have been identified that are associated with an increased likelihood of death at home: (1) presence of direct care in the home, (2) a high intensity of home care services (frequency of visits from home health or hospice staff), (3) living with relatives especially spouse/long-term partner, (4) the presence of extended family support above and beyond what is available in the home (additional family or friends as caregivers), and (5) support for the family or extended network of care persons from social services or hospice providers (Horsfall et al., 2017; Nuño-Solinís, 2014).

Family members have an active role in all aspects of care, including medication administration for symptom management (Lee et al., 2019), often with very little prior experience, training, or ongoing support, especially those in rural and remote communities (Campbell et al., 2021)

Patients and their families need support from the interprofessional palliative care team from diagnosis to end of life. However, community resources are not available until the last weeks or months.

CHALLENGES PROVIDING PATIENT-CENTERED CARE FOR DIVERSE COMMUNITIES

As noted earlier, the earliest adopters of the model of palliative care started at St. Christopher's Hospice in London were white women with cancer (Buck, 2011). Although palliative care providers do provide services to a great variety of diagnoses, they often are not providing direct care and services to people who are members of racial/ethnic minorities. African Americans and Hispanics are less likely to receive primary palliative care services (Rising et al., 2018; Sloan et al., 2021).

Lesbian, gay, bisexual, transgender, and queer or questioning (LGBTQ) elders from the baby boom cohort are aging and must reach out to the health care system for care and needed services at a time of great physical, emotional, and spiritual vulnerability (Acquaviva, 2017). LGBTQ elders are not confident that health and social care services will provide sensitive EOL care to meet their needs (Stein et al., 2020). This generation of elders has not always been welcomed with compassionate, loving care by hospice and palliative care providers (Campbell & Catlett, 2019; Stein et al., 2020).

Patients and families (biological and chosen) of LGBTQ people may experience a lack of communication, conflict, and dissatisfaction with health care providers. Areas of concern are the unwillingness of providers to consider needs related to sexual orientation and gender identity, to provide safe spaces for the patient and family, to embrace non-heteronormative ideas about family/constellations of care, and to support the expression of spirituality. Conflicts can arise while the patient is alive, at the time of death, or during bereavement.

In summary, four barriers to palliative care have been identified as lack of an educated palliative care workforce, late referrals, lack of community support for care at home, and poor access for racial/ethnic or sexual minorities (sexual orientation and gender identity). These barriers prevent patients with advanced illness from accessing particularly important palliative care services when people are at their most vulnerable physically, emotionally, financially, and spiritually. Roshi Joan Halifax, an expert in EOL care, has a vision for a "radical and practical shift" within our health systems so more people can have access to palliative care (Upaya Zen Center, 2021). Transformation will start with different models of education for the palliative care workforce. The chapter will conclude with best practices to provide education to increase the capacity to provide hospice and palliative care.

BEST PRACTICES TO INCREASE THE CAPACITY TO PROVIDE HOSPICE AND PALLIATIVE CARE

This excerpt from Dr. Atul Gawande's book *Being Mortal: Medicine and What Matters in the End* illustrates eloquently the fantastic opportunity that is within our grasp: "We have the opportunity to refashion our institutions, our culture, and our conversations in ways that transform the possibilities for the last chapter of everyone's lives" (Gawande, 2014, p. 243). One of the four areas of recommendation in the American Academy of Nursing's Expert Panel report is to integrate palliative care education into nursing curricula (Rosa et al., 2021).

Lippe et al. (2018) evaluated preidentified knowledge and attitude learning outcomes in educational interventions for EOL care across multiple health care professions from 2001 until the present. Further research is needed to address self-efficacy, comfort, and communication skills competencies in health profession educational programs.

EDUCATED PALLIATIVE CARE WORKFORCE

The American Association of Colleges of Nursing's (AACN's) new curriculum to educate undergraduate nursing students, and Upaya Zen Center's *Being With Dying* program for education of the interprofessional team represent two exemplar programs that prepare nurses and other health care providers for palliative care roles.

In 2017, the AACN introduced new competencies and recommendations for educating undergraduate graduate nursing students. Under the leadership of Betty Farrell, the End-of-Life Nursing Education Consortium (ELNEC) was developed. The ELNEC curriculum has been used for continuing education and staff development in palliative care education around the world. The ELNEC curriculum provides the foundation for an online self-directed curriculum to educate undergraduate nursing students. The curriculum is designed to provide basic palliative care education over the course of their education to meet 17 competencies (Box 21.1). The modules are (1) Introduction to Palliative Care; (2) Communication; (3) Pain Assessment and Management; (4) Symptom Management; (5) Loss, Grief, and Bereavement; and (6) Care of the Imminently Dying Patient and Family. View the ELNEC Undergraduate/New Graduate Hall of Fame (https://www.aacnnursing.org/Portals/42/ELNEC/PDF/ELNEC-hall-of-fame.pdf) institutions with 10 or more students enrolled from 2019 to 2022.

Although the modules are designed to educate an undergraduate cohort, all of the modules are robust enough to be used for continuing education for nurses in the early years of their career or for experienced nurses who may be new to palliative care. Three of the modules that are particularly salient for novice palliative care nurses are Communication; Loss, Grief, and Bereavement; and Care of the Imminently Dying Patient and Family (Ferrell et al., 2018).

Upaya Zen Center in Santa Fe, New Mexico, has created a powerful interprofessional learning experience called Being With Dying: The Professional Training Program for Clinicians in Compassionate Care of the Seriously Ill and Dying. Roshi Joan Halifax, who is the Abbot of the Zen Center, is the founder and project director. Since 1970 this program has been educating clinicians from all disciplines, including nursing, medicine, pharmacy, alternative and complementary therapists, spiritual care providers, artists, and healers through a week-long intensive program. Through the exploration of personal beliefs, the introduction to resilience practices for the clinician, and the application of skills in the ethical, existential, and spiritual aspects of illness and dying, participants develop skillful means to care for people who are dying (Upaya Zen Center, 2021). The program is innovative in two respects. First, it has an interprofessional group of learners using a common curriculum to develop a skill set. The skills transcend any specific discipline. The disciplines or professions of the learners are not revealed until the final day. A true learning community is developed. Second, participants are learning not only to examine their own beliefs about death and dying but also start to unbundle some of the practices within their own systems that are barriers to EOL care. The in-person Being With Dying program was placed on an indefinite hiatus during the first year of the COVID-19 pandemic; however, it resumed in an online format in the spring of 2021 (Upaya Zen Center, 2021).

University of Virginia's School of Nursing is committed to creating a compassionate community ready to meet the complex needs of people living with a life-limiting illness. To bring this vision to life, the School of Nursing has collaborated with University of Virginia Health System, the School of Medicine, and a community-based hospice to send more than 70 clinicians, faculty members, staff, and graduate students to Being With Dying. Table 21.1 provides a list of on-line resources related to hospice and palliative care.

BOX 21.1 Selected Competencies From the AACN Palliative CARES Document

- Perform a comprehensive assessment of pain and other symptoms common in serious illness.
- Educate and communicate effectively and compassionately with patient, family, health care team members, and public about health issues.
- Collaborate with members of the interprofessional team to improve palliative care for patients with serious illness, enhance the experience and outcomes from palliative care, and ensure coordinated and efficient palliative care for the benefit of communities.
- Elicit and demonstrate respect for patient and family values, preferences and goals of care, and shared decision making during serious illness and end of life.
- Provide competent, compassionate, and culturally sensitive care for patients and their families at the time of diagnosis through end of life.
- Realize the need to seek consultation (from advanced practice nursing specialists, specialty palliative care teams, and ethics consultant) for complex patient and family needs.

Modified from: American Association of Colleges of Nursing (AACN). (2016). *CARES: Competencies and recommendations for educating undergraduate nursing students: Preparing nurses to care for the seriously ill and their families.* https://www.aacnnursng.org/Portals/42/ELNEC/PDF/New-Palliative-Care-Competencies.pdf

TABLE 21.1   Resources for Hospice and Palliative Care

Organization	Description
End-of-Life (EOL) Nursing Education Consortium https://www.aacnnursing.org/ELNEC	Comprehensive resource for EOL nursing education
E-hospice http://www.ehospice.com/	International news source on EOL care
Hospice and Palliative Care Nursing Association (HPNA) https://www.advancingexpertcare.org/	Nursing organization whose mission is to advance expert care in serious illness through education, competence, advocacy, leadership, and research
National Hospice and Palliative Care Organization (NHPCO) https://www.nhpco.org/	Resources for staff education, patient-family care and services, and bereavement
National Health Care Decisions Day (NHDD) http://www.nhdd.org/	Resources about advance directives and guidance through the advance care planning process

SUMMARY

Palliative care is an interprofessional model of care to support patients with advanced disease and their circle of support. A nurse has a vital role to play in palliative care as a member of an interprofessional team, a leader, coordinator, educator, and direct care provider for body, mind, and spirit. Although there are great benefits to the patient and family, many racial/ethnic minorities may not have access to hospice or palliative care. Moreover, members of the LGBTQ communities are concerned that hospice and palliative care providers will not be responsive to their needs at the end of life. One key to transformation is developing an educated palliative care workforce who will have the tools to guide change within the health care system to improve access to palliative care for all who need this important service.

SALIENT POINTS

- Palliative care should be integrated throughout the disease course.
- The patient and family (as defined by the patient) are the unit of care.
- Palliative care is available across settings of care.
- Family members receive support for caregiving such as education, hands-on-caregiving, emotional support, and spiritual care.
- An educated palliative care workforce is a fundamental element for providing high-quality care.

CRITICAL REFLECTION EXERCISES

1. What are the barriers and facilitators of integrating the palliative care philosophy across the disease course for persons and their caregivers for someone with cancer?
2. What are the barriers and facilitators of integrating the palliative care philosophy across the disease course for a person and the caregivers for someone with dementia?
3. What factors contribute to the lack of racial/ethnic diversity of people using hospice or palliative care programs? Within your organization what changes could be made?
4. Reflect upon your wishes for a death with dignity. How would you describe this to your family or a close friend? What images come to mind? What do you imagine your last days and weeks of life will be like? Where will you be living? Who will be providing care for you?

REFERENCES

Acquaviva, K. (2017). *LGBTQ-inclusive palliative care: A practical guide to transforming professional practice*. Harrington Park Press.

American Association of Colleges of Nursing. (2016). *CARES: Competencies and recommendations for educating undergraduate nursing students: Preparing nurses to care for the seriously ill and their families*. https://www.aacnnursing.org/Portals/42/ELNEC/PDF/New-Palliative-Care-Competencies.pdf

Bakitas, M., Lyons, K. D., Hegel, M. T., Balan, S., Brokaw, F. C., Seville, J., Hull, J. G., Li, Z., Tosteson, T. D., Byock, I. R., & Ahles, T. A. (2009). Effects of a palliative care intervention on clinical outcomes in patients with advanced cancer: The project ENABLE II randomized controlled trial. *Journal of the American Medical Association, 302*(7), 741–749. https://doi.org/10.1001/jama.2009.1198

Buck, J. (2011). Policy and the re-formation of hospice: Lessons from the past for the future of palliative care. *Journal of Hospice and Palliative Nursing, 13*(6), S35–S43. https://dx.doi.org/10.1097/NJH.0b013e3182331160

Campbell, C. L., & Catlett, L. (2019). Silent illumination: A case study exploring the spiritual needs of a transgender-identified elder receiving hospital care. *Journal of Hospice and Palliative Nursing (JHPN): The Official Journal of the Hospice and Palliative Nurses Association, 21*(6), 467–474. https://doi.org/10.1097/NJH.0000000000000596

Campbell, C. L., Kelly, M., & Rovnyak, V. (2017). Pain management in home hospice patients: A retrospective descriptive study. *Nursing & Health Sciences, 19*(3), 381–387. https://doi.org/10.1111/nhs.12359

Campbell, C., Ramakuela, J., Dennis, D., & Soba, K. (2021). Palliative care practices in a rural community: Cultural context and the role of community health worker. *Journal of Health Care for the Poor and Underserved, 32*(1), 550–564. https://doi.org/10.1353/hpu.2021.0040

Chochinov, H. M., Hack, T., McClement, S., Kristianson, L., & Harlos, M. (2002). Dignity in the terminally ill: An empirical model. *Social Science & Medicine, 54*(3), 433–443. https://doi.org/10.1016/S0277-9536(01)00084-3

Connor, S. R. (Ed.). (2020). *Global atlas of palliative care* (2nd ed.). Worldwide Hospice Palliative Care Alliance (WHPCA) and World Health Organization (WHO). http://www.thewhpca.org/resources/global-atlas-on-end-of-life-care

Diamond, E. L., Russell, D., Kryza, M., Bowles, K., Applebaum, A., Dennis, J., DeAngelis, L. M., & Prigerson, H. G. (2016). Rate and risks for late referral to hospice in patients with primary malignant brain tumors. *Neuro-Oncology, 18*(1), 78–86. https://doi.or/10.1093/neuonc/nov156

Dionne-Odom, J. N., Azuero, A., Taylor, R. A., Wells, R. D., Hendricks, B. A., Bechthold, A. C., Reed, R. D., Harrell, E. R., Dosse, C. K., Engler, S., McKie, P., Ejem, D., Bakitas, M. A., & Rosenberg, A. R. (2021). Resilience, preparedness, and distress among family caregivers of patients with advanced cancer. *Supportive Care in Cancer: Official Journal of the Multinational Association of Supportive Care in Cancer, 29*(11), 6913–6920. https://doi.org/10.1007/s00520-021-06265-y

Doorenbos, A. Z., Jansen, K., Oakes, R. P., & Wilson, S. A. (2017). Palliative care for dignified dying: International Classification for Nursing Practice (ICNP®) catalogue. *International Council of Nurses*. https://www.icn.ch/sites/default/files/inline-files/Palliative_Care.pdf

Duff, J. M., & Thomas, R. M. (2017). Impact of palliative chemotherapy and travel distance on hospice referral in patients with stage IV pancreatic cancer: A retrospective analysis within a Veterans Administration medical center. *Journal of Hospice and Palliative Care, 35*(6), 875–881. https://doi.org/10.1177/1049909117746390

El-Jawahri, A., Greer, J. A., Park, E. R., Jackson, V. A., Kamdar, M., Rinaldi, S. P., Gallagher, E. R., Jagielo, A. D., Topping, C., Elyze, M., Jones, B., & Temel, J. S. (2021). Psychological distress in bereaved caregivers of patients with advanced cancer. *Journal of Pain and Symptom Management, 61*(3), 488–494. https://doi.org/10.1016/j.jpainsymman.2020.08.028

Ferrell, B., Malloy, P., Mazanec, P., & Virani, R. (2016). CARES AACN: New competencies for educating undergraduate nursing students to improve palliative care. *Journal of Professional Nursing: Official Journal of the American Association of Colleges of Nursing, 32*(5), 327–355. https://doi.org/10.1016/j.profnurs.2016.07.002

Ferrell, B., Mazanec, P., Malloy, P., & Virani, R. (2018). An innovative end-of-life nursing education consortium curriculum that prepares nursing students to provide primary palliative care. *Nurse Educator, 43*(5), 242–246. https://doi.org/10.1097/NNE.0000000000000497

Gawande, A. (2014). *Being mortal: Medicine and what matters in the end*. Metropolitan Books, Henry Holt & Company.

Horsfall, D., Leonard, R., Rosenberg, J. P., & Noonan, K. (2017). Home as a place of caring and wellbeing? A qualitative study of informal carers and caring networks lived experiences of providing in-home end-of-life care. *Health & Place, 46*, 58–64. https://doi.org/10.1016/j.healthplace.2017.04.003

Kennard, C. (2016). Undying hope. *Journal of Palliative Medicine, 19*(2), 129–130. http://doi.org/10.1089/jpm.2015.0331

Lee, M., Ryoo J. H., Campbell, C., Hollen, P. J., & Williams, I. C. (2019). Exploring the challenges of medical/nursing tasks in home care experienced by caregivers of older adults with dementia: An integrative review. *Journal of Clinical Nursing, 28*(23–24), 4177–4189. https://doi.org/10.1111/jocn.15007

Lippe, M., Johnson, B., Stephanie, B. M., & Kyle, R. K. (2018). Palliative care educational interventions for prelicensure health-care students: An integrative review. *American Journal of Hospice and Palliative Care, 35*(9), 1235–1244. https://doi.org/10.1177/1049909118754494

National Hospice and Palliative Care Organization. (2021). *2021 Hospice facts and figures*. https://www.nhpco.org/hospice-care-overview/hospice-facts-figures/

Nipp, R. D., Horick, N. K., Qian, C. L., Knight, H. P., Kaslow-Zieve, E. R., Azoba, C. C., Elyze, M., Landay, S. L., Kay, P. S., Ryan, D. P., Jackson, V. A., Greer, J. A., El-Jawahri, A., & Temel, J. S. (2022). Effect of a symptom monitoring intervention for patients hospitalized with advanced cancer: A randomized clinical trial. *JAMA Oncology, 8*(4), 571–578. https://doi.org/10.1001/jamaoncol.2021.7643

Nuño-Solinís, R. (2014). Integrated end of life care: The role of social services. *International Journal of Integrated Care, 14*(1), 1–3. http://doi.org/10.5334/ijic.1537

Richmond, C. (2005). Dame Cicely Saunders. *BMJ, 331*(7510), 238. https://doi.org/10.1136/bmj.331.7510.238

Rising, M. L., Hassouneh, D. S., Lutz, K. F., Lee, C. S., & Berry, P. (2018). Integrative review of the literature on Hispanics and hospice. *American Journal of Hospice and Palliative Care, 35*(3), 542–554. https://doi.org/10.1177/1049909117730555

Rosa, W. E., Buck, H. G., Squires, A. P., Kozachik, S. L., Huijer, H. A., Bakitas, M., Boit, J. M., Bradley, P. K., Cacchione, P. Z., Chan, G. K., Crisp, N., Dahlin, C., Daoust, P., Davidson, P. M., Davis, S., Doumit, M., Fink, R. M., Herr, K. A., Hinds, P. S., … Ferrell, B. R. (2021). American Academy of Nursing Expert Panel consensus statement of nursing's roles in ensuring universal palliative care access. *Nursing Outlook, 69*(6), 961–968. https://doi.org/10.1016/j.outlook.2021.06.011

Schroeder, K., & Lorenz, K. (2018). Nursing and the future of palliative care. *Asia-Pacific Journal of Oncology Nursing, 5*(1), 4–8. https://doi.org/10.4103/apjon.apjon_43_17

Siegel, M., Critchfield-Jain, I., Boykin, M., & Owens, A. (2021). Actual racial/ethnic disparities in COVID-19 mortality for the non-Hispanic Black compared to non-Hispanic White population in 35 U.S. states and their association with structural racism. *Journal of Racial and Ethnic Health Disparities*, 1–13. https://doi.org/10.1007/s40615-021-01028-1

Sloan, D. H., Gray, T. F., Harris, D., Peters, T., Belcher, A., Aslakson, R., & Bowie, J. (2021). Church leaders and parishioners speak out about the role of the church in advance care planning and end-of-life care. *Palliative & Supportive Care, 19*(3), 322–328. https://doi.org/10.1017/S1478951520000966

Sloan, D. H., Peters, T., Johnson, K. S., Bowie, J. V., Ting Y., & Aslakson, R. (2016). Church-based health promotion focused on advance care planning and end-of-life care at Black Baptist churches: A cross-sectional survey. *Journal of Palliative Medicine, 19*(2), 190–194. https://doi.org/10.1089/jpm.2015.0319

Stein, G. L., Berkman, C., O'Mahony, S., Godfrey, D., Javier, N. M., & Maingi, S. (2020). Experiences of lesbian, gay, bisexual, and transgender patients and families in hospice and palliative care: Perspectives of the palliative care team. *Journal of Palliative Medicine, 23*(6), 817–824. https://doi.org/10.1089/jpm.2019.0542

Temel, J. S., Greer, J. A., El-Jawahri, A., Pirl, W. F., Park, E. R., Jackson, V. A., & Ryan, D. P. (2017). Effects of early integrated palliative care in patients with lung and GI cancer: A randomized clinical trial. *Journal of Clinical Oncology, 35*(8), 834–841. https://doi.org/10.1200/JCO.2016.70.5046

Temel, J. S., Greer, J. A., Muzikansky, A., Gallagher, E. R., Admane, S., Jackson, V. A., & Lynch, T. J. (2010). Early palliative care for patients with metastatic non–small-cell lung cancer. *New England Journal of Medicine, 363*(8), 733–742. https://doi.org/10.1056/NEJMoa1000678

Unsar, S., Erol, O., & Ozdemir, O. (2021). Caregiving burden, depression, and anxiety in family caregivers of patients with cancer. *European Journal of Oncology Nursing: The Official Journal of European Oncology Nursing Society, 50*, 101882. https://doi.org/10.1016/j.ejon.2020.101882

Upaya Zen Center. (2021). *Being with dying.* https://www.upaya.org/being-with-dying/

Vernon, E., Hughes, M. C., & Kowalczyk, M. (2022). Measuring effectiveness in community-based palliative care programs: A systematic review. *Social Science & Medicine, 296*, 114731. https://doi.org/10.1016/j.socscimed.2022.114731

Wang, X., Knight, L. S., Evans, A., Wang, I., & Smith, T. J. (2017). Variations among physicians in hospice referrals of patients with advanced cancer. *Journal of Oncology Practice, 13*(5), e496–e504. https://doi.org/10.1200/JCO.2016.34.15_suppl.10027

22

The Wisdom of Self-Care, Well-Being, and Resilience in Nursing

Regina M. DeGennaro, DNP, CNS, AOCN, CNL

http://evolve.elsevier.com/Friberg/bridge/

OBJECTIVES

At the completion of this chapter, the reader will be able to:

- Articulate principles and strategies for health and well-being, including stress management.
- Identify coping strategies and relaxation techniques.
- Describe the concept of resilience.
- Define the characteristics of a resilient person.
- Explain how nurses could benefit from resilience training.
- Describe mindfulness/meditation as it relates to resilience.
- Describe belly breathing as it relates to resilience.
- Describe cognitive restructuring as it relates to resilience.
- Describe expressive writing/journaling as it relates to resilience.
- Describe the benefits of physical exercise as it relates to resilience.
- Describe wisdom principles to optimize well-being.
- Discuss principles of integrative nursing and holistic self-care.
- Describe opportunities for optimizing well-being outcomes.

INTRODUCTION

Nurses face a wide range of stressors on the job, including heavy workloads, long hours, time pressures, and multi-tasking. They have long been subjected to human pain and suffering, which can lead to burnout and posttraumatic stress–like symptoms. The novel coronavirus disease (COVID-19) pandemic represented an unprecedented trial for health care systems across the world (IBISWorld, 2020). The devastating spread of the disease in late 2019 and early 2020 overwhelmed many health care systems and clinicians struggled to provide intensive care unit beds, ventilators, and personal protective equipment (PPE) for health care team members and patients. The unprecedented pandemic provided the unwelcome opportunity for nurses to navigate a perfect storm of situations that threatened their health, well-being, and ability to perform and optimize clinical outcomes (Neto et al., 2020).

Reports from many of the world's COVID trouble spots, including the United States, documented extreme levels of exhaustion, physical discomfort from long working hours with face masks and other PPE, fear of contagion, and emotional distress in nurses. This combination of physical and emotional strain on an already stressed and burdened nursing workforce has become a hallmark of the COVID-19 pandemic (Colombini, 2020; Neto et al., 2020; Plaisance & Warren, 2022). Professional organizations have determined that it is critical to study nurses' experiences and well-being during and in the aftermath of the crisis and to identify risk groups for ill health, mitigation strategies, and potential sources of organizational intervention (ANA, 2021; Drick, 2016; Dryden et al., 2021; Stephens, 2019). The nursing profession requires this attention and care (ANA, n.d., 2021; Dyrbye et al., 2017; National Academies of Sciences, Engineering, and Medicine [NASEM], 2021).

How can nursing and health care bounce back from a worldwide pandemic? To be honest, nursing as a profession was challenged before the pandemic. Many of the news headlines focused on substantial political, racial, and human issues, while mental health and wellness experts were communicating serious concerns regarding issues of mental health and work-life balance. With 2 years of lockdowns, social distancing and isolation have only expanded these problems. While the impact of the COVID pandemic will take years to examine, the implications on mental and physical health already exist. Exhaustion, burnout, fatigue, and anxiety are all emotions that are reported in nursing and in the general population. Perhaps a way forward might be to create a new normal with healthier routines and behaviors. Resilience has become a popular term. The American Psychological Association (APA, October 26, 2021) press release on the report *Stress in America 2021* (https://www.apa.org/news/press/releases/stress/2020/report-october) reported stress as issue compromising the lives of countless Americans. In evaluating the unpredictability and volatility the world has gone through during this recent pandemic, reflection on our resilience skills is required for our health and well-being. Resilience conveys the ability to "bounce-back" and requires self-compassion.

A survey examined nurses' perceptions of working during early stages of the pandemic in the United States and shared that greater than 50% of respondents reported symptoms of depression and anxiety, and nearly one-third had symptoms of posttraumatic stress disorder (PTSD) (Arnetz et al., 2020). The daily and compounded stress that nurses face can affect their health, well-being, and ability to care for their patients effectively. Several themes emerged from the survey analysis and the literature: exposure/infection-self; illness/death-others; workplace; PPE/supplies; unknowns; opinions/politics (Arnetz et al., 2020). Additional themes included pandemic-related restrictions and feelings of inadequacy and helplessness regarding patients and treatment (Arnetz et al., 2020). Health care and professional organizations are recognizing the need to provide opportunities for nurses to mitigate the stress they are experiencing, provide support, and recommend workplace adaptations to address stress and burnout potential. Providing nurses with the resources they need to strengthen their resilience is required for their health and well-being. This impacts and influences the health care system and provides rationale for the importance of resilience in nursing practice.

The American Psychological Association (APA, 2022) defines *resilience* as the process and outcome of successfully adapting to difficult or challenging life experiences, especially through mental, emotional, and behavioral flexibility and adjustment to external and internal demands (https://dictionary.apa.org/resilience). The literature identifies additional predictors of resilience specific to health care professionals. These predictors include the ability to laugh and find humor, the capacity for self-reflection and insight, the ability to find meaning in beliefs and spirituality, and the willingness to embrace a professional identity. Although multiple definitions of resilience exist, experts in the field agree that core principles can be taught because they involve behaviors, thoughts, and actions that can be modified. The APA believes that factors such as maintaining good relationships, accepting situations that cannot be changed, and having a hopeful outlook contribute to resilience. A gold standard for measuring resilience has not yet been widely agreed upon. With increasing complexity in the health care system, resilience is a necessity for nurses to thrive and remain professionally engaged.

Burnout may be described as a public health crisis, negatively affecting individuals, organizations, patients, and communities. Enhanced personal resilience can be combined with strategies to build resilient teams to examine causes of moral distress and burnout, which may arise from organizational and systems failures and lack of leadership. Personal resilience can be developed through education, support, and experiential training to improve nurses' ability to manage the challenges of a chaotic health care environment (Stephens, 2019).

Despite the physical and emotional demands of the nursing profession, there are methods described in the literature to improve resilience and well-being in the nursing profession. High role expectations and difficult working conditions place some nurses at risk for burnout and stress-related illness. Nurses continue to deliver high-quality patient care, remain resilient, and advance professionally despite some of the challenges of the health care environment. Some organizations can describe methods that are used to enhance the well-being of nurses individually and organizationally (Brennan, 2017; Dryden et al., 2021).

Professional nursing organizations such as the American Nurses Association (ANA), the American Holistic Nurses Association (AHNA), and the American Association for Critical-Care Nurses (AACN) have described the need for wellness for nurses over the years (AACN, 2016; AHNA, n.d.; ANA, 2021). Matney et al. (2016) described a plan for *wisdom in action* and reviewed the wisdom literature of other disciplines to help nurses demonstrate wisdom in practice as they provide nursing care and teach new generations of nurses the process of becoming wise. *Becoming wise* includes recognizing one's strengths, stating one's needs to sustain safe practice, and enjoying well-being while practicing in professional nursing environments.

Resilience and Health

By studying people who cope with stress exceptionally well, early researchers into stress management defined what they call the stress-hardy personality. Research into the stress-hardy personality set the groundwork for today's understanding of resilience.

Kobasa's (1979) classic work at the University of Chicago Stress Project compared two groups of executives in high-stress positions and found those who stayed healthy had a significantly different way of viewing the world. The healthy managers viewed change as inevitable, not as "good" or "bad." They made practical use of optimistic thinking and thought they could control the impact of problems. Rewards for this kind of thinking were substantial. Managers with a more optimistic worldview experienced half the illnesses of those in the nonhardy or non-resilient group. The researchers concluded that stress-hardy people feel in control of their lives, view stress as a challenge instead of a threat, and embrace commitments with enthusiasm instead of a sense of dread. Kobasa defined these traits—*commitment, control, and challenge*—as "the three Cs" of the stress-hardy personality.

D'Ambrosia (1987) completed a study of oncology nurses and found that hardiness factors were a strong predictor of burnout. He found that a sense of control versus powerlessness was especially important in reducing burnout in nurses. Simoni and Patterson (1987) conducted a similar study on hardiness in nurses and found that hardiness reduced burnout and improved nurses' career satisfaction. Rich and Rich (1987) concluded that hardiness allowed stress resistance in female staff nurses, which prevented or reduced burnout.

Jennings et al. (2017) examined results of resilience training designed to improve nurses' mental health. The study relied on acceptance and commitment therapy (ACT), which emerged out of the cognitive behavioral therapy (CBT) field (Hayes, 2016). The goal of ACT is to cultivate mindfulness and acceptance by encouraging participants to act according to their values rather than being controlled by their thoughts and emotions. The training provided participants with the necessary tools to identify their values and become more attuned to their attitudes and behaviors relative to those values. The study findings revealed significant improvements in the nurses' general health after participation in the training. Nurses learned to be less reactive and to recover more quickly from stress. They also gained a greater ability to adhere to their personal values and make choices about their responses to stress. After completion of the training, many of the nurses reported the program allowed them to focus more on self-care. The training increased nurses' awareness of the conflicting pressures and the need for self-care activities.

We now understand that the major traits of the resilient personality have been identified and can be taught. It is incumbent upon nursing leaders and health care administrators to advocate for evidence-based programs that support resilience education for their nursing staff. Starting with Kobasa's (1979) concept of the three C's of the stress-hardy personality, we can consider a framework for effective resilience programs specifically for nurses. The world needs more people to enter the nursing field and more

nurses as quickly as possible (Keypath Education, 2021; NASEM, 2021).

Commitment. A strong sense of commitment supports good coping mechanisms and resilience. Nursing leaders and administrators can use this insight as a guide to nurturing collaborative work environments that foster a sense of belonging, meaning, and commitment. Such an environment would include a healthy work-life balance that honors the nurse's need for strong interconnections with family, colleagues, community, friends, and faith (Dyrbye et al., 2017; Smith et al., 2020). These represent basic, human values to support nurses and the important work they do every day in all health care settings.

Benson (1975), a pioneer in the field of stress research, observed that people who maintain close relationships and a strong support system are much less likely to fall prey to stress-related illnesses. Strong relationships and a sense of belonging can be encouraged through a workplace that proactively supports social interactions between coworkers and their families. Providing community space conducive to gathering solidifies relationships and creates a strong sense of belonging. Programs and policies that support commitment and connectedness include onsite nursing support groups, nursing wellness and resiliency programs, philanthropy benefits, generous maternity leave, time off to participate in community outreach programs, opportunities for nurses to socialize across departments, onsite gyms and yoga studios, orientation events that encourage connection with colleagues through "buddy programs," and special events that include family and friends.

Control. Studies show that how we perceive the amount of control we have over a stressor directly influences our ability to cope with it. How nurses experience their sense of control can be influenced at both the personal and institutional levels. Health care settings that demand a lot from their nurses *and* give them little or no control over their performance create an environment conducive to stress and burnout. This type of environment may create a condition identified as *learned helplessness*, described more than 50 years ago by Martin Seligman, founder of Positive Psychology (Seligman, 2006). When people believe they have no control over their environment, they often give up. Characteristics of learned helplessness include decreased effort, diminished persistence, reduced ability to learn, belief that one's actions make no difference, and anxiety or depression. These findings suggest the need to create environments that offer nurses a sense of control, including the opportunity to participate in shared governance professionally, the ability to contribute to quality improvement projects and the chance to play a role on hospital decision-making committees relevant to their jobs.

Behavioral/cognitive programs can offer nurses a greater sense of control by helping them understand their thinking processes. Kobasa (1979) identified two basic ways people perceive control: internally and externally. Nurses with an internal locus of control know they cannot influence all external events in their lives, but they have a sense of empowerment and believe they have influence. Nurses with an external locus of control believe that they have little or no control over their lives because of fate or influences "outside of themselves." Implementation of integrative resilience programs can guide nurse recognition of whether they perceive control to be unavailable so they can shift their thinking and perhaps serve them better. Through cognitive restructuring and reframing programs, nurses can develop a greater internal focus, which can increase their sense of empowerment and resilience.

Challenge. Individuals view life events on a continuum from threat to challenge. Resilient, stress-hardy people view change as a challenge, not as a threat. They see it as an inevitable part of life and an opportunity to learn and grow. Helping nurses embrace challenge can be accomplished through cognitive restructuring and reframing programs. When nurses learn to change their perceptions of their work and work environments, they can change their experience. Integrating opportunities for healthy challenge into the health care environment can help nurses practice resilience skills. Activities to help nurses embrace challenge with positivity include leadership development programs, shared governance opportunities, professional development, and graduate school and specialty organizations. The professional burnout that occurs when nurses are constantly witnessing devastating situations can lead to stress and negative attitudes in nurses who have enjoyed their nursing careers. They may not realize how harmful this can be to mental health. The National Academy of Medicine's (NAM) Action Collaboration on Clinician Well-Being and Resilience (https://nam.edu/initiatives/clinician-resilience-and-well-being/) launched in 2017 is a collaboration of 200 organizations committed to reversing the trend of clinician burnout in the United States by raising awareness of the risks and symptoms of burnout so that self-care practices and well-being can be prioritized. Taking care of the health care worker is as important as taking care of the patient. The collaborative issued a draft National Plan for Health Workforce Well-Being in June 2022 (https://nam.edu/initiatives/clinician-resilience-and-well-being/national-plan-for-health-workforce-well-being/) identifying the high demand for about 200,000 nurses

each year through 2026. The profession, health care organizations, administrators, and nurses new to the profession, will need to recognize and address this professional workforce gap with measures that allow them to continue to practice to the full scope of their license. This is no small feat. It is possible to compassionately care for patients and continue to be an excellent nurse while also practicing compassionate care of self. Sinsky et al. (2020) describe the need for health care organizations to move resilience planning forward by prioritizing workforce well-being in a concentrated effort: through commitment to assessment and reporting of burnout; by sharing accountability across roles in leadership; by evaluating policies regularly, through measurement and improvement of the work environment and with creation of a culture of clinician connection and support (Sinsky et al., 2020).

RESILIENCE PRACTICES

A number of evidence-based programs have increased resilience. These include implementing mindfulness/meditation/breathing technique programs, resilience/stress management programs, cognitive restructuring, expressive writing/journaling, exercise/walking programs, animal-assisted therapy, and more. There is not a one-size-fits-all approach when it comes to boosting resilience. Nursing is a caring profession and nurses need to understand that they can grow from adversity and use the wisdom they have gained to recognize weaknesses and vulnerabilities to improve systems and situations (AHNA, n.d.; Kitson, 2020). Each nurse will gravitate toward the program that aligns best with his or her comfort level and preferred learning style (visual, aural, verbal, or physical).

Meditation, acupuncture, massage therapy, jogging, and even breathing deeply can trigger marked physiological changes conducive to a more positive attitude and a more resilient outlook. Many health care facilities have already developed programs to support resilience, including drop-in yoga, tai chi, and mindfulness classes. Resiliency practices need not take an inordinate amount of time. If a nurse is too busy to attend a 45-minute meditation, exercise or yoga class, many activities can be woven into a busy day. For example, fun walk-the-steps competitions can be established with the help of fitness trackers and exercise apps. Facilities also can establish designated quiet zones for meditation and reflection; or they can partner with contributors to establish indoor and/or outdoor meditation labyrinths. Virtual training and classes have expanded during the pandemic, allowing the option of taking part in some resilient activity from the comfort of home.

MODALITIES

Resiliency and Stress Management Programs

Rich and Rich (1987) reported that nurses who participated in a hardiness-learning program improved their resistance to stress through a renewed commitment to themselves and to their jobs. They gained a sense of greater control over their lives and learned to view unexpected events more as challenges than as stressors. By learning resilience and stress management strategies, nurses can influence how events affect them and impact their response. They may not have control over certain stressors, but they have control over their thoughts and therefore over their physiology.

Tarantino et al. (2013) implemented a resilience program called the Healing Pathway Program to reduce burnout in health care professionals in a medical school. The researchers observed that nurses who participated in the program experienced reduced stress and improved coping and mindfulness. They reported that nurses who invest time in self-care techniques such as body movements, Reiki, yoga, and meditation improved their overall well-being and may have provided higher-quality patient care.

Meditation and Breathing Techniques

Benson (1975), founder of Harvard's Mind/Body Medical Institute and director emeritus of Mass General's Benson-Henry Institute for Mind Body Medicine (BHI), is largely credited with bringing meditation into the mainstream. In the 1960s and 1970s, Benson conducted quantifiable research that showed meditation offered a variety of psychological and physiological benefits. He also renamed meditation "the relaxation response." Benson's research showed that just 20 minutes of meditation eased muscle tension, reduced blood pressure, lowered resting heart rate, decreased oxygen consumption, slowed respiratory rate, and produced a relaxed, alert state. Benson described the relaxation response as a deep state of relaxation and described that regular practice provided an effective treatment for a wide range of stress-related disorders. According to Benson, more than 60% of all visits to health care providers are related to stress. Stress triggers the "fight or flight" hormones to flow into the bloodstream. This, in turn, provokes additional symptoms, including headaches, insomnia, hypertension, irritable bowel syndrome, and chronic low back pain, as well as heart disease, stroke, and cancer.

Another stress-reducing practice related to meditation is mindful breathing. Harvey Alexander (2017) recommends belly breathing for relieving stress and eliciting the relaxation response. Belly breathing is a technique that involves easy, relaxed breathing with a focus on the abdominal region. The technique requires that you mindfully expand your belly as you inhale and allow the belly to contract as you exhale. As the belly expands and contracts, practitioners use the inhale pause to notice the effects of the breathing and the exhale pause to rest. Inviting the mind to focus on sensation and follow body and belly movements allows the mind to let go of thoughts and just rest. This is therapeutic by bringing the person back to the body.

The beauty of belly breathing is that it can be practiced lying down or anywhere you happen to be, such as the hospital cafeteria, the elevator, or in traffic on the way to work. Once the simple practice is learned, nurses can use it whenever they need to relax their bodies, focus their minds, aid digestion, or shift into a more positive state of mind.

Mindfulness

Jon Kabat-Zinn, a scientist and mindfulness teacher defines *mindfulness* as the intention to focus on each moment at a time without judgment. As the founder of the Center for Mindfulness in Medicine, Health Care, and Society, Kabat-Zinn introduced mindfulness to the mainstream in 1979. Practitioners often use the term "beginner's mind" to describe a state of mindfulness. Those who cultivate the beginner's mind encounter the world with a sense of curiosity and wonder, much like a child, without judgments or assumptions.

Kabat-Zinn (2009) developed a technique known as Mindfulness-Based Stress Reduction (MBSR) to help people tap into their inner resources to cope better with stress, pain, and illness. Kabat-Zinn recommends the use of mindfulness as a complementary treatment for a wide range of conditions, including anxiety, major depression, mood disorders, stress disorders, sleep disorders, asthma, gastrointestinal disorders, high blood pressure, cancer, and more. He believes every human has the capacity for mindfulness. Like any new and learned behavior, mastery requires practice.

Nurses can cultivate mindfulness through a variety of practices, such as yoga, tai chi, and chi gong, but most of the scientific literature has focused on mindfulness meditation. Walsh and Shapiro (2006) share that an important skill to master is the ability to focus your attention enough to control your mental processes. This then nurtures general mental well-being, calmness, clarity, and concentration.

As mindfulness has grown in popularity over the years, so have opportunities to learn mindfulness techniques. From local onsite classes to live-streaming events, individuals interested in the topic enjoy a wide range of choices. The Compassionate Care Initiative (CCI) at the University of Virginia School of Nursing historically sponsored a public radio documentary series called *Resilient Nurses,* where nurses examine how they are facing the challenges of their profession, and this has included discussions of mindfulness practices (https://www.humanmedia.org/product/nurses/).

Expressive Writing/Journaling

Progoff (1975), a psychologist and former Director of the Institute for Research in Depth Psychology at Drew University, found clients were able to work through their psychological issues more quickly when they wrote about them in a journal. This insight led him to develop an Intensive Journal method in the mid-1960s and 1970s. Workshops based on this technique still thrive today through the Progoff Intensive Journal Program for Self-Development (http://intensivejournal.org/index.php). The technique guides participants to gain insights into personal relationships, careers, special interests, body, and health. The program offers specialized journaling programs to support resilience in nurses. Reflection and journaling are recognized widely in schools of nursing. The Josie King Foundation (n.d.) has completed research and produces journals with prompts (https://josieking.org/jkf-tools/nurses-journal/).

Expressive writing, which grew out of Progoff's classic work, is a technique that involves writing down your deepest feelings and emotions related to a traumatic or upsetting experience (Progroff, 1975). This form of writing requires the participant to write continuously for 15 to 20 minutes, disregarding spelling errors and grammar. The practice is done for 3 to 4 consecutive days. Expressive writing has been used effectively to treat anxiety, depression, and PTSD.

Pennebaker and Beal (1986) reported that people who wrote about traumatic events and their deepest feelings related to those events experienced improvement in their health 2 to 3 months after writing. These findings were based on both self-reports and testing for physiological markers. Subsequent studies drew a correlation between expressive writing and improvements in minor and major mental health disorders and acute and chronic diseases. It seems that telling stories positively affects immune function, skin conductance, blood pressure, and heart rate, and it even reduces visits to the physician.

Researchers (Pennebaker et al., 1988) report that expressive writing has been observed to influence stress hormones. People under stress often experience higher levels of cortisol and epinephrine (adrenaline). Cortisol suppresses immune activity, and adrenaline increases blood pressure. When you reduce major internal conflicts, you reduce these powerful stress hormones and improve the feeling of well-being.

Journaling and expressive writing is an option for most people. The point of journaling is reflection and to become aware of events that might require processing consciously. Because nurses face pain and suffering daily, journaling or expressive writing could serve as a powerful tool to foster resilience.

Exercise

Studies suggest that exercise helps reduce fatigue, improve alertness, reduce stress, boost concentration, improve sleep, and increase overall cognitive function. Researchers originally believed that exercise reduced stress by boosting the production of endorphins, opiate-like feel-good substances in the brain. Scholars now believe exercise reduces stress by boosting norepinephrine, serotonin, and dopamine, which are strongly linked to mood. Norepinephrine is especially interesting to investigators because half of the brain's supply is produced in an area that connects to other regions of the brain involved in regulating stress response. Although researchers do not fully understand how antidepressants work, they know that some boost levels of norepinephrine in the brain. Investigators have found that exercise forces the body's physiological systems (cardiovascular, renal, muscular, and others) to communicate more closely with each other, which improves stress response (Dishman et al., 2013).

Allen et al. (2018) found that exercise can change microbes in your gut. People who exercise had an increased level of specific microbes proven to reduce inflammation, fight insulin resistance, and bolster metabolism. The study found that when people stopped exercising, their microbiomes reverted to preexercise levels within 6 weeks.

A meta-study (Gordon et al., 2017) observed that resistance training significantly improves anxiety symptoms among both healthy participants and participants with a physical or mental illness. Greater benefits were observed in healthy participants compared with those with physical or mental illnesses, although reduced levels of anxiety were observed in both groups (Gordon et al., 2017).

Although the research established an evident relationship between exercise and the reduction of anxiety, there is a need for further research into the mechanisms behind this correlation. Supporting resilience in nurses, however, it is enough to know that the relationship exists and that it provides a powerful tool for increasing resilience. Simply parking the car farther from the building or taking the steps instead of the elevator throughout the day may suffice. Activity and body movement is helpful and supportive overall.

Cognitive Reframing and Restructuring

Cognitive restructuring is the therapeutic process of identifying and challenging irrational thoughts. Cognitive restructuring is a form of CBT introduced in the 1950s by Albert Ellis (1987) and further refined and studied in the 1960s and 1970s by Aaron T. Beck (1976, 1997).

Beck found that his depressed patients experienced a spontaneous flood of negative thoughts about themselves, the world, and their futures. By helping his patients identify and evaluate these thoughts, he helped them correct their cognitive distortions. Examples of cognitive distortions include all-or-nothing thinking, magical thinking, overgeneralization, magnification, and emotional reasoning. For example, a nurse who relies on emotional reasoning might conclude, "My supervisor is going to fire me because I feel anger toward her," even if her supervisor had shown her nothing but respect.

Another example of a cognitive distortion, called all-or-nothing thinking, would be the thought, "I won't get that promotion because I always fail." The words "never" and "always" are red flags that a cognitive distortion is in play. Reivich and Shatte (2002) reported that resilience can be boosted by changing thoughts about adversity. Some of their suggestions for changing how you think include:

- *Be aware of your self-talk* when faced with adversity so you can gain insight into how your thoughts affect your feelings and behavior.
- *Avoid thinking traps* such as blaming yourself, jumping to conclusions, and assuming you can read others' thoughts.
- *Identify deep, unconscious themes* and figure out when they help or hurt.
- *Find new problem-solving/thinking strategies* to avoid pursuing the wrong solutions.
- *Stop thinking about "what if"* and perceiving every failure as a catastrophe.

- *Stay calm and focused* when overwhelmed by stress or emotion.
- *Change your counterproductive thoughts* into more resilient ones. If you have certain thoughts that repeat, learn to identify them, and stop them.

A review of meta-analyses in 2013 validated much of Beck's work and reported that the evidence base for CBT is strong (Hofmann et al., 2012). This research describes that the major pathways through which stress exerts its damaging effects are greatly influenced by thoughts and perceptions. CBT and several other forms of therapy rely on cognitive restructuring to leverage the link between thoughts, feelings, and behaviors. A variety of techniques fall within the category of cognitive restructuring, offering nurses multiple cognitive-based resources to support resiliency (Hofmann et al., 2012).

In 2017, Rushlau described self-care practices that Victoria Maizes spoke about at the Integrative Healthcare Symposium conference in New York. Self-care practices have been articulated for decades as important for nurses and care providers, and Nightingale, in her wisdom, wrote about them. The recommendations include beginning with a self-assessment in key wellness areas, including movement, mind-body, food, environment, relationships, sleep, and spirituality (Rushlau, 2017). The American Holistic Nursing Organization (AHNA) has addressed the need for practitioners to be aware of managing their physical activity, diet, stress, environmental exposures, sleep, relationships, and spirituality throughout their careers and lives. The premise is that once nurses or caregivers address their own health and self-care, they are prepared to offer caregiving and well-being to clients.

SUMMARY

Nurses work in high-stress environments that expose them to pain and suffering and a wide range of institutional stressors daily. To help nurses cope with their demanding profession and avoid burnout, it is incumbent upon health care leaders and administrators to foster resilience in their nursing staff. The evidence is clear that resilience can be fostered and taught. Starting with Kobasa's concept of the stress-hardy personality, we can begin to build a framework for effective resilience programs for nurses.

To foster resilience, administrators must advocate for an environment that honors commitment, offers personal control, and provides healthy challenges. They can offer nurses a toolbox of evidence-based resilience resources, including resilience stress management, mindfulness/meditation, breathing techniques, cognitive restructuring, expressive writing/

journaling, physical exercise, and more. Providing nurses with the resources they need to increase resilience is paramount to their health and well-being, and ultimately to the effectiveness of the health care system itself. As we are observing with the immeasurable stress that the pandemic has delivered to patients, families, and the health care settings, nurse well-being and retention is paramount to recovery. Taking care of nurses on the job is a benefit that everyone must consider. It is a necessity so that nurses are supported in their ongoing efforts to care and advocate for patients with high-level expertise and mastery. It is time for *nurses* to advocate for nurses and for them to self-advocate. The well-being of the nurse providing the care is critically important.

Everyone has choices to make. With time, experience, education, and continued learning opportunities, people can begin to discern and continue to develop life-long wisdom. Sustained development of "discernment" and "wisdom" will allow people to consider choice in coping with difficult situations. Resilience, research, practice, and lifelong learning point the way.

It is incumbent on each nurse to embrace personal resilience activities that promote well-being. As professional nurses, we possess invaluable information on how to deal effectively with public health issues. Nurses should not be afraid to voice those issues. At this time of great uncertainty, the "voice of the nursing profession" needs to be heard by the world, not only in the battle against COVID-19 but also in preparation for the next major health challenge. Globally, public health depends upon it.

SALIENT POINTS

- Nurses work in high-stress environments that make them vulnerable to stress and burnout.
- Resilient nurses are less likely to suffer from extreme stress and burnout.
- Researchers have defined environmental attributes and personal characteristics that foster resilience and safeguard against stress.
- Studies show resilience can be fostered and taught.
- By creating an environment conducive to resilience and by teaching nurses to be more resilient, nursing leaders can foster greater resilience and reduce burnout in their nursing staff.
- Resilience leads to improved job satisfaction and a greater ability for nurses to care for themselves and their patients.
- Clinician well-being optimizes patient and clinician relationships and outcomes.

CRITICAL REFLECTION EXERCISES

1. Discuss how the nursing population would benefit from resilience training.
2. Describe environments that have fostered your resilience.
3. Examine opportunities for the integration of resilience programs in a health care setting familiar to you.
4. Describe ways to overcome identified barriers to implementing resilience programs in a health care setting familiar to you.
5. Describe a nurse you know who exhibits resilience and explain why.
6. Explain how resilient nurses benefit patients.
7. Brainstorm strategies not mentioned in this chapter that could foster resilience in nurses.
8. Describe how clinicians can advance evidence-based, multidisciplinary solutions to optimize patient care by advocating for systematic solutions to raise awareness of burnout and recognize and value clinicians and their professional expertise.
9. Provide an example of specific information and/or strategies presented in this chapter that you could implement to increase your personal and professional resilience.

REFERENCES

Alexander, H. S. (2017). *Learning to breathe, learning to live: Simple tools to relieve stress and invigorate your life*. Balboa Press.

Allen, J. M., Mailing, L. J., Niemiro, G. M., Moore, R., Cook, M. D., White, B. A., Holscher, H. D., & Woods, J. A. (2018). Exercise alters gut microbiota composition and function in lean and obese humans. *Medicine & Science in Sports & Exercise*, 50(4), 747–757. https://journals.lww.com/acsm-msse/Fulltext/2018/04000/Exercise_Alters_Gut_Microbiota_Composition_and.14.aspx

American Association of Critical-Care Nurses. (2016). *AACN standards for creating and sustaining healthy work environments: A journey to excellence* (2nd ed.). https://www.aacn.org/wd/hwe/docs/hwestandards.pdf

American Holistic Nurses Association. (n.d.). *Resources to enhance practice: Self-care modalities*. https://www.ahna.org/resources

American Nurses Association. (October, 2021). *Year four highlights 2020–2021*. https://www.healthynursehealthynation.org/~4a9f4b/globalassets/hnhn-assets/all-images-view-with-media/about/hnhn-oct21-issue-921.pdf

American Nurses Association. (n.d.). *Work environment-health & safety: Combating stress*. https://www.nursingworld.org/practice-policy/work-environment/health-safety/combating-stress/

American Psychological Association. (2021, October 26). *Stress in America™ 2020* [Press release]. Accessed January 19, 2023. https://www.apa.org/news/press/release/stress/2020/report-october

American Psychological Association. (2022). *Definition of resilience*. https://dictionary.apa.org/resilience

Arnetz, J. E., Goetz, C. M., Arnetz, B. B., & Arble, E. (2020). Nurse reports of stressful situations during the COVID-19 pandemic: Qualitative analysis of survey responses. *International Journal of Environmental Research and Public Health*, *17*(21), 8126. https://doi.org/10.3390/ijerph17218126

Beck, A. (1976). *Cognitive therapy and emotional disorders*. International Universities Press.

Beck, A. (1997). The past and future of cognitive therapy. *Journal of Psychotherapy Practice and Research*, *6*(4), 276–284. https://www.ncbi.nlm.nih.gov/pmc/articles/PMC3330473/pdf/jp64276.pdf

Benson, H. (1975). *The relaxation response*. Harper Collins.

Brennan, E. J. (2017). Towards resilience and wellbeing in nurses. *British Journal Nursing*, *26*(1), 43–47. https://www.magonlinelibrary.com/doi/abs/10.12968/bjon.2017.26.1.43

Colombini, S. (2020). *Florida health care workers feeling strain of coronavirus surge*. Health News Florida. https://health.wusf.usf.edu/health-news-florida/2020-07-22/florida-health-care-workers-feeling-strain-of-coronavirus-surge#stream/0

D'Ambrosia, S. J. (1987). *A study to examine if there is a relationship between burnout and hardiness of nurses working with oncology patients* (Unpublished Doctoral Dissertation). Temple University.

Dishman, R., Heath, G., & Lee, I-Min. (2013). *Physical activity epidemiology* (2nd ed.). Human Kinetics.

Drick, C. A. (2016). Self-care: Finding time and balance. *Beginnings*, *36*(4), 6–7. https://www.cpgh.org/wp-content/uploads/2022/02/2016_August_Beginnings.pdf

Dryden, E. M., Bolton, R. E., Bokhour, B. G., Wu, J., Dvorin, K., Phillips, L., & Hyde, J. K. (2021). Leaning into whole health: Sustaining system transformation while supporting patients and employees during COVID-19. *Global Advances in Health and Medicine*, *10*, 21649561211021047. https://doi.org/10.1177/21649561211021047

Dyrbye, L. N., Shanafelt, T. D., Sinsky, C. A., Cipriano, P. F., Bhatt, J., Ommaya, A., West, C. P., & Meyers, D. (2017). *Burnout among health care professionals: A call to explore and address this underrecognized threat to safe, high-quality care*. NAM Perspectives [Discussion Paper]. National Academy of Medicine, Washington, DC. https://doi.org/10.31478/201707b

Ellis, A. (1987). *Reason and emotions in psychotherapy*. Carol Publishing.

Gordon, B. R., McDowell, C. P., Lyons, M., & Herring, M. P. (2017). The effects of resistance exercise training on anxiety: A meta-analysis and meta-regression analysis of randomized controlled trials. *Sports Medicine*, *47*(12), 2521–2532. https://link.springer.com/article/10.1007%2Fs40279-017-0769-0

Hayes, S. (2016). Acceptance and commitment therapy, relational frame theory, and the third wave of behavioral and cognitive therapies [Republished article]. *Behavior Therapy*, *47*(6), 869–885. https://doi.org/10.1016/j.beth.2016.11.006

Hofmann, S. G., Asnaani, M. A., Imke, J. J., Vonk, M. A., Sawyer, M. A., & Fang, M. A. (2012). The efficacy of cognitive behavioral therapy: A review of meta-analyses. *Cognitive Therapy Research*, *36*(5), 427–440. https://link.springer.com/article/10.1007%2Fs10608-012-9476-1

IBISWorld. (2020, April 16). *Special report: Effects of COVID-19 on global healthcare systems*. https://www.ibisworld.com/blog/covid19-effects-global-healthcare-systems/99/1133/

Jennings, T., Flaxman, P., Egdell, K., Pestell, S., Whipday, E., & Herbert, A. (2017). A resilience training programme to improve nurse's mental health. *Nursing Times*, *113*(10), 22–26.

Josie King Foundation. (n.d.). *Nurse's Journal*. https://josieking.org/jkf-tools/nurses-journal/

Kabat-Zinn, J. (2009). *Full catastrophe living: Using the wisdom of your body and mind to face pain, stress and illness*. Random House.

Keypath Education. (2021). *Future of Nursing: Twelve trends to watch in the coming years*. [Blog]. https://globalhealtheducation.com/article/future-nursing

Kitson, A. (2020). Rising from the ashes: Affirming the spirit of courage, community resilience, compassion and caring. *Journal of Clinical Nursing*, *29*(15–16), 2765–2766. https://doi.org/10.1111/jocn.15182

Kobasa, S. (1979). Stressful life events, personality, and health: Inquiry into hardiness. *Journal of Personality and Social Psychology*, *37*(1), 1–11. https://psycnet.apa.org/doi/10.1037/0022-3514.37.1.1

Matney, S. A., Avant, K., & Staggers, N. (2016). Toward an understanding of wisdom in nursing. *The Online Journal of Issues in Nursing*, *21*(1). https://doi.org/10.3912/OJIN.Vol21No01PPT02

National Academies of Sciences, Engineering, and Medicine. (2021). *The future of nursing: Charting a path to achieve health equity: Summary*. https://doi.org/10.17226/25982

National Academy of Medicine. *Action collaborative on clinician well-being and resilience*. https://nam.edu/initiatives/clinician-resilience-and-well-being/

Neto, M. L. R., Almeida, H. G., Esmeraldo, J. D., Nobre, C. B., Pinheiro, W. R., De Oliviera C. R., Sousa I. D. C., Lima, O. M. M. L., Lima, N. N. R., Moriera, M. M., Lima, C. K. T., Junior, J. G., & da Silva, C. G. L. (2020). When health professionals look death in the eye: The mental health of professionals who deal daily with the 2019 coronavirus outbreak. *Psychiatric Research*, *288*, 112972. https://www.ncbi.nlm.nih.gov/pmc/articles/PMC7152886/

Pennebaker, J. W., & Beal, S. K. (1986). Confronting a traumatic event: Toward and understanding of inhibition and disease. *Journal of Abnormal Psychology*, *95*(3), 274–281. https://psycnet.apa.org/doi/10.1037/0021-843X.95.3.274

Pennebaker, J. W., Kiecolt-Glaser, J., & Glaser, R. (1988). Disclosures of traumas and immune function: Health implications for psychotherapy. *Journal of Consulting and Clinical Psychology*, *56*(2), 239–245.

Plaisance, S., & Warren M. (2022, July 23). *Pandemic taking a toll on mental health of hospital workers*. Associated Press. Accessed January 17, 2023. https://apnews.com/fadf6ae2b898341833d063c7bc8923a4

Progoff, I. (1975). *At a journal workshop: The basic text and guide for using the intensive journal process*. Dialogue House.

Reivich, K. W., & Shatte, A. (2002). *The resilience factor: Seven essential skills for overcoming life's inevitable obstacles*. Broadway Books.

Rich, V. L., & Rich, A. R. (1987). Personality hardiness and burnout in female staff nurses. *Journal of Nursing Scholarship*,

19(2), 63–66. https://psycnet.apa.org/doi/10.1111/j.1547-5069.1987.tb00592.x

Rushlau, K. (2017, March 3). *Seven self-care tips for practitioners and patients.* Integrative Practitioner. https://www.integrativepractitioner.com/about/integrative-healthcare-symposium/seven-self-care-tips-for-practitioners-and-patients

Seligman, M. (2006). *Learned optimism.* Alred A. Knopf.

Simoni, P., & Patterson, J. (1987). Hardiness, coping, and burnout in the nursing workplace. *Journal of Professional Nursing, 13*(3), 178–185. https://www.sciencedirect.com/science/article/abs/pii/S8755722397800695?via%3Dihub

Sinsky, C. A., Daugherty Biddison, L., Mallick, A., Legreid Dopp, A., Perlo, J., Lynn, L., & Smith, C. D. (2020, November 2). *Organizational evidence-based and promising practices for improving clinician well-being. NAM Perspectives.* [Discussion Paper]. National Academy of Medicine. https://doi.org/10.31478/202011a

Smith, G. D., Ng, F., & Li, W. H. C. (2020). COVID-19: Emerging compassion, courage and resilience in the face of misinformation and adversity. *Journal of Clinical Nursing, 29*(9–10), 1425–1428. https://doi.org/10.1111/jocn.15231

Stephens, T. (2019). *Building personal resilience.* American Nurse. https://www.myamericannurse.com/building-personal-resilience/

Tarantino, B., Earley, M., Audia, D., D'Adamo, C., & Berman, B. (2013). Qualitative and quantitative evaluation of a pilot integrative coping and resiliency program for healthcare professionals. *Explore (NY), 9*(1), 44–47. https://doi.org/10.1016/j.explore.2012.10.002

Walsh, R., & Shapiro, S. (2006). The meeting of meditative disciplines and western psychology. *American Psychologist, 61*(3), 227–239. https://psycnet.apa.org/doi/10.1037/0003-066X.61.3.227

Select National Initiatives for Quality and Safety: Quality Chasm Series (National Academy Press, Washington, DC)

PHASE I—BURDEN OF HARM

Institute of Medicine (IOM). (1997). *National Roundtable on Health Care Quality.* https://doi.org/10.17226/9439
- "The quality of health care can be precisely defined and measured with a degree of scientific accuracy comparable with that of most measures used in clinical medicine. Serious and widespread problems exist throughout American medicine. These problems, which may be classified as underuse, overuse, or misuse, occur in small and large communities alike, in all parts of the country, and with approximately equal frequency in managed care and fee-for-service systems of care. Very large numbers of Americans are harmed as a direct result. Quality of care is the problem, not managed care. Current efforts to improve will not succeed unless we undertake a major, systematic effort to overhaul how we deliver health care services, educate and train clinicians, and assess and improve quality" (p. 10. Abstract). http://www.nap.edu/catalog/9439.html
- Committee on the Quality of Health Care in America (1998).
- Continually reduce the burden of illness, injury, and disability, with the aim of improving health status, functioning, and satisfaction of the American people.

PHASE II—VISION FOR TRANSFORMATION

Institute of Medicine (IOM). (2000). To Err is Human: Building a safer healthcare system. https://doi.org/10.17226/9728
- Human beings in all lines of work make errors. Errors can be prevented by designing systems that make it hard for people to do the wrong thing and easy for people to do the right thing (p. ix).
- At least 44,000 Americans die each year as a result of medical errors. Total national costs (lost income, lost household production, disability, and health care costs) of preventable adverse events are estimated to be between $17 and $29 billon of which health care costs represent over one-half.
- Established the connection between quality and safety.
- Concepts introduced: safety, error, adverse event, culture of safety (vs. culture of blame), framework/roadmap for safety.

Institute of Medicine (IOM). (2001). *Crossing the quality chasm: A new health system for the 21st century.* https://doi.org/10.17226/10027
- Health care today harms too frequently and routinely fails to deliver its potential benefits. Between the health care we have and the care we could have lies not just a gap, but a chasm (p. 1).
- Quality is a system property. The current system has significant safety flaws that impede the workforce's ability to do the right thing.
- Improvement Aims for a **21st-Century Health Care System: Safe**, **Effective**, **Patient-centered**, **Timely**, **Efficient**, **Equitable**.
  - Process design: System design using the 80/20 principle (Pareto Principle)
- National Quality Report
- New care environment:
  - Applying evidence to health care delivery (clinical practice guidelines, clinical decision support systems, evidence-based practice, making information available on the Internet, defining quality measures).
  - Using information technology
  - Aligning payment policies with quality improvement
  - Preparing a workforce (education, regulation, liability systems)
  - Design for safety, make errors visible and mitigate for harm from errors

PHASE III—BLUEPRINT FOR TRANSFORMING HEALTH PROFESSIONS EDUCATION FOR 21ST-CENTURY HEALTH CARE SYSTEM

Institute of Medicine (IOM). (2003). *Health professions education: A bridge to quality.* https://doi.org/10.17226/10681

- **Core Competencies** for ALL Health Professions (common language):
  - Provide patient-centered care
  - Work in interdisciplinary teams
  - Employ evidence-based practice
  - Apply quality improvement
  - Utilize informatics
- Use oversight processes (accreditation, certification and licensure) to drive curriculum and practice reform to demonstrate competency (competency-based approach).
  - Remove geographic barriers such as restrictive licensure requirements across states as well as separate or sometimes conflicting state scope-of-practice acts.
  - Partnerships between practice and education to create 'learning centers'.
  - Explore alternative ways of paying clinicians.
  - Leadership for change.
  - Biennial interdisciplinary summits.

Institute of Medicine (IOM). (2003). *Priority areas for national action: Transforming health care quality.* https://doi.org/10.17226/10593

- We have extraordinary knowledge and capacity to deliver the best care in the world, but we repeatedly fail to **translate** that knowledge and capacity into clinical practice (p. 2).
- Using a systems approach and consumer-oriented framework, identified a total of 20 priority areas with 17 priority areas across the continuum of care and lifespan. Staying Healthy (preventive care), Getting Better (acute care), Living with Illness/Disability (chronic care), and Coping with End-of-Life (palliative care); one emerging priority area (obesity); and two cross-cutting systems interventions (**care coordination** and **self-management**).
- National Healthcare Quality Report

Institute of Medicine (IOM). (2004). *Patient safety: Achieving a new standard for care.* https://doi.org/10.17226/10863

- Established a need for a national health information infrastructure to provide immediate access to complete patient information and decision-support tools as well as the development of data interchange standards and clinical terminologies for collection, coding, and classification of patient safety information as a building block for that infrastructure.
- Concepts introduced: **near miss, adverse event analysis, root-cause analysis (RCA), errors of commission, errors of omission, electronic health record (EHR), serious reportable events, de-identification, data protection, primary and secondary uses of data.**

Institute of Medicine (IOM). (2005). *Quality through collaboration: The future of rural health.* https://doi.org/10.17226/11140

- About a fifth of the US population resides in Rural America and possesses unique strengths and creativity to apply the newest tools available such as information and communication technology (ICT) to the work of delivering high-quality health care in rural settings that vary by density and remoteness.
- **Core health care services**: Primary care, emergency medical services, hospital care, long-term care, mental health and substance abuse services, oral health care, and public health services.
- Recruitment and retention of health care professionals.
- Telehealth

The Future of Nursing 2011 and 2021

INSTITUTE OF MEDICINE'S FUTURE OF NURSING 2010–2020: LEADING CHANGE, ADVANCING HEALTH.

Summary of the four key messages and eight recommendations:

Key Message #1: The Need to Transform Practice

Nurses should practice to the full extent of their education and training.

Key Message #2: The Need to Transform Education

Nurses should achieve higher levels of education and training through an improved education system that promotes seamless academic progression.

Key Message #3: The Need to Transform Leadership

Nurses should be full partners, with physicians and other health professionals, in redesigning health care in the United States.

Key Message #4: The Need for Better Data on the Health Care Workforce

Effective workforce planning and policy making require better data collection and improved information infrastructure.

> **Recommendation 1**: Remove scope-of-practice barriers.
>
> **Recommendation 2**: Expand opportunities for nurses to lead and diffuse collaborative improvement efforts.
>
> **Recommendation 3**: Implement nurse residency programs (transition-to-practice programs).
>
> **Recommendation 4**: Increase the proportion of nurses with a baccalaureate degree to 80% by 2020.
>
> **Recommendation 5**: Double the number of nurses with a doctorate by 2020.
>
> **Recommendation 6**: Ensure that nurses engage in lifelong learning.
>
> **Recommendation 7**: Prepare and enable nurses to lead change to advance health.
>
> **Recommendation 8**: Build an infrastructure for the collection of an analysis of interprofessional health care workforce data.

Adapted from Summary, Institute of Medicine. (2011). *Future of nursing 2010-2020: Leading change, advancing health.* The National Academies Press. https://doi.org/10.17226/12956

****

NATIONAL ACADEMY OF MEDICINE'S FUTURE OF NURSING 2020–2030: CHARTING A PATH TO ACHIEVE HEALTH EQUITY

Summary of the nine recommendations:

Recommendation #1: Creating a Shared Agenda

> Addresses activities nursing organizations can take both internally across nursing organizations and externally to nursing organizations to create a shared agenda that addresses social determinates of health (SDOH) and achieves health equity. This includes assessing and eliminating racists and discriminatory policies; leveraging expertise of public health nursing; care coordination and care management; developing mechanisms for nurse's well-being; amplifying health-equity issues; increasing the number and diversity of nurses; and establishing awards recognizing contributions in achieving health equity.

Recommendation #2: Supporting Nurses to Advance Health Equity

> By 2023, regardless of practice setting, initiate substantive actions to enable the nursing workforce to address SDOH and health equity more comprehensively. This includes increasing expertise in health equity and in specialty areas with current shortages (public and community health, behavioral health, primary care, long-term care, geriatrics, school health and maternal health) through public health education and traineeships; direct funding to increase gender, geographic, and racial diversity; nurse loan and scholarship programs; prioritizing longitudinal community-based learning opportunities through

academic-community-based partnerships; supporting socioeconomically disadvantaged student's academic progression; establishing a National Nursing Workforce Commission; quantifying nursing expenditures related to health equity and SDOH; including nursing expertise in health-related multisector policy reform; providing sustainable state and federal funding to prepare sufficient numbers of baccalaureate, APRN, and PhD nurses to advance health equity and SDOH; and employer support for nurses in playing a leading role in achieving health equity.

Recommendation #3: Promoting Nurse's Health and Well-Being

By 2021, nursing education programs, employers, nursing leaders, licensing boards, and nursing organizations implement systems, structures, and evidence-based interventions to promote nurses' health and well-being. This includes integrating health, well-being, and self-care content into nursing education programs; protecting students most at risk for behavioral health challenges; employer resourcing of sufficient human and material resources (including PPE) to enable nurses to provide high-quality care effectively and safely; establishing a culture of physical and psychological safety in the workplace; protecting nurses from retaliation; supporting diversity, equity, and inclusion across the nursing workforce; employer investment in health interventions for nurses; strengthening nurses' contribution to improving design and delivery of care and decision making in the workplace; reducing the stigma associated with mental and behavioral health treatment for nurses; and collecting systematic data to understand the health and well-being of the nursing workforce, mitigate burnout, fatigue, and the development of behavioral and mental health problems.

Recommendation #4: Capitalizing on Nurses' Potential

All organizations, including state and federal entities and employing organizations, should enable nurses to practice to the full extent of their education and training by removing barriers (regulatory and public/private payment limitations, restrictive policies and practices, and other legal, professional, and commercial impediments) that prevent them from more fully addressing social needs or SDOH and improving health care access, quality, and value. **By 2022**, all APRN and RN expanded scope of practice, telehealth eligibility, insurance coverage, and service payment parity policies or laws adopted in response to COVID-19 should be made permanent. Federal authority should be used where available to supersede restrictive state laws and the Nurse Licensure Compact should be adopted nationwide. The Health Care Regulator Collaboration should advance interstate compacts and adoption of model legislation.

Recommendation #5: Paying for Nursing Care

All public and private payers and public health agencies should establish sustainable and flexible payment mechanisms that support nurses in health care, public health and school nursing to address social needs, SDOH, and health equity. Including reforming fee-for-service payment models, CPT codes, relative value units (RVUs), value-based payment models, alternative payment models describing and reimbursing nurse-led services like case management, care coordination, and team-based care; reimbursement of school nursing; nurse telehealth services; nursing interventions; disparities-sensitive measures; and adequately fund school and public health nursing. Additionally, create a National Nurse Identifier to recognize and measure the value of nurse provided services.

Recommendation #6: Using Technology to Integrate Data on SDOH into Nursing Practice

Incorporate nursing expertise in designing, generating, analyzing, and applying data to support initiatives focused on SDOH and health equity using diverse digital platforms, artificial intelligence (AI), and other innovative technologies. Including building a nationwide infrastructure to integrate SDOH data into electronic health records (EHRs) and closing the 'digital divide', ensuring the existing public/private health equity collaboratives (Gravity Project8) encompass nursing-specific care processes' visualization of SDOH data associated with nurse decision-making and personalization of preference-based care. Additionally, resource the facilitation of telehealth by nurses.

Recommendation #7: Strengthening Nursing Education

Assure that nurses are prepared to address SDOH and health equity through nursing education curriculum, continuing education opportunities, accreditation, certification, and licensure processes by including content on social needs; SDOH; population and environmental health; trauma-informed care (TIC); nurse's well-being and self-care; disaster preparedness; competencies in use of data to plan, implement, and evaluate care; and health policy/advocacy/civic engagement. **By AY 2022 to 2023**, assess individual student access to technology, virtual-learning, and multisector-simulation engagement. Promote inclusion, diversity, and equity across students, staff, and faculty. Increase academic progression through academic partnerships.

Recommendation #8: Preparing Nurses to Respond to Disasters and Public Health Emergencies

Federal agencies and other stakeholders (employers) should strengthen and protect the nursing workforce to ensure a knowledgeable and resourced national nursing workforce prepared to respond to disasters and public health emergencies and coordinated employer-based emergency response plans to support families, behavioral health, and protect nurses' health and well-being.

Recommendation #9: Building an Evidence Base

Develop and support a public/private nursing, public health and health care research agenda, and evidence base describing the impact of nursing interventions including multisector collaboration and team approaches on SDOH, environmental health, health equity, and nurses' health and well-being. Use evidence-based approaches to increase number and diversity of students from disadvantaged groups; eliminate structural racism and implicit biases to strengthen culturally competent care; and use technology to identify and integrate health and social data to improve nurse's capacity for support.

Adapted from Chapter 11, National Academies of Science, Engineering, and Medicine. (2021). *The future of nursing 2020-2030: Charting a path to achieve health equity.* The National Academies Press. https://doi.org/10.17226/25982

INDEX

Note: Pages followed by b, t, or f refer to boxes, tables, or figures, respectively.